The Fundamentals of
Clinical Neuropsychiatry

The Fundamentals of Clinical Neuropsychiatry

MICHAEL ALAN TAYLOR, MD

Professor of Psychiatry
Finch University of Health Sciences / The Chicago Medical School

New York   Oxford
OXFORD UNIVERSITY PRESS
1999

Oxford University Press

Oxford   New York
Athens   Auckland   Bangkok   Bogotá   Buenos Aires   Calcutta
Cape Town   Chennai   Dar es Salaam   Delhi   Florence   Hong Kong   Istanbul
Karachi   Kuala Lumpur   Madrid   Melbourne   Mexico City   Mumbai
Nairobi   Paris   São Paulo   Singapore   Taipei   Tokyo   Toronto   Warsaw

and associated companies in
Berlin   Ibadan

Published by Oxford University Press, Inc.,
198 Madison Avenue, New York, New York 10016

Oxford is a registered trademark of Oxford University Press.

Library of Congress Cataloging-in-Publication Data
Taylor, Michael Alan, 1940–
The fundamentals of clinical neuropsychiatry /
Michael Alan Taylor.
p.   cm.   Includes bibliographical references and index.
ISBN 0-19-513037-5
1. Neuropsychiatry.   I. Title.
[DNLM: 1. Mental Disorders—physiopathology.   2. Neuropsychology.
3. Nervous System—physiopathology.
WM 140 T244f 1999]   RC341.T388   1999
616.8—dc21   DNLM/DC   for Library of Congress   98-55497

9 8 7 6 5 4 3 2 1

Printed in the United States of America
on acid-free paper.

To Max Fink, who got this all started years ago;
to residents whose interest and questions keep it going;
and to patients and their good care, who, after all,
are the reason for it all

Acknowledgments

Nutan Atre-Vaidya critically read most of the early manuscript of this book and gave sound advice to improve it. Lori Moss, Max Fink, and Steve Dinwiddie also helped. Small parts of the book come from a nonpublished manuscript that was co-authored with Fred Sierles, and those sections are as much his as mine. Georgette Pfeiffer prepared all the many manuscript versions, completed references, obtained copyrights, and accomplished all the unheralded things without which books do not get written. Any errors that remain are mine, not their's.

Preface

In the past 20 years psychiatry and behavioral neurology have experienced an information explosion. Textbooks about general psychiatry, neuropsychiatry, and related topics have grown in number and size. Some of these books are excellent, and I often make reference to them. Their wealth of information, however, is also their limitation. Experienced and inexperienced clinicians alike are faced with almost daily new revelations about neurotransmitters. They are barraged with study after study reporting startling findings of brain dysfunctions in many psychiatric conditions, novel drugs of all sorts (atypical antipsychotics, specific reuptake-inhibiting antidepressants, autoreceptor enhancers), and new relationships (co-morbidities) found between disorders that make each new diagnostic system outdated in some areas before publication. Synthesis is needed. We need to make sense of it all.

Over the years I have been forced to try and do that in my lectures, seminars, and teaching rounds. Most students and residents are as well read as I and do not need a recitation of what is in reference textbooks. They need some guidance in how to put it all together and then to be taught the principles of diagnosis and treatment so that they can use the latest information in a reasoned way when taking care of their patients. I have tried to write that book.

Because students and residents, and most of us, learn best from plain speaking, I have also tried to make the writing less formal than the typical textbook, and I use language as I might on rounds or in a seminar. I begin each topic with the basics and then build the complexity upon that. I emphasize the fundamentals of how the brain is organized to generate behavior (its main *raison d'être*) and the principles of evaluation and treatment.

Because I am not a renaissance man, I have written about things I know something about and that reflect my clinical experience. If a reader finds some glaring omission (there is no chapter on child psychiatry, for example) it is not missing because I do not think the topic important, but rather because it is best left to those who have had to make sense of that topic in the care of their patients and in their teaching of students and residents.

Although I incorporate *Diagnostic and Statistical Manual of Mental Disorders* (DSM) terminology and classification into the discussion of many syndromes, the DSM is imperfect, and I organize some conditions from a different perspective. For example, I include some of the DSM impulse control disorders (e.g., trichotillomania, kleptomania) with obsessional syndromes because most research points to that association, and when treated as having a variant of obsessive compulsive disorder patients with these conditions often get better. I have included dissociative disorders with epilepsy because these clinical features often co-occur, and many documented dissociative states result from a seizure disorder. In Chapter 16 I include conditions that do not have common pathophysioliogies, but that do have similar diagnostic challenges. Although each condition deserves a book of its own, I discuss them briefly because their omission would be glaring in a general book about neuropsychiatry.

The old saying "those who can, do; those who can't, teach" certainly does not apply to clinical medicine. The best teachers in my experience are those who have something to teach, have a passion for it, and are themselves learning daily from their patients. I have had the added advantage of learning from my colleagues, residents, and students. If this book even approximates that experience, I'll consider it a success.

Neuropsychiatry provides the perspective that has made most sense to me in my efforts to synthesize the neurosciences and clinical psychiatry. Neuropsychiatry is now a major theme in psychiatry, and there is now widespread recognition that many patients with major psychiatric disorders (e.g., the DSM's axis I conditions) have something wrong with their brains and that the necessary element of treatment for these patients is biological. It is also now widely recognized that behavioral change is a common expression of many general medical conditions (e.g., hyperthyroidism, hypertension) and of what is still called *neurologic disease* (to artificially separate it from mental illness). Indeed, the main premise of this book is that psychiatry and neurology are one field; that is, in its broadest sense, neuropsychiatry is the theoretical and practical approach to psychiatric patient care that recognizes the brain as the organ of the mind and that mental illness is, in fact, not "mental" at all, but the behavioral disturbances associated with brain dysfunction and disease.

Because of this broad view of neuropsychiatry, I include discussions of "classic psychiatric" disorders (e.g., depression, obsessive compulsive disorder) along with traditional "neurologic" conditions (e.g., stroke, headache). To me they all represent dysfunction of the brain. I have also included a long chapter on personality because there is a neurology underlying personality just as there is a neurology underlying all behavior, no matter how complex, and because understanding personality is important in providing good patient care.

This broad view of neuropsychiatry leads to the logical conclusion that psychiatry and neurology are parts of the same thing. No matter where you start, you end up at the same place; abnormal behavior results from brain dysfunction and brain dysfunction leads to abnormal behavior. For example, if you examine "neurologic " patients with brain diseases, you find that the most common expression of that disease is behavior change, not an abnormal reflex or other "neurologic" signs. This is true for disease almost anywhere in the brain, but it is particularly true when disease affects anterior brain circuits (prefrontal cortex, basal ganglia, thalamus) or the limbic system (particularly the amygdala and hippocampus). The accompanying table displays some conditions affecting anterior brain circuits and their commonly observed behavioral changes. The striking thing about these

Some Behavioral Syndromes Associated With Anterior Brain Lesions

Condition	Personality	Mania	Depression	Obsessive Compulsive Disorder
FRONTAL CORTEX				
Dorsolateral prefrontal cortex trauma	Yes	No	Yes	No
Orbitolateral prefrontal cortex trauma	Yes	Yes	No	No
BASAL GANGLIA				
Parkinson's disease	Yes	Yes	Yes	No
Huntington's disease	Yes	Yes	Yes	Yes
Stroke	Yes	Yes	Yes	Yes
Carbon monoxide poisoning	Yes	No	No	Yes
THALAMUS				
Stroke	Yes	Yes	No	Yes

relationships is that it is not the pathophysiology that is most important, but rather the area of the brain that is involved. Anterior brain systems have more to do with behavior than with anything else. Disease in this system almost always produces behavioral change, and most commonly that behavioral change is a disturbance in mood and affect or in personality.

A reasonable alternative interpretation of the association between the diseases in the accompanying table and depression is that "who wouldn't feel depressed with a disease like that?!" However, of the 30% of Huntington's disease patients who become depressed, most do so *before* they know they have the condition. Among the 50%–70% of Parkinson's disease patients who become depressed, there is little correlation between the degree of neurologic impairment and the degree of the depression. Only convoluted theorizing could try to explain why the same group of illnesses can also cause an elevated mood as in mania or why obsessive compulsive disorder apperars more likely if the nondominant basal ganglia are involved and depression more likely when the dominant basal ganglia are involved.

In addition to brain lesions producing syndromes we usually think of as "psychiatric" (e.g., depression, obsessive compulsive disorder), brain lesions also can produce classic psychopathology. The following vignettes from Macdonald Critchley's famous monograph on the parietal lobe* illustrate this point:

*Macdonald Critchley, *The Parietal Lobes,* Hafner Press, New York, 1953.

"I had a terrible shock this morning when I touched my left hand; I thought it was the head of a reptile." Asked where her left arm was, she said: "I don't know. Where is it? I don't feel it." When confronted with her left hand, she said: "That is someone else's hand." "Whose is it?" "It is not mine. It's a reptile."

One patient insisted that a board had been inserted in place of the left side of the trunk and the left limbs. Of her left limbs, she said: ". . . that's an old man who stays in bed all the time." Asked if she had any objection, she replied: "Yes, I don't want any spirits in bed with me." A second patient thought her daughter was in bed with her because there was a strange arm across her chest.

In both vignettes, the patient expresses a delusional idea based on an experience that a body part actually belongs to another creature (a reptile) or to another person. These are *experiences of alienation* and in the psychiatric literature are termed *first rank symptoms* (see Chapter 3). They are common in several psychoses. Without specific evidence that the above patients had suffered nondominant parietal lobe strokes, they surely would have been hospitalized in a psychiatric hospital and labeled "psychotic." Only their other "neurologic" features led to the recognition that they suffered strokes and were "neurological."

The artificial nature of the separation of neurology and psychiatry is also illustrated by what follows in this book: Many patients with classic, primary psychiatric disorders, nevertheless, show evidence of brain disease or dysfunction. For example, schizophrenics have enlarged cerebral ventricles and cerebral cortical atrophy. They, and manics, and many depressed patients have decreased cerebral metabolism. Patients with obsessive compulsive disorder have visuospatial and visual memory problems. These and patients with other psychiatric conditions are as much "neurologic" as are Critchley's stroke patients. The neurology is just different.

Chicago, Ill.   M.A.T.

ADDITIONAL READINGS

Pincus JH, Tucker GJ: *Behavioral Neurology* (3rd ed). Oxford University Press, New York, 1985.

Reynolds EH, Trimble MR (eds): *The Bridge Between Neurology and Psychiatry*. Churchill Livingstone, Edinburgh, 1989.

Sano M: Basal ganglia and depression. *Neuropsychiatry, Neuropsychology and Behavioral Neurology* 4:24–35, 1991.

Contents

The Fundamentals of
Clinical Neuropsychiatry

Brain Organization and Neurobehavioral and Neurocognitive Function

The functional organization of the brain has specific diagnostic and treatment implications. Chapters 3 and 4 describe specific behavioral and cognitive assessments of this organization. Three overlapping frameworks of brain functional organization are

1. *Left and right systems* motorically controlling and perceptually responding to the contralateral side of the rest of the body and two different information-processing styles and patterns of cognitive specializations of the dominant and nondominant cerebral hemispheres
2. *An action brain system* (anterior brain structures and the cerebellum-pons) and a *perceptual-integrating brain system* (temporo-parietal-occipital cortices and their related subcortical structures)
3. A brain stem to neocortical *tripartite phylogenetic system* (old vertebrate, social mammal and primate, and uniquely human structures)

LEFT AND RIGHT BRAIN SYSTEMS

Hemisphere Specialization

The cerebral hemispheres in humans have different specializations and information processing styles (Table 1.1). Knowing these different processing styles helps determine the side of a brain lesion because the different processing styles and specializations affect behavior differently. A helpful metaphor for hemisphere specialization is a train station. Think of the left hemisphere as a train station with one track, so that only one train at a time can enter the station. This forces the left hemisphere to look into each train car (in which metaphorical information is

TABLE 1.1. Information Processing Styles of the Left and Right
Cerebral Hemispheres

Left	Right
1. Sequential processing	1. Parallel processing
2. Analytic, syllogistic	2. Intuitive, impulsive, emotional, rapid scanning, holistic
3. Focal and discreet	3. Diffuse
4. High frequency	4. Low frequency

being carried), one car at a time. Tedious and focused, the left hemisphere is very good at detail and is able to analyze and make inferences from that information. For example, if car one has 2 bits of information and car two 4 bits, the functioning left hemisphere will reason that car three is likely to have 6, 8, or 16 bits and, based on what that car actually has in it, the left hemisphere will then know the rule (adding twos, doubling or squaring the number). In contrast, the right hemisphere is like a train station into which several trains can enter simultaneously. Although the right hemisphere can be forced to look at each car in the sequential fashion of the left, it is not good at this. It is best at rapid scanning of information to detect broad patterns, or gestalts (for example: the trains are coming in fast or slowly or there are many trains, or only a few).

The train station metaphor suggests the two hemispheres are constructed ("hard wired") differently (Table 1.2), and there are left–right cerebral hemisphere differences consistent with the left being a discrete processor suited for language-related information (e.g., specific structures are larger) and the right hemisphere being a holistic processor of broad patterns of information (e.g., uniformly more white matter and dendritic communication).

Because of their structural differences, each hemisphere focuses on different physical attributes of the information being processed. For example, Figure 1.1 shows the letter H in high and low frequency forms. High frequency refers to dense information (or signal) per unit time or area; low frequency refers to less information per unit time or area. Although the letter H is a language symbol and should be processed better by the hemisphere organized for language (usually the left), this is only true when the H is presented as a high frequency stimulus. When presented as a low frequency stimulus, it is processed better by the right hemisphere because it is visually more ambiguous, and might represent several different things e.q. a goalpost or a street map. Figure 1.2 shows this even more dramatically. Information can be initially presented to only one hemisphere. This is done with an instrument termed a *tachistoscope,* which flashes stimuli into one or the other hemivisual fields. Because of the visual system's organization, left hemivisual field information goes to the right hemisphere first, and right hemivisual field information goes to the left hemisphere first. When information like that in Figure 1.2 is presented to each hemisphere, the left "sees" H, the high frequency stimulus, while the right "sees" S, the low frequency stimulus. Each hemisphere

TABLE 1.2. Anatomic Cerebral Hemisphere Asymmetries

Favoring Left	Favoring Right
Cerebral hemisphere larger and denser	Larger frontal area
Larger planum temporale (the posterior roof of the temporal lobe and an extension of Wernicke's area).	Greater dendritic arborization
Longer sylvian fissure and lateral ventricle	Relatively more white matter
Relatively more gray matter	Greater concentration of serotonergic neurons
Larger posterior temporal/parieto-occipital regions	
Greater concentration of dopaminergic neurons	

also differentially responds to other physical attributes of stimuli (e.g., luminescence, geometric shape, linearity). Because language and symbolic related stimuli are loaded with high frequency physical attributes, the left hemisphere, hard wired to handle the high frequency physical attributes of information, is activated when presented with such stimuli, and processes them, and so we think of it as "the language hemisphere."

In the real world, stimuli include both high and low frequency information, and the two hemispheres work together. As you read this book your nondominant hemisphere is processing the patterns. You can tell at a glance, even if you turn the book upside down, that the page has printed letters on it that form words and that the type of lettering is immediately recognizable as a Western European language. From the big picture provided by the nondominant hemisphere, the dominant hemisphere deals with the details, and you "read" what is written. The corpus callosum integrates these different forms of information processing, as well as being an interhemispheric communication bridge. For example, lesions in

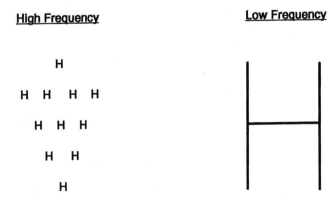

Figure 1.1. The frequency of the stimulus determines which hemisphere best processes it.

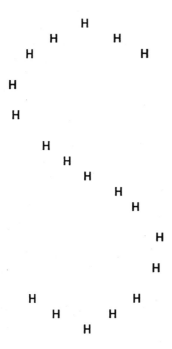

Figure 1.2. The left hemisphere processes the high frequency information and "sees" H. The right hemisphere processes the low frequency information and "sees" S.

the anterior corpus callosum can disconnect lexical language from the emotional content of language leading to a loss of emotional expression while reading aloud and speaking, but spontaneous emotional expression remains intact.

Although most people are left hemisphere dominant for language and right hemisphere specialized for visuo-spatial function (Table 1.3), specific language and nonlanguage tasks are variably lateralized in the same person. Thus, when trying to lateralize a lesion, always look for the pattern. Do not hang your diagnostic hat on one cognitive or behavioral peg. Other chapters describe the behaviors of dominant and nondominant cerebral hemisphere lesions in detail. Some classic dominant hemisphere syndromes are Broca's and Wernicke's aphasias and Gerstmann's syndrome. Some classic nondominant hemisphere syndromes are motor and receptive aprosodia, left spatial neglect, and misidentification syndromes (Capgras and Fregoli's).

Handedness

Primates prefer using one hand over the other for fine motor tasks. The preference distribution runs 50–50. Ninety percent of humans, however, primarily use the right hand for fine motor tasks. Hand preference roughly correlates with cerebral hemisphere organization for language. Assess each patient for handedness when looking for localized brain lesions.

TABLE 1.3. Some Specific Functions of the Left and Right
Cerebral Hemispheres

Left	*Right*
1. Language	1. Visuospatial
2. Verbal learning and memory	2. Visual learning and memory
3. Verbal reasoning and planning	3. Nonverbal reasoning and planning
4. Complex fine motor function	4. Facial recognition

Determine handedness by asking patients to demonstrate the use of objects and by writing their name or a sentence. Patient self-report is not reliable (i.e., which hand they say they use for a task is not always the hand they actually use). Demonstrations include using a knife to cut bread, pouring liquid from a bottle, threading a needle, and brushing one's teeth. Pure right handers consistently do these things and write with the right hand. Their language hemisphere is the left. Pure right-handed women have more bilateral representation of cognitive functions than do men, but they are also primarily left hemisphere "dominant" for language. Among left handers and persons with mixed handedness (i.e., they do several things with each hand) there is less certainty which hemisphere is dominant for language. The odds, however, still favor the left. Combined with an assessment of behavior and cognition, knowing the handedness of a patient helps in lateralizing lesions to the right or left.

Because only 10% or so of the population is left handed, left handers are deviant. For some left handers this deviance is familial and may be associated with creativity and better performance on some cognitive tests. For example, there is a disproportionately high number of left handers among persons with PhDs. For other left handers, their deviance may reflect prenatal or perinatal neural developmental problems. Thus, left handedness is also associated with developmental disorder, alcoholism, bipolar mood disorders, and numerous other neurologic conditions.

Eye and foot preferences are not correlated with cerebral organization. Nevertheless, children with mixed eye, foot, and hand preferences (e.g., right or mixed handed, left footed, right eyed) are more likely to have behavioral and school problems.

THE PERCEPTUAL-INTEGRATING BRAIN

The temporal, parietal, and occipital lobes of the cerebral hemispheres and related subcortical structures organize and make sense of the world around us. The perceptual-integrating brain may also subserve consciousness because it recognizes the distinction between ourselves and the external world—literally where we end and where the rest of the world begins. The perceptual-integrating brain tells us where we are in three-dimensional space vis à vis other objects and then stores this information as memory. Alzheimer's disease is a classic disease of the perceptual-integrating brain.

Parietal Lobes

The parietal lobes are roughly divided into two functional units: an anterior unit (the primary sensory cortex and its unimodal sensory associational cortex) *and a posterior heteromodal association unit (the inferior parietal lobule including the angular and supramarginal gyri, and the superior parietal lobule). The parietal lobes function as the primary and associational cortices of the thalamus.

Parietal lobe functions are (1) awareness of three-dimensional space and the relationship of the self to that space; (2) integrating semantic and visual sensory stimuli (e.g., vision to language); (3) linking somatosensory perception to motor performance and guidance of motor behavior in three-dimensional space; (4) manipulating spatial coordinates of abstract stimuli (e.g., mathematics); and (5) focused attention. Specifically, the parietal lobes are needed when we do calculations, simple motor and constructional tasks, read aloud, locate objects in space, pay attention to areas of the space surrounding us, and make abstract constructions.

Occipital Lobes

The occipital lobes process movement, color, and shape and begin organizing visual stimuli. The occipital lobes have no heteromodal cortex.

Temporal Lobes

Temporal lobe functions are (1) auditory sensory processing (recognizing and understanding speech and environmental sounds); (2) auditory and visual perception (facial recognition, reading); (3) providing affective tone (emotions) to sensory input; (4) new learning and long-term storage of sensory input (memory); and (5) triggering flight/fight behaviors and their physiologic changes. Specifically, the temporal lobes function in understanding speech, recognizing environmental sounds, generating emotion, learning new things, storing old perceptions and experiences for future reference, focusing our attention on sound, recognizing danger or potential danger, and initially and rapidly responding to danger.

Thalamus

The thalamus is the "pentium chip" of the brain. All somatosensory routes to the cerebral cortex pass through the thalamus. The thalamus (1) directly relays somatosensory information from the external world to the appropriate parietal primary sensory cortical homunculus so that body image is maintained; (2) through feedback projections, synchronizes visual and auditory information with the rest

*See below for details of cerebral cortex organization.

of the perceptual-integrating system; (3) organizes all sensory information so that, rather than experiencing the world in parts, we perceive it as an integrated whole; (4) integrates sensory information in conjunction with a special heteromodal cortical area in the temporal lobes (near the insula); and (5) provides tone to the frontal circuits and modulates attentiveness, wakefulness, and sleep.

Sensory experience is not a kaleidoscope but an integrated experience. The feel and weight of this book, the temperature of the room you are in, the ambient noise and light, the words on the page each are independently delivered to its respective primary sensory cortex. Because of integrating oscillations of the thalamus, and the further integration within the special heteromodal cortical area in the temporal lobes, you experience the entire integrated scene you are now in.

The thalamus is part of the perceptual-integrating brain *and* the action brain (see below). It links the posterior part of the action brain (the cerebellar-pontine unit) to the anterior part (the frontal loops). It is the feedback unit of the five left and five right functional frontal lobe circuits described below. Because of its connections to the reticular activating system it provides tone to the frontal circuits. It is one of the frontal circuitry connections to the limbic system.

Thalamic lesions can cause (1) frontal lobe syndromes (particularly avolition and eye tracking problems); (2) disturbances in emotion; (3) perceptual disturbances of disintegration (including hallucinations); (4) speech and language problems; (5) coordination and balance problems; (6) analgesia, hyperesthesia, and pain syndromes; (7) disturbances in body image; and (8) parietal lobe features (e.g., Gerstmann's syndrome, astereognosia).

Thalamic stroke and its effect on speech and language is a model for formal thought disorder, a classic feature of schizophrenia. Because of its multiple and integrating functions, the thalamus has been implicated as a major site in the pathophysiology of schizophrenia.

THE ACTION BRAIN

The perceptual-integrating brain makes sense of the world. The action brain responds. The action brain roughly includes the frontal lobes and their related subcortical structures, the cerebellum and pons, and the motor system between these anterior and posterior units. Inattention and *modest* altered arousal (low or high) have only moderate impact on the perceptual-integrating brain. Even small problems with attention and arousal can adversely affect action brain functioning. Structures of the limbic system involved in emotional expression and memory recall (e.g., amygdala, anterior hippocampus) can also be considered part of the action brain. The basic functions of the action brain are generating ideas, problem solving, emotional expression, and motor behavior (including speech).

The action brain also performs "executive" functions. These include planning, initiating actions, monitoring actions and self-correcting, verifying the planned action is being carried out correctly, and terminating the action when it is completed. Working memory (the brief holding of information in your mind's eye while you do something with that information, e.g., dial a phone number just said to you), recall of memory, and willed action are also basic to action brain functions.

The anterior part of the action brain is organized into five left and five right parallel circuits that can operate independently of each other. Figure 1.3 illustrates a generic anterior circuit. Information in the circuit only flows in one direction. The limbic system has its own frontal circuit (the anterior cingulate circuit) and also connects to the other parallel circuits via the globus pallidus and striatum. Thus, the action brain is greatly influenced by emotion. The prefrontal cortex also interacts with other heteromodal cortices via cortico-cortical fibers. The five parallel circuits are

1. *The motor circuit*: The primary and secondary motor cortex (areas 4, M2-medial surface anterior to area 4), the supplementary motor area (area 6), and some somatosensory fibers send afferents to the putamen that in turn sends information to the globus pallidus and substantia nigra. The globus pallidus sends information to the thalamus, which sends feedback to the primary and secondary motor cortices. Deficits in this system cause problems with sequential movement, movement initiation, self-correction, and learning of new motor sequences (particularly when area 6 is involved). Schizophrenics have problems with these functions.

2. *Oculomotor circuit*: The frontal eye fields and prefrontal cortex project to the caudate, globus pallidus, and substantia nigra. The globus pallidus then sends information to the thalamus,which sends feedback to the cortical areas that began the circuit. Lesions in this circuit can result in deficits in eye-tracking of moving objects. Schizophrenics and some of their first-degree relatives have eye-tracking problems.

3. *Dorsolateral prefrontal circuit*: Brodmann areas 9 and 10 project to the head of the caudate. The caudate connects to the globus pallidus and

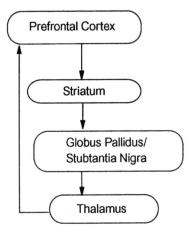

Figure 1.3. Anterior "action" brain parallel loop.

substantia nigra. The globus pallidus sends information to the thalamus, which sends feedback to the dorsolateral prefrontal cortex. Lesions in this circuit cause deficits in executive function. Patients cannot generate new ideas or shift cognitive set. They have no fluency or flexibility of thought. They have problems with organizational strategies for learning, poor construction strategies, and problems with motor programming (alternating and reciprocal motor tasks). The classic syndrome is termed the *dorsolateral frontal lobe syndrome,* and behaviorally these patients are avolitional (see Chapter 3). Chronic schizophrenics also have this syndrome. Pick's disease begins with this syndrome.

4. *Lateral orbitofrontal circuit*: The inferior lateral prefrontal cortex (Brodmann area 10) projects to the caudate. The caudate connects to the globus pallidus and substantia nigra with subloops to the globus pallidus externa and subthalamic nucleus. The globus pallidus and substantia nigra connect to the thalamus, which sends feedback to the lateral orbitofrontal cortex. Lesions in this circuit may lead to the classic *orbitofrontal (or disinhibition) syndrome* characterized by irritability, Witzelsucht (a silly, shallow mood), a coarsening of the personality with loss of social graces and tactlessness, echo phenomena,* and utilization behavior (they see an object and must touch it and use it). Chronic and atypical manics have this syndrome.

5. *Anterior cingulate circuit*: Brodmann area 24 projects to the striatum, nucleus accumbens, and the olfactory tubercle. The ventral striatum (or limbic striatum) also receives fibers from the hippocampus, amygdala, and entorhinal and perirhinal cortices. The ventral striatum then projects to the globus pallidus and substantia nigra. These connect with the subthalamic nucleus, ventral tegmental area, habenula, hypothalamus, amygdala, and thalamus. The thalamus then sends feedback to the anterior cingulate cortex. Lesions in this circuit can produce akinetic mutism, stupors with incontinence, and profound generalized analgesia. Catatonic patients can have these features.

Basal Ganglia

The basal ganglia form an integral unit of the frontal parallel circuits. They also have afferent and efferent connections with the limbic system. If the thalamus is the "pentium chip" of the brain, the basal ganglia is the crossroad of the brain. The frontal circuits and limbic system send information to it, and it sends feedback information to these systems. The brain's mesolimbic dopaminergic reward system (see Chapter 13) connects to it. The basal ganglia (1) fine-tune motor behavior and provide procedural memory programs of learned motor sequences (like riding a bike) to the frontal lobes; (2) help in self-monitoring of speech dur-

---

*Echolalia, the patient repeating your words; *echopraxia,* the patient repeats your movements. These are also catatonic features.

ing conversation; (3) participate in hand and facial expression during conversation and spontaneous emotion; and (4) participate in cognitive tasks (e.g., attention, working memory, new learning; particularly sensorimotor and visuomotor sequencing).

Classic basal ganglia syndromes include Parkinson's and Huntington's diseases. Obsessive compulsive disorders and Gilles de la Tourette's syndrome also involve the basal ganglia. Disease of the basal ganglia typically leads to problems with *motor* function, *mood*, and *memory*. The basal ganglia are the 3M Company of the brain.

Cerebellum

The cerebellum and pons are part of the motor system and, therefore, part of the "action" brain. This "unit" works in concert with the prefrontal cortex. There is direct functional reciprocal interaction between contralateral cerebellar and frontal neocortices. Anatomic connection is via corticopontine and cortico-olivary projections and lateral thalamic nuclei. Vermal connections to the thalamus are ipsilateral.

The cerebellum functions beyond motor coordination. It also modulates limbic system activation. This is an important consideration in diagnosing a person with what appears to be psychosensory (partial complex) epilepsy with irritability (see Chapter 10) because although the patient's symptoms may at first suggest a lesion in the temporal lobes, the pathology may actually be in the cerebellum. Your assessment of cerebellar motor signs helps differentiate these possibilities.

The cerebellum is also involved in (1) motor planning: trial and error planning with a motor output, (e.g., learning carpentry, solving a puzzle that requires moving objects into a pattern); (2) new learning: procedural motor responses that can be rapidly and automatically begun without having to "think" about it (e.g., learning martial arts, dance steps); and (3) speech and language: using action verbs, helping organizing motoric language

Cerebellar lesions can result in (1) loss of learned movement sequences (e.g., knitting, playing a musical instrument); (2) the inability to learn new movement sequences (practice does not help); (3) deficits in the ability to be classically conditioned (the conditioned stimulus—e.g., a tone is linked to an unconditioned stimulus such as a puff of air to the cornea that causes eyeblink, so that after a while the tone produces the blink); and (4) speech problems in which verbs are no longer used properly (incorrect tense, e.g., "I wanted to going to the store") and fluency is impaired (trouble linking action verbs and nouns).

THE TRIPARTITE PHYLOGENETIC SYSTEM

Almost 30 years ago Paul McLean described the triune brain: an old reptilian brain, a newer paleomammalian system, and the new primate neocortex. Each of these systems has its neuroanatomy and characteristic behaviors. Compared with our closest primates, the human brain differs most in the size of the prefrontal cortex, the parietal lobe heteromodal cortex, and the neocortex of the cerebellum. Although oversimplified, McLean was making the following points:

1. Human behavior and the brain systems that subserve it are products of human evolution. A full understanding of human behavior is within an evolutionary context.
2. Evolution is a great conservator; it typically does not discard structures, it reuses them in modified ways.* Thus, human behavior includes aspects of our phylogeny.
3. Human behavior is not simply a function of the neocortex; subcortical structures and older cortex also play major roles in generating human behavior.

The left–right view of brain behavior relationships has heuristic value, but it is two-dimensional. When put together with the tripartite, phylogenetic three-dimensional view of the brain, the combined concepts tell us that lateralized cognitive function (e.g., the "left brain" does this, the "right brain" does that) is limited. The left and right sides of the oldest parts of our brains do not process information differently and do not have specialized "talents." Only the neocortex and specific nuclei in some subcortical structures (in the basal ganglia and thalamus) are lateralized this way. This understanding of the limits of lateralization helps when you try to localize lesions or hypothesize the pathophysiology of a behavioral syndrome.

The Reptilian Brain

Many parts of our brains have changed very little from those of reptiles. The anatomy of this system is brain stem, related vestibular system, thalamus, hypothalamus, basal ganglia, some forebrain nuclei, the amygdala, and the hippocampus.

This system is primarily responsible for arousal, activation, balance, information input and output, homeostatic and procreative drives, and flight/fight. Lesions in this system have generalized cognitive and behavioral effects, usually due to problems with arousal. Lesions in this system (usually bilateral) can result in stuporous states, catatonia, and anxiety disorders.

The Paleomammalian Brain and Limbic System

This system is primarily the limbic system, and it phylogenetically develops in earnest among social mammals where subtleties in emotion and good memory are helpful in maintaining the social structure of a relatively small group of individuals (as opposed to a herd of thousands). The anatomy of this system is the mammillary bodies, fornix, corona radiata, hippocampus, parahippocampus,

---

*For example, the basal ganglia participate in flight/fight motor actions (reptilian), fine tune hand and facial movement and expression (primates), and are involved in conversational speech (humans).

amygdala, hypothalamus, entorhinal cortex and pathways, septal nuclei, and the cingulate gyrus. The limbic system modifies appetitive drives and flight/fight. It generates emotion and provides emotional tone to perceptions. It is important in new learning and memory.

Although there is some evidence that some social emotions (nostalgia, shame, guilt, disgust) are related more to left hemisphere activity, this may be an artifact of attribution verbalized in language systems (i.e., what we feel guilty or shameful about depends on what we have culturally learned), and this is embedded in our language. So-called primary emotions—anger, fear, happiness, sadness—are seen in other primates and are less lateralizeable. Not surprisingly, there are no consistent findings for lateralized dysfunction in patients with primary mood or anxiety disorders.

Disorders of the limbic system produce numerous forms of psychopathology. Disease of mesial structures (mesial orbitofrontal and diencephalon) can result in disinhibition, depression, mania, anxiety, and panic. Disease of the mesial amygdala and hypothalamus can cause rage; disease of the lateral amygdala and temporal lobe pole can lead to extreme placidity as part of the Kluver-Bucy syndrome.* Disease of the anterior cingulate can cause apathy and stupor. Psychotic features are also commonly seen with limbic system disease.

The Neomammalian Brain

The newest system of our brain includes the cerebral hemisphere heteromodal associational cortices, the cerebellar neocortex, and large parts of the corpus callosum. The neomammalian brain is part of the action brain *and* the perceptual-integrating brain. Lesions in this system can lead to specific behaviors that can be linked to the left or right.

Cerebral Hemisphere Cortex Functional Organization

In addition to left–right specializations, the cerebral cortex is divided into five zones: limbic cortex, paralimbic cortex, primary sensory and motor cortices, unimodal association areas, and heteromodal associational areas.

The *primary sensory cortices* receive afferentation (incoming information) from the external environment. This information is initially modality specific, that is, each primary sensory cortex can accept only one type of input (e.g., the primary occipital cortex can only process visual information; the primary auditory cortex in the temporal lobes can only process sounds). This "unimodal" information is then correlated with other sensory information.

Each primary sensory area is connected to a *unimodal sensory association area.* These secondary cortices organize sensory information into recognizable patterns (perceptions). For example, information of patterns of light and shadow from the primary visual cortex are further organized in the unimodal associational visual

---

*Bilateral temporal lobe disease causing placidity, increased oral behavior (compulsive chewing and biting; swallowing of foreign bodies), hypersexuality, and visual agnosia.

cortex to form an image so that the light and shadow on this page become recognizable as organized groups of black symbols representing words. Even if the symbols were in an unfamiliar language you would recognize the group of pages as a book.

Heteromodal association areas are in the inferior and superior parietal lobule, the temporal lobe neocortex, and the prefrontal cortex. The occipital lobe does not have heteromodal association cortex. These areas synthesize sensory information from different unimodal sensory association areas and with the limbic system produce integrated, language-relevant perceptions. Names are put to objects. Images on a page are given specific meaning.

The *primary motor cortex* in the frontal lobes subserves the brain's response to sensory information. It gives rise to the internal capsule, and the corticospinal and corticobulbar tracks, the former conveying motor impulses down the spinal cord to the skeletal musculature for movement. The primary motor cortex recruits motor neurons to perform movements.

Unimodal motor association areas contain motor programs for complex movements (e.g., typing, writing, speaking, playing golf). The motor program contains the central representation of all the combinations of pools of motor neurons needed to perform the task. A neuron may be in more than one pool, because there are many more complex motor movements (programs) than there are motor neurons. The motor programs guide the primary motor cortex in selecting the correct pools of motor neurons to do the task. The unimodal motor association areas in turn are guided by sensory information. For example, to hit a golf ball the motor neuron pools called upon for each sequence of the stance and swing must be guided by where the head and torso and the arms and legs are located through each phase of the swing. What each part of the body is doing, where it is precisely located in three-dimensional space at each moment in time, is needed sensory information to guide motor sequencing.

The *limbic cortex* modulates the internal milieu (homeostasis), provides emotional coloring to experience, modulates drives and instincts, and participates in memory and learning. The limbic cortex is in the temporal lobes, particularly the hippocampus.

The *paralimbic cortex* forms a rough link between the rest of the limbic system and cortical heteromodal association areas. It includes orbitofrontal cortex, insula, the temporal pole, parahippocampal gyrus of the temporal lobes, and the cingulate gyrus that curves over the corpus callosum and forms part of the mesial aspects of the frontal and parietal lobes.

NEUROCHEMICAL ORGANIZATION

Many behavioral disorders have been related to the brain's specific neurochemical systems. Some of these systems are distributed more or less evenly throughout the brain. Others have more anatomic and behavioral specificity. Understanding neurochemical neuroanatomy helps in understanding behavior, diagnosing and localizing brain disease, and guiding pharmacologic treatments. Several chapters in this book describe the neurochemical–neuroanatomic relationships of particular conditions (e.g., anxiety disorder, substance abuse), behaviors (e.g., violence), and treatments (e.g., the pharmacodynamics of psychotropic drugs). This section gives an overview of these relationships.

Table 1.4 displays the typical steps in pre- and post-synaptic neuron neurotransmitter activity. Different psychotropic drugs work at different steps in these processes. For example, specific serotonin reuptake-inhibiting antidepressants (SSRIs) such as fluoxetine work on presynaptic Step 5, keeping more neurotransmitter in the synaptic cleft. The increased neurotransmitter, serotonin in this case, is now more available to post-synaptic receptors *and* to presynaptic autoreceptors. Changes in these receptors, reduced (downregulation) or increased (upregulation) numbers, or sensitivity of receptors, is thought to account for the pharmacodynamic behavioral effects of these drugs. Pindolol, in contrast to reuptake inhibitors, is an antagonist of presynaptic serotonin autoreceptors (presynaptic Step 4) inhibiting the presynaptic terminal from slowing the production of serotonin. When given with an SSRI, pindolol permits continued serotonin synthesis and release despite the SSRI keeping more serotonin in the synaptic cleft, which would normally trigger autoreceptors to slow production. This neurochemical "enchancement" is the rationale for pindolol's use as an SSRI antidepressant enhancer (therapeutic effect is uncertain). A different example is lithium, which works on postsynaptic neurons affecting second-messenger systems (post-synaptic Step 2). Monoamine oxidase inhibitors work intracellularly to prevent the presynaptic neuron from breaking neurotransmitters so more is available (presynaptic Step 6).

Table 1.5 displays the different types of neurotransmitters. Neurotransmitters include monoamines, peptides, and amino acids. Receptors, ion channels, and second messengers respond to these transmitters. Hormones and other substances modulate the response. Table 1.6 displays the neuroanatomy and significance of the neurotransmitters presently considered most important to neuropsychiatry.

TABLE 1.4. Generic Steps in Neurotransmitter Action

Presynaptic Terminal	*Post-synaptic Terminal*
1. Transmitter synthesis from a *precursor*	1. Transmitter binding with receptors
2. Transmitter storage in a *vesicle*	a. *Ligand-binding receptor* opens *ion channel*, permitting ions through cell membrane
3. Transmitter release into *synaptic cleft*	
4. Transmitter interaction (binding) with presynaptic *autoreceptors* to regulate synthesis and release (by inhibiting presynaptic membrane activity or through presynaptic *second-messenger* systems)	b. *G protein–coupled receptor* initiates post-synaptic intracellular sequences via a *second-messenger* substance
	2. Ion exchanges through membrane and second-messenger cascades (e.g., cyclic AMP activity) lead to post-synaptic neuron inhibition or excitation
5. *Reuptake* of transmitter by presynaptic terminal	
6. Reuse of transmitter or breakdown of transmitter by *monoamine oxidase*	3. Enzymes degrade the transmitter or transmitter is transported back to presynaptic neuron for reuptake

TABLE 1.5. Neurotransmitters and Modulators

Monoamines	Peptides	Amino Acids	Second Messengers	Hormones
Dopamine	Endorphins	Excitatory Glutamic acid Aspartic acid	Cyclic AMP	Testosterone and other androgenic steroid hormones
Norepinephrine	Enkephalin (beta-, leu-, met-)	Inhibitory Glycine Gamma- aminobutyric acid (GABA Tacrine Proline	Phosphatidyl- linositol cycle	Estrogens
Serotonin	Dynorphin			Progesterone
Adenosine	Tachykinins			Cortisol and related steroid hormones
Acetylcholine	Substance P			
	Somatostatin			
	Cholecystokinin			
	Angiotensin			
	Oxytocin			
	Vasopressin			
	Prolactin			
	Interleukins			
	Neuropeptide Y			
	Neurotensin			

Dopamine is concentrated in the core of the central nervous system and mediates tone (but not arousal), the processes of the action brain, and the hedonistic reward system. Too much dopamine activity usually results in increased motor behavior, mood changes (euphoria and irritability), and disrupted frontal circuit function. Too little dopamine activity usually results in apathy, motor movement disorder, depressive-like syndromes, and poor working memory. Norepinephrine activity is fundamental to flight/fight. Its distribution begins in the pons and then bifurcates into each side of the limbic system and into the cerebral hemispheres. Too much norepinephrine activity usually results in anxiety and defensive or attack behavior. Serotonin distribution begins centrally in the brain stem. Its distribution then splits, one branch paralleling dopamine and the other paralleling norepinephrine. Becuse it interacts with several neurotransmitter systems, abnormalities in serotonin activity result in a wide variety of behavioral changes. Dopamine, norepinephrine, and serotonin are monoamine neurotransmitters. Monoamine oxidase degrades them all.

Endogenous opiates are neuropeptides that usually work as a co-transmitter with some other neuroactive compound. Other neuropeptides are tachykinins,

Table 1.6. Neurotransmitters

Neuroanatomy	Significance

DOPAMINE (DA)

1. DA receptors are G-protein linked; D_1 (post-synaptic) stimulate cyclic AMP, D_2 (presynaptic) and D_4 (post-synaptic) inhibit cyclic AMP	1. Provides tone to the brain core and via the thalamus to frontalcircuits
2. DA neurons are located in the brain stem, midbrain, and forebrain	2. The most important transmitter in the action brain, involved in movement and cognition
3. Subsystems include	3. The neurotransmitter of hedonistic reward (pleasure); all drugs of abuse affect DA
a. Nigrostriatal (D_1, D_2)	
b. Tubulofundibular (D_1, D_2)	4. Underlies hypothalamic–pituitary–end organ axes
c. Mesolimbic (D_2, D_4)	
d. Mesocortical (D_4, D_1, D_2 low)	5. Underlies personality traits of behavioral activation (e.g., exploratory behavior, impulsivity)
4. The lateral hypothalamus, ventral tegmental area, and nucleus accumbens linked by the medial forebrain bundle is the brain's hedonistic reward system	
5. Mediates some pain sensation via dorsal horn spinal cord projections	

NOREPINEPHRINE (NE)

1. NE receptors are G-protein coupled; alpha receptors inhibit cyclic AMP; beta receptors stimulate cyclic AMP: $alpha_1$ (throughout the brain) are post-synaptic, $alpha_2$ (cortex and locus ceruleus) are pre- and post-synaptic; beta (throughout the brain) are post-synaptic	1. Regulation of blood pressure, cardiovascular tone, lung airway dilation, intestinal motility
2. Major transmitter of the post-synaptic sympathetic nervous system	2. Mediates arousal
3. Spinal cord projections involved in muscle tone	3. Underlies flight/fight system
4. Major source is the locus ceruleus in dorsolateral pons, projects to	4. Involved in new learning and mood (e.g., fear, anxiety, anger)
a. Cerebellum (few)	5. Underlies behavioral maintenance trait behaviors
b. Median forebrain bundle to the hypothalamus, thalamus, basal ganglia, amygdala, hippocampus, and cerebral cortex	

SEROTONIN (5-HT)

1. Origin in a series of midline brain stem nuclei: raphe nuclei	1. Major homeostatic neurotransmitter; regulates gut, brain stem arousal, and sleep
2. Multiple receptors: $5\text{-}HT_1$, $5\text{-}HT_2$, $5\text{-}HT_4$ are G-protein linked; $5\text{-}HT_3$, in periphery only, is ligand gated; some	2. Modulates NE and DA actions

Table 1.6. (*continued*)

Neuroanatomy	Significance

SEROTONIN (5-HT) (continued)

receptors are post-synaptic, others are presynaptic

3. Projections include:

    a. Descending spinal cord in pain modulation

    b. Dorsal raphe nucleus projections parallel DA projections (forebrain–frontal circuits reward system)

    c. Median raphe nucleus projections parallel NE projections (limbic system, flight/fight system)

3. Low levels implicated in impulsiveness, violence; high levels implicated in anxiety

4. Underlies behavioral inhibition trait behaviors

OPIATES

1. Distribution of opiate-related peptides (endorphin, enkephalin, dynorphin) and receptors (mu, delta, kappa) is widespread; some areas of concentration are

    a. Amygdala and hypothalamus

    b. Ventral tegmental area and n. accumbens

    c. Basal ganglia

    d. Hippocampus

    e. Cerebral cortex

2. Receptors are ligand binding

3. Receptors located at different sites than peptides (!?)

1. Pain, pleasure, and reward systems modulated by opiate system

2. Opiates modulate monoamine neurotransmitter systems

GAMMA-AMINOBUTERIC ACID (GABA)

1. GABA widespread throughout the brain, released presynaptically

2. GABA is the only output neurotransmitter of the cerebellar Purkinje cell system, the caudate putamen, and n. accumbens

3. Other GABA concentrations include other basal ganglia structures, the thalamus, and the hippocampus

4. GABA$_A$ receptor, located with GABA neurons, is a ligand-gated chloride ion channel (hyperpolarizes post-synaptic neuron). Benzodiazepines modulate these channels even if GABA is absent

5. Benzodiazepine receptors: "peripheral" is on mitochondrial transporter and

1. The predominant fast-acting inhibitory neurotransmitter

2. The inhibitor of the action brain

3. Antikindling drugs work on GABA-mediated ion channels

Table 1.6. Neurotransmitters (*continued*)

Neuroanatomy	Significance

Gamma-aminobuteric acid (GABA) (*continued*)

has nothing to do with GABA; "central"
type 1 is anxiolytic, type 2 is sedative
and antiseizure

6. $GABA_B$ receptor, located on presynaptic
non-GABA neurons and on post-synaptic GABA neurons, is G-protein linked
and inhibits cyclic AMP

Glutamate

1. Widespread; particularly action brain

2. "Internal" triangle functional relaton-
ship: presynaptic release, glial uptake
and re-release, and presynaptic
reuptake

3. Several types of ion channel–related
receptors: *AMPA* (alpha-amino-3-
hydroxy-5-methylisoxazole-4-propionic
acid) works on sodium channels, particularly in the action brain; *NMDA* (N-
methyl-D-aspartate) works on calcium
channels, particularly in hippocampus
and cerebral and cerebellar neocortices;
kainate works on sodium channels in the
neocortex; *metabotropic* G-protein–
linked receptors in cerebellum, thalamus, basal ganglia, hippocampus,
cortex

1. Brain's main excitatory amino acid
neurotransmitter

2. Function appears to be CNS homeostasis
and facilitating new learning

3. Too much release occurs in response to
toxins and is implicated in seizure focus
spread; phencyclidine binds to the
NMDA receptor

Glycine

1. Widespread on inhibitory spinal cord
inter neurons and at NMDA sites

2. Post-synaptic inhibitory receptors and a
second receptor that is part of the glutamate NMDA receptor required for that
receptor to work

1. Inhibitory amino acid, needed for
NMDA activation

Acetylcholine (Ach)

1. Six types of Ach neurons in CNS with
distribution in spinal cord motor ventral horn and brain stem motor nuclei

2. Projections to motor system and peripheral nervous system

3. Projections from pons to basal ganglia as
part of the Reticular Activating System

4. The nucleus basalis of Meynert projects
to other forebrain areas and then to the

1. Major transmitter of the peripheral
motor system

2. Major transmitter of the presynaptic autonomic nervous system

3. Major post-synaptic transmitter in sweat
glands and the entire parasympathetic
nervous system

4. As part of Reticular Activating system
(RAS) regulates sleep/wake cycles

Table 1.6. (*continued*)

Neuroanatomy	Significance

ACETYLCHOLINE (ACH) (continued)

entire cerebral neocortex, hippocampus, and amygdala 5. *Nicotinic receptor* linked to ion channels (sodium and calcium) mostly in presynaptic neurons in CNS and sympathetic ganglia; *muscarinic receptors* mostly on post-synaptic parasympathetic neurons (influence heart, gut, sweat glands). A CNS muscarinic post-synaptic receptor (M_1) is G-protein linked, an M_2 version is an autoreceptor	5. Hippocampal and cortical projections involved in new learning; Ach neuronal degeneration in nucleus basilis of Meynert implicated in Alzheimer's disease; Ach neuronal degeneration in basal ganglia implicated in Parkinson's disease

substance P, and somatostatin, concentrated in the medulla, hypothalamus, and hedonistic reward system. Amino acid neurotransmitters include GABA and glycine (both inhibitory), glutamate (excitatory), and acetycholine (the prime transmitter of the peripheral nervous system as well as a fundamental central nervous system transmitter).

ADDITIONAL READINGS

Alexander GE, Crutcher MD: Functional architecture of basal ganglia circuits: Neural substrates of parallel processing. *TINS* 13:266–271, 1990.

Alexander GE, Crutcher MD, De Long MR: Basal ganglia–thalamocortical circuits: Parallel substrates for motor, oculomotor, "prefrontal" and "limbic" functions. In Ulyings HMB, Van Eden Cg, De Bruin JPC, Corner MA, Feenstra MA (ed): *The Prefrontal Cortex: Its Structure. Function and Pathology. Progress in Brain Research*, vol 85. Elsevier, Amsterdam, 1990, pp. 119–146.

Alexander GE, De Long MR: Strict parallel organization of functionally segregated circuits linking basal ganglia and cortex. *Annu Rev Neurosci* 9:357–381, 1986.

Banich MT: The missing link: The role of interhemispheric interaction in attentional processing. *Brain Cogn* 36:128–157, 1998.

Barker WW, Yoshii F, Loewenstein DA, Chang JY, Apicella A, Pascal S, Boothe TE, Ginsberg MD, Duara R: Cerebrocerebellar relationship during behavioral activation: A PET study. *Journal of Cerebral Blood Flow and Metabolism* 11:48–54, 1991.

Boni S, Valle G, Cioffi RP, Bonetti MG, Perrone E, Tofani A, Maini CL: Crossed cerebello-cerebral diaschisis: A SPECT study. *Nucl Med Commun* 1:824–831, 1982.

Bryden MP: *Laterality. Functional Asymmetry in the Intact Brain.* Academic Press, New York, 1982.

Campbell R: The lateralization of emotion: A critical review. *Int J Psychol* 17:211–229, 1982.

Contreras D, Destexhe A, Sejnowski TJ, Stervade M: Control of spatiotemporal coherence of a thalamic oscilllation by corticothalamic feedback. *Science* 274:771–774, 1996.

Crosson B: Subcortical functions in language: A working model. *Brain Lang* 25:257–292, 1985.

Crosson B, Huges CW: Role of the thalamus in language: Is it related to schizophrenic thought disorder? *Schizophr Bull* 13:605–621, 1987.

Davidson M: Neuropeptides. In Davis K, Klar H, Coyle JT (eds): *Foundations of Psychiatry*. WB Saunders, Phildelphia, 1991, pp 92–98.

DiPellegrino G, Wise SP: A neurophysiological comparison of three distinct regions of the primate frontal lobe. *Brain* 114:951–978, 1991.

Doyan J, Gaudreau D, LaForce R Jr, Castonguay M, Bedard PJ, Bedard F, Bouchard J-P: Role of the striaum, cerebellum, and frontal lobes in the learning of a visuomotor sequence. *Brain Cogn* 34:218–245, 1997.

Fein D, Waterhouse L, Lucci D, Pennington B, Humes M: Handedness and cognitive functions in pervasive developmental disorders. *J Autism Dev Dis* 15:323–333, 1985.

Frith C: Positron emission tomography studies of frontal lobe function: Relevance to psychiatric disease. In Ciba Foundation Symposium 163: *Exploring Brain Functional Anatomy With Positron Tomography*. Wiley, Chichester, 1991, pp 181–197.

Iaccino JF: *Left Brain–Right Brain Differences, Inquires, Evidence, and New Approaches*. Lawrence Erlbaum Associates, Hillsdale, NJ, 1993.

Geschwind N: *Selected Papers on Language and the Brain*. D Reidel, Boston, 1974.

Geschwind N: The anatomical basis of hemisphere differentiation. In Diamond S, Beaumont J (ed): *Hemisphere Function in the Human Brain*. Halstead Press, New York, 1977, pp 7–24.

Goldman-Rakic PS: Development of cortical circuitry and cognitive function. *Child Dev* 58:601–622, 1987.

Graybiel AM, Aosaki T, Flaherty AW, Kimura M: The basal ganglia and adaptive motor control. *Science* 265:1826–1831, 1994.

Kim SG, Ashe J, Hendrich K, Ellermann JM, Merkle H, Ugurbil K, Georgopoulos AP: Functional magnetic resonance imaging of motor cortex: Hemispheric asymmetry and handedness. *Science* 261:615–617, 1993.

Kolb B, Whishaw IQ: *Fundamentals of Human Neuropsychology* 4th ed., WH Freeman, New York, 1996.

LaMendola NP, Bever TG: Peripheral and cerebral asymmetries in the rat. *Science* 278:483–486, 1987.

Levander M, Schalling D, Levander SE: Birth stress, handedness and cognitive performance. *Cortex* 25:673–681, 1989.

Lidsky TI: Neuropsychiatric implications of basal ganglia dysfunction. *Biol Psychiatry* 41: 383:385, 1997.

Llinas R: Is dyslexia a dyschronia? *Ann NY Acad Sci* 682:48–56, 1993.

MacLean PD: In *A Triune Concept of the Brain and Behavior*. University of Toronto Press, Toronto, BC, 1973.

MacLean PD: *The Triune Brain in Evolution, Role in Paleocerebral function*. Plenum Press, New York, 1990.

Mega MS, Cummings JL, Salloway S, Malloy P: The limbic system: An anatomic, phylogenetic and clinical perspective. *J Neuropsychiatry Clin Neurosci* 9:315–330, 1997.

Mesulam MM: *Principles of Behavioral Neurology*. FA Davis, Philadelphia, 1985

Metter EJ, Kempler D, Jackson MA, Hanson WR, Riege WH, Camras LR, Mazziotta JC, Phelps ME: Cerebellar glucose metabolism in chronic aphasia. *Neurology* 37:1599–1606, 1987.

Mind and Brain, Readings from Scientific American. WH Freeman, Salt Lake City, UT, 1993.

Murphy M, Deutsch SI: Neurophysiological and neurochemical basis of behavior. In Davis K, Klar H, Coyle JT (eds): *Foundations of Psychiatry*, WB Saunders, Philadelphia, 1991, pp 67–86.

Penny JB Jr: Neurochenical neuroanatomy. In Fogel BS, Schiffer RB, Rao SM (eds): *Neuropsychiatry*. Williams & Wilkins, Baltimore, 1996, pp 145–171.

Powell DA: The prefrontal–thalamic axis and classical conditioning. *Integr Physiol Behav Sci* 27:101–116, 1992.

Proverbio AM, Zani A, Avella C: Hemispheric asymmetries for spatial frequency discrimination in a selective attention task. *Brain Cogn 34*:311–320, 1997.

Sackeim HA, Greenberg MS, Weiman AL, Gur RE, Hungerbuhler JP, Geschwind N: Hemisphere asymmetry in the expression of positive and negative emotions. *Arch Neurol 39*: 210–218, 1982.

Sandson TA, Daffner KR, Carvalho PA, Mesulam M-M: Frontal lobe dysfunction following infarction of the left-sided medial thalamus. *Arch Neurol 48*:1300–1303, 1991.

Satz P, Orsini DL, Saslow E, Henry R: The pathological left-handedness syndrome. *Brain Cogn 4*:27–46, 1985.

Scheibel AB: The thalamus and neuropsychiatric disease. *J Neuropsychiatry Clin Neurosci 9*:342–353, 1997.

Scheibel AB, Wechsler AF (eds): *Neurobiology of Higher Cognitive Function.* Guilford Press, New York, 1990.

Sergent J: Influence of luminance on hemispheric processing. *Bull Psychonomic Soc 20*:221–223, 1982.

Smith CUM: Evolutionary biology and psychiatry. *Br J Psychiatry 162*:149–153, 1993.

Smith GS, Dewey SL, Brodie JD, Logan J, Vitkun SA, Simkowitz P, Schloesser R, Alexoff DA, Hurley A, Cooper T, Volkow ND: Serotonin modulation of dopamine measured with [^{11}C] raclopride and PET in normal human subjects *Am J Psychiatry 154*:450–456, 1997.

Stahl SM: *Essential Psychopharmacology.* Cambridge University Press, Cambridge, England 1996.

Szelies B, Herholz K, Pawlik G, Karbe H, Hebold I, Heiss W-D: Widespread Functional effects of discrete thalamic infarction. *Arch Neurol 48*:178–182, 1991.

Thach WT: On the specific role of the cerebellum in motor learning and cognition: Clues from PET activation and lesion studies in man. *Behav Brain Sci 19*:411–431, 1996.

Vogel SA: Gender differences in itelligence, language, visual-motor abilities, and academic achievement in students with learning disabilities: A Review of the literature. *J Learn Disabil 23*:44–52, 1990.

Yamamoto T, Yoshida K, Yoshikawa H, Kishimoto Y, Oka H: The medial dorsal nucleus is one of the thalamic relays of the cerebellocerebral responses to the frontal association cortex in the monkey: Horseradish peroxidase and fluorescent dye double staining study. *Brain Res 579*:315–320, 1992.

2

Neuropsychiatric Evaluation

Neuropsychiatric evaluation is the medical examination of the brain. The *mental status examination*, and the *psychiatric interview* are terms from the era of a mind–body dichotomy. There is no "mental" to it. The mind, in a neuroscience sense, is a shorthand metaphoric term for summing up what our brains do that reaches our awareness (e.g., internal speech subserved by the dominant hemisphere, emotional experience generated by the limbic system, body image and its physical limits subserved in part by the parietal lobes, and memory acquisition, storage, and recall subserved by several brain systems). When you assess "mental functions" and behavior you are assessing brain functions.

In examining for brain disease or dysfunction, behavior changes are the patient's signs and symptoms. Your questions and comments are your osculation and percussion. The evaluation, however, is of the brain, and the examination follows all the rules for the evaluation of any body organ. The evaluation includes the examination itself (the present state of the patient), the history, and laboratory studies. An analogy is the examination of the digestive tract with its different components (e.g., stomach, gallbladder, large intestine). Each component has its pattern of signs and symptoms, and each component is vulnerable to different diseases. The brain also has component parts or systems with different signs and symptoms (e.g., left, right, action vs. perceptual-integrating brain) and different disease vulnerabilities (e.g., herpes has an affinity for the temporal lobes). Knowing the brain's different components and their behavioral signs and systems helps to structure your examination.

EXAMINATION GOALS

Neuropsychiatric examination requires skill in interacting with people. It is mostly done without touching the patient and begins when you first meet the patient. The goals are to establish a reasonable doctor–patient relationship (essential for correct diagnosis and treatment) and determine probable diagnosis.

Keep historical information separate from behavioral observations made during the examination. Past information is needed for diagnosis, but behaviors can change as the illness changes: Bipolar patients can shift from stupor to excitement to depression within hours or minutes; suicidal feelings may fluctuate. You may need to examine an acutely ill patient several times daily, and confusion results if you mix historical with physical findings.

The examination also gathers information needed to plan laboratory testing (e.g., neuropsychological testing, brain imaging, electrophysiologic measures) and treatment. For example, knowing a patient's hobbies and interests may not be helpful for diagnosis, but it may provide clues about cognitive strengths and weaknesses that could affect treatment outcome. In such a situation neuropsychological testing might help vocational planning following recovery. Some personal information has no diagnostic importance (e.g., names and interests of the patient's children), but, because treatment is often long-term, this information helps you maintain an interest in the patient's life, reinforces the doctor–patient relationship, and increases compliance with treatment.

EXAMINATION STYLE

The style of the examination depends on your personality. You can facilitate the examination by establishing a conversational manner and interactive relationship with the patient (i.e., the tone and style of the examination) and reinforcing this interactive relationship with personal and supportive comments.

A metaphor for the examination style is a kitchen conversation with a neighbor who comes to you for advice. In that situation, many people would invite the neighbor into the kitchen (more homey and relaxing than the living room), ask the neighbor to sit, and perhaps share some coffee. There would be "small talk" while the coffee is brewing, and finally the reason for the visit would be raised. In the form of a medical evaluation, the patient is invited in and made to feel comfortable. You determine the setting and you initiate the "small talk." Doing this controls the situation and begins subtly establishing the doctor–patient relationship.

This process begins when you first see the patient. Greet the patient outside the office, and chat with him during the walk to the office and as he sits. This introduction often sets the tone for the rest of the examination. Put the patient at ease by commenting about the weather, or a recent inpatient activity, or the trip to the clinic or office. Patient uncooperativeness usually results from anxiety, suspiciousness, or irritability.

Additional examination style strategies are to

1. Sit kitty-corner to the patient, not behind a barricading desk (face to face is too aggressive and anxiety provoking for many patients).
2. Assume a relaxed posture (rather than sitting stiffly like a "judge").
3. Avoid jargon. Use colloquialisms and idioms whenever possible so that terms such as *episode, hospitalization,* and *diagnosis* become phrases such as "when you were sick before," "when you last stayed overnight in a hospital," and "did your doctors tell you what they thought was

the problem (did they give it a name)?" Specific words and phrases you use are important. "Hi" is less formal than "hello"; "chat" is more relaxing than "examine" or "talk."

4. Use appropriate humor. Patients also say and do things that are humorous; do not be afraid to laugh or also say something humorous.

5. Be forthright. Even the awkwardness of having to complete clinical forms while examining the patient can be minimized by comments such as "I'll be taking a few notes to keep things straight in my mind" or "to be thorough to make sure I don't forget to check on things that may be important."

6. Use supportive comments to put the patient at ease, and give him the sense that you are interested in him as a person and not just as a clinical entity. Manic patients, for example, often become cooperative following positive comments about their colorful dress. Dysphoric depressed patients are more willing to relate their experiences following empathic comments about their obvious distress rather than "how are you feeling" type comments.

THE EXAMINATION STRUCTURE

The conversational tone of the examination is its style. Despite this seeming informality, the examination should not be haphazard. Structure is important. Questions and testing procedures should proceed logically while remaining responsive to the patient's behavior. Cover every area of the examination in a standardized manner. Use open-ended questioning at the beginning of the assessment of each topic area and then focus on the details. Maintain a sequence of topics and approach for each symptom area. The examination structure follows the logical steps underlying the diagnostic and treatment planning process.

Step 1: Determine the syndrome by establishing the patient's fundamental chief complaint. The fundamental chief complaint is not simply the first thing the patient tells you about why he is seeing you. It is the minimum amount of information needed to generate an initial differential diagnostic list. For example, the patient says he is "anxious." Such a statement usually becomes *the* chief complaint in a medical history. The fundamental chief complaint, however, puts this initial statement into some context. The fundamental complaint is a word picture suggesting diagnostic ideas to you. "Anxiety and headaches" has different but overlapping diagnostic implications from "anxiety and loss of interest." The first would generate a list of diagnostic choices that would include pheochromocytoma; the second would generate a list that included major depression. When looking for the pattern, focus on the basic big picture features of the signs and symptoms. When considering diagnostic choices also remember that the most important diagnostic information is age, gender, and then type of illness onset (e.g., acute vs. insidious). For example, if the patient is female you do not have to worry about testicular disease. The odds are also against antisocial personality disorder, Gilles de la Tourette's disease, and most alcohol-related conditions. These are not absolutes, but probabilities. The diagnostic choices are also different (although overlapping) for different age groups (e.g., under 40 or over 70 years). Complaints of anxiety and tremor in the latter would have Parkinson's disease high on the differential list, while in the former anxiety disorder would be high on the list.

An illustration combining age, gender, and onset is that of a 70-year-old man who became confused at a party and then fainted. Upon awakening he was frightened and did not recognize his neighbor. Put more precisely, a 70-year-old man had a sudden neurologic-like event. The same patient described a bit differently presents a clearer picture, and you think immediately of stroke or a TIA or RIND*.

Once you begin thinking of the differential diagnosis of the patient's fundamental chief complaint, you then ask a screening question for each of your choices. If the patient endorses a screening question, pursue the details to see if the patient in fact has that condition. As you proceed, you may think of additional diagnostic possibilities, and you also screen for these. At the end of this step you should reach your conclusion: the syndrome.

Step 2: decide if the syndrome is primary (idiopathic) or secondary to some classic neurologic (e.g., stroke) or general medical condition (e.g., hypothyroidism). This step is necessary for assessing prognosis and for determining specific treatments.

Step 3: Gather other information and identifying co-occurring conditions needed to shape acute and long-term management (e.g., other conditions the patient may have that increase drug side effect risks, premorbid personality traits that can hinder or help rehabilitation).

The above diagnostic steps apply to all branches of medicine. For example, a patient complains of a cough and feeling tired and feverish. You think of pneumonia, and the physical examination confirms it. That is Step 1. You next try to determine etiology: viral, bacterial, toxic. That is Step 2. Lastly, you gather additional information necessary for treatment, for example, is the patient asthmatic or immunologically compromised. That is Step 3.

Although generic to medical diagnosis, these steps are particularly important in diagnosing behavioral syndromes because the etiology and specific pathophysiology of these disorders remain elusive. Present-day classification is also a "best guess" approximation, and many patients do not clearly fit into the a diagnostic category. Within category heterogeneity is also likely. Knowing *how* to diagnose is more important than knowing every set of diagnostic criteria in the

---

*TIA, transient ischemic attack, usually lasts less than 24 hours; RIND, reversible ischemic neurologic deficit, usually lasts less than a week. Neurologic deficits related to a vascular event that last beyond 2–3 weeks define stroke.

Diagnostic and Statistical Manual of Mental Disorders (DSM). Criteria and categories change, but the logic of the diagnostic process does not.

Procedures for examining the brain need to be overlearned, just as procedures for examining the heart or lungs must be overlearned. Learn a flexible script or pattern of inquiry for each area of psychopathology or historical topic. Sample questions are:

> *Introducing topic areas:*
> "Sometimes when people feel the way you do now they also have (or experience). . . ." "I knew someone who had the same thing happen to him, and he also had. . . ." "You said you've had some difficulties with your memory. Is it the kind of difficulty that. . . ."

> *Screening questions:*
> "Has there ever been a time when for weeks or even longer you were feeling down, sad, depressed, or without energy or interest in things?" "Have you ever felt the opposite of being depressed, where you were full of energy, excited, or really hyper for more than a few minutes or hours?

"Occasionally, patients remain uncooperative or difficult to examine despite your efforts to put them at ease. Table 2.1 lists some of the more common examination problem situations and techniques that help resolve them.

Thus, to be a good examiner you must know the examination structure, know the script of questions, and have an examination style that puts patients at ease and gets them to talk. You also must understand how to generate a useful differential diagnostic list and know how to describe and organize examination observations so that they make sense.

THE DIAGNOSTIC PROCESS (FIGURING OUT THE SYNDROME)

Most clinicians diagnose by pattern recognition (interpretation of EEG and most x-rays are done this way). Pattern recognition is the hallmark of residency training: See a few, remember what they looked like and what treatments worked, and if you see it again reach the same conclusion and do the same thing again. All well and good, but consider the following:

It is Saturday night and a middle-aged man stumbles into your busy urban emergency room. His speech is slurred, and his eyes are blood shot. He is irritable and loud. Most clinicians are trained to recognize this word picture (this pattern) as possible alcohol intoxication because the odds are good that the patient is intoxicated. The man might even have had a drink, and so his breath smells of alcohol. But, of course, other conditions must be considered: He might have diabetic hypoglycemia, be an epileptic who just had a seizure outside the hospital and is now in a post-ictal state, or be suffering from a hit to the head while having a drink in a local bar. Only an understanding of the diagnostic process and how to use it will result in the correct diagnosis for this patient. Thus, as long as the patient has a typical syndrome or is well known to the physician, using pattern recognition to diagnose is helpful. Pattern recognition diagnosis can be very accurate, but it has only modest reliability (e.g., the degree to which a group of clinicians would agree on the diagnoses of a group of patients). Table 2.2 displays some neuropsychiatric patterns. However, additional methods are necessary for diagnosis because there are no pathognomonic laboratory tests for psychiatric illness, and many patients do not fit the DSM patterns. The method that is the basis for all medical diagnosis is the probabilistic process of exclusion and inclusion.

A patient's most likely diagnosis is selected from many possibilities. For example, Patient A arrives for evaluation and treatment. Without additional information (e.g., age, gender, chief complaint), every condition in the *International Classification of Disease* is equally probable. With additional information, however, the probability that Patient A is suffering from some conditions diminishes, eventually reaching zero, while the probability favoring other diagnoses increases. Eventually, this continuing process of exclusion and inclusion leaves you with the most likely diagnosis. This is the process you use in Step 1 of the examination structure. To illustrate further, if Patient A is female, the possibility of prostate disease is zero. If Patient A is a 23-year-old sexually active woman who has missed two periods, the possibility of pregnancy becomes a strong probability, while the probability of most other conditions decreases, many to virtually zero. More information is obviously needed for furthering the exclusion/inclusion process, but if you do it properly you will reach the most likely diagnosis.

The process of exclusion/inclusion by probability requires you to (1) know the possibilities (i.e., the available diagnostic choices); (2) know the information that discriminates patient groups (i.e., which clinical data change the probabilities and which do not); (3) be able to elicit signs and symptoms (the psychopathology that alters the probabilities); and (4) be able to identify and properly organize signs and symptoms.

Additional guidelines are

1. *The duck principle*, which states that "If it looks, walks and quacks like a duck, it most likely is a duck." This is pattern recognition. For example, a 68-year-old man complains of concentration and memory problems and his wife says he is not himself and he is losing his mind. He is also despondent and apprehensive, having trouble sleeping, is not eating and is losing weight, and says he wants to die. This "duck" is melancholia.

2. *Sutton's law*, which is based on the vignette that when Willy Sutton, a famous U.S. bank robber in the 1950s, was asked by a reporter why he robbed banks, he replied incredulously "Because that's where the money is!" Applied to diagnosis, Sutton's law tells you the most likely condition under the particular circumstances of the situation is probably the correct diagnosis. A corollary to this is, when you hear hoofbeats in the United States they are from horses, not zebras. The above melancholic man also had problems concentrating and with his memory. His wife said he was losing his mind. He is 68. Alzheimer's dis-

TABLE 2.1. Difficult Examination Situations and How To Resolve Them

Situation	Resolving Techniques
	DEPRESSION
A. Psychomotor retardation	1. Slow down rhythm of questions, reduce number of questions, ask more closed-ended, concrete questions.
	2. Interview in several 10–15 minute segments rather than one long interview.
	3. Interview in late afternoon when retardation may be less due to diurnal pattern of symptoms
B. Continuous ruminations	1. The approach is the same as for mania, C, but at a much reduced rate
	MANIA
A. Agitated, pacing patient	Walk with the patient and have an examination "conversation" "on the go"
B. Irritable, tendency to dismiss the question as stupid, to tell examiner to read the information in the chart	1. Address the least emotionally laden topics first.
	2. If the patient has a constant theme, use it to introduce questions on other topics that must be assessed, even if the sequence strains logic.
	3. Do not get insulted.
	4. Remain firm but nonjudgmental and matter of fact
C. Overtalkative with press of speech; circumstantial speech or flight-of-ideas	1. Increase interview structure, use more closed-ended questions, and speed up rhythm of questions.
	2. Repeatedly come back to a topic so that the interview content does not "get away."
	3. If the patient is interruptible without producing unacceptable irritability, stop the flow of speech and say such things as. "I'd like to know more about that later, but right now. . . .

ease is a reasonable consideration. Sutton's law, however, also picks melancholia because in persons 65–70, depression is four times as common as Alzheimer's, which typically does not fully express itself until the mid-70s.

3. *The rule of parsimony* tells you to try to explain the patient's many complaints and clinical features by as few underlying pathophysiologic processes as possible—one being the best. Looking for parsimony is looking for the common underlying theme. In the melancholic man above, you find out he has some cortical atrophy and ventricular en-

TABLE 2.1. *(continued)*

Situation	Resolving Techniques
	4. If flight-of-ideas is uncontrollable, use the patient's distractibility by switching with great show to questions related to specific diagnostic criteria, or have a third party in the room to which you address your questions (e.g., "how old did you say he was?"), perhaps stimulating the patient to interrupt you with the answer (e.g., "48").
	5. Begin to ask questions in so soft a voice that the patient becomes distracted by it and asks you what you said. The examiner raising his voice rarely helps
	SCHIZOPHRENIA
A. Persecutory delusions and extreme suspiciousness	1. Start with the least emotionally laden topics.
	2. Orient the wording of all questions about present episode and psychopathology to the patient's viewpoint.
	3. Avoid all judgmental sounding phrases
B. Avolitional patient with paucity of speech and content	1. The approach is the same as for depression.
	2. Patient may be willing to do paper and pencil cognitive tests and cooperate with general medical examination.
	3. The latter can be used as a structure for assessing behavior
C. Patient with severe formal thought disorder	1. The approach is the same as with an avolitional patient.
	2. Some information may also be obtained by focusing on visual and pictorial tasks rather than verbal tasks

largement on magnetic resonance imaging (MRI) and diffuse cognitive impairment. You could conclude that he has both depression and Alzheimer's, but the MRI and cognitive findings are also consistent with depression and so all his problems can be explained by that single pathophysiologic process. Parsimony facilitates good treatment.

Diagnostic choices are discussed throughout the rest of this book. Discriminating data for each are presented. A good examination style and structure helps you to elicit important information. The phenomenologic clinical method (see below) helps you to organize psychopathology and other information that relates to specific conditions. This organizing helps you formulate a recognizable clinical pattern.

TABLE 2.2. Some Diagnostic Patterns Seen by the Neuropsychiatrist

Pattern	Most Likely Diagnosis
Hallucinations, delusions fluctuating language disturbance, loss of emotional expression, loss of drive and ambition, no history indicating traditional neurologic disease (e.g., stroke, tremor)	Schizophrenia
Typical depressive features (e.g., insomnia, anorexia, psychomotor retardation), but without profound unremitting sadness or dysphoria (the words, but not the "music" of depression)	Secondary depression A. With increased muscle tone and bradykinesia: parkinsonism B. With renal stones: parathyroid disease C. With paresis: stroke
Altered mood (irritability or euphoria), rapid/pressured speech, hyperactivity	
A. Broad affect, no traditional neurologic disease	Bipolar mood disorder, mania
B. Shallow mood, avolitional, chronic course	Frontal lobe disinhibited syndrome
Transient and episodic perceptual disturbances and delusions with altered responsivity, but no affective blunting at other times	Seizure disorder
Anxiety or obsessive compulsive features beginning after age 35 years in a male patient	General medical condition (e.g., endocrinopathy, hypertension), traditional neurologic disease
Altered or fluctuating level of arousal, agitation, diffuse cognitive impairment, rambling speech	Delirium
Clear consciousness; diffuse cognitive impairment, particularly affecting memory; organizational and problem-solving difficulties	Dementia
Dementia with ataxia and urinary incontinence	Normal-pressure hydrocephaly

THE PHENOMENOLOGIC CLINICAL METHOD

The phenomenologic clinical method incorporates (1) objective observation of signs and symptoms; (2) description using precise terminology; and (3) assessment of the form of behavior separately from its content.

Objective observation of signs and symptoms means first observe, then interpret. For example, if a patient is loudly mumbling to himself, you might interpret this as hallucinating, and some patients do subvocalize while they are experiencing auditory hallucinations. But what if this patient is not hallucinating and instead has frontal lobe disease and is no longer able to monitor his own behavior? Most of us talk to ourselves, but we do it in private. We have learned to monitor our behavior to keep it socially acceptable. A hallucinating patient is psychotic, and that suggests a number of diagnostic possibilities. A patient who cannot self-monitor from frontal lobe disease reflects a different group of possibilities. Treatments for these two groups often differ. Because no single behavior is pathognomonic, the best approach is to describe each behavior accurately and see if the descriptions fit into a recognizable pattern.

A corollary of observation before interpretation is observation before treatment. Treating a patient means you have already made several important decisions: The patient is ill and needs treatment (a very big decision indeed), and the patient has a particular condition likely to respond to the treatment choice.

Sometimes treating immediately (e.g., the patient is hallucinating, give him an antipsychotic) works, but many times it masks important clinical features (e.g., are those tremors from the neuroleptic drug, or does the patient have basal ganglia disease that caused the behavioral symptoms?). Rushing to treatment may also make some patients worse. For example, some antipsychotics can lower seizure thresholds so that some patients with post-ictal psychosis can be made more irritable (and possibly dangerous) by giving them an antipsychotic for their psychosis rather than an anticonvulsant.

Precise terminology is important because imprecise terms fail to discriminate disorders. For example, the term *confusion*, could refer to an altered state of consciousness (as in delirium), disorientation in clear consciousness (as in dementia), unintelligible speech (as with a dominant hemisphere stroke), or it could describe a patient who gets easily lost or who cannot find his way about the hospital unit (as with some nondominant hemisphere strokes). Each of these conditions has a different diagnostic implication that goes unrecognized when each is subsumed under the vague term *confusion.*

Terms such as *incoherent or irrelevant speech* or *looseness of associations* are also imprecise. Does looseness of associations mean jumping from topic to topic, uttering nonsequiturs, speaking in word salad, having fluent paraphasic speech, or rambling? The speech of some aphasic patients is incoherent and at times irrelevant to the topic, as is the speech of some schizophrenics and some manics. If you think in and use imprecise terms, you will not discriminate aphasia from schizophrenic formal thought disorder or from manic flight-of-ideas, and misdiagnosis may occur. *Paranoid* is imprecise: Does it mean delusional, having persecutory delusions, being suspicious, being uptight, being crazy? The precise term helps in the diagnostic process. The imprecise term usually leads down a diagnostic dead end.

Form separated from content is difficult. The form of psychopathology reflects the illness process (what you are trying to identify). The content of psychopathology most often reflects the person and his experience. What a patient is talking about, the words spoken by a hallucinated voice, and the specifics of a delusional idea are content. The linkage of speech and word usage, the clarity and duration of a hallucination, and whether the delusional idea derives from other psychopathology or appears suddenly and fully formed are form. The content of psychopathology varies dramatically across cultures; the form of psychopathology does not. For example, melancholic patients from rural African villages and from industrialized western cities share the characteristic profound apprehensiveness, gloominess, insomnia, anorexia, psychomotor retardation, and feelings of guilt. What varies is the content of the guilty ideas and ruminations.

USING THE DSM SYSTEM

The DSM system is easy. The criteria for individual syndromes, however, are complicated, and very few clinicians know all the criteria for all the syndromes. The system fits with the examination structure previously described: (1) diagnose the syndrome; (2) decide if the syndrome is primary (idiopathic) or secondary (to a knowable neurologic pathophysiology or a general medical condition); and (3) identify other co-morbid conditions. The rest of the evaluation is done either to confirm these three steps or to gather additional information necessary for treatment and management.

However, knowing some diagnostic criteria is important, because you use diagnostic criteria at the beginning *and* at the end of the diagnostic process. At the beginning, the DSM provides the list of choices (i.e., the possibilities). In the DSM system these possibilities are axis I (the primary and secondary states of illness) and axis II (the personality disorders). A working knowledge of specific sets of diagnostic criteria is also needed, so when the patient endorses a screening question, or you strongly suspect a condition and need to know the details, you know what to ask and look for. For example, if the chief complaint suggests depression, you ask a screening question for depression. If the patient endorses this, you must know the basic diagnostic criteria for depression to ask further questions (e.g., about sleep, appetite, changes in libido). Criteria help shape the structure of the evaluation from its beginning. Once you have collected all the information you need, knowledge of diagnostic criteria is again used to evaluate what has been collected. You do this to determine if the patient's signs and symptoms and historical information meet criteria.

The DSM system's complexity of criteria does not ensure their specificity. Many criteria, are not operationally defined. For example, the diagnosis of dysthymia requires the vaguely defined criteria "low energy" or "fatigue," "poor concentration," and "difficulty making decisions"; the criteria for generalized anxiety disorders include "feeling keyed-up or on edge" and "having difficulty concentrating." The DSM does not define these terms. There are specific tests, however, of concentration and more precise ways of describing various other criteria, but these procedures cannot all be incorporated into the DSM system. You must have your definitions to become a precise diagnostician. The scientific literature provides some data suggesting what constitutes an abnormal "this" or a deviant "that" and how to go about measuring them. Succeeding chapters will focus on these suggested operational definitions.

THE NEUROPSYCHIATRIC HISTORY

A good psychiatric history is the basis of a good neuropsychiatric history. If there is a difference, it is of emphasis. For example, a good psychiatric history must determine if the behavioral syndrome is secondary to some classic neurologic or general medical condition. The neuropsychiatric history does this too, but also focuses on psychopathology as indicators of specific brain dysfunction (e.g., action vs. perceptual-integrating brain disease) that may respond to more specific treatments rather than just information to determine if DSM criteria are met. For example, you assess a patient's avolition to see if he meets criteria for schizophrenia or depression. The neuropsychiatrist also wants to know if this avolition is due to action brain dysfunction that might respond to a dopamine agonist such as methylphenidate. The neurologic implications of historical information about psychopathology are covered throughout this book. Historical areas to assess when determining if a behavioral syndrome is primary or secondary are displayed in Table 2.3.

THE TRADITIONAL NEUROLOGIC SCREENING EXAMINATION

No psychiatric evaluation is complete without a traditional neurologic examination. The traditional neurologic examination includes an assessment of gait, balance, coordination, motor strength, reflexes, and cranial nerve and sensory function. Table 2.4 describes a screening neurologic examination that takes about 20 minutes to complete.

Many patients with behavioral syndromes have normal traditional neurologic examination findings, but nevertheless, have *soft neurologic signs.* These are expressions of brain dysfunction, but with less localizing power than the neurologic signs described in Table 2.4. Some soft neurologic signs are advantitious motor overflow, Gegenhalten, and stereotypes (see Chapter 3—motor behavior). Also included is soft signs are palmomental reflex, and double simultaneous discrimination)*. When a patient has a behavioral syndrome and specific neurologic features, assume the behavioral syndrome is secondary until proven otherwise. Chapters on syndromes describe specific relationships. The presence of soft signs, however, is consistant with a primary syndrome.

LABORATORY ASSESSMENT

To use laboratory tests well, several principles and strategies are followed. Other than tests required by hospital or clinic policy, there are no routine laboratory tests. Every test costs time and money and may inconvenience or discomfort the patient. Have a specific reason for ordering every test. Some basic reasons are as follows:

To confirm or eliminate a suspected etiology for the patient's behavioral syndrome is the main reason for ordering laboratory tests. To get the highest yield

---

*The *palmomental reflex* is induced by scratching the fleshy base of the thumb causing a downward movement at the corners of the mouth. The reflex indicates dysfunction only when repeated stimulation continues to produce a response. The frontal lobes are usually involved when the reflex fails to extinguish. *Double simultaneous discrimination* (the face–hand test) is tested by having the patient close his eyes and then lightly stroking him on the cheek and dorsal surface of the hand ipsilaterally and contralaterally. Failure to perceive the hand being stimulated or one side of the face or hand (left or right) indicates dysfunction usually in the frontal or parietal lobes.

TABLE 2.3. Historical Antecedents of Secondary Behavioral Syndromes

Antecedent	Most Likely Secondary Syndrome(s)
Cardiovascular disease	
Hypertension	Generalized anxiety disorder, subcortical dementia
Atherosclerosis	Focal stroke syndrome, vascular dementia
Acute heart failure	Delirium with psychosis
Chronic heart failure	Personality change, frontal lobe dementia, atypical depression
Lung disease	
Acute infection	Delirium with psychosis
Chronic obstructive pulmonary disease	Personality change, frontal lobe dementia, atypical depression
Kidney disease	
Infection or acute renal failure	Delirium
Chronic renal failure	Personality change, frontal lobe dementia, atypical depression
Diabetes	Vascular dementia, hypoglycemic delirium, stroke syndromes
Other neurologic disease	
Viral encephalitis	Dementia, generalized anxiety disorder, adult-onset attention deficit disorder
Head injury	Many syndromes, including personality change, dementia, focal brain syndromes
Epilepsy	Many syndromes, including depression, psychosis, and panic disorder
Multiple sclerosis	Anxiety disorder, nonmelancholic depression
Other conditions	
Lupus erythematosis	Mood disorders
AIDS	Nonmelancholic depression, subcortical (white matter) dementia
Carcinoma	Depression, subcortical (white matter) dementia
Gestational, labor, and delivery problems	Developmental disorders, schizophrenia
Drug Abuse	
Acute	Delirium, psychosis
Chronic	Psychosis, dementia
Endocrinopathies	
Hyperthyroidism	Anxiety disorders, delirium
Hypothyroidism	Depression, dementia
Cushing's disease	Depression, bipolar mood disorders, generalized anxiety disorder, delusional disorder

TABLE 2.4. Screening Neurologic Examination

Examination Area	Techniques	Some Important Findings
Inspection	Looking with educated eyes	1. Dysplasia* 2. The triangular-shaped head and face with large ears, lips, and nose of fragile-X syndrome 3. Short stature, webbed neck of Tuner and Noonan (male Turner) syndromes 4. Short stature and facial features of Down syndrome 5. Asymmetry of facial features, trunk, and limb muscle groups from atrophy
Gait	Free walk and tandom walking (about 12 feet). Standing with feet together, eyes closed for 1 minute (Romberg sign if the patient is unsteady)	1. Loss of secondary arm movements in Parkinson's disease 2. Broad-based gait in cerebellar disease 3. Shuffling gait of anterior brain disease 4. Hemiplegias 5. Ataxia
Motor strength (rest of motor examination is covered elsewhere)	Flexion, extension, rotation of head; shrugging shoulders, flexion, extension abduction of limbs and fingers all to resistance; sitting up from a prone position standing on one leg and then the other for 10 seconds each; simplest routine is to do motor examination in rostral to caudal order	1. Weakness in both legs, or both legs and arms, indicates spinal cord problem 2. Weakness in lower face, arm, and leg on one side indicates damage in contralateral cerebral hemisphere or brain stem. 3. Weakness in distal part of limb indicates peripheral neuropathy
Deep tendon stretch reflexes (DTRs)	Dorsum of arms, triceps, knee "jerk," ankle, and plantar muscle tendons tested; must be relaxed and under maximum gravity effect	1. Asymmetry is more important than absolute rating of reflex, intensity can be altered by many factors (e.g., anxiety, drugs) 2. DTRs are hyperactive with corticospinal damage, and are hypoactive with peripheral nerve damage 3. If patient has an atypical depression always check for sluggish reflexes of hypothyroidism 4. Extension of the big toe to plantar stimulation (Babinski sign) seen with brain or spinal cord damage (upper motor neuron)

TABLE 2.4. Screening Neurologic Examination (*continued*)

Examination Area	Techniques	Some Important Findings
Somatosensory function (excluding the face)	Pain and touch: Stimulate the skin with the sharp and blunt ends of a safety pin in random order covering dorsum and soles of hands and feet Vibratory sense: Apply vibrating tuning fork to bony eminences (the malleoli, distal ends of radii) of each limb	The main purpose of somatosensory testing in a neuropsychiatric setting is to assess for peripheral neuropathy due to alcoholism, thiamine deficiency, and diabetes
Cranial Nerves		
Olfactory (I)	Any strong odor-producing substance will do. Test one nostril at a time. Most overlooked area of examination.	1. Unilateral and bilateral anosmia not due to pharyngeal disease is ominous. Look for olfactory groove meningioma (unilateral), optic atrophy and optic nerve tumor (unilateral), and frontal lobe masses 2. Frontal head trauma shearing olfactory nerves is most common cause of anosmia. Change in olfaction can cause poor appetite and changes in food preferences and sexual behavior. Associated with frontal lobe dysinhibition syndrome
Optic (II)	Always look at the optic nerve and test for visual acuity; carry a pocket eye chart or have one in the examining room.	1. Normal fundus is yellow, flat, and clearly demarcated from surrounding red retina. Vessels are clear and not tortuous 2. "Salt and pepper" pigmentation seen in thioridazine overexposure and complaints of night vision problems 3. Poor light reflex and pale fundus seen in optic neuritis (think of multiple sclerosis) 4. Blurred and raised optic disc with retinal vessel pulses visible indicate increased intracranial pressure.
	Visual fields tested just before testing range of ocular movement. Face the	Patterns of visual field loss 1. Unilateral central: Migraine, optic neurotics, nerve damage

TABLE 2.4. *(continued)*

Examination Area	Techniques	Some Important Findings
	patient and stand 50 cms apart. Have him stare at your nose. Have the patient cover one eye with his hand. Hold your index finger just outside your peripheral field in the inferior quadrant equidistant between you and the patient. Wiggle finger slowly and move it toward center field until the patient sees it. Repeat in all quadrants, and then repeat with other eye	2. Bitemporal upper quadrant: Lesion in the optic chiasm, such as pituitary adenoma or craniopharyngioma 3. Bitemporal hemianopsia: Advanced optic chiasm lesion 4. Homonymous hemianopsia (same sides of visual fields): Contralateral cerebral lesion such as stroke 5. Homonymous upper quadrant anopsia: Contralateral temporal lobe lesion
Oculomotor (III), trochlear (IV), and abducens (VI)	Range of ocular movement: Tell the patient to follow your finger with his eyes without moving his head. Then, holding your finger 50 cms in front of the patient, move it from the center of the patient's presumed visual field to the right, left, up, and down positions. At the extremes of these check for nystagmus.Then have the patient follow your finger to the tip of his nose	1. Impairment: Dilated pupil, ptosis, outward deviation of eye (III) 2. Eye deviated inward (superior oblique). Look for midbrain lesion (IV) 3. Inturning of the eye (lateral rectus muscle) but no ptosis or pupil changes. Look for pontine lesion. Classic sign of Wernicke-Korsakoff constellation (VI) 4. Diplopia results from dysconjugate gaze from III or VI lesion. 5. Basilar artery syndrome: Brain stem lesion causing diplopia, contralateral hemiparesis, or ataxia
Trigeminal (V)	Touch and sharp–dull testing of three divisions: forehead, cheek, jaw Corneal reflex tested with a wisp of cotton on cornea producing a blink While feeling the muscle, have patient clench jaw, protrude jaw, and push jaw left and right against your hand pressure Jaw jerk: While patient's jaw is relaxed, place your index finger under lower lip and tap it with wide end of reflex hammer	1. Damage causes facial analgesia, poor corneal reflex, hypoactive jaw jerk, and jaw deviation to side of lesion 2. Nasopharyngeal tumor, gun shot wounds, acoustic neuroma (unilateral hearing loss) 3. Hyporeflexic in bulbar palsy, 4. Hyperreflexic in pseudobulbar palsy (associated with dysarthria, dysphagia, and emotional lability) 5. Upper motor neuron lesions

TABLE 2.4. Screening Neurologic Examination (*continued*)

Examination Area	Techniques	Some Important Findings
Facial (VII)	Observe expressions; test taste with diluted salt or sugar solution if patient complains or other signs indicate need	1. Poor facial expression (muscles of the face are paretic) 2. Can chew (V) but cannot taste (glossopharyngeal posterior $\frac{1}{3}$ of tongue for taste, facial anterior $\frac{2}{3}$) 3. Upper facial muscles bilaterally innervated; lower facial muscles contralaterally innervated 4. Lyme disease can mimic Bell's palsy (idiopathic inflammatory disease), with unexpected crying or laughing.
Acoustic (VIII)	Whisper into each of the patient's ears while covering the other, or use tuning fork beginning at same distance you can hear it. Weber test: Tuning fork on vertex, mastoid	Unilateral deficit in men usually hereditary and benign. Can be due to sudden noise, virus, Meniere's disease, or acoustic neuroma (rare) Nerve problem, air and bone conduction of sound poor and from vertex, sound louder on less impaired side. Conduction problem, sound louder on more impaired side
Glossopharyngeal (IX), vagus (X), spinal accessory (XI), Hypoglossal (XII)	Listen to the patient's speech, look for uvula deviation, induce gag reflex with tongue depressor, feel patient's throat as he swallows, have patient stick out tongue, swallow, cough	1. Bulbar group nuclei in brain stem caudal to III, IV, and VI 2. Look for pontine and medulla lesions 3. Dysarthria, dysphagia, hypoactive jaw, and gag reflexes in pseudobulbar palsy

*Dysplasia refers to body parts disproportionate in size or shape and deviant in location (e.g., low-set or malformed ears, eyes too widely spaced apart, arms or legs too short for torso).

from these tests, be specific. For example, if you order an EEG, the patient should have a suspected condition likely to produce an abnormal EEG. EEG is helpful if epilepsy, delirium, or a focal brain injury is suspected. EEG is usually not helpful in distinguishing the pseudodementia of depression from Alzheimer's disease. Other laboratory tests are more discriminating. Specific laboratory testing is described in chapter sections on differential diagnosis. The principle, however, is to be specific in what tests you order and link them to specific choices on your differential diagnostic list or to determine whether a syndrome is secondary to a suspected pathophysiology (e.g., you think the patient's depression is due to hypothyroidism and so you order thyroid studies).

Monitoring treatment often requires laboratory testing. In neuropsychiatry, medication blood levels are frequently obtained to guide pharmacotherapy. Renal, heart, and liver functions are assessed to make sure a drug is not contraindicated. Baseline values are determined in case drug-induced changes occur later on (e.g., thyroid function prior to giving lithium).

Gaining knowledge is often a good reason to order a laboratory test, particularly when that knowledge directly helps the patient or his family. During training, almost all laboratory tests have something to teach: A positive test correlating with a syndrome or specific psychopathology teaches you about the pathophysiology of these behaviors and sharpens your clinical skills in future diagnosis.

Defending oneself is a sad, but necessary, reason for ordering some laboratory tests. Thirty years ago the aphorism was "under every patient's bed is a lawyer." Today, under every patient's bed are two lawyers and a third one is outside the room waiting to finish you off if the first two do not. Today, people sue doctors for bad outcomes more than for bad practice. Defensive medicine is a necessary evil, but it should not be consuming—do not order everything "just to be on the safe side." Be prudent. In neuropsychiatry, for example, the frequent ordering of lithium blood levels is more for legal than patient care purposes.

Screening tests are also frequently used in medicine. Every child born in a hospital in the United States has a drop of blood taken to screen for phenylketonuria. In neuropsychiatry we do a cognitive screening test on most patients.

SOME FREQUENTLY USED LABORATORY TESTS IN NEUROPSYCHIATRY

Specific uses of laboratory tests are described in the chapters on syndromes. Below is an introduction to the commonly used tests. Some guidelines for their use are as follows:

1. *Behavior* is the most sensitive measure of brain function, and no laboratory test replaces a thorough behavioral examination.
2. *Cognitive function* is the next most sensitive measure of brain function, but it is less specific than imaging and some electrophysiologic findings.
3. *Electrophysiologic studies* (EEG and evoked potential) are sensitive measures of brain dysfunction: EEG when assessing patients suspected of having circumscribed cortical disease (e.g., injury, seizure disorder) and evoked potentials when assessing subcortical structures (e.g., multiple sclerosis), cranial nerves, and thalamic lesions.
4. *Metabolic imaging* is helpful in looking for localized or circumscribed dysfunction, but its sensitivity is affected by the patient's present mood and cognitive state.
5. *Structural imaging* with computed tomography scans, limited to looking for suspected hemorrhagic lesions or gross cortical atrophy and

TABLE 2.5. Typical EEG Findings in Some Common Neuropsychiatric Disorders

Disorder	EEG Findings
Schizophrenia	50% normal; 50% diffuse, mild slowing, choppy wave forms
Mood disorder	Two-thirds or more normal; about one-third diffuse, mild slowing, choppy waveforms; right posterior predominance of findings
Complex partial epilepsy	Unilateral or bilateral discharges of spike and slow waves; diffuse or focal; usually in temporal or fronto-temporal areas; multiple examinations may be needed to demonstrate abnormalities
Generalized epilepsy	Rapid rhythmic onset with decreasing (tonic/clonic) frequency and increasing amplitude slow and spike waves in clonic phase
Tumors	Focal delta and thetawaves; regional decrease in amplitude and loss of organization of normal frequencies and background activity (alpha or beta); focal sharp or spike waves
Stroke	Local, but nonspecific increase in slow activity, decreased fast activity, loss or reduction in amplitude of normal background rhythms; occasional epileptiform patterns (sharp or spike waves). If deep stroke, no EEG findings; if associated with depression, EEG changes may be in left frontal areas
Metabolic and toxic encephalopathies	Nonfocal, slowing of alpha, increased theta; polymorphic waveforms, delta or rhythmic frontal delta, if severe; in chronic state decreased voltage and slow activity; in addition, more specific sharp or spike waves in renal failure, triphasic high voltage slow waves in hepatic encephalopathy, anoxia, urema, hypercalcemia

ventricular enlargement, and MRI, helpful for all other types of lesions and the imaging of choice if hemorrhage or calcified lesions are not likely. MRI also permits the determination of the volume of structures that may be reduced in some neuropsychiatric conditions (e.g., temporal lobe reduction in chronic temporal lobe epilepsy, thalamic reduction in schizophrenia).

Electroencephalogram

EEG measures electrical activity (in microvolts) across the scalp. It is an indirect measure of electrical potentials from deep brain structures. Electrodes are attached to the scalp in a standard pattern (the 10–20 international system), and the electrical activity is recorded from 16–21 leads or channels. The pattern of relationships among the leads (the montage) can be changed to maximize identification of abnormalities. Reference electrodes are positioned on the ears for patients

TABLE 2.5. (*continued*)

Disorder	EEG Findings
Acute encephalitis	Slow activity, frontal high-voltage delta in coma; epileptiform activity
Slow virus encephalitis (subacute panencephalitis, Creutzfeldt-Jakob disease)	periodic bursts of 1–2 seconds high-voltage, sharp and slow waves every 5–15 seconds, associated random bursts of theta and delta
Herpes simplex encephalitis	Focal sharp and slow discharges bitemporally
AIDS (and other leukoencephalopathies)	Focal or diffuse background slowing, some increased delta and theta
Alzheimer's disease	Initially normal, progresses through decreasing voltage and alpha with increasing theta and then delta; some sharp activity, asymmetries, and sleep spindles and K-complexes may diminish
Huntington's chorea	Initially normal, progresses to low-voltage and no organized rhythms
Parkinson's disease	In patients with dementia: Mild background changes similar to Alzheimer's disease
Multiple sclerosis	50% normal, 50% have nonspecific, focal, or generalized slowing
Normal pressure hydrocephalus	Initially normal, may progress to mild nonspecific slowing
Head injury	Ranges from normal to severely abnormal, from mild increased theta to focal slow activity or bursts of slow and sharp waves
Migraine headaches	Usually normal; in complex migraine can be generalized, or unilateral high-voltage polymorphic slowing

with tardive dyskinesia, as the usual reference placement on the jaws can cause muscle artifacts in these patients. Recordings can be made by ink on paper or directly into a computer.

EEG frequencies range from 0.5 cycles per second (or Hertz [Hz]) to about 35 Hz. Frequencies above 35 Hz often represent muscle activity. Frequencies are separated into delta, 0.5–3.5 Hz; theta, 4–7 Hz; alpha, 7.5–12 Hz; and beta, 12.5 and above. A normal, alert individual in a resting state (with eyes closed) should have a symmetrical EEG pattern with little delta or theta activity, minimal beta activity, and predominantly alpha activity particularly at the electrodes attached to the back half of the head. When a normal, alert person is asked to concentrate on something, alpha activity, diminishes and beta predominates. When a normal, alert person becomes sleepy, alpha activity diminishes and delta and theta activity increases.

EEG abnormalities generally fall into six categories. These include abnormalities in amplitude, frequency, pattern of amplitude and frequency, waveform, some combination of the first four, or an abnormality in EEG activity over time (usually related to sleep stage disturbances). Amplitude deviation can be high (as in delirium or epilepsy) or low (as in dementia). Frequency can be slow (as in any lesion resulting in cell loss or diminished function), or fast (as in hyperarousal states and delirium tremens). Waveform can be abnormal, as in the bi- and triphasic waves of encephalopathies. Patterns can be abnormal as in epilepsy (e.g., spikes and sharp waves, paroxysms of slow waves, three per second sharp and slow wave complexes). Amplitude and frequency can be abnormally distributed (e.g., resting alpha diminished or high amplitude slow waves each circumscribed to a particular scalp region). Waveforms can also be abnormally affected by stimulation such as flashes of bright light leading to spike activity. When ordering an EEG, consider the above limitations and relationships. Be specific and state your diagnostic hypothesis. This specificity can determine the procedures (e.g., flashing light, nasopharyngeal leads for deep temporal lobe foci) and montages that are used.

Seizures are usually transient, and several assessments may be needed. Sleep deprivation prior to EEG or sedation helps the patient to fall asleep while being recorded. Epileptic foci are occasionally revealed during this drowsy state. Twenty-four hour telemetry (similar to EKG halter monitoring except that the electrodes are on the scalp under an electrode cap) can sometimes pick up transient seizure activity. Table 2.5 displays the typical EEG findings of some neuropsychiatric disorders. Many medications also influence the EEG (Table 2.6). Always tell the electroencephalographer what medications a patient has recently taken. Whenever possible, EEGs should be performed when the patient is unmedicated.

Topographic EEG is computer-enhanced EEG information. The computer interpolates likely voltages and frequencies between electrodes. Thus, rather than only 16–21 points (channels) of information, the computer creates many additional points generating an electrical voltage map within each frequency band across the scalp. The computer also counts more numbers faster than a human, and so all these points (real and created) can be determined for each half Hertz from 0.5 to 35 Hz for each second (or milliseconds) of recording. All this information can be color-coded, creating a colored map of electrical activity (i.e., the higher the voltage [now termed *power* as filters transform it], the redder the color). In addition to making combinations of frequency, amplitude, and waveform deviations more recognizable as patterns, topographic EEG also provides pictures for each time period that can be cartooned, creating a dynamic moving picture of electrical activity, occasionally revealing relationships that might be obscured by events occurring at different times and locations.

The biggest problem whith an EEG is artifacts (i.e., electrical activity resulting from sources other than the brain). Common artifact sources include scalp and jaw muscle activity that causes bilateral fast activity and "spikes" bitemporally, eye and eyelid movement that causes "frontal slowing," and faulty electrodes and electrode contact with the scalp that produce "abnormal" waveforms. A second problem in interpretation is that the normative pattern is based on an individual who is alert, eyes closed, thinking of nothing, but not falling asleep, and who is unmedicated. Psychiatric patients rarely meet this standard so that their mental, as well as their muscle, activity can falsely distort the EEG.

One way to minimize the above problems is to standardize the EEG examina-

TABLE 2.6. Medications Commonly Used or Encountered in a Neuropsychiatry Practice and Their EEG Effects

Substance	EEG Finding
Neuroleptics	Increased background theta and delta, slowing of alpha (to its lower range)
Benzodiazepines	Increased beta, speeding of alpha (to its higher range), increased amplitude
Barbiturates	Increased beta, speeding of alpha (to its higher range, increased amplitude
Alcohol	Increase alpha (single dose), increased beta, and reduced amplitude with withdrawal
Lithium	Increased theta, sharp waves
Nonspecific and partially specific monoamine reuptake-inhibiting antidepressants	Increased background theta and delta, increased beta and decreased amplitude
Monoamine oxidase inhibitors	Decreased alpha, some increased beta and decreased amplitude
Anticonvulsants (phenytoin, carbamazepine, valproic acid)	In therapeutic doses: Suppression of spike activity, increased normal voltages At high or toxic doses: Slowing of alpha, increased background slowing, high amplitude, diffuse theta and delta
Anticholinergics	Same as nonspecific and partially specific monoamine reuptake-inhibiting antidepressants
Opiates (in analgesic doses)	Increased alpha
Hallucinogens (LSD, mescaline, psilocybin)	Increased beta, decreased amplitude
Stimulants (amphetamine, cocaine, methylphenidate)	Increased beta, decreased amplitude
Specific Monoamine Reuptake-Inhibiting Antidepressants	
Sertraline, zimelidine, and fluoxetine	Similar to partially specific monoamine reuptake inhibitors
Bupropion,	Increased beta, decreased amplitude, decreased alpha and speeding of alpha, spiking in high doses
Paroxitine	Little effect
Venlafaxine	Similar to but less effect than partially specific monoamine reuptake drugs

tion situation by asking for EEGs with all patients sedated, or receiving a standard dose of a drug, or doing a standard, verifiable mental task (e.g., mental math). When these techniques are not practical, an alternative method of assessment is evoked potential.

Magnetoencephalography is a new technique that measures magnetic intracranial currents arising from ion movements in nerve cells. Its goal is to provide better localization of lesions than either EEG or evoked potential because both of these techniques can only measure the end product of all potentials being generated by the brain as they appear on the scalp. Magnetic fields are less distorted by other tissues, and specific brain structures have specific magnetic "signatures." Magnetoencephalography is available at only a few medical centers.

Finally, if you take the trouble and someone's expense to order the EEG, make sure you read the details of the report, not just its conclusions. Some electroencephalographers underread EEGs, and the "normal EEG" conclusion may accompany a description of an abnormality exactly in the area you suspected.

Evoked Potential

Evoked potential assessment stimulates the patient's brain, evoking brain electrical activity (i.e., potentials). Each potential is time-locked to the stimulus (i.e., it only occurs immediately following the stimulus). These potentials are too small to be seen on the typical EEG. However, the EEG represents a series of randomly occurring (not time-locked), approximately equal positive and negative waveforms that, when averaged, equal zero. This averaging is done by computer, and what is left are the time-locked (nonrandom) potentials evoked by the stimulus. Many of these potentials are then averaged to enhance them, and the electrical waveform that is produced represents brain cell responses to the stimuli. The anatomic sources of the various components of this evoked, averaged waveform have been roughly determined and can be followed from the peripheral nerve to the cortex. Topographic evoked potential permits the response to be followed across the cortex and even across the corpus callosum. Stimuli can be auditory (tones), visual (flashes of light, patterns, or words), or somatosensory (electrical).

Evoked potentials are used to study the way the brain processes information. Visual and auditory evoked potentials are important for diagnosing multiple sclerosis (delayed and abnormal waves due to demyelinating axonal conduction problems). Evoked potentials are normal in patients with hysteria or who are malingering. Brain tumors can compress surrounding axons and produce prolonged interwave periods. Gliomas, acoustic neuromas, and chiasmic lesions can cause localized or lateralized evoked potential abnormalities. Postconcussion syndrome also produces prolonged interwave periods, whereas ischemic lesions lead to low amplitude waves without changes in when they occur. In addition, dementias can also result in abnormal evoked potentials with wave-onset delays (Parkinson's dementia) or decreased wave amplitude (Huntington's and Alzheimer's diseases). Brain stem evoked potentials help determine the degree of coma and whether brain death has occurred. Finally, many neurosurgical procedures are performed under evoked potential monitoring to guard against cranial nerve compression and stretching.

Neuropsychological Testing

Experimental neuropsychology focuses on the relationships between brain structure and information processing and cognition. It is one of the disciplines conceptually underlying neuropsychiatry. Clinical neuropsychology uses this database to develop strategies and measuring instruments for assessing the cognitive function of patients. The Halstead-Reitan and Luria-Nebraska test batteries, and even the Weschler Adult Intelligence Scale (WAIS), used as a measure of intelligence, can discriminate brain-damaged patients from the healthy.

Neuropsychological testing is used to assess specific cognitive functions in great detail to confirm or eliminate a diagnostic possibility (e.g., circumscribed right hemisphere or frontal lobe lesion). Neuropsychological testing is also used to plan long-term patient care. Once the patient is recovered from an acute episode, knowing that patient's cognitive strengths and weaknesses helps in vocational and social rehabilitation. This assessment can also provide information about a patient's thinking ability and, along with personality testing, helps guide psychotherapy.

Neuroimaging

Computer-enhanced tomography (CT) measures the attenuation of an x-ray beam as it passes through the brain. The computer divides the brain into serial "slices," each slice further divided into tiny cubes, or voxels. The greater the number of voxels per area, the higher the resolution of the image. The degree of attenuation of the x-ray beam is measured through each voxel and each measurement is coded on a scale of shading from white through gray to black. The shading pattern forms the picture of the structures being scanned. The x-ray beam is least affected as it passes through cerebrospinal fluid which appears darkest in the picture. Bone, and then white matter attenuate the x-ray beam the most, and appear the lightest. Scanning is limited to the transverse or transaxial plane. CT abnormalities have been found in many psychiatric patient groups. None of these abnormalities is pathognomonic. Use CT if your diagnostic choices are: acute hemorrhagic stroke, subdural hematoma, calcified lesions (such as Fahr's disease with bilateral basal ganglia calcifications, or cryptococcosis), or bone disease. For the rest, use MRI.

Structural and Functional Magnetic Resonance Imaging

MRI and functional MRI (FMRI) have several advantages over CT: (1) images are of much greater resolution; (2) images can be obtained in all planes; (3) a relatively safe magnetic field and radio waves are used to generate an image rather than x-rays; (4) bone artifacts are not a problem; and (5) FMRI combines high spatial resolution with images of neural activity.

MRI works by placing the patient in a magnetic field that slightly realigns hydrogen protons. The patient is then bombarded with a radiofrequency signal that "jiggles" the protons. The computer measures the original changes in realignment through changes in the magnetic field and, following the radiofrequency signal bombardment, the relaxation of the protons in various dimensional planes (T_1 and T_2 longitudinal and transverse relaxation times, respectively). Patients with metal aneurysm clips, skull plates, and pacemakers that can shift in the magnetic field cannot be evaluated by MRI. Because patients are placed in a tubular structure, some (10%) become claustrophobic. Minimize this by preparing the patient or having him wear a sleep mask.

FMRI uses the magnetic signal from hemoglobin as it releases oxygen to create an image of neural activity within the resolution of MRI. It combines the structural resolution of MRI with the principle of cerebral blood flow: Increased neural activity requires increased neuronal fuel (glucose and oxygen) that is differentially brought by small blood vessels to the brain areas doing the work. As the oxygen is released to these working areas, the magnetic signal is created.

FMRI is a new technique available at only a few medical centers. MRI is readily available and generally preferable to CT. Coronal images permit visualization of structures of particular interest to the neuropsychiatric clinician: basal ganglia, amygdala, and hippocampus. T_1-weighted scans are best for visualizing these structures. Posterior fossa structures are also best visualized with MRI, and bony artifact is avoided. T_2-weighted scans are particularly good for visualizing tumors, multiple sclerotic plaques, and microinfarcts. However, because of its high resolution, patient movement produces MRI artifacts.

Single Photon Emission Computer Tomography

Single photon emission computer tomography (SPECT) is a technology available at many medical centers. Positron emission tomography (PET) is limited to some university centers. SPECT uses isotopes that emit single photons to measure cerebral blood flow. These isotopes are stable and have relatively long half-lives. SPECT can be used for repeated assessments of the same patient over a short period of time. Images can only be made in the transaxial plane. Resolution is low compared with MRI.

The principle underlying SPECT and PET is similar to FMRI: Blood is diverted to brain regions that are actively processing information. Patients can be measured when at rest or when performing various cognitive tasks related to different cognitive/anatomic systems, and then their SPECT pattern can be compared with those observed in normal persons under the same conditions.

Clinically, SPECT is potentially helpful in further clarifying lesions that affect blood flow or that produce a pattern of neuronal damage or dysfunction that results in more or less neuronal activity and, thus, more or less blood flow to that region. Imaging time varies between 10 and 45 minutes.

As SPECT does not have the resolution of either CT or MRI, it is not as helpful in identifying and characterizing static structural lesions. SPECT can be helpful, however, in documenting clinically ambiguous strokes. Some patients with AIDS demonstrate patchy areas of decreased perfusion in the early stages of CNS involvement. Caffeine and nicotine produce generalized decreases in cerebral perfusion, whereas anxiety states are associated with a generalized increase. Excitatory lesions (i.e., seizure foci) produce a localized increase in perfusion during ictus and reduced or normal perfusion interictally. SPECT is also useful in differentiating Alzheimer's disease from pseudodementia depression and from vascular dementia and in identifying basal ganglia disease (e.g., Huntington's disease), brain tumors, and systemic lupus erythematosus. The specifics are discussed throughout the rest of the book.

ADDITIONAL READINGS

Andreasen NC (Section Editor): Brain Imaging. In Oldham JM, Riba MB, Tasman A (eds): *Review of Psychiatry,* vol. 12. American Psychiatric Press, Washington DC, 1993.

Bleuler E, Zinkin J (Trans): *Dementia Praecox or the Group of Schizophrenias.* International Universities Press, New York, 1950.

De Myer W: *Technique of the Neurologic Examination. A Programmed Text,*(3rd ed). McGraw-Hill, New York, 1980.

Fink M: EEG profiles and bioavailability measures of psychoactive drugs. In Itil TM (ed): *Psychoactive Drugs and Human EEG.* Basal, Karger, 1974, pp 76–98.

Hamilton M (ed): *Fish's Clinical Psychopathology: Signs and Symptoms in Psychiatry, Revised Reprint,* John Wright and Sons, Bristol, England, 1974.

Kaufman DM: *Clinical Neurology for Psychiatrists* (4th ed). WB Saunders, Philadelphia, 1995.

Tyner FS, Knott JR, Mayer WB Jr: *Fundamentals of EEG Technology,* Raven Press, New York, vol 1, 1983; vol 2, 1989.

3

Psychopathologic Phenomena

.

To practice neuropsychiatry well, you need to be able to recognize and elicit psychopathology. You use the patient's psychopathology to make a DSM diagnosis. If you understand the neurologic implications of these and other behaviors, you also can determine which brain systems are dysfunctional. This awareness helps shape treatment. How a patient sits in a waiting area, greets you, and interacts with other patients or staff on the inpatient unit are some of the behaviors that reveal how that patient's brain is working.

Behavior is the most sensitive measure of brain function. No technology can tell if a person is happy or sad. A positron emission tomography (PET) scan can show a metabolic pattern consistent with reading aloud, but it cannot tell you if the person reading fully understands and likes what is being read. Obviously you can know all these things, sometimes by just observing the person's body language. In fact, a computed tomography (CT) scan without infusion cannot tell if the person in the machine is alive or recently dead! EEG results, evoked potentials, and cognitive functioning are the next most sensitive measures of brain function.

Because behavior is our most sensitive measure of brain function, and because there is no specific laboratory test for any psychiatric disorder (no serum mania level or panic disorder antibodies), getting a careful history and doing a thorough examination is the best way of finding out if a patient has a brain illness. The most diagnostically important parts of the examination are appearance (inspection in "physical examination" terms), motor behavior, and affect. This information provides the pattern of many syndromes. Motor behavior also helps localize lesions. General areas of psychopathology are described in this chapter. Additional psychopathology and patterns of behavioral disturbance are described in the chapters on individual syndromes.

Appearance

Obvious aspects of general appearance, that is, age, gender, level of consciousness (i.e., arousal or alertness) are often the most helpful in diagnosis. Women have greater risks than do men for mood disorder and some anxiety disorders; stroke is more common in the elderly than in the young; full alertness rules out delirium.

Evaluate the patient's appearance first. Interviewing or testing the patient is not necessary to do this. Greet the patient outside the examination room and walk with him to that room. What the patient does or does not do in the inpatient unit dayroom or at meals may be diagnostically as important as his behavior during the examination. Deliberately consider the patient's apparent age, gender, race/ethnicity, nutrition, personal hygiene, and level of consciousness. Table 3.1 lists some of the diagnostic implications of some general appearance findings.

MOTOR BEHAVIOR AND THE ORGANIZATION OF THE MOTOR SYSTEM

Observations of motor behavior also begin upon meeting the patient (Table 3.2). Consider gait, coordination, smoothness and frequency of movement, rhythm, speed, and any abnormal movements. Some examples are the wide-based or ataxic gait of the alcoholic, the hesitant gait of the Huntington's patient, the stooped shuffle of the patient with frontal lobe disease, and the manneristic hopping and tiptoe gaits of catatonia.

Examining the motor system is often the best way of circumscribing or localizing suspected brain lesions. Table 3.3 displays a conceptualization of the motor system that maximizes anatomic localization of lesions resulting in behavioral change.

Left versus Right

The left versus right system is traditionally taught in medical school: The left side of the motor system interacts with the right side of the rest of the body, whereas the right side of the motor system interacts with the left side of the rest of the body. Check for asymmetric motor function. Except for the cerebellar vermus, which is ipsilaterally linked within the motor system, asymmetry of motor behavior implies lateralized, usually contralateral brain pathology.

Anterior versus Posterior

The anterior versus posterior view of the motor system is also taught in medical school, but is rarely stressed as such. The anterior part of the motor system includes the frontal lobes and their related subcortical structures (i.e., the basal ganglia and thalamus). The posterior part of the system includes the cerebellum and pons. The motor system, of course, is also the oldest part of the action brain.

Anterior Motor Signs Indicating Frontal Lobe Circuit Disease

Bradykinesia is reduced and slow movement. It is typically seen in Parkinson's disease and frontal lobe dementias.

TABLE 3.1. Some General Appearance Findings and Their Diagnostic Implications

Findings	Implications
Poor personal hygiene (dirty, unkempt)	Chronic illness, such as schizophrenia, dementia, chronic drug-induced psychosis
Altered arousal	
a. Reduced	Delirium, sedative-hypnotic drug intoxication, depressive or catatonic stupor, epilepsy (the seizure or post-ictal period), head injury
b. Increased	Anxiety, mania or hypomania, frontal lobe disinhibited syndrome, stimulant drug intoxication
Odd dress (gaudy decorations, multiple layers of clothes, scant clothing)	Mania
Odd manner	
a. Suspicious and hostile	Delusional condition, mania, drug abuse, antisocial personality, personality change due to epilepsy or chronic alcoholism
b. Intrusive and importunate	Mania, frontal lobe disinhibited syndrome, agitated depression
General medical signs	Papular rash around mouth and nose with inhalant abuse, scarring over veins with intravenous drug abuse, rhinophyma with alcoholism
Dysplastic body signs	Small head circumference and large ears; nose and lips of fragile-X syndrome; malformed ears, teeth, and hair whorls of developmental disorder

Flexed posture refers to forearms slightly raised (as if carrying several pieces of fire wood), slight forward bending at the waist, knees slightly bent, and shuffling gait. When accompanied by increased muscle tension, basal ganglia are usually involved; when associated with reduced tone (floppy limbs), the frontal lobes are likely involved.

Resting tremor is a hand tremor, often coarse, that disappears when the patient uses the hand. Resting tremor is associated with contralateral basal ganglia disease.

Poor motor sequencing is the inability to perform simple motor tasks in a continuous sequence, such as placing the side of a fist on a table, lifting the fist, coming down with the side of the open hand on the table, lifting the hand, and coming down again with the palm on the table. The sequence is fist, up, edge of open hand, up, palm, up. The sequence is repeated five times with each hand. Perseverations, errors in the sequence, and inability to continue performing the sequence despite prodding (motor impersistence) are some examples of sequencing abnormalities seen in frontal lobe disease, particularly involving the motor and dorsolateral circuits.

Poor finger tapping is having difficulty drumming one's fingers on the table in

TABLE 3.2. Some Important Motor Behaviors To Look For

Behavior	Definition	Implications
Agitation	Increased frequency of nongoal-directed movement, including pacing, hand wringing (suggesting depression), head rubbing, fidgeting in a chair, playing with one's fingers (suggesting anxiety), picking at bed sheets (suggesting delirium)	An expression of intense mood or changes in arousal as in delirium or some intoxications, melancholia, psychosis, anxiety state
Hyperactivity	Doing too many things simultaneously or in a short period of time, resulting in decreased function. When severe patient appears in a frenzy and activities are not completed	Seen in mania, stimulant drug intoxications, frontal lobe disinhibited syndrome
Hypoactivity	Reduced activity that, when severe, results in long period of inactivity and unresponsiveness. Along with slow thinking, defines psychomotor retardation	Seen in depression, frontal lobe dementia, some deliria, intoxication with sedating drugs, strokes, and, other conditions that reduce arousal
Dyskinesias	Involuntary, repetitive, and sometimes distorted movements of muscle groups not due to tremor. Includes choreoathetoid finger movements, oral-buccal movements, pelvic thrusts, head twisting or overextension, and rocking movements.	Tardive dyskinesia, diseases of the basal ganglia, e.g., Parkinson's disease, Huntington's chorea
Tremor	Involuntary dysregulation of opposing muscle groups	
	a. Resting hand tremor	Basal ganglia disease, psychotropic drug side effect
	b. Intention tremor	Cerebellar disease, anxiety, psychotropic drug side effect, benign essential tremor
Dyspraxias	Despite understanding the task and having adequate motor strength and sensory function, the inability to perform simple motor tasks (e.g., demonstrating the use of an imagined key; putting on an article of clothing; mimicking the examiner's hand posture)	Many psychotic conditions in which the dysfunction includes the parietal lobes or the left frontal lobe; ablating lesions of the parietal or frontal lobes

Table 3.3. The Motor System

Functional Organization Viewpoint	Clinical Findings
Left and right	Contralateral: Paralysis, paresis, upper motor neuron reflexes, dyspraxias, tremor. Diagnostically lateralizing when sign(s) unilateral
Anterior and posterior	Anterior motor signs include bradykinesia, flexed posture, resting tremor, increased muscle tone or floppy limbs, poor motor sequencing, poor finger tapping, adventitious motor overflow, motor impersistence or perseverations, dysarthria
	Posterior motor signs include intention tremor, past-pointing, dysmetria, poor alternating movements, poor coordination, poor tandem gait
Top and bottom	Top motor signs: include cortical signs of frontal or parietal lobe dysfunction. See anterior motor signs for frontal
	Parietal motor signs are ideomotor, kinesthetic, dressing apraxias.
	Bottom motor signs refer to the basal ganglia.

some sequence, such as from index to little finger. Awkwardness, perseverative movements with one or several fingers, and slapping rather than tapping are some abnormal features seen in patients with motor and dorsolateral frontal circuit disease.

Adventitious motor overflow refers to choreiform movements, usually associated with basal ganglia disease. Ask the patient to hold his arms out in front of himself with palms down. Look for sudden, brief finger or hand twisting movements. Choreiform movements can also be seen during finger tapping, with tapping-like movements in the hand not doing the task being the overflow. Sticking the tip of your tongue out while writing is another adventitious movement, but it has no clinical significance.

Motor impersistence is the inability to maintain a simple position, such as making a fist, shutting one's eyes, or sticking out one's tongue for 15 seconds. Three different positions need to be tested for good reliability (i.e., the test results will be reproducible). Test this when assessing for other motor signs. Impersistence is seen in disease of the lateral orbitofrontal circuit.

Perseveration refers to making unnecessary repetitions of words, ideas, or movements. It can be observed while testing for other motor signs and is associated with disease of the motor and dorsolateral circuits.

Dysarthria refers to distortions of speech sounds. Alcohol intoxication is the most common cause. The muscles used in speech cannot form the proper sounds because of brain dysregulation.

Stereotypy refers to automatic repetitive mundane movements such as tapping, gesturing, and grooming.

Posterior Motor Signs Indicating Cerebellar-Pontine Disease, Such as From Multiple Sclerosis, Degeneration From Chronic Alcoholism, or Stroke

Intention tremor refers to a coarse hand tremor when moving a limb, but no tremor at rest.

Past pointing (dysmetria) is difficulty putting the index finger directly onto a target, with the finger missing and going passed the target. Ask the patient to touch your finger while you move it to high, low, left, and right positions. The patient touching your finger and then his nose is a variation.

Poor coordination refers to awkward, jerky movements and, when severe, ataxia (gait, trunk, head)

Ataxia refers to head- or body-weaving movements. It can be observed or tested by asking the patient to heel/toe walk with eyes open for 12 feet. *Dystaxia* is observed when the patient is standing erect with feet together and eyes open. The patient sways or staggers in reaction to a slight push to his back.

Poor tandem gait refers to the patient being unable to walk a straight line, heel to toe.

Dysdiadochokinesia is the inability to perform rapid, alternating movements (20 trials) such as pronation and supination of the hands (placed on thighs). Mistakes in placement, breaks in movement, and jerky irregular movements can occur. Another test is having the patient rapidly touch the tip of his thumb with the tip of each finger in sequence (both hands palms up, fingers fully extended on thighs for 15 trials).

Asynergy is the inability to smoothly perform simple movements. Ask the patient to put his arms at his sides and, with eyes open, to touch his nose with one and then the other hand, five times with each hand. Loss of speed and fluidity, jerky movement, and performance in stages as if a robot are abnormal responses. Past-pointing (dysmetria) or intention tremor may also be observed at this time.

Top versus Bottom

The top and bottom view of the motor system overlaps with the anteroposterior and left–right perspectives. Together these three viewpoints help triangulate lesions.

The *top* of the top–bottom view is the frontal and parietal heteromodal cortices. Frontal motor features are described above as part of the anterior view. Dyspraxia is the most striking parietal lobe motor feature. *Dyspraxia* is defined as the inability to perform a simple previously learned motor task despite adequate motor strength and sensory control and an understanding of the task. Dyspraxias include the following.

Dressing dyspraxia is the inability to properly arrange clothes on one's body. Test this by asking the patient to put on a hospital robe or a lab coat. Patients with large parietal lobe lesions cannot visualize the three-dimensional nature of the robe or coat and cannot rotate that mental image to fit their body orientation and limb location.

Kinesthetic dyspraxia is the patient's inability to mimic your hand and limb postures (use several for better reliability) when you ask him to "Do with your left hand what I do with my left hand, and do with your right hand what I do with my right hand, without looking at your hands." Mirrored movements reflect frontal lobe problems (stimulus-bound echopraxia). Parietal lobe dysfunction can cause contralateral hand positioning problems.

Ideomotor dyspraxia occurs when the patient cannot link the idea with the movement. The patient will be awkward or use a hand or fingers as the object rather than showing you how the object must be held. The patient will have difficulty showing you how to use a hammer, key, scissors, comb, or toothbrush.

Constructional dyspraxia is the inability to copy simple geometric shapes (see Chapter 4).

The *bottom* of the top–bottom view is the basal ganglia. Some features of basal ganglia disease are discussed as part of the anterior motor system because the three views of the motor system overlap. Basal ganglia features include (1) flexed posture *with increased muscle tone* (a form of dystonia); (2) difficulty in locomotion: unsteadiness in turning, lurching gait, difficulty stopping, small rapidly increasing strides (festination), loss of arm swing; (3) tremor: resting and postural, pill rolling being an extreme form; and (4) dyskinesias: chorea (irregular muscle jerks of arms, face [grimacing], tongue), dysarthria, athetosis, hemiballismus, tics.

Table 3.4 displays some motor patterns and their implications. Examples of how to use these patterns in diagnosis follow.

A patient has become inefficient at work. He has difficulty planning his activities and has become impulsive. His moods alter between mild irritability and shallow good humor. These behavioral changes suggest the frontal lobe dysinhibited syndrome (action brain disease). A frontal–basal ganglia–thalamic loop stroke is suspected. The motor examination, however, reveals the patient to have an intention tremor, mild past-pointing, and dysdiadochokinesia indicating involvement of the posterior part of the motor system. Magnetic resonance imaging reveals cerebellar-pontine degeneration. Because the prognosis, treatment, and management of cerebellar-pontine degenerations differ from those for stroke, the anteroposterior distinction becomes important in the care of this patient.

A 76-year-old man becomes increasingly avolitional, suggesting action brain disease. He is not depressed. Except for some word-finding problems and repeating old stories he has no speech or language difficulty. He is not dyspraxic. The lack of these features suggest that the problem is not cortical (top). He has a right-hand resting tremor, but no bradykinesia and no increased muscle tone. These symptoms suggest basal ganglia (bottom) stroke (on the left) rather than Parkinson's disease. He has an anterioral action brain, left, subcortical (bottom) lesion. Methylphenidate substantially relieves his avolitional frontal lobe circuit syndrome.

Catatonia

Catatonia is a syndrome characterized by specific motor behaviors and by periods of extreme hypoactivity. The specific motor behaviors, however, can occur inde-

TABLE 3.4. Motor Patterns and Some Associated Behavioral Syndromes Helpful in Circumscribing Brain Pathology

Dominant (Left) Frontal Cortex (Top)	Lateral Orbitofrontal Cortex (Top)	Nondominant (right) Frontal Cortex (Top)
Perseveration	Motor impersistence	Perseveration
Poor verbal fluency	Echophenomena	Poor left finger tapping
Poor right motor sequencing	Hyperactivity	Poor left motor sequencing
Psychomotor retardation without gloominess	Logorrhea (too much speech)	*Motor aprosodia* (inability to express emotion in language)
Flexed slow gait with normal tone	*Catatonia*	
Poor right finger tapping or overflow	*Mania*	
Dementia		
Schizophrenia-like syndrome		
Left Basal Ganglia (Bottom)	**Bilateral Basal Ganglia (Bottom)**	**Right Basal Ganglia (Bottom)**
Dysarthria	Parkinsonism (bilateral resting tremor with increased muscle tone, bradykinesia, slow shuffling gait)	Left-hand resting tremor with normal muscle tone
Right hand resting tremor with normal muscle tone		*Obsessive compulsive disorder*
Frontal circuit avolitional syndrome	Overflow	*Mania*
Depression	*Subcortical dementia pattern*	
	Depression	
	Catatonia	
Dominant (Left) Parietal Lobe (Top)	**Cerebellum (Back)**	**Nondominant (Right) Parietal Lobe (Top)**
Ideomotor dyspraxia	Nystagmus	Constructional dyspraxia
Right-hand kinesthetic dyspraxia	Intention tremor	Left-hand kinesthetic dyspraxia
Dysgraphia (poor hand writing)	Past-pointing (dysmetria)	Dressing dyspraxia
	Ataxia and poor tandem gait	*Mania*
Unilateral right catatonia	Poor coordination	
	Dysdiadochokinesia	*Depression*
	Mild "frontal lobe" syndrome Impulse control disorder with irritability	*Impulse control disorder with irritability*
		Unilateral left catatonia
		Anosognosia (not recognizing one's illness)
		Nonaffective positive symptom psychoses

pendently of the full syndrome. Between 25% and 50% of patients with catatonic features have mood disorder, and about 15% to 20% of bipolar mood disorder patients have catatonic features. Remember the aphorism: "To scratch a catatonic is, often, to tickle a manic."

Mood disorder patients with catatonic features are indistinguishable from mood disorder patients without catatonia in their demographic characteristics, psychopathology, treatment response, and prevalence and pattern of psychiatric illness in their first-degree relatives. Although 5%–10% of catatonics are schizophrenic, catatonia generally has a favorable treatment response. About 10% of acutely ill psychotic inpatients will have two or more catatonic features.

Table 3.5 lists the catatonic features. Mutism and stupor are characteristic of catatonia, but are not pathognomonic. Other motor behaviors should be present, and most patients have several features. Most catatonics speak and move about. Mutism, negativism, and stupor occurring together indicate negativistic stupor (i.e., akinetic mutism or coma vigil secondary to orbitomesial frontal lobe damage, third ventricle tumors, or lesions of the reticular activating system and caudal hypothalamus). Mutism, stereotypy, catalepsy, and automatic obedience also occur together and represent the classic description of catatonia associated with mania. Catatonia is often associated with frontal lobe dysfunction, and the frontal lobe signs of pathologic inertia (difficulty initiating motor acts or stopping them once started) and stimulus-bound behavior (motor response to stimuli despite instructions to the contrary) may underlie catatonic features.

Test for catatonia when a patient does any of the following: walks with an odd gait inconsistent with a known neurologic disease (e.g., tiptoe walking, hopping), stands in one place for prolonged periods, holds arms up as if carrying something, shifts position when you shift position, repeats most of your questions before answering, responds to most of your questions with the same question (e.g., You: How old are you? Patient: How old are you?), makes manneristic hand or finger movements that are not typically dyskinetic, performs inconspicuous repetitive actions (e.g., making a series of clicking sounds before or after speaking, taps or automatically touches objects or body parts while walking about), is mute, or is bradykinetic, speaks with progressively less volume until his speech is a nonunderstandable mumble (prosectic speech).

Patients displaying one or more of the above features while conversing with you may allow themselves to be placed in odd postures, may be unable to resist your moving their arms despite your instructions to the contrary, or may be unable to resist shaking your proffered hand despite your instructions to the contrary (automatic obedience).

The DSM diagnostic criteria for catatonia put too much stress on mutism and stupor, which occur in other conditions. Table 3.6 lists another set of criteria. The differential diagnosis of catatonia (its etiology) includes (in order of most to least likely): bipolar mood disorder, depression, an identifiable action brain condition (e.g., stroke, vascular malformation), drug-induced state (e.g., neuroleptic overdosing, neuroleptic malignant syndrome, phencyclidine intoxication), metabolic disorders, epilepsy, and schizophrenia.

TABLE 3.5. Catatonic Features

Feature	Description
Mutism	A state of verbal unresponsiveness, not always associated with immobility
Stupor	Extreme hypoactivity and reduced or altered arousal in which the patient is mute, immobile, and unresponsive to painful stimuli
Gegenhalten (negativism)	Patient resists examiner's manipulations, light or vigorous, with strength equal to that applied, as if bound to the stimulus of the examiner's actions
Catalepsy	Maintenance of postures for long periods. Includes facial postures, such as grimacing, *Schnauzkrampf* (lips in an exaggerated pucker), and body postures such as *psychological pillow* (patient lying in bed with his head elevated as if on a pillow), lying in a jackknifed position, sitting with upper and lower portions of body twisted at right angles, holding arms above the head or raised in prayer-like manner, and holding fingers and hands in odd positions
Waxy flexibility	The examiner's experience of the patient offering initial resistance before gradually allowing himself to be postured, similar to bending a candle
Stereotypy	Often striking, nongoal-directed, repetitive motor behavior. The repetition of phrases and sentences in an automatic fashion, similar to a scratched record, termed *verbigeration*, is a verbal stereotypy. The neurologic term for the same behavior is *palilalia*
Echophenomena	Includes *echolalia*, in which the patient constantly repeats the examiner's utterances, and *echopraxia*, in which the patient spontaneously copies the examiner's movements or is unable to refrain from copying the examiner's test movements despite instruction to the contrary
Automatic obedience	Despite instructions to the contrary, the patient permits the examiner's light pressure to move his limbs into a new position (posture), which may then be maintained by the patient despite instructions to the contrary
Ambitendency	The patient appears motorically "stuck" in an indecisive, hesitant movement, resulting from the examiner verbally contradicting his own strong nonverbal signal, such as offering his hand as if to shake hands while stating, "Don't shake my hand, I don't want you to shake it."
Mannerisms	Odd, purposeful movements, such as holding hands as if they were six-shooters, saluting passersby, or exaggerations or stilted caricatures of mundane movements

TABLE 3.6. Diagnostic Criteria for Catatonia

1. Immobility, mutism, *or* stupor of at least 1 hour duration, if associated with at least one of the following, which can be observed or elicited on two or more occasions: - catalepsy, automatic obedience, posturing

2. In the absence of immobility, mutism, or stupor, at least two of the following, which canbe observed or elicited on two or more occasions: stereotypy, echophenomena, catalepsy, automatic obedience, posturing, negativism or Gegenhalten, ambitendency

Other Spontaneous Abnormal Movements

Abnormal movements have been described in psychiatric patients for centuries, and all the motor disturbances attributed to psychotropic drugs were observed in the predrug era. Stereotyped movements among the chronically psychiatrically ill are common (e.g., rocking, flicking and licking of the tongue, rubbing, picking, kneading, tapping). Also observed are ballistic arm movements; athetoid finger and hand movements; uncoordinated, stiff, and fragmented movements with a loss of normal smooth-transition movements; continuous grimacing and twisting of facial features; and making snorting, guttural, and clicking sounds. Kraepelin, who formulated the concept of dementia praecox (the old term for schizophrenia), believed that choreiform movements of the face and fingers were common in his patients, and he and Bleuler (a Swiss psychiatrist who coined the term schizophrenia) each described dementia praecox patients as exhibiting tremor, diadochokinesia, and ataxia ("the cerebellar form of dementia praecox"). The true prevalence of these behaviors then and now is unknown. When they occur, however, they do not change in character or frequency over time, although they occur more often during stress.

Drug-Induced Abnormal Movements

Most psychotropic agents in therapeutic doses affect motor function. Nonspecific and partially specific monoamine reuptake-inhibiting antidepressants (e.g., imipramine and desipramine, respectively) and lithium can produce persistent, fine, and rapid tremors and coordination difficulties that can impair fine motor performance. Coarse tremors, ataxia, and myoclonus can occur at toxic levels. Monoamine oxidase inhibitors may induce agitation. Benzodiazepines, in large doses, can cause ataxia, tremors, and myoclonus. Benzodiazepine withdrawal can produce obsessive compulsive–like behaviors. Neuroleptics have the most profound effect on motor behavior, although they differ widely in potency.

Parkinsonism is a common side effect of drugs with substantial dopamine (D_2) blocking properties. *Bradykinesia*, the earliest and most common feature of drug-induced parkinsonism, is characterized by an expressionless face, slow initiation of motor activity, and loss of secondary movements (such as arm swing). When severe, the patient looks stiff and frozen. Handwriting becomes small and choppy (micrographia), and having a patient on a neuroleptic write his signature every few days provides an easy, highly sensitive measure of the extrapyramidal effects of the drug.

Bradykinesia is associated with muscle weakness and fatigue, muscle rigidity of the neck, trunk, and extremities, and cogwheeling, that is, as you flex and extend the patient's arm at the elbow, you feel the arm move in short, stop-and-go arcs, as if periodically stopped by the gears of a wheel.

Postural difficulties also occur, including a flexed posture and deficits in righting responses, and a shuffling, propulsive gait. Tremor at rest and during voluntary actions, pill rolling at rest (uncommon in drug-induced states), and a fine perioral tremor (the rabbit syndrome) can occur. Drug-induced parkinsonism usually begins within a few days of drug administration and seldom occurs for the first time after 3 months of treatment independent of some other event (e.g., stroke, the addition of another psychotropic drug, sudden dramatic improvement in a psychosis associated with receptor hypersensitivity). Depending on the neuroleptic administered and the dosage, upward of 50% of patients may develop these extrapyramidal side effects. The very young, the very old, and women may be most susceptible.

Dystonias, sudden muscle spasms, usually begin within the first few days of neuroleptic treatment. They are dramatic, frightening to the patient, often painful, and may recur over several days before they are controlled. Young patients are most vulnerable. Common dystonias are spasms of the muscles of the face, jaw, neck, throat, and tongue (e.g., oculogyric crisis, blepharospasm, respiratory stridor with cyanosis, torticollis, and opisthotonos). *Acute dyskinesias* without severe muscle spasm can also occur early in treatment (e.g., tongue protrusion, lip smacking, chewing movements, blinking, athetosis of the fingers and toes, shoulder shrugging, and myoclonic movements of the head, neck, and extremities). The incidence of dystonias rises with the increased usage of high-potency neuroleptics or the atypical neuroleptics with high serotonergic receptor affinity.

Akathesia is a state of motor restlessness in which the patient is unable to sit or be still. It is usually associated with a subjective feeling of jitteriness and may be mistaken for anxiety or an exacerbation of psychoses, although patients often say they are not anxious, "just restless." Akathesia usually begins after several days of drug administration and increases in incidence during the first several months of treatment. Its severity and duration are variable. Akathesia occurs in about 20% of neuroleptic-treated patients, particularly those receiving low to moderate doses of high potency neuroleptics or the atypical neuroleptics with high serotonergic receptor affinity. At high doses, high potency neuroleptics, produce more lethargy and less akathesia.

Tardive dyskinesia (TD), characterized by a variety of abnormal movements, occurs in 30%–50% of patients exposed to prolonged neuroleptic treatment. Onset is usually after months of treatment and may appear only after dose reduction or discontinuation of neuroleptics. Elderly patients, those with preexisting brain disease, and bipolar mood disorder patients are most vulnerable. In some patients who have dystonias and other extrapyramidal side effects during acute neuroleptic treatment, TD may occur after a relatively brief exposure (3–6 months) to the drug. Features of TD include the buccolingual-masticatory syndrome (vermicular movements of the tongue on the floor of the mouth; protruding, twisting, and curling tongue movements combined with sucking, pouting, and bulging of the cheeks), choreiform movements of the extremities (particularly the fingers), ballistic arm movements, gait and postural abnormalities (shifting of weight, lordosis, rocking and swaying, pelvic thrusting, and rotary movements), grunting vocalizations, respiratory dyskinesias and chest heaving resulting in stridor and cyanosis, and dysphagias. Spasms and weakness of esophageal muscles can lead to aspiration pneumonia. Symptoms are exacerbated by stress, but many patients seem unaware of their abnormal movements.

Severe TD can incapacitate. Like naturally occurring basal ganglia disease, TD is associated with cognitive impairment. Typical problems are a general slowing of cognitive functioning (bradyphrenia), poor attention and working memory, and poor new learning (verbal and nonverbal). This cognitive impairment may be one reason why chronic bipolar mood disorder seems to be more prevalent today than in the past. The use of stimulant street drugs, particularly cocaine, which as a class also affect basal ganglia dopamine systems, is another reason for chronicity (see Chapter 8 for detailed discussion). Because of the terrible motor and cognitive problems that prolonged use of neuroleptics can cause, make them your last resort, and limit their use to the shortest possible time.

Drug-induced abnormal movements are strikingly similar to spontaneous abnormal movements, and discriminating these two is difficult but important because the spontaneous movement disorders provide critical diagnostic information. Drug-induced parkinsonism (i.e., bradykinesia with stiffness and tremor) is usually associated with other neuroleptic side effects (e.g., anticholinergic-induced signs, greasy sweat, dry mouth, sluggish pupillary accommodation, constipation, and urinary difficulty in older men). Because drugs affect the brain bilaterally, unilateral abnormal movements, particularly those of the nonpreferred hand, are usually due to the disease and not to psychotropics (early TD is an exception often seen first as choreoathetoid finger movements in the preferred hand). Lithium can also produce a mild unilateral tremor, typically in the nonpreferred hand. Sudden onset of fully formed abnormal movements is almost always drug induced, unless paroxysmal (think of epilepsy) or following a neurologic-like event (think of stroke or head trauma).

MOOD AND AFFECT

Many behavioral syndromes are characterized by some disturbance in affect. *Affect* refers to the regulation and expression of emotion. *Mood* refers to the emotion of the moment: sadness, happiness, anger, anxiety. Mood has a cognitive (the subjective feeling) and an arousal component. Mood intensity and arousal correlate, and mood intensity predicts pulse, heart rate, blood pressure, and pupillary dilation. The more intense the mood, the greater the arousal.

Normal emotional expression requires an integration of brain structure and function bilaterally. Thus, patients with primary mood disorder do not have lateralized brain dysfunction on laboratory testing. Patients with secondary mood disorders, however, may have lateralized or localized laboratory abnormalities (usually the nondominant hemisphere for irritability, left anterior circuits for avolitional or apathetic depressions, and frontal orbital circuits for manic-like syndromes).

Mood influences motor behavior (e.g., agitation, gestures, facial expression), manner, tone of speech, thought processes, thought content, and, when extreme, the development of delusions and perceptual disturbances. When assessing these features you are assessing *emotional expression.* Emotional expression can be abnormally intense (as in mania and depression), low (as in schizophrenia), unvarying (expressing only one mood as in depression), unstable (lability of mood as in mania), or inappropriate (laughing in sad circumstances). Inappropriateness of mood is not pathognomonic and may reflect normal anxiety (e.g., gallows humor), as well as serious illness. It has limited diagnostic importance. Also, test emotional expression by asking the patient about the usual emotion-related aspects of life: family, friends, good and bad life events, personal interests.

Loss of emotional expression is similar to the neurologic concept of *motor aprosodia.* In motor aprosodia there is an impairment in the emotional expression of language. Speech is bland or monotoned; gestures are reduced or lost; facial expression is lost. When severe, you cannot tell what, if anything, the patient is emotionally experiencing.

The nondominant hemisphere subserves prosody, the expression of emotion and emotional gesturing in speech, and the understanding of the emotion in the speech of others. Patients with normal dominant hemisphere functioning but with lesions in the nondominant hemisphere have normal spontaneity, clarity, and comprehension of speech, but may have impairments of range, modulation, and melody of voice, of gesturing with speech, or of comprehension of the emotional tone of the speech of others. These abnormalities are analogous to aphasic disturbances due to dominant hemisphere dysfunction. For example, in an anterior (nondominant frontal) prosodic disturbance, there is impaired spontaneous emotionality and gesturing when speaking; in a posterior (nondominant temporal parietal) prosodic disturbance there is impaired comprehension of the prosody and gesturing of others. Motor prosody is tested when you assess emotional expression and emotional blunting. The only difference between the motor aprosodia of schizophrenia (i.e., loss of emotional expression or blunting) and motor aprosodia due to stroke or injury is that the stroke or injury patient is often aware of the problem and tries to compensate for it by adding gestures (e.g., shaking a fist) or words (e.g., profanity, emotional words) to signal what mood they are feeling, but are unable to express.

Receptive prosody is tested by standing behind the patient so that only your tone of voice can be interpreted and then asking him to determine the emotion in an emotionally neutral sentence ("The boy went to the grocery store.") in a sad, happy, angry, and emotionally neutral voice. Assessing receptive prosody is analogous to assessing receptive language.

Volition refers to that aspect of personality and cognition related to planning, drive, ambition, and desires. Patients with frontal lobe lesions, particularly in the dominant dorsolateral circuit, often are avolitional. In its severest form, loss of volition extends to grooming and hygiene, and avolitional patients often appear slovenly.

Assess volition by asking the patient what he thinks about his present situation and what are his future plans. Ask about past, present, and future work, willingness to stay in the hospital for a prolonged period, plans for having a family, and what he does for fun. Ask the patient what his typical day is like. Loss of volition and emotional expression are signs of action brain disease.

Emotional blunting is a combination of loss of emotional expression and avolition. It is a core feature of schizophrenia. Schizophrenics have an unvarying affect, have decreased mood intensity, and are apathetic. They are expressionless, monotone, seclusive, and indifferent to their surroundings. They express little feeling for their families and are unconcerned about their present situation. They are devoid of libido. They are without future plans or desires. They are content to remain hospitalized for many years. If they want to leave the hospital, it is to go to a nursing home or a halfway house that lets them watch TV all day. In the hospital, they lie on the floor, stand in a corner, or sit alone. They have little interest in hospital activities and prefer to smoke and drink soda pop. Outside the hospital they have no friends, rarely see their family, do not work, and have no hobbies or interests. When asked "What would you do if you won ten million dollars in the lottery?" they are at a loss, and, beyond saying, "I'd put it in a bank or give it to charity," they can think of nothing they would like to do. Occasionally patients with emotional blunting will make silly jokes and will express a fatuous but shallow mood, incongruous to the situation. This is *Witzelsucht* (German, meaning "searching for wit") and is associated with the lateral orbitofrontal syndrome. A married, working person with some interests is unlikely to be schizophrenic, no matter how psychotic.

Depression is sometimes confused as emotional blunting. The two patterns, however, are different. Depressed patients have decreased affective range, but their mood is often profound and intense. They are gloomy, dysphoric (irritable and gloomy), or apprehensive. Their emotional expression is not lost; they have not lost motor prosody, it is just stuck in one gear. Their facial expression is despondent or apprehensive. Their tone of voice also suggests sadness or worry. They are usually highly concerned about their predicament. Those depressives who are not psychotic want to get better and resume their lives. Those depressives who are psychotic may be convinced they are bad or are going to die or that they should kill themselves, but these are not the thoughts of someone who is indifferent to his situation or surroundings. If a patient has many features of depression (e.g., loss of interest, feeling guilty, worthless, or helpless), but not the above mood, and is instead emotionally blunted, consider the depression secondary until proven otherwise.

SPEECH AND LANGUAGE

Odd communication is a common feature of several behavioral disorders. Different patterns of odd communication are associated with different behavioral disorders and dysfunction in different brain regions. Most speech and language problems reflect dysfunction in dominant brain structures.

Speech content primarily reflects cultural and personal life experiences and is less diagnostically important than the form of word usage and organization. Exceptions are the thoughts of suicide, guilt, and hopelessness often expressed by depressed patients or the grandiose ideas of some manics. This content is the verbal expressions of their abnormal mood. Strange or "bizarre" ideas are not diagnostic and occur in many conditions.

Table 3.7 lists the forms of speech and language to examine. If during the taking of the history and other parts of the evaluation the "conversation" with the

TABLE 3.7. Speech and Language Assessment

Area To Assess	Abnormality	Implications
Turn-taking	Intrusive with press of speech	Mania, stimulant drug intoxication
	Paucity of speech	Depression, sedating drug intoxication, schizophrenia, metabolic states causing reduced arousal, some ictal and post-ictal states, transcortical motor aphasia, left basal ganglia, and thalamic strokes
Spontaneity	Overly spontaneous (usually with distractibility)	Mania, stimulant drug intoxication, some hallucinogen intoxications
	Reduced spontaneity	Sedating drug intoxication, metabolic states causing reduced arousal, Broca's and transcortical motor aphasias, left basal ganglia and thalamic strokes, depression, schizophrenia, some ictal and post-ictal states
Fluency of speech	Reduced (few words when speaking)	Depression, transcortical motor aphasia, schizophrenia
	Reduced and halting	Broca's aphasia, some ictal states
	Increased (too many words)	Mania, stimulant drug use, anxiety
Distractibility of speech	Increased (jumping from topic to topic)	Mania (flight-of-ideas), stimulant drug intoxication, some deliria (rambling speech), substantial anxiety (distractibility will be mild)
	Decreased	States of reduced arousal, melancholia with stupor
Language organization (syntax, word usage, logic)	Disorganized with paraphasias	Schizophrenia, hallucinogenic drug-related psychosis, dominant frontotemporal seizure focus, thalamic aphasia, receptive aphasia (Wernicke's, transcortical sensory, mixed aphasias)

patient appears normal, that is, you do not notice anything odd about it, then the patient probably has no speech or language problem. This may seem superficial, but, in fact, you are an expert in conversations—you have had thousands of them and know a bad one when you hear it. If the conversation appears odd in some way, specific evaluation needs to be done. Some definitions follow.

Flight-of-ideas is speech that jumps from topic to topic. The patient is distracted by his own associations and surrounding stimuli. Flight-of-ideas produces many words, many rapidly shifting topics during which the patient has poor turn-taking, making interrupting him difficult. Most patients said to have "looseness of associations," in fact, have flight-of-ideas. Flight-of-ideas is observed in mania, stimulant drug intoxications, and the frontal disinhibited syndrome.

> Example:
> Q. "What type of work do you do?"
> A. "I've been working in New York for over 20 years. The city is too crowded and dirty. Bacteria are everywhere and antibiotics don't work anymore. I had a friend who died from it. He was a high school teacher. Boy, do they have a tough job. Do you know about the murder rate in schools?"

Circumstantial speech is tightly linked associations but with extra, nonessential details interspersed. Speech takes a circuitous route before reaching the goal. Circumstantial speech is observed with mania and chronic epilepsy, in chronic drug users in whom limbic system sensitization occurs (stimulants, alcohol), and in some elderly persons.

> Example:
> "How long have I been working in Atlanta? Let me tell you it hasn't been easy. All that political stuff, then the recessions. My own health problems added to that, you know, but after all this time things have finally turned out okay. It took a long time, however, and now I've been with the company 25 years."

Rambling speech is nongoal-directed, distractible speech occurring during delirium and intoxications. Meaningful connections between phrases and sentences are lost, but the syntax and meaning of the fragments remain generally intact. It differs from flight-of-ideas in the degree of jumping from topic to topic (less topics but bigger jumps) and in number of words spoken (less).

> Example:
> "It's too cold, turn it off, turn it off . . . who's that person? . . . I'm not a victim . . . did it happen?"

Formal thought disorder (FTD) does not mean faulty thinking. It was assumed to reflect faulty thinking, and so the name, but what it really refers to is aphasic-like speech and language problems that are seen in some psychiatric patients, particularly schizophrenics. The elements of FTD are similar to those observed in several forms of fluent aphasia. The pattern of FTD is similar to that found with lesions involving the dominant basal ganglia or thalamus. Some elements of FTD are

1. *Word approximations* (in class semantic paraphasias) are substitute words that have a close (thus "in class") but not the precise meaning of the correct word that should be used. Word approximations are observed in anterior subcortical and posterior cortical aphasias and in schizophrenia.

Example:
Using the word *writer* for *pen,* the phrase *book collection building* for *library.*

2. *Private word usage* (out of class semantic paraphasias) is the idiosyncratic use of words or phrases making their meaning obscure. Private word usage occurs in schizophrenia and with dominant basal ganglia or thalamic strokes.

Example:
"I can't be responsible for the *linear reduction* of his actions."

3. *Neologisms* are new words formed by the improper use of the sound of the words (phonemic paraphasias) or by the meaningless combination of two or more words (a portmanteau word).

Example (Sound):
Flober for *flower.*

Combination:
Combining *parallel* and *circumstantial* into *parastantial.* Neologisms occur in Wernicke's and mixed aphasia and in subcortical aphasias involving dominant basal ganglia or thalamic lesions.

4. *Perseveration* is the repetition of stock words and phrases automatically placed into the flow of speech. It often occurs with subcortical anterior lesions affecting frontal lobe function.

Example:
"I've been intellectually involved for years. The intellectual flow of thoughts is manifest. My intelligence, your intelligence are all part of the academic intellectual community." Some non-ill elderly persons use stock words as substitutes for their inability to elaborate on their ideas (e.g., "and so on and so forth").

5. *Verbigeration* (*palilalia* is the "neurologic" term) is a verbal stereotype, the patient automatically repeating associations, particularly at the

end of a thought. Verbigeration may take the form of clang associations, that is, associations by the sound rather than the meaning of the words ("I started in the lumber, tumbler, number business"). Verbigeration or palilalia occurs with some basal ganglia lesions, and in catatonia, frontal dysinhibited syndromes, and secondary and chronic mania.

Example:
"I've been working in New York for 20 years, 20 years, 20 years, years, years. I been working for 20 years."

6. *Driveling (jargon) speech* refers to associations that are tightly linked and appear to follow grammatical rules, but the meaning (content) of the speech is lost, as if the patient's language were unfamiliar to you. Driveling is similar to double talk. Word salad (no two consecutive words are meaningfully connected) is its most severe form. Driveling occurs in Wernicke's aphasia, anterior subcortical aphasias, schizophrenia, and some chronic drug-induced psychoses. In Wernicke's aphasia the driveling is fairly constant, whereas in subcortical aphasia and schizophrenia the driveling is typically sporadic and of short duration when it occurs.

Example:
"I'm not boxed by electric door frame stations, don't you?"

7. *Derailment* is the sudden, disrupted switch from one line of thought to a new parallel line of thought. Mild derailment (sometimes termed *cognitive slippage*) is observed in some patients with schizotypal personality disorder. More severe forms are observed in patients with anterior subcortical aphasia, cerebellar neocortical lesions, schizophrenia, and some chronic drug-induced psychoses.

Example:
"I started in construction, but earthquakes do a lot of damage."

8. *Nonsequiturs* are responses that are totally unrelated to the previous comment or question. In the absence of flight-of-ideas, or severe psychomotor slowing (where the timing of the patient's responses is off), nonsequiturs are observed in Wernicke's aphasia because of poor auditory comprehension, and in schizophrenia. Nonsequiturs are also observed in patients with nondominant frontal lobe lesions.

Example:
Q. "How old are you?
A. "I'm a very practical person."

9. *Elliptical* speech is tightly linked associations that skirt the point, but never get to the point. Responses are vague, but the general subject matter is usually related to the question. It differs from flight-of-ideas in which associations move progressively further away from the point. Elliptical speech occurs in anterior subcortical aphasias and in schizophrenia.

Examples:
Q. "What type of work do you do?"
A. "I work in Dallas."
Q. "Yes, but what do you do in Dallas?"
A. "I've been there a year."
Q. "And what have you been working at for that year?"
A. "It's hard work."

Patients with FTD, and those with some aphasias, have strikingly similar speech and word usage, although the neurologic and psychiatric terms sometimes differ (Table 3.8). *Circumoculatory speech* refers to the patient referring to an object, event, or person by phrases related to function or physical characteristic rather than by its name. For example, a pen becomes "the thing you write with." It is similar to elliptical speech in that the patient appears to have understood the subject being discussed and what information he is being asked to communicate, but he cannot precisely communicate that information. What is uttered is vague and allusive or around the point (circumoculatory speech).

Despite the fact that schizophrenics with FTD and patients with posterior aphasia have similar abnormalities of speech, the two speech patterns differ. Table 3.9 displays the observed differences in speech patterns between the two patient groups.

TABLE 3.8. Aphasia and Formal Thought Disorder

Language Disorder	Neurologic Term	Psychiatric Term
Semantic disorders	Jargon agrammatism	Driveling
	Paragrammatism	Derailment
	Nonsequitur	Nonsequitur
	Semantic paraphasia (out of class)	Private word usage
	Portmanteau word (combination)	Neologism
Nominal disorders	Verbal paraphasias (in class)	Word approximation
	Anomia	Word finding problems
	Circumloculatory speech	Elliptical speech
Phonemic disorders	Phonemic paraphasias (literal)	Clanging
	Neologism	Neologism

Table 3.9. Schizophrenic and Aphasic Language

Feature	Language	
	Schizophrenics	Wernicke's Aphasics
Fluency	OK	OK
Spontaneity	Poor	Adequate
Repetition	OK	Poor
Auditory comprehension	OK	Poor
Use of complex words	OK	Very poor
Word-finding problems	Poor	Very poor
Reduced nouns	Poor	Very poor
Private words	present	not present
Aphasic elements	present	present

Aphasia

Because patients with fluent aphasia, but no paralysis, are sometimes mistaken as psychotic (those with past psychiatric problems are most at risk), speech and language assessment sometimes requires specific assessment for aphasia. Most aphasias are due to stroke and involve specific parts of the language system (Table 3.10). The variables to assess are spontaneity of speech, fluency of speech, organization of speech, auditory comprehension, and repetition. Table 3.11 lists some aphasia patterns.

The function of speech and language localizes primarily to the parasylvian areas of the frontal, temporal, and parietal lobes of the dominant (for words and word usage) and nondominant (for prosody) hemispheres. In the dominant hemisphere this includes Broca's area, the frontal cortex deep to Broca's area, the supplementary motor cortex, the arcuate fasciculus connecting Broca's to Wernicke's area, Wernicke's area and adjacent temporal lobe structures, and the supramarginal gyrus of the parietal lobe.

Nonfluent Aphasias

Broca's aphasia results from damage to the dominant posterior interior frontal gyrus, adjacent areas of the operculum and insula, and sometimes to the anterior parietal lobe and underlying frontal lobe white matter. Auditory comprehension is intact, but these patients are unable to express themselves fluently and are occasionally mute. They struggle to get words out. They often omit small words, such as "the," to," or "a." Their speech seems "telegraphic." They are often dysarthric, with labored or mispronounced syllables. Dysarthric speech can also occur from isolated lesions in the dominant precentral gyrus of the insula, a cortical area beneath the frontal and temporal lobes. This area seems to be specialized for the motor planning of speech.

TABLE 3.10. Brain Language Areas and Their Clinical Correlations

Language Area	Clinical Correlations
Broca's area (inferior posterior lateral aspect of the dominant frontal lobe)	Broca's (motor) aphasia; nondominant hand and facial ideomotor apraxis; contralateral hemiparesis, dysarthria
Wernicke's area (posterior part of the superior dominant temporal lobe gyrus)	Wernicke's (receptive or sensory) aphasia with normal motor functioning
Arcuate fasciculus (fiber tract between Wernicke's and Broca's areas)	Mixed aphasia
Watershed areas	
a. Portions of dominant frontal lobe near to Broca's area and the dorsal mesial frontal cortex	a. Transcortical motor aphasia, contralateral hemiparesis, ipsilateral hand ideomotor dyspraxia
b. Portion of medial and lateral parietal lobe	b. Transcortical sensory aphasia
Anterior brain subcortical structures (dominant basal ganglia and thalamic nuclei)	Subcortical aphasia, frontal lobe apathetic syndrome
Cerebellar neocortex (contralateral to dominant hemisphere)	Word-finding problems (action verbs, complex words) dysarthria, mild verbal fluency problems
Dominant parietal lobe heteromodal cortex and related corpus callosum	Word-finding problems (nouns), difficulties with symbolic lexical relationships, dyslexia with dysgraphia
Dominant occipital lobe unimodal cortex and related corpus callosum	Dyslexia without agraphia
Nondominant structures homologous to Broca's and Wernicke's areas, arcuate fasciculus, watershed areas, and basal ganglia and thalamic nuclei	Aprosodias: motor, sensory, mixed, transcortical, subcortical, respectively

Sometimes a mild motor aphasia is not immediately recognizable, but can be tested by having the patient repeat sentences or phrases containing small words (e.g., "No ifs, ands, or buts"), or phrases difficult to pronounce (e.g., "Methodist Episcopal," "Massachusetts Avenue"). Repetitive language also involves decoding and phonemic expression, so dysfunction in posterior language areas must be ruled out if a patient has difficulty repeating phrases.

Because of the extent and type of brain damage producing Broca's aphasia, other problems often co-occur. These include (1) ideomotor dyspraxia using the ipsilateral hand, (2) buccolingual dyspraxia (the patient may have trouble puffing out his cheeks, or blowing out a match), (3) weakness or paralysis of the contralateral extremities, and (4) dysgraphia using the ipsilateral (and sometimes the contralateral) hand. In general, many patients with aphasia of any type cannot compensate for the aphasia by writing. Learned facial motor skills (e.g., whistling) may also be impaired. Some patients have preserved ability to fluently sing, use profanity, or say overlearned sequences such as the days of the week or months of

TABLE 3.11. Patterns of Speech Variables in the Aphasias

	Speech and Language Function				
Type of Aphasia	Spontaneous Speech	Speech Fluency	Auditory Comprehension	Repetition	Speech Organization (Syntax/Grammar Word Usage)
Broca's	Poor (labored and dysarthric)	Nonfluent	Reduced, but globally adequate	Labored and telegraphic, but can repeat some words	Telegraphic (some word-finding problems, but otherwise intact)
Transcortical motor	Poor (no dysarthria)	Nonfluent	Adequate	Can repeat some words, better performance than Broca's	Paucity of speech, but organization adequate. Difficulty reading aloud
Transcortical sensory	Normal	Normal	Poor	Adequate (biggest difference from Wernicke's)	Paraphasic and agrammatical; poor naming, reading, and writing
Wernicke's	Normal	Normal	Poor	Poor	Paraphasic and agrammatical; poor naming, reading, and writing

the year, suggesting that the storage of language is not exclusively cortical.

Transcortical motor aphasia results from damage to the dominant mesial frontal lobe, the supplementary motor cortex, white matter anterior and lateral to the frontal horn of the lateral ventricles, and occasionally the lenticular nucleus of the basal ganglia. In this type of aphasia there is a paucity of spontaneous speech. Speech is labored, as with Broca's aphasia, but it is not telegraphic. Because posterior language structures are intact, auditory comprehension and repetition are usually preserved.

Global aphasia is uncommon and is characterized by poor verbal output and problems with comprehension, naming, writing, and reading. It usually results from middle cerebral artery occlusion, but may occur without hemiparesis.

Fluent Aphasias

If the patient's speech is fluent, next decide if the speech is understandable, if words are appropriately used, and if comprehension is good. Fluent, nonunderstandable speech with poor comprehension suggests Wernicke's aphasia.

Wernicke's aphasia is caused by a lesion in or around Wernicke's area, the posterior one third of the superior temporal gyrus. Sometimes lesions extend into the head of the caudate and internal capsule. It is characterized by fluent jargon-filled speech and impaired comprehension of the speech of others. Repetition of speech is poor. As with Broca's aphasia, writing is usually aphasic.

Wernicke's aphasia patients have poor auditory comprehension, and they inappropriately respond to simple requests (e.g., "Fold this paper three times."). Sometimes they respond properly to simple, but not to complex requests ("Point to all the pictures that show something you'd find in the kitchen.").

On occasion, a small lesion of the middle one third of the superior temporal gyrus will produce a solitary defect of auditory comprehension (pure word deafness). Here the patient's speech is fluent, clear, and understandable, but the patient has grossly impaired comprehension of the speech of others.

Broca's aphasics have nonfluent speech and problems with repetition. Fluent aphasias with repetition problems include Wernicke's and conduction aphasias. Conduction aphasics have reasonably intact comprehension, but have word-finding problems, and they make phonemic paraphasic errors. Reading aloud, naming, and writing to dictation are impaired. Although speech is fluent, verbatim repetition is markedly impaired. The arcuate fasciculus between the dominant parietal and frontal lobes is usually involved.

Fluent aphasics with no repetition problems include anomic aphasics and transcortical sensory aphasics. Transcortical sensory aphasics are similar to patients with Wernicke's aphasia, but repetition is preserved. They can repeat complex sentences, but cannot understand them. Spontaneous speech is empty, circumlocutory, and paraphasic. Reading and auditory comprehension are impaired. The angular gyrus and the mesial surface of the dominant parietal lobe are usually involved. The thalamus may also be involved.

Other Abnormalities of Fluent Speech

Test naming (anomic aphasia) by asking the patient to name simple objects you show him, i.e., naming to confrontation (e.g., pen, watch, paper clip). Then ask the patient to point to objects you name (e.g., "Show me a collar."). Pick items consistent with the patient's level of education. Dysnomia can result from a dominant temporal or dominant parietal lesion. It has no clearer localizing significance. In severe anomic aphasias speech is spontaneous, but empty. It is filled with circumlocutions, vague phrases, and indefinite references. Pronouns rather than nouns make up the content. Fluency of speech can be interrupted with multiple pauses, resulting in a stumbling verbal output. Repetition and comprehension are usually intact, but reading and writing disturbances can occur. Anomic aphasia is often a residual syndrome following improvement from other aphasic states.

Reading, writing, and reading comprehension are language functions assessed with the screening test described in Chapter 4. Occasionally, silent reading and reading comprehension are intact, but the patient is unable to read aloud. This suggests a lesion in the arcuate fasciculus disconnecting Wernicke's and Broca's areas. If a patient can write but cannot read, the disconnecting lesion is between the occipital lobes and Wernicke's area.

Dominant thalamic lesions can result in aphasia. Thalamic aphasia is fluent, but with reduced spontaneity and sometimes a paucity of speech. Repetition is adequate. Comprehension may be variably impaired. Reading aloud, writing, and naming are impaired, and utterances can be paraphasic. The syndrome is often transient and is associated with attentional problems, avolition, and perseverative behavior. This pattern is similar to FTD observed in blunted schizophrenics. Dominant basal ganglia lesions (particularly the head of the caudate) can also produce a fluent aphasia, with dysarthric and paraphasic speech, poor comprehension, and variable repetition ability.

Also pay attention to how the patient gestures while he speaks. Some hand gestures are cultural signals (e.g., holding your arm out straight, with palm of hand facing out signals "stop"; opposing your index finger and thumb tips forming a circle while extending the other three fingers signals "okay"). Hand gestures during speech, however, are integral parts of communication. They include gestures that define the spatial and lexical relationships and content of what is being said. They also function to help the speaker, not the person being addressed. These hand gestures are an expression of the self-monitoring function of the action brain. Think of people gesturing while speaking with someone on the phone. They cannot see each other, but they gesture anyway. Patients with self-monitoring deficits tend not to gesture when they speak. This is typical of patients with language problems involving the thalamus or basal ganglia and of schizophrenics with FTD.

DELUSIONS

A delusion is a false or arbitrary idea developed without adequate proof and is not consistent with the person's social and cultural background. The false idea may be fixed or fleeting. Delusions are nonspecific, and 30%–40% of severely ill psychiatric patients are delusional. Delusions occur with equal frequency in patients with bipolar mood disorder, schizophrenia, and drug-induced psychosis.

Delusions can develop from altered moods that distort the patient's thinking, leading to false conclusions (e.g., a euphoric mood leading to feelings of great power and then to the conclusion of being divine). Delusions also develop from hallucinatory and other psychopathological experiences that are thought by the patient to be real, thus providing the "evidence" to support the delusion (e.g., the hallucinated voices warn against danger, and the patient accepts these voices as real and therefore there is a plot against him). When a delusional idea develops from other psychopathology (e.g., altered mood, hallucinations) it is termed a *secondary delusional idea*.

Primary delusional ideas evolve without obvious development from other psychopathology. Usually they develop over time as "evidence" builds up. For example, a patient thought a co-worker was in love with him because he saw several women in different places near his home who looked like her, and then the woman went to a staff dinner knowing he was going to be there. This patient's sequence of thought, although arbitrary, has some understandable connection, and you can follow how he reached his conclusion. Sometimes a delusional idea develops suddenly and is fully formed (*autochthonous delusional idea*). Autochthonous delusional ideas suggest a secondary psychosis from epilepsy or drug abuse.

Delusional perceptions are ideas in which you cannot connect the "evidence" to the conclusion. Delusional perceptions are based on real perceptions that are then given great significance and personalized by the patient. For example, a patient concluded that there was a plot to kill him because the lights were left on overnight at a store near his house. Delusional perceptions are primary delusions because they do not develop from other obvious psychopathology.

Delusional mood, the simplest delusional experience, is characterized by the intense and persistent "feeling" that "something is wrong," that "things are not right" and perhaps sinister. It is like the feeling of being watched or the common experience of self-consciousness when you enter a noisy room full of people who, for the moment, become quiet to observe you. Delusional moods are observed in many primary psychotic disorders and can be intensely experienced following viral illnesses, drug intoxications, and epilepsy.

Ideas of reference refers to the more specific conclusions reached by some patients with a delusional mood. Apparently developing from their general unease and suspiciousness, these patients begin to feel that people (even strangers in the street) are looking at them, watching them, or talking about them.

Many patients readily relate their delusional ideas because they feel them to be obvious to everyone. Others are guarded because they know that others will think them crazy. When a patient expresses a delusional idea, take immediate interest and get more specific information about the situation. In a nonconfrontational manner, ask the patient for proof, for example, "How did you learn about these things?"

When examining for delusions, ask about trouble with neighbors, co-workers, or relatives. Use the patient's other psychopathologic experiences. For example, ask the patient who hears voices if the voices or the sources of the voices try to harm him in any way. More direct questions include "Have you had the experience that people are plotting against you (or trying to hurt you, poison you, spy on you)? Have you had the experience that you saw or heard something that other people felt was unimportant, but you knew was a message just for you, or a signal?"

OVERVALUED IDEAS

Delusional ideas evolve from arbitrary or illogical thinking. However, patients with severe obsessive compulsive disorder or hypochondriasis also express ideas that are fixed, clearly false, and derive from what appears to be arbitrary or illogical thinking. An overvalued idea is another example of a thought (usually associated with an intense mood) that takes precedence over all other ideas. It becomes the main theme in the patient's life.

Obsessions, hypochondriacal notions, and overvalued ideas are difficult to distinguish from some primary delusions (other than autochthonous or delusional perception). Some distinguishing features of overvalued ideas are that their expression is usually isolated, without other features of psychosis; their content is typically mundane (e.g., contamination, health, litigation about money owed) rather than odd or sinister as in many delusions (e.g., poison plots, aliens from Mars); and at least in the early expression of obsessions, the patient, though committed to them, is aware that the idea is unfounded or exaggerated.

Overvalued ideas, by definition, cause the patient difficulties because they consume all his time and energy, leading to job or interpersonal problems. The patient usually understands this, but thinks it is the inflexibility or lack of appreciation of the employer or family members that is the problem. Overvalued ideas are observed in persons with some personality disorders (e.g., schizotypal), persons whose personalities make them culturally deviant (the "flower child" who is consumed with herbalism, mysticism, alternative medicine), and persons with chronic temporolimbic disease (epilepsy, some chronic drug abusers).

PERCEPTUAL DISTURBANCES

Perceptions without any external stimuli (*hallucinations*) and misperceptions of real external stimuli (*illusions*) are common experiences among patients with brain disease. Hallucinations can occur in all sensory modalities—visual, auditory, olfactory, gustatory, tactile, and visceral—and can occur in a variety of non-pathologic conditions, such as fatigue, distractibility, and when falling asleep or awakening. In non-ill persons, illusions are associated with an intense mood. For example, a person is walking down a dark street at night, the wind is howling, he is apprehensive, and he mistakes a swaying bush for a lurking mugger. When illusions are not the result of an intense mood, consider a hallucinogen drug-induced state, epilepsy, or schizotypal personality disorder.

Other perceptual distortions include *dysmorphopsia,* objects perceived as changing in shape; *dysmegalopsia,* objects perceived as changing in size; *hyper- and hypoacusis,* sound perceived as unusually loud or low, respectively; and *synesthesias,* stimuli in one sensory modality trigger a perception in another sensory modality (e.g., seeing sound).

Perceptual distortions are typically experienced in drug-induced states, epilepsy, and mood disorder, particularly bipolar mood disorder. Table 3.12 displays the different forms of perceptual disturbances, their definition, and the disorders to which they best correlate. None is pathognomonic. Perceptual disturbances are expressions of perceptual-integrating brain dysfunction.

Hallucinatory experiences are elicited in a manner similar to delusions: "Do you overhear conversations about you? Do the people bothering you say things to you through electronic devices, such as the TV or radio? Have you seen them following you or plotting against you? Can they touch you even when they are not in the room? Can you feel them? Do they do anything to your food? Do they try to harm you with gas that smells bad? Have you ever experienced hearing someone talking to you or about you, but no one was there with you? Have you ever heard

TABLE 3.12. Perceptual Disturbances

Form	Definition	Correlations
Illusion	Misinterpretation of a real stimulus	Can occur in non-ill persons in intense mood states or when fatigued, drug intoxications, epilepsy, and schizotypal personality disorder
Pseudohallucination	Any vague, poorly formed hallucination	Can occur in non-ill persons, drug intoxications, withdrawal states, and depression
Hypnagogic/hyponopompic hallucination	Pseudohallucinations occurring, respectively, upon falling asleep and awakening	Can occur in non-ill persons and in narcolepsy
Incomplete auditory hallucination	Most common perceptual disturbance. A muffled or whispered voice limited to a few words.	Any psychosis
Complete auditory hallucination	Most common first-rank symptom. A clear, sustained voice perceived as originating from an external source	Any psychosis
Elementary hallucination	Unformed hallucinations such as flashes of light, unidentified sounds, smells, and tastes	Toxic and epileptic states, migraine
Functional hallucination	A hallucination that occurs only immediately after ordinary stimulation in that particular sensory modality (e.g., hearing voices only when the water faucet is turned on)	Toxic and epileptic states, schizophrenia and mood disorder, particularly depression
Extracampine hallucination	A hallucination outside the normal sensory field (e.g., seeing people behind you, hearing people talking in another country)	Toxic and epileptic states, schizophrenia
Panoramic visual hallucination	Hallucinating entire scenes of action as if watching a movie	Epilepsy

voices in the air, but no one was around? Have you ever had the experience where you smelled something odd or illogical, but there was no usual explanation for it? Have you ever had the experience where you saw something odd or unusual or frightening that other people didn't see?"

Also helpful is "I have spoken with other people with experiences [feelings, situations] similar to yours and they also experienced. . . ." Examples of delusions and hallucinations can then be given, and many patients will respond with "Yes, I've had that happen to me, too." Some chronic patients will respond to the direct "You've heard many patients here complain about being bothered by voices. Has that ever happened to you?" However, it is always best to relate questions about a specific area of psychopathology back to the patient's complaints and concerns.

If a patient asks you your opinion about his delusional ideas or hallucinatory experiences, the best response is, "I understand what you're saying and I know you are experiencing these things, but I think it is because you are ill." If the patient says, "No, you're wrong," go on to the next logical topic. Do not argue. Even if the patient gets angry at you, many patients will trust a truthful examiner far more than one who is condescending, appeases them, or disregards their feelings and debates the validity of their experiences.

First-Rank Symptoms

Kurt Schneider, a German psychiatrist, was the first to systematically describe clinical phenomena that he termed *first-rank symptoms* because he considered them pathognomonic of schizophrenia. First-rank symptoms occur in 60%–75% of schizophrenics, but other psychotic patients also experience them. Complete auditory hallucinations are most common, but the precise frequency of each phenomenon is unclear. Delusional perceptions are described above. Other first-rank symptoms include the following.

Complete auditory hallucinations are sustained hallucinated voices that occur in clear consciousness, are clearly audible, and are experienced as coming from some source external to the patient. These voices continually comment on the patient's actions, multiple voices discuss the patient among themselves, or a voice repeats the patient's thoughts (thought echo).

Thought broadcasting is uncommon and refers to the patient literally experiencing his thoughts escaping from his head into the external world. Secondary delusional ideas involving telepathy, electronic surveillance, or metaphysical intervention often co-occur.

After asking about delusional ideas, test for thought broadcasting by asking, "Do you feel people know what you're thinking? Can others really hear your thoughts? You mean, if I were standing next to you, I could hear your thoughts coming out of your head, as loud as my voice? You mean to say it's as if your head were a radio, and everyone here can hear what you're thinking?" When a patient expresses the feeling that others can read his mind or says he believes people know what he's thinking by the expression on their faces, he most probably has delusional ideas. However, only endorsing the above questions satisfies a strict definition of thought broadcasting.

Experience of influence is described as one's sensations, feelings, impulses, thoughts, and actions experienced as being controlled and manipulated by an outside force that cannot be resisted. Secondary delusional ideas often co-occur. Ask the following: "Have people been trying to hypnotize you, turn you into a puppet or a robot? Do they use electronics or other energy to make you do things against your will? Do you actually feel them moving you . . . forcing you to think those thoughts?" Patients often (and at times correctly) feel that others (family, doctors, and nurses) are trying to control them or influence their thinking. However, to be a first-rank symptom the influence must be physically experienced, perceived as irresistible, and attributed to a controlling mechanism that is delusional: either fantastic (e.g., ozone rays from the stratosphere) or manifestly improbable (e.g., neighbors beaming microwaves through the cable TV box).

Experience of alienation is the patient's internal perception that his mental activity, actions, or body parts literally belong to someone else. Some patients with large parietal lobe lesions will also deny any relationship to certain of their body parts (usually those contralateral to the lesion). First ask about secondary delusional ideas, and then ask, "Have you ever had the experience where you were literally forced to think someone else's thoughts? Where the thoughts in your head belonged to another person? Where your arms or your legs were not yours, but belonged to someone else?"

PSYCHOSENSORY SYMPTOMS

Psychosensory symptoms, typical of complex partial epilepsy, also occur in mood disorders and some drug-induced psychoses. These features overlap in form with some of the perceptual disturbances previously described. In addition, they include visceral hallucinations, depersonalization and derealization, deja vu and jamais vu experiences, paroxysmal autonomic and emotional states, and emotional incontinence. Questions to elicit these phenomena include the following.

"Have you ever experienced the feeling that there was a foreign object inside your body or a cold, empty, or warm feeling inside your belly that pushes up into your chest?" (visceral hallucination)

"Have you ever experienced hearing sounds as unnaturally too loud or too soft even though other people didn't notice?" (dysacusia)

"Have you ever had the experience, when awake and going about your business, that suddenly you felt detached from yourself, as if you were floating above yourself and watching yourself going through the motions?" (depersonalization)

"Have you ever had the experience when awake that you suddenly felt as if you were put into a dream or that the world became suddenly flat, like a cartoon?" (derealization)

"Have you ever had the experience where you went to a new place and had the strong feeling that you had been there before and had said and done before the things you were really doing for the first time?" (deja vu)

"Have you ever had the experience where you went to a place where you had been to many times, but it all seemed unfamiliar, and you didn't recognize the place or the people?" (jamais vu)

"Have you ever had the experience of suddenly feeling very cold or very hot for just a few minutes, but it wasn't because of the temperature in the room or outside? Or suddenly feeling your heart beating very fast or heavily, even though you weren't scared or doing any exercise?" (autonomic paroxysms)

"Have you ever had the experience of being in your usual health when suddenly, for no reason, you felt intensely sad (or happy), and, after lasting for a few seconds or minutes, this feeling went away?" (emotional paroxysm)

"Have you ever had the experience where you weren't feeling sad (or happy), but you suddenly found yourself crying (or laughing) for no reason or thought and were embarrassed or frightened by it? (emotional incontinence)

Positive answers to several of the above questions suggest that the patient has a temporolimbic disorder. If epilepsy can be ruled out, the patient, particularly if he has a mood disorder, may respond to anticonvulsants such as valproic acid and carbamazepine.

Diagnostic Implications of Patterns of Psychopathology

Specific patterns of psychopathology are discussed in the chapters on syndromes. One approach to using patterns of psychopathology is to determine if a pattern fits with one of the DSM diagnostic choices. A second approach is also to consider if the pattern fits with the functional organization of the brain. The second approach helps to identify secondary behavioral syndromes and can help guide management.

For example, a 20-year-old student became suspicious that unknown persons were plotting to kill him. He "overheard" their conversations about him. He was unable to continue in school and stopped seeing his friends. He had no features of mania and, other than being subdued, no features of depression. He was diagnosed schizophrenic. His psychosis quickly resolved with risperidone, but he remained avolitional and modestly suspicious and was referred for long-term care. Although he met DSM criteria for schizophrenia, he had adequate emotional expression. He also had motor problems: bradykinesia without stiffness or tremor, stilted overly formal speech, and difficulty starting simple motor sequences. Because he had no aphasia, dyspraxia, or anomia, a subcortical action brain lesion was suspected, and single photon emission computed tomography revealed thalamic and bilateral basal ganglia hypoperfusion. The former resolved with improvement in the psychosis. Some contaminant in the marijuana he had used heavily the year prior to his psychosis was suspected. His resperadone was stopped, and lorazapam, a benzodiazspine with an intermediate-length half-life begun. This resolved his motor features. The treatment plan then focused on education for the family and the patient to the fact that he has a chemically induced brain lesion that could improve but that should not worsen if there was no further drug abuse. Vigorous motor and cognitive rehabilitation to maintain and improve present function and the *avoidance* of neuroleptics that might further damage his basal ganglia were also part of the treatment plan. The DSM diagnosis was changed to psychosis, not otherwise specified (NOS) secondary to drug abuse.

ADDITIONAL READINGS

Bleuler E: *Dementia Praecox or the Group of Schizophrenias*. International University Press, New York, 1950.

Bleuler E: *Textbook of Psychiatry*. Arno Press, New York, 1976.

Crosson B: Subcortical functions in language: A working model. *Brain and Language* 25:257–292, 1985.

Crosson B, Hughes CW: Role of the thalamus in language: Is it related to schizophrenic thought disorder? *Schizophr Bull* 13:605–621, 1987.

Hamilton M (ed): *Fish's Clinical Psychopathology, Signs and Symptoms in Psychiatry*. John Wright and Sons, Bristol, 1974.

Jankovic J: Tardive syndromes and other drug-induced movement disorders. *Clinical Neuropharmacology* 18:197–214, 1995.

Kahlbaum KL: *Catatonia*. The Johns Hopkins University Press, Baltimore, 1973.

McNeill D: *Hand and Mind: What Gestures Reveal About Thought*. University of Chicago Press, Chicago, 1992.

Owens DG, Johnstone EC, Frith MA: Spontaneous involuntary disorders of movement: Their prevalence, severity, and distribution in chronic schizophrenics with and without treatment with neuroleptics. *Arch Gen Psychiatry* 39:452–461, 1982.

Rogers D: The motor disorders of severe psychiatric illness: A conflict of paradigms. *Br J Psychiatry* 147:22–132, 1985.

Ross ED: The aprosodias, functional–anatomic organization of the affective components of language in the right hemisphere. *Arch Neurol* 38:561–569, 1981.

Ross ED, Harney JH, deLacoste-Utamsing C, Purdy PD: How the brain integrates affective and propositional language into a unified behavioral function: Hypothesis based on clinicoanatomic evidence. *Arch Neurol* 38:745–748, 1981.

Schneider K: *Clinical Psychopathology*. Hamilton MW (trans). Grune & Stratton, New York, 1959.

Taylor MA: Catatonia: A review of a behavioral neurologic syndrome. *Neuropsychiatry, Neuropsychol Behav Neurol* 3:48–72, 1990.

Wade JB, Taylor MA, Kasprisin A, Rosenberg S, Fiducia D: Tardive dyskinesia and cognitive impairment. *Biol Psychiatry* 22:393–395, 1987.

4

The Cognitive and Behavioral Neurologic Examination

The neuropsychiatric evaluation detailed in Chapters 2 and 3 provides information needed to make a DSM diagnosis *and* to identify dysfunctional systems in the brain. The relationship between diagnosis and treatment is obvious. Knowing which brain systems are involved is equally important for treatment because it (1) identifies specific syndromes now grouped together in the DSM "not otherwise specified" (NOS) categories; (2) identifies subgroups of patients who, despite meeting criteria for a DSM category, are still atypical in some way that suggests that they have a different underlying pathophysiologic process (i.e., they have a secondary syndrome); and (3) determines medication choices and areas needing rehabilitation.

The following vignettes illustrate these points.

> A 65-year-old man complains of loss of interest and lack of energy. He thinks he may be depressed and expresses feelings of helplessness. He thinks his life is over because he "can't do anything." He sleeps over 10 hours and is still tired. He does not enjoy eating, but has not lost any weight. He appears subdued more than sad and can occasionally joke.

This patient is atypical because, although he has some symptoms that suggest depression (loss of interest and energy, feeling helpless, saying he is depressed), he has other features that are not consistent with depression (sleeping too much, no weight loss, able to joke). He could be diagnosed depression, NOS, and begun on an antidepressant. In fact, he was, but his symptoms did not improve. From a neuropsychiatric perspective, however, atypical always means "secondary until proved otherwise." Loss of interest and energy but still able to joke, means avolition and apathy, not depression. Combined, these clinical indicators suggest an action brain syndrome (apathy and depressive-like features), and further evaluation revealed this man to have had several small left basal ganglia infarcts. Because the infarcts occurred in a dopaminergic system and produced symptoms consistent with disruption of that system, he was treated with methylphenidate, a modest dopamine agonist, and substantially improved.

> A 33-year-old man was hospitalized for schizophrenia. He was experiencing complete auditory hallucinations on and off for almost a year. On examination he spoke in a stilted manner as if a robot. He showed no emotional expression except irritability. Over the past year he had several unprovoked outbursts of severe anger during which he destroyed household objects, frightening his wife. He had no past or present features of a mood disorder. He never used street drugs, was a tea-toteler, and never before was ill with anything other than mild colds. He never had a head injury. He worked steadily all his adult life until 3 months prior to hospitalization. He met criteria for DSM schizophrenia. Nevertheless he is atypical: married, working steadily (suggesting no prepsychosis avolition), late onset of illness (most schizophrenics become psychotic between ages 15 and 25 years), severe angry outbursts (rather than being irritable only when prodded to do something). Further evaluation revealed this man to have a seizure disorder. Because his psychotic features were directly linked to his fits, an anticonvulsant drug controlled his seizures and stopped the psychoses.

> A 23-year-old man was hospitalized for a drug-induced psychosis. He was treated for this, and all his symptoms resolved. He was a college graduate and very articulate and personable. The unit staff was hoping he would enter a psychotherapy program and go back to school to finish a Master's course. However, in conversation his thinking seemed vague. Cognitive testing revealed a substantial loss of abstract thinking, problems with new learning, and some visuo-spatial dysfunction. The degree of his impairments suggested that he could not at present succeed in the original plan. Instead, he entered a cognitive rehabilitation program (as if he had suffered a traumatic brain injury, which of course he had on the molecular level). He received counseling rather than the originally planned psychotherapy that would have required more abstract thinking on his part. He was eventually able to get a job and stay off drugs.

Although the correlations are not perfect, several patterns of psychopathology suggest dysfunction in particular brain systems. These patterns are discussed throughout the book.

Cognitive and behavioral neurologic assessment is also used in diagnosis and to determine dysfunction in specific brain systems. The cognitive examination can conceptually be divided into five stages:

1. Determining level of arousal
2. Assessing attention and concentration
3. Assessing speech and language
4 Screening for diffuse impairment
5. Doing additional specific testing based on all previous findings (e.g., history; behavioral, neurologic, and general medical examinations; and cognitive assessment).

The goal of the cognitive examination is to get the patient's best performance. Thus, administer the examination in a quiet room without distractions. Provide the patient with an adequate surface on which to write. Make sure your instructions are clear. Learn them like other instructions you know for examining other organ systems. Administer the tests the way they are designed, and always administer them the same way so you maintain their reliability (i.e., their precision). Only with reliability can you have confidence that the tests are measuring what you think they are measuring and that the results mean what you think they mean. Take into account the patient's motivation in interpreting his performance. Encourage him if needed throughout the examination. Your constant prodding and encouragement tells you that you need to interpret the test results cautiously. Emotionally blunted patients, severe melancholics, and unstable manics are the most difficult to test. Remember that cognitive tests assume adequate motor strength to perform; sensory processing to see, hear, and feel; and understanding of the instructions. Fatigue also reduces performance.

Cognitive testing requires the patient to be alert, not overly distracted, and reasonably motivated to cooperate. When testing cognition, maintain the rules and style of the rest of the evaluation. Keep it conversational. Do not refer to it as a "test" or "questions that I have to ask," or as "routine." Try to link the cognitive examination to the patient's complaints and endorsements of psychopathology. The following introductions to cognitive testing are helpful.

> "You were telling me about [your difficulties concentrating, your memory problems, etc.]. I need to know more about that. I'd like you to do something for me now. . . ."
>
> "With all the things that have been happening to you recently, have they affected your concentration or memory?" Even if the response is "no," you can say "that's good, but I need to check that out, so I'd like you to do something for me now. . . ."

STEP 1: DETERMINING LEVEL OF AROUSAL (CONSCIOUSNESS)

Cognitive function depends on the degree of arousal (Table 4.1). *Alert* means a person's level of arousal is neither lowered (coma being the most severe level of lowered arousal) nor elevated (manic excitement being the most severe level of elevated arousal).

Determining level of arousal begins when you meet the patient. If the patient is reasonably alert (not too low or high in arousal),* further testing may be done reliably and with good validity. If the patient is not reasonably alert, then poor performance on cognitive tests cannot be interpreted.

STEP 2: ASSESSING ATTENTION (CONCENTRATION)

Many cognitive functions depend on attention. Attention is easily assessed by a letter cancellation test (Fig. 4.1).

---

* When reasonably alert a person (1) will respond to your comments and requests promptly, unless aphasic; (2) will focus his attention on you as you speak or on the task you ask him to do; (3) will not be distracted by ambient room noise; (4) will keep to the topic of conversation, and (5) will not doze.

TABLE 4.1. Altered Arousal

Reduced Arousal	Elevated Arousal
MILD	
The patient looks fatigued; sluggish, or hesitant in responsiveness	Somewhat distractible, restless; speech usually fast
MODERATE	
Appears sleepy; eyes only focus on strong stimuli with effort; speech content may wander from the topic; responses slow; some rambling speech; occasionally fails to obey examination requests	Appears excited, agitated, hyperactive; easily distracted; mild to moderate flight-of-ideas; speech rapid and pressured; may fail to obey some examination requests
SEVERE	
Appears as if in a trance, lethargic, somnolent, or comatose. Lethargy can be associated with agitation, fearfulness, and rambling speech. Eyes rarely focus on examiner; some generalized analgesia. In coma, analgesia profound	Hyperactivity and excitement can be extreme; the patient is moving and talking continuously. The patient may shout; flight-of-ideas may be extreme; speech rapid to the point of being unintelligible. General analgesia can be significant

Instruct the patient as follows: "I am going to read a series of letters to you. Every time you hear the letter A, I want you to tap the desk with this pencil." Then, in a clear, sufficiently loud, monotoned voice, read the series of letters at the rate of one letter per second, and record all errors of omission (the patient not responding when the letter A is read, usually associated with lowered arousal) and comission (the patient responding to letters other than A, usually a sign of distractibility or perseveration). If more than five errors occur, further cognitive testing will probably be invalid.

The A test and the behavioral assessment of arousal should be considered two

L T P E A O A I C T D A L A A

A N I A B F S A M R Z E O A D

P A K L A U C J T O E A B A A

Z Y F M U S A H E V A A R A T

Figure 4.1. Letter cancellation test: The A test.

doors through which the patient must first pass before further cognitive testing is done. Because the A test is very sensitive to arousal and thus delirium, it is an inexpensive fast, and easy way to assess arousal in a medical or surgical inpatient with behavioral changes. Alternative tests, e.g., serial 7s and spelling a five letter word backwards (e.g., *World*) are not as good as letter cancellation. The former requires calculating ability, so the meaning of early mistakes in subtracting is unclear. The latter is not long enough to adequately test sustained attention. Because you can substitute any letter for A (as long as you place it in the same positions as shown in Fig. 4.1), the A test is resistant to improved performance from practice (termed a *practice effect*), and thus can be used repeatedly with the same patient.

STEP 3: SPEECH AND LANGUAGE TESTING

Because most cognitive testing depends on the patient understanding your instructions and then verbally responding, aphasic patients often do poorly on the relatively simple tests used at the bedside. Your testing of language in the behavioral examination is a third door through which the patient must pass. Always consider the patient's language functioning before proceeding with further cognitive testing (see Chapter 3 for details).

STEP 4: SCREENING FOR DIFFUSE COGNITIVES IMPAIRMENT: THE MINI-MENTAL STATE

There are a number of screening tests for diffuse cognitive impairment. Figure 4.2 displays the Mini-Mental State (MMS) test with instructions for its administration. The MMS has important limitations (see below), and, although used to screen for diffuse impairment and thus dementia, several dementias have characteristic patterns of impairment that are not technically diffuse (see Chapter 12). Nevertheless, the MMS has become the most widely used cognitive screening test in many countries and will be generally familiar to many recently trained clinicians. It is presented here not as a definitive test, but as only one step in the process of cognitive assessment.

The MMS takes about 15–20 minutes to administer. It has a top score of 30. Most non-ill persons get 30 points. Non-ill persons with little education can score between 22 and 26. Among persons with primary axis I syndromes, scores of 27–29 are common, reflecting their problems with attention and mood and the fact that many have brain dysfunction. Normal persons over 80 years average 25. For patients under 70 years who have a high school or better education and who are literate and fluent in English, there are three important MMS scores to remember: 30, 25, and 22. A 30 indicates that the patient is probably not demented. A score of 25 or less indicates that the patient's behavioral syndrome may be secondary and that further testing (see Step 5, below) is definitely needed. A score of 22 indicates that the patient is probably demented because, prior to administering the MMS you determine that arousal and concentration were adequate (thus no delirium), and the patient could understand your instructions, and still he missed many MMS items.

Record MMS findings objectively; record any error as an error. Thinking that, "Well, he got that wrong only because he was tired, so I won't report it" is making an interpretation, not an observation, and interpreting individual items as normal may lead you to miss a clear pattern of mild abnormalities. You must be prepared to "judge" the normal speed and correctness of the patient's responses against some normal standard, usually your own performance. The patient may require supportive comments from you, for example, "Try your best; there's no penalty if you make an error." Be patient with persons whose brain dysfunction makes them slow to reply. Remember, the goal of testing is to determine the best, not the worst, performance.

Unfortunately, the MMS alone is not sensitive to many frontal lobe and nondominant cerebral hemisphere lesions. This is so because only two items, spelling *world* backward and the three-stage command, are directly influenced by frontal lobe functions, and these items are relatively easy; and because only one item, copying the intersecting pentagons, relates to visuospatial (nondominant hemisphere) function. Thus, a score of 30 only tells you that the dysfunction is not diffuse and, therefore, the patient is probably not demented (i.e., he does not have diffuse or substantial cognitive impairment with adequate arousal). Because the behavioral assessment of level of arousal and the A test are done first, a patient cannot be delirious (delirious patients also do poorly on the MMS) because the MMS is not given unless arousal and concentration are adequate.

Because the MMS is not sensitive to frontal lobe and nondominant cerebral hemisphere dysfunction, you need to compensate for these test limitations. This is done in two ways. First, pay attention to the way the patient performs and not just to the final result. Because the frontal lobes subserve executive functions, frontal lobe dysfunction often results in difficulties planning a test-taking strategy, starting and stopping the actions planned, and recognizing and self-correcting errors. Suggestive frontal lobe behaviors to look for during testing include perseveration (unnecessarily repeating responses or motor actions), difficulty starting a task (hesitancy, unexplained unusual slowness, automatically saying "I can't do it" without first considering the task), and making obvious errors and not recognizing or correcting the errors.

Second, do more testing of visuo-spatial motor coordination. Having the patient copy intersecting pentagons begins to test this. Figure 4.3 displays the intersecting pentagons and three different responses. In response 1 the patient's first attempt is poor (it would lose him a point on the MMS). At this point ask the patient to compare his copy with the original. Does he recognize his poor performance? Nonrecognition suggests frontal or nondominant dysfunction and denial of illness, termed *anosognosia*. Whether he recognizes his poor performance or not, encourage him to try again. "Try to copy it again. I think you can do better" usually works. In response 1 the second effort is clearly better, and the patient should be encouraged to try once again. Remember, you want to see the patient's best performance. On the third try, he does well enough that had it been his first effort he might have gotten a point for it. This tells you that the patient has the ability to

MiniMental LLC

NAME OF SUBJECT_____ Age _____

NAME OF EXAMINER _____ Years of School Completed _____

Approach the patient with respect and encouragement.
Ask: "Do you have any trouble with your memory?" ☐ Yes ☐ No   Date of Examination_____
"May I ask you some questions about your memory?" ☐ Yes ☐ No

SCORE	ITEM

5 ( ) TIME ORIENTATION

Ask:

"What is the year_____(1), season_____(1),

month of the year_____(1), date_____(1),

day of the week _____(1)"?

5 ( ) PLACE ORIENTATION

Ask:

"Where are we now? What is the state_____(1), city_____(1),

part of the city_____(1), building_____(1),

floor of the building_____(1)?"

3 ( ) REGISTRATION OF THREE WORDS

Say: "Listen carefully. I am going to say three words. You say them back after I stop.
Ready? Here they are... PONY (wait 1 second), QUARTER (wait 1 second), ORANGE (wait one
second). What were those words?"

_____(1)

_____(1)

_____(1)

Give 1 point for each correct answer, then repeat them until the patient learns all three.

5 ( ) SERIAL 7s AS A TEST OF ATTENTION AND CALCULATION

Ask: "Subtract 7 from 100 and continue to subtract 7 from each subsequent remainder
until I tell you to stop. What is 100 take away 7 ?"_____(1)

Say:

"Keep Going."_____(1),_____(1),

_____(1),_____(1),

3 ( ) RECALL OF THREE WORDS

Ask:

"What were those three words I asked you to remember?"

Give one point for each correct answer._____(1),

_____(1),_____(1),

2 ( ) NAMING

Ask:

"What is this?" (show pencil) _____(1). "What is this?" (show watch)_____(1).

For more
information or
additional copies
of this exam,
call (617)587-4215

© 1998 MM, LLC

O   V   E   R

Figure 4.2. The Mini-Mental State Examination; Mini Mental LLC, Boston MA.

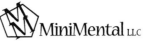

1 ( )   **REPETITION**

Say:

"Now I am going to ask you to repeat what I say. Ready? 'No ifs, ands, or buts.'

Now you say that." _____ (1)

3 ( )   **COMPREHENSION**

Say:

"Listen carefully because I am going to ask you to do something:

Take this paper in your left hand (1), fold it in half (1), and put it on the floor." (1)

1 ( )   **READING**

Say:

"Please read the following and do what it says, but do not say it aloud." (1)

Close your eyes

1 ( )   **WRITING**

Say:

"Please write a sentence." If patient does not respond, say: "Write about the weather." (1)

_____

_____

1 ( )   **DRAWING**

Say: "Please copy this design."

TOTAL SCORE _____   Assess level of consciousness along a continuum

Alert	Drowsy	Stupor	Coma

	YES	NO
Cooperative:	☐	☐
Depressed:	☐	☐
Anxious:	☐	☐
Poor Vision:	☐	☐
Poor Hearing:	☐	☐
Native Language:		

	YES	NO
Deterioration from previous level of functioning:	☐	☐
Family History of Dementia:	☐	☐
Head Trauma:	☐	☐
Stroke:	☐	☐
Alcohol Abuse:	☐	☐
Thyroid Disease:	☐	☐

FUNCTION BY PROXY

Please record date when patient was last able to perform the following tasks.
Ask caregiver if patient independently handles:

	YES	NO	DATE
Money/Bills:	☐	☐	___
Medication:	☐	☐	___
Transportation:	☐	☐	___
Telephone:	☐	☐	___

Model

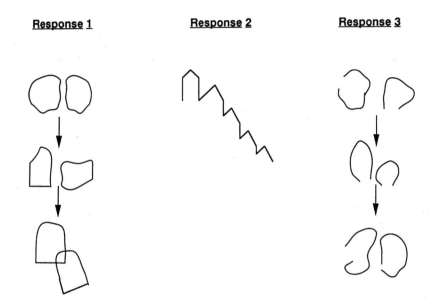

Figure 4.3. Copying geometric figures.

do the task, but not the ability to monitor and self-correct his performance. That suggests frontal lobe dysfunction.

In response 2, the patient gets stuck in a movement and repeats it. This is perseveration and, along with an inability to monitor and self-correct one's performance, is typical of patients with substantial frontal lobe disease.

In response 3, however, despite repeated tries, the patient's performance does not improve. This suggests nondominant hemisphere dysfunction. To be sure of this, two additional things need to be done. First, ask the patient to copy the pentagons with his other hand. Tell him it is not a test of drawing so he need not be concerned about that. He should just do his best. Figure 4.4 shows why this strategy is necessary. To produce the copy with the right hand (assuming it is the preferred hand) the brain representation of the problem, that is, the pentagons, must be sent across the corpus callosum to the contralateral parietal heteromodal cortex. From there the information is sent to the frontal heteromodal cortex, then to the secondary and primary motor cortices, and finally into the right hand. A corpus callosum lesion, disconnecting the left and right hemispheres, a left parietal

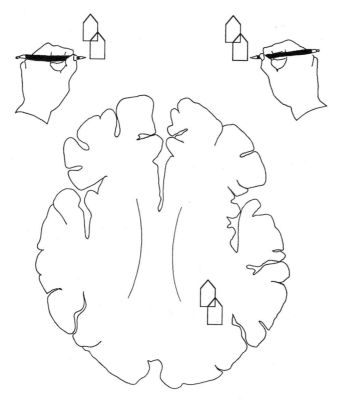

Figure 4.4. Testing for a disconnection syndrome.

lesion or disconnection between the left parietal and frontal cortices could each prevent the right hand from "knowing" how to do the task. By having the patient try it with his nonpreferred hand, the representation from the right parietal lobe only has to go to the right prefrontal cortex and then the right motor strip to get to the left hand, thus circumventing the other connections. A nonpreferred hand performance that is substantially better than the performance of the preferred hand indicates a disconnection. If both hands perform poorly (nonpreferred typically worse than the preferred) the dysfunction is likely to be in the nondominant hemisphere. To be sure of this, then ask the patient to copy additional shapes (see below).

Step 5: Additional Specific Testing

If all information from the history, behavioral examination, A test, and MMS combined indicate no knowable, traditional neurologic disease, then further testing may not be needed. If further testing is needed, it is not a good idea to shorten the examination by reducing the number of trials per test (this strategy will reduce reliability) or the number of tests per cognitive function (this strategy will reduce validity). A better strategy is to consider the following.

1. If the evaluation to that point suggests a localized or circumscribed disorder (e.g., stroke, injury, tumor), review or expand on the motor examination previously described, looking for a pattern that can narrow the disorder to the anterior frontal circuits or the posterior cerebellar-pontine unit, the left or the right motor system, or the frontal or parietal cortex (top) or a subcortical (bottom) structure. If the motor evaluation indicates a specific brain system is involved, do additional cognitive tests of that system to confirm it.

2. If the evaluation following the MMS suggests an action brain (frontal) disorder (e.g., alcohol frontal lobe syndrome, basal ganglia stroke, frontal lobe injury), do additional frontal lobe testing to confirm this suspicion.

3. If the evaluation following the MMS suggests a perceptual-integrating or a diffuse cognitive problem (e.g., dementia), consider which dementia is most likely for that patient and test for that. For example, if you suspect Alzheimer's disease, look for a parietotemporal pattern of impairment; if you suspect vascular dementia, look for a patchy or frontal lobe pattern of impairment or for bradyphrenia. Chapter 12 details the diagnostic steps in assessing dementia.

FRONTAL LOBE TESTING

Because anterior brain disease (the action brain) typically results in behavioral changes, frontal lobe testing is the next specific area to consider after motor behavior (which of course also relates to the action brain). The action brain generates ideas, solves problems, expresses emotions, and produces motor behavior (including speech). It also performs "executive functions." These functions can all be tested. In addition, each frontal cortex–basal ganglia–thalamic circuit produces its own typical syndrome. The combination of cognitive testing and behavioral assessment can give a remarkably clear picture of anterior brain function.

First, decide if the patient has one or more of the anterior circuit syndromes (see Chapter 1). If the patient does not have any of these behaviors, anterior brain pathology is unlikely. If the patient has one discrete syndrome, the lesion is most likely cortical. If the patient has a mixture of symptoms from several circuit syndromes, the lesion is either subcortical within the basal ganglia or thalamus where the "wiring is crammed together in a small space" so that a small lesion (e.g., infarct) can result in a diffuse picture, or the disease process is diffuse or scattered throughout the anterior brain. Motor functioning can help determine if the lesion is localized. For example, if the mixture of symptoms is associated with a resting tremor and increased muscle tone, then the lesion is subcortical (basal ganglia). When the syndrome itself seems circumscribed, patchy, or unclear, cognitive testing can help localize or verify anterior brain dysfunction.

The first step in frontal lobe testing is to review the information that has already been gathered. The following examples all suggest anterior action brain dysfunction:

1. Broca's, transcortical motor, or subcortical motor aphasia (dominant hemisphere–related structures)
2. Avolition (dominant dorsolateral frontal loop)
3. Loss of emotional expression (i.e., emotional blunting, or motor aprosodia—nondominant frontal areas)
4. Catatonia (particularly when features include echo phenomena, Gegenhalten, and stereotypies)
5. Witzelsucht
6. Basal ganglia and frontal lobe motor signs and symptoms
7. Secondary obsessive compulsive disorders (bilateral basal ganglia involvement, nondominant more than dominant)
8. Poor judgment in solving problems of daily living because of impulsivity, inability to recognize one's shortcomings and responses of others to one's abnormal behavior, or inability to make a realistic plan
9. Inappropriate social behaviors, such as being intrusive, being dirty and unkempt, coming too close when speaking with others, talking loudly to oneself in public
10. Perseverative thought content, word usage, and actions.

If the patient shows none of these behaviors, an action brain disorder is unlikely.

To plan and carry out the plan successfully, a person must be able to generate ideas, form a problem-solving strategy, and shift gears to self-correct as the plan is being put into effect. These functions are tested as follows.

Testing the Generation of Ideas

The generation of ideas is tested by assessing verbal fluency. If the patient has a speech and language disorder, these tests cannot be used. Although the patient may have adequate fluency of spontaneous speech, his fluency of ideas may be impaired. The brain areas that generate words and ideas are different from the brain areas necessary to say the words. Test verbal fluency by asking the patient to name as many words as he can think of in 1 minute that begin with a particular letter (A or S are usual). Instruct the patient not to repeat words, not to include proper names such as "Alice" or "Saturday," and not to repeat portions of words, such as in *every*one, *every*time, *every*place. Begin with words that start with A. Write down the patient's responses, recording number of responses and number of repetitions. Each correct word is scored as 1 point. Do not count repeated and restricted words. Give people over 65 years of age a 3-point bonus and people with less than a high school education a 4-point bonus. A score of 19 points or less is abnormal.

Testing Strategy

Fluency of ideas can also be tested by asking the patient to name in 1 minute as many animals as he can think of or as many categories of products he could find in a supermarket. These tests are more difficult than naming words that begin with A or S, and, in addition to the score (less than 15 is abnormal), the way the patient tries to solve the task is important. That is, does he follow some logical sequence, starting with farm animals, switching to birds and then marine animals, or does he name animals randomly? The latter suggests action brain dysfunction, regardless of the number of animals named, although the number will likely be low.

Testing Problem Solving

A patient's judgment regarding situations in his life is an indirect but clinically useful global measure of problem solving. Ask the patient to comment on specific problems or opportunities about family relationships, job, or plans for the future. More structured testing of problem-solving ability involves mathematical word problems, such as:

> "If I had three apples, and you had four more than I, how many apples would you have?"
> "If you had 18 books and had to put them on two shelves so that one shelf had twice as many books as the other, how many books would you put on each shelf?"

Calculating ability is tested before asking mathematically based problems. Assess calculating ability by asking the patient to solve in his head simple problems such as $23 - 8 = ?$ A poor performance on arithmetic tasks is termed *dys-* or *acalculia* and is associated with dominant hemisphere (often parietal) dysfunction.

Testing Thinking

Verbal concept formation can be tested by asking the patient to state how two items are similar. For example, "In what way are an airplane and a bicycle similar? In what way are paint and concrete the same?" Although there are many possible "abstract" responses to such questions, correct answers are those that reveal the most important, usually functional, characteristics of the items. For example, the answer "The plane and the bicycle are both means of transportation" is better than "Both have wheels."

Verbal reasoning (items modified from the Stanford-Binet Intelligence Scale) can be tested by asking the patient to listen to a statement and state what is "foolish" about it. Such statements include (1) A man had pneumonia twice. The first time it killed him, but the second time he quickly got well; (2) In the year 1999, many more women than men got married in Canada; and (3) Most train accidents involve the first and last cars; to reduce the number of accidents, we should remove the first and last cars.

Visual reasoning can also be tested by asking the patient to look at a picture depicting a logical absurdity and then tell you what is "foolish" about the picture (Fig. 4.5).

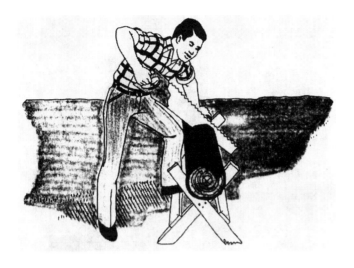

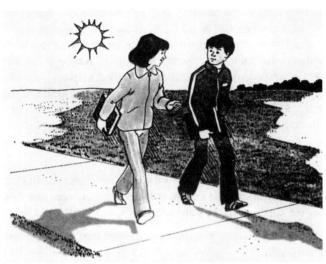

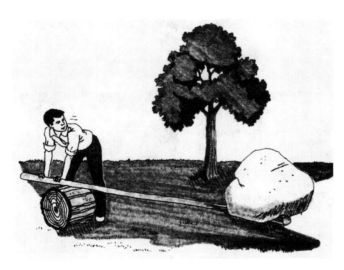

Figure 4.5. Test of visual reasoning, depicting logical absurdities. (After Mesulam, 1985, pp. 86–90).

Testing Shifting Gears

To successfully solve real-life problems, you must be cognitively flexible. You must be able to change assumptions as new information is obtained and self-correct your performance. This flexibility is assessed by testing a patient's ability to change set.

Trail-making tests A and B (Fig. 4.6, 4.7), measure the ability of the patient to shift sets. To be valid, the patient must have basic motor skills and the ability to count and know the alphabet. Trail A is straightforward and is used to familiarize the patient with the task. Trail B requires the patient to shift between alternating numbers and letters.

Trail-making tests can discriminate the brain injured from normal individuals with hit rates of about 85%. Normal performance for Trail A is below 60 seconds with no errors; for trail B, below 90 seconds with no errors.

Ask the patient to connect as quickly as possible the circles for sample A beginning at number 1 on up to number 7. If the patient can do the sample correctly, have him do the test page. If the patient fails to complete the sample correctly, the errors are explained. For example, you might say, "You did not complete the circles in order. You need to go from 1 to 2 to 3 rather than from 1 to 2 to 4." If the subject cannot complete the sample even after explanation, Trails A and B cannot be done.

When the actual test for Trail A begins, repeat the instructions, and then tell the patient to begin. Watch and time the patient. When a mistake is made, immediately tell the patient, allowing him to continue from the point where the error was made. For example, you might say, "You skipped a number" or "You failed to draw your line all the way to the last circle." The test is completed when the patient correctly reaches the last circle. Persons with altered arousal, poor concentration (both previously assessed), slowed thinking or movement, or with neglect of space will do poorly on Trail A.

After Trail A is completed, give the patient the sample for Trail B. Tell the patient to connect the circles by going from 1 to A to 2 to B, doing first a number, then a letter, then a number again. The patient does the sample. If it is correctly performed, he does Trail B. If an error is made, follow the same procedures described for Trail A. Except for the change in basic tasks, Trail B is done exactly as Trail A. Scoring for both parts is identical. If the patient is unable to complete Trail B after 300 seconds, stop testing.

PARIETAL LOBE TESTING

The diagnosis of dementia is a major concern in neuropsychiatry. Cognitive testing is important in the diagnosis. A person who behaviorally appears alert, makes less than five errors on the A test, and scores below 23 on the MMS may be demented. Alzheimer's dementia is a common concern. It can also be detected early in the disease process (see Chapter 12 for details). Cognitive testing shows a temporoparietal pattern of dysfunction in early Alzheimer's disease.

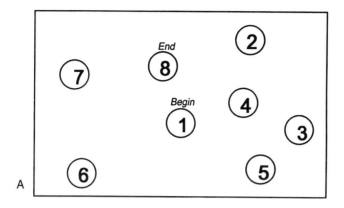

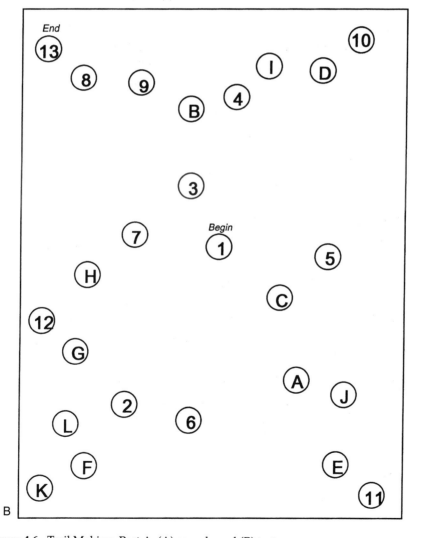

Figure 4.6. Trail Making, Part A, (A) sample and (B) test.

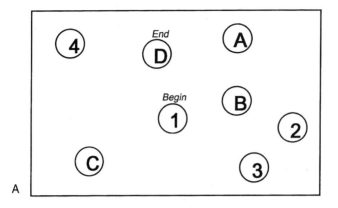

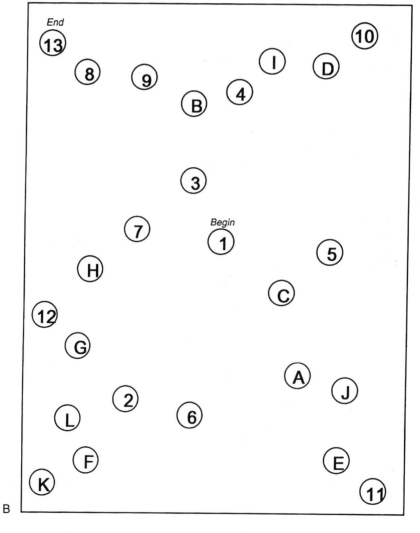

Figure 4.7. Trail Making, Part B, (A) sample and (B) test.

Classic tests of parietal lobe function include stereoagnosia and graphasthesia; calculating; left–right orientation; writing; reading aloud; spatial recognition; recognizing one's illness; and copying geometric shapes.

Doing simple mental calculations in which numbers must be carried over in one's mind's eye (e.g., 17 – 9 = ? 83 – 17 = ?), reading aloud when the visual information from the page must link with language and be given symbolic meaning, and writing a sentence when visuomotor control of the preferred hand is linked to language are all tests of dominant parietal lobe function. Ask the patient to write a sentence in long hand because this is more difficult and thus a more sensitive test than printing. Then ask him to read a sentence aloud.

Orientation to left and right is also a task assessing the dominant parietal lobe. First determine if the patient knows right from left by asking him to point to his right hand, left hand, right ear, left ear. Then ask him to do right–left tasks requiring him to cross his midline: "Put your left hand on your right ear; put your right hand on your left elbow; put your right hand on your left knee; put your left hand on your right elbow." Continued hesitation in doing these tasks or inability to carry them out suggests dominant parietal lobe dysfunction.

Awareness of one's symptoms and problematic behavior is termed *insight*. The neuropsychiatric term for a patient being unable to recognize his serious medical disabilities is *anosognosia*. For example, in Babinski's agnosia a patient with hemiparalysis may attempt to get out of bed and walk (and is very prone to an accident) despite evidence of paralysis from repeated failures to walk and despite instructions from staff and visitors not to walk. In Anton's syndrome, a blind patient believes he is able to see. Other phenomena routinely described as "denial" are actually mild forms of anosognosia, the product of nondominant hemisphere or frontal lobe dysfunction.

Some patients with intact left–right orientation nevertheless pay no attention to the left side of their body or to objects in their left visual field. Left spatial nonrecognition, or *spatial neglect,* is seen with lesions of the nondominant parietal lobe. Signs of it include not shaving the left side of one's face, bumping into objects on the left, reading only the right side of printed materials, or writing only on the right side of the page. Patients with left frontal lobe lesions may have the same kinds of neglect for the right side of space. In addition to the signs of spatial neglect, any paper and pencil test described in this chapter can be used to assess patients' awareness of left and right space (i.e., they fail to use that part of the paper). Other examples of spatial neglect are shown in Figure 4.8 in which the patient was asked to draw the face of a clock with the hands indicating 10 minutes past 11 and where the patient is asked to cross all the lines he sees.

Tests for *Graphesthesia* and *stereognosis,* assess the parietal lobe contralateral to the hand being tested and the connections between the two cerebral hemispheres when the nonpreferred hand is tested. To test for graphesthesia, tell the patient that you are going to trace some letters, one at a time, on the palms of his hands. Use a closed pen. After drawing each letter ask the patient to name it. If the patient experiences difficulty, try drawing numbers. The inability to recognize and name these symbols is termed *agraphesthesia*. Test the nonpreferred hand first so that you simultaneously test corpus callosum function; that is, can the informa-

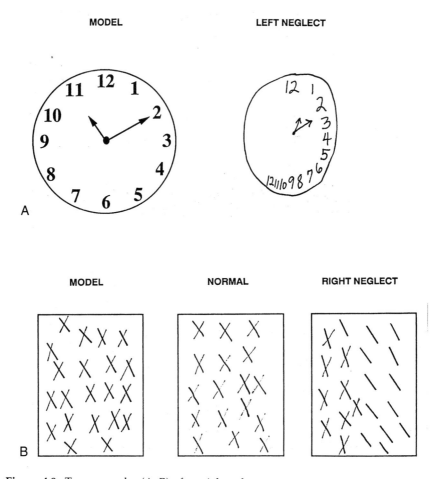

Figure 4.8. Two examples (A, B) of spatial neglect.

tion from the nonpreferred hand (usually the left) be organized in the contralateral parietal lobe and then be sent to the dominant parietal lobe (usually the left) to be connected with language and given a name (e.g., the letter or number you traced on the palm).

If the patient has no anomia, graphesthesia in only the nonpreferred hand indicates dysfunction in the contralateral parietal lobe or in the corpus callosum. Other testing would be needed to determine which possibility is more likely.* Graphesthesia in the preferred hand usually reflects dysfunction in the dominant parietal lobe.

To test stereognosis, tell the patient that you are going to place several objects, one at a time, in his palms. Ask the patient to supinate his hands and close his eyes, and then place, one at a time on the palm, several items (e.g., a key, several coins of different sizes, the cap of a ballpoint pen—all items that make no noise

---

*Another test for corpus callosum function is to position the fingers of one of the patient's hands and have the patient duplicate the positions in his other hand with his eyes closed.

when palpated). Begin with the nonpreferred hand. After each placement have the patient feel the object with his fingers and then name it. If the patient has no anomia, an inability to name the objects could be due to dysfunction of the contralateral parietal lobe (in this case, the nondominant) or of interhemispheric connections such as the corpus callosum. If the patient has astereognosis in the preferred hand, the abnormality is probably in the contralateral (dominant) parietal lobe. Constructional tasks (e.g., copying shapes, such as the intersecting pentagons on the MMS, testing for apraxias and somatosensory functions) also assess parietal lobe function.

Digit Span and Digit Symbol Substitution

Digit span and digit symbol substitution are also used to test for Alzheimer's disease. They tap temporoparietal and frontal functions.

Digit span is a measure of immediate auditory memory. Digits backward, which requires the ability to reverse sequencing, also assesses spatial function and working memory. It is particularly sensitive to dominant hemisphere disease, including temporoparietal lobe dysfunction, and so it is useful in screening for signs of early dementia. Digit span (particularly digits forward) is also sensitive to anxiety, and patients who are depressed or substantially anxious will do poorly.

To assess *digit span,* tell the patient that you will say some numbers, and you want him to repeat them exactly as you say them. Start with three digits and work up until the patient misses a series. If a series is missed, give a second series of the same length. If this is done correctly, go on; if not, stop. The maximum number to test is 9.

Digits backward is given much the same way, but the patient repeats the numbers given in the reverse order. The maximum tested is 8 numbers. Most patients who are not depressed or anxious and who have good temporoparietal functioning can do five to six numbers backwards.

Digit symbol substitution is a timed subtest of the Weschler Adult Intelligence Scale (WAIS). It tests basic learning skills and the ability to associate a symbol with a number. Visual memory and the ability to maintain a course of rapid action against the clock are also tested. Very anxious or depressed patients will do poorly on this test. Test performance also declines with normal aging, but not to the degree observed in Alzheimer's disease. It is very sensitive to diffuse cognitive decline and, therefore, is a good screening test for dementia.

Digit symbol substitution requires the patient to match empty spaces under the numbers 1 to 9 with symbols assigned to those numbers in a table at the top of the work page. Figure 4.9 shows a simulated version. The actual test can be obtained as a subtest of the WAIS-R*. Describe the task to the patient, and then go over the first three items, showing him what to do. Have the patient do seven additional sample items. These 10 items serve as the practice portion of the test. Then tell the patient that the task is timed, and you will stop him after 90 seconds. Tell the patient to fill in as many squares as he can as fast as possible *without skip-*

*WAIS, revised, copyright 1955, 1981, by The Psychological Corporation.

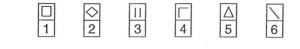

Figure 4.9. Simulated digit symbol substitution.

ping any items. If the patient skips an item, restate that he should do them in order without skipping. Stress that perfect reproduction of figures is not necessary. Tell him to go to the second line as soon as he finishes the first line. Tell him not to erase, just to write over any error.

In the actual test there are 100 squares to fill. Ten are samples, and thus the top score is 90. Teenagers and young adults on average score 60. Middle-aged persons on average score 50. Persons over 70 years on average score in the low 30s. Because left handers may cover the symbol table as they do the test, they may score a few points lower for their age group. Persons with temporoparietal dysfunction score 10–15 or more points below the average for their age group.

MEMORY

Assessing a patient's memory is always necessary. Memory storage can be divided into five stages.

In *stage 1*, information is registered without requiring any focused attention by the primary sensory cortex and is held in a sensory memory "store." If not attended to within 1 to 2 seconds, this information is not remembered.

Stage 2 involves information being immediately organized into patterns by the secondary sensory cortex and attention paid to it. Stages 1 and 2 are not formally tested, but these are necessary to carry on a conversation (i.e., to remember the last sentence so that the next one fits in sequence). Delirious patients cannot do this because of reduced arousal, and so their speech is fragmented (i.e., rambling).

In *stage 3*, Seven to eight items can be "held" or "retained" if the patient concentrates or makes an effort. This short-term or working memory holds information for about 20 seconds unless processed further. Stage 3 of memory is tested with digit span or immediate recall of words or diagrams.

In *stage 4*, memory becomes consolidated if some effort is made to remember (e.g., rehearsing). This is new learning and takes place within 30 seconds to 30 minutes. It has a verbal and visual component, and both are tested. New verbal learning can be tested by asking the patient to learn a series of nine words by repeating the list until it is memorized. Recall after 20 minutes confirms that new

TRAIN	STATION	WAGON
HOLLOW	FILL	FINANCE
SWALLOW	EMPTY	MONEY

Figure 4.10. Test of new verbal learning.

learning has occurred. Figure 4.10 displays one such list, but any nine words will do as long as they cannot be linked into an easily remembered sentence or two such as *tree, apple, cat, old, big, orange, bird, black, little,* or *the big orange cat chased the little black bird up the old apple tree.* Remembering short paragraph stories as in the Wechsler memory test* is another good test of new verbal learning. You tell the patient you are going to read a little story to him, and he should try to remember it as closely as possible to the way you say it so he can tell you everything you read. Each story has 25 bits of specific information (e.g., the name of a person, where she lives, what her job is, where she goes). Most persons without brain dysfunction can immediately recall 15–17 items and after 20 minutes two-thirds of their original score.

A good test of new visual learning is the copying and recall of the Rey-Osterrieth complex figure (Fig. 4.11). This test kills two cognitive birds with a sin-

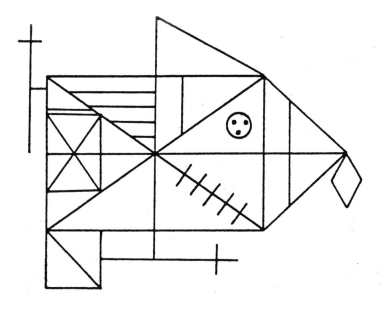

Figure 4.11. The Rey-Osterrieth complex figure.

*Wechsler Memory Scale, 3rd ed, 1997, The Psychological Corporation.

gle test stone: It assesses visual memory and constructional ability. Show the patient the figure and ask him to copy it. Watch how he does it. Getting the overall shape of the figure and the shape of its big parts is equivalent to but harder than the copying of the intersecting pentagons of the MMS. It is constructing the gestalt, and it is sensitive to nondominant hemisphere problems. After the "big picture" is copied, the details come next. Getting the details correct often involves verbal self-cuing and is sensitive to dominant hemisphere function (e.g., "the circle has three dots, the lower right rectangle diagonal has five cross hatches, whereas the upper left rectangle has four horizontal lines"). After the patient copies the figure, remove the model and the copy and ask the patient to immediately reproduce the figure from memory. Encourage the patient to get as much of the figure as possible (e.g., "Do you remember what went here? How many lines were there?"). When finished, show the patient the model and compare it with the recalled drawing, pointing out what is missing. Then do other testing. Twenty minutes later ask the patient to try and recall the figure. Loss of details but adequate gestalt reproduction on recall suggests dominant hemisphere temporoparietal dysfunction. If the gestalt is lost but the details are mostly preserved, nondominant hemisphere temporoparietal dysfunction is suggested. If the details and the gestalt are both lost, the dysfunction is likely bilateral.

Stage 5 is long-term memory. Information here is remembered beyond 30 minutes and sometimes for a lifetime. This information is probably stored in secondary and tertiary cortical areas and other structures throughout the brain, and it is grossly tested by asking the patient about his personal history, childhood, and present life (e.g., the clinical history). In addition to the usual questions about school and jobs, also ask about public events and celebrities during various periods in the patient's life: names of favorite TV shows, movies, or athletes. Abnormal responses range from failure to recognize names of people, shows, and events and being vague without providing details, to being unable to give any meaningful information.

Storage of memory (encoding) and *retrieval* of memory (recall) are different processes involving different brain areas. New learning is subserved by parahippocampal cortex (posterior mesial-temporal regions) and the cerebellar neocortex (if motor responses are involved). Storage is subserved by the hippocampus and amygdala, cerebellum, and cerebral hemisphere neocortices. Recall is subserved by anterior mesial-temporal areas. Patients with anterior mesial temporal lobe or frontal lobe dysfunctions (e.g., Parkinson's dementia) have difficulty spontaneously recalling information but can be successfully cued and can recognize recently learned information (e.g., nine words they were asked to memorize) among novel information (e.g., nine additional words not included in the original memory task). Patients with posterior mesial temporal lobe disease (e.g., Alzheimer's disease) will also have problems with new learning, but this will be with storage, so cuing and recognition tasks do not help with recall.

Problems with recall (as in "the patient is a poor historian") are of two types; The patient cannot remember details or sequences of events (anterior mesial temporal); and the patient remembers details but confuses or combines sequences (e.g., the chapters of his life have some details, but the chapters are in the wrong

TABLE 4.2. Cognitive Tests Used in Clinical Examination

Area Assessed	*Functions Measured*
	STEP 1
Appearance of alertness	Level of arousal
	STEP 2
A test	Arousal and ability to sustain attention
	STEP 3
Speech and language testing	Does the patient understand the instructions? Is the patient aphasic?
	STEP 4
Mini-Mental State	Screening for diffuse cognitive impairment. When modified as discussed in the text, it can also help assess frontal lobe and nondominant cerebral hemi sphere function
	STEP 5
Specific testing: Motor examination	To circumscribe and localize suspected lesions. Can be divided into frontal versus cerebellar-pontine, left versus right, or cortex (frontal and pareital) versus subcortical (basal ganglia) patterns
Specific testing: Frontal (action brain) lobe testing	Evaluating for frontal psychopathology, the ability to generate ideas using verbal fluency tasks, problem-solving ability, and ability to shift gears using trails A and B
Specific testing: Temporoparietal functions*	Testing for stereoagnosia and graphesthesia assesses the ability to link tactile information to language (BL, D > ND); reading aloud (D) tests the ability to link visual information to language; calculating and left–right orientation (D) tests symbolic spatial ability; assessing for anosognosia (ND) and copying geometric shapes (ND) test constructional ability and visual memory; digit span (BL, D > ND) assesses immediate auditory memory and the ability to reverse sequencing; digit symbol substitution (BL, D > ND) assesses basic learning and visual memory; learning a list of words or remembering a paragraph story (D) tests new learning; getting a history assesses long-term memory

*D, dominant; ND, nondominant; BL, bilateral.

order or past and present events are combined). The latter is usually due to poor executive functioning from frontal lobe dysfunction.

The two patterns detailed above are: Recall is an anterior frontotemporal function (action brain), and storage is a posterior temporal parietal (perception integrating brain) function except for motor-related information, which is stored in the cerebellum and basal ganglia. Language and symbolic information is primarily stored in the dominant hemisphere, and visuo-spatial information is primarily stored in the nondominant hemisphere.

Long-term memory is also divided into *procedural memory* (e.g., remembering and being able to demonstrate skills like riding a bicycle) and *declarative memory* (e.g., remembering the names of the 50 U. S. states). Declarative memory is what is mostly assessed on memory tests like the ones described above. Because procedural memory remains intact in most amnestic patients, it is not routinely tested. Always ask, however, if a patient has procedural skills (playing a musical instrument, typing, driving, playing a particular sport) and whether those skills are intact. If you have any concerns, then ask the patient to demonstrate that skill. Patients with basal ganglia and cerebellar lesions can have adequate declarative memory, but a loss of some procedural memory.

Table 4.2 displays the complete menu of clinical cognitive tests. Stages 1–4 are almost always done The tests in stage 5 are selected to clarify what you suspect from previous behavioral and cognitive assessments. Chapters on syndromes provide additional details for fine-tuning cognitive and behavioral neurologic diagnoses.

ADDITIONAL READING

Folstein MF, Folstein SW, McHugh PR: "Mini-Mental State": A practical method of grading the cognitive state of patients for the clinician. *J Psychiatr Res* 12:189–198, 1975.

Gabrieli JDE, Brewer JB, Desmond JE, Glover GH: Separate neural bases of two fundamental memory processes in the human medial temporal lobe. *Science 276*:264–266, 1997.

George MS, Parekh PI, Rosinsky N, Ketter TA, Kimbrell TA, Heilman KM, Herscovitch P, Post RM: Understanding emotional prosody activates right hemisphere regions. *Arch Neurol 53*:665–670, 1996.

Kolb B, Whishaw IQ: *Fundamentals of Human Neuropsychology*, 4th ed. WH Freeman, New York, 1996.

Lezak MD: *Neuropsychological Assessment*, 3rd ed. Oxford University Press, New York, 1995.

Mesulam MM: *Principles of Behavioral Neurology*. FA Davis, Philadelphia, 1985.

Ross ED: Nonverbal aspects of language. *Behav Neurol 1*:9–23, 1993.

Spreen O, Strauss E: *A Compendium of Neuropsychological Tests, Administration, Norms, and Commentary*, 2nd ed. Oxford University Press, New York, 1998.

Squire LR: Neuropsychological effects of ECT. In Abrams R, Essman WB (eds): *Electroconvulsive Therapy: Biological Foundations and Clinical Applications*. Spectrum, New York, 1982, pp 169–185.

Squire LR: *Memory and Brain*. Oxford University Press, New York, 1987.

Yudofsky SC, Hales RE (section eds): The neuropsychiatry of memory. In Oldman JM, Riba MB, Tasman A (eds): *A Review of Psychiatry*, vol 12. American Psychiatric Press, Washington DC, Chapters 24–29, 1993.

5

Patient Management

The principles of management apply equally to biological and interpersonal treatments. Whether you prescribe psychotherapy or electroconvulsive therapy (ECT), do not begin treatment until you have made your best diagnostic effort and you have considered factors that influence treatment (e.g., the patient's personality and likelihood of compliance, cognitive function and intelligence, interpersonal and job situations, general medical health, and specific strengths and weaknesses in each domain). The need to diagnose before treatment is obvious. Sometimes, however, this is not fully accomplished, and targeted symptoms (e.g., psychosis, excitement, trouble keeping a job) get treated rather than the processes underlying the symptoms. The problems with this "target symptom" approach are discussed in the pharmacology section of this chapter.

Dosage and duration of treatment are also critical. Commonly, medications are underdosed. This leads to delayed or incomplete responses. Rather than raising the dosage, additional medications are often added, complicating treatment rather than maximizing improvement. "Dosages" of psychotherapy must also be determined: How often and for how long does the patient need to be seen? You need to consider all of these variables before treatment is started. Do not start or change treatments in an erratic fashion; follow a planned course of action with periodic taking stock of progress. Most importantly, whatever the treatment modality, remember that you are treating a patient and, therefore, that patient's overall health concerns, personality, and life circumstances, as well as specific behavioral illnesses. They all need attention.

Table 5.1 lists the information categories needed to plan and carry out effective treatment. For example, lithium is effective for mania, but if the patient has poor kidney function or is a noncomplier, lithium may not be the best medication choice. If the patient has substantial abstract thinking and planning problems because of a head injury or substance abuse, psychotherapy that relies on the ability to generate and use abstract ideas is not appropriate. If a patient needs a dopamine agonist but does not have adequate funds or insurance to pay for the medication, methylphenidate may be a better choice than the more expensive bromocriptine because compliance will likely be better. Note that all the other as-

TABLE 5.1. Assessment Necessary for Effective Treatment

Area	Influence on Treatment
Axis I syndrome and etiology, if knowable	Guides biologic treatments and suggests prognosis
Personality	In addition to axis II co-morbidity, a dimensional assessment of personality (see Chapter 6) guides rehabilitation and psychotherapy strategies, helps in setting goals, predicts other co-morbidities and compliance, and helps select some biologic treatments
Cognition	Helps determine etiology of behavioral syndrome, suggests prognosis, helps predict compliance, and helps guide rehabilitation and psychotherapy
Education, areas of skill, knowledge and general intelligence	Overlaps with cognition in helping guide rehabilitation and psychotherapy
General medical health	DSM axis III helps determine etiology of behavioral syndrome, helps guide biologic treatments and rehabilitation
Environmental context	The patient's social, interpersonal, and job situations; helps to set goals, predicts prognosis, and guides biological, psychotherapy, and rehabilitation therapeutics; learning about the patient's personal and social history adds to your understanding of his present environmental context and gives you things to talk about other than symptoms and drug side effects
Strengths and weaknesses	In addition to resolving the axis I condition, the goal of treatment is to rehabilitate. Rehabilitation (be it a broken leg or psyche) works to improve weaknesses by using strengths and safeguarding those strengths

sessment areas have as much (or more) influence on treatment as making a syndromal diagnosis. The biggest mistake in assessment is thinking that for some patients (e.g., psychotic inpatients) you need to mostly know their axis I diagnosis, whereas for other patients (e.g., clinic or community based, nonpsychotic patients) you mostly need to know their environmental context. To give good care, you need to know as much as you can about the patient in both of these areas.

INTERPERSONAL MANAGEMENT AND BEHAVIORAL GUIDELINES

The most important factor in patient management is the doctor–patient relationship. If this relationship is bad or problematic in some way, compliance will be poor, advice and counseling will be ignored, and the patient's feelings, thoughts, and psychopathologic experiences will be withheld or denied. The most powerful predictor of psychotherapy outcome (good and bad) is the patient's perception of the relationship with the therapist. Directly or indirectly this is true for all treatments: Surgery will remove the clot in the blocked artery, but the patient may refuse treatment because he does not trust the surgeon. Pilocarpine is very effective in treating glaucoma, but the patient may not always take it because the ophthalmologist does not seem to take an interest in the patient other than in his eyes, and even then the doctor is not enthusiastic, so why should the patient be? ECT may be the best treatment for melancholia, but the patient must have great confidence in his physician to consent to having electricity shot into his brain to induce a grand mal seizure.

At a minimum, your interpersonal efforts should try to achieve the following: (1) Convince the patient and, when necessary, his family of the correctness of your diagnosis and treatment through persuasion, education, explanation, reassurance, and force of personality. (2) Maximize compliance with treatment. (3) Advise the patient and, when necessary, his family about how to deal with the illness (e.g., what to tell family members, friends, and employers about the condition and its treatment; the limitations, if any, to all areas of function; specifics of rehabilitation). (4) Be a "sounding board" and offer *limited* advice regarding important changes or stresses in the patient's life.

After concerns about the direct effects of illness on the patient's cognitive skills, self-image, and interpersonal and job circumstances, the most likely areas of focus in talking therapy are sex and love, parents and children, job or school, and money. Common sense is the best rule to follow, but beware of your biases. For example, you might be someone who could divorce or have an abortion, but what counts for a patient in these situations is the patient's best interests given *his* attitudes. Your attitudes will influence what you say to a patient, but if your attitudes cannot be subservient to the patient's needs, you should not care for that person.

Saying "no" to a patient is sometimes part of your job. If you know your attitudes may interfere with the care of a patient, you need to discuss this problem with him and perhaps refer him to someone else. Sometimes a patient (or his family) has strong opinions about treatment that may substantially conflict with what you think is best for the patient. If, despite your efforts to convince them of your point of view, they still do not accept your treatment advice, you have two choices: Come up with a reasonable alternative, or, if no alternative is acceptable to you, tell the patient (and his family) that for you to be his doctor he needs to accept your advice in this situation. If he cannot, his best interests are for you to refer him to a doctor in whom he may have more confidence. This is an uncommon situation, and most patients faced with the choice will want to stay with you. Their confidence in you will often go up, because they will recognize your commitment to them and your treatment. For the few patients who still will not accept your advice, as long as you ensure a smooth referral, there will be no issue of patient abandonment. Some additional treatment guidelines are:

1. Be the patient's main advocate. This means directing and participating in placements or referrals to other physicians or agencies and explaining the patient's difficulties and needs to family members.
2. When the patient is faced with a difficult life situation, first obtain the details. Then help the patient to clarify the situation and explore his

options. This is often sufficient for many patients to make a decision. If you see options that the patient does not, tell him.

3. When advising, find out what the patient really wants to do. If you agree that action is in the patient's best interest, say so. "Giving your blessing" is often all the patient really needs to carry out a decision.

4. When a patient is intellectually or emotionally unable to make a decision that you believe is in his best interest, particularly a medical decision, offer your opinion. This is best done in the presence of a concurring family member or guardian.

5. If you do not know what should be done, but you believe something must be done, find out or refer the patient to an expert in that area.

6. All the guidelines for talking therapy apply to families as well as to the individual patient. The patient's family is often helpful in treatment. Their role may include persuading the patient to accept needed treatment, visiting and comforting the patient in the hospital, and monitoring the patient's treatment following discharge. Do not keep relatives at a distance during the treatment process; make them participants. Establish a cordial relationship with one or more family members whenever possible. The majority of patients want some explanation provided to relatives. When preparing to discuss the patient's condition with the family, first ask the patient if there is anything he does not want you to mention, and if at all possible maintain that confidentiality. In a life-threatening situation requiring contact with a relative, you can breach the patient's confidentiality. When a relative acts maliciously or when hospitalization is extremely embarrassing to the patient, keeping the family at a distance may be necessary.

How to Establish a Good Doctor–Patient Relationship

Table 5.2 lists the requirements for a good doctor–patient relationship. There is no magic in getting it right. You have many life experiences interacting with people—use them. Know your personality, and use your strengths so that you can be more natural and relaxed in your interactions with patients. If you are shy, try modeling yourself after a physician who you think is good at establishing a doctor–patient relationship. Use that person's behaviors and when and how he interacts with his patients. Be skilled in comforting, educating, and advising patients. Spend time with them. Help them resolve situational and interpersonal problems, and they will perceive the doctor–patient relationship as a good one.

All interactions with patients are important to the patient. Your tone of voice, manner, and choice of words are each important whether on the inpatient unit, in an outpatient setting, or in an unexpected meeting in public.

Patients often focus on the specific words spoken to them rather than on the basic message of the statement. For example, a depressed, irritated patient might be further angered if asked "How are you feeling?" rather than "Would you tell

TABLE 5.2 Requirements for a Good Doctor–Patient Relationship

Requirement	How To Achieve It
The patient has confidence in you	Know your stuff. Practice the principles of diagnosis and patient management well. Know how to do the behavioral examination well. Know the databases of diagnosis and treatment. Be good at educating the patient and, when necessary, his family about the patient's illness and treatment and what to expect over the years.
	The patient gets better. Nothing succeeds like success. Know what works and use it logically
The patient believes you care	*Every* interaction with a patient no matter how short, no matter if the patient is hospitalized, in your office, on the phone, or met by chance in a public place, should include showing respect, sympathy, empathy, patience, and interest. Private conversations with the patient should also include education about the illness and treatments, clarification of illness, and personal issues of concern to the patient
The patient trusts you	Do not lie to the patient unless you feel the truth will put you in immediate danger (e.g., while alone in an emergency department interviewing room telling an angry psychotic person you are going to put him in the hospital against his will, or when you are not going to do what a malingering person wants)
	Be patient and empathic. Educate the patient about his illness and treatments. Within limits, encourage the patient and, when appropriate, family members to participate in planning management and carrying out the plan. Make sure that the things you tell the patient are accurate; thus, they happen, and a cycle of trust is built: The more you are right the more likely you will be right again
The patient is comfortable with you	Do not use jargon. Do not speak above, below, or down to the patient. Do not patronize. Be friendly, relaxed, warm, funny, interested. Listen more than you talk

me what's happened to upset you?" Nonjudgmental expressions ("How come?" rather than "Why?") and more implicitly empathic phrasings work best.

INPATIENT UNIT AND INPATIENT BEHAVIOR MANAGEMENT

The acute treatment psychiatric inpatient unit is analogous to a critical care unit. On both types of units, the physician has the ultimate professional responsibility and liability for treatment, but most patient care is carried out by other professionals (nurses, aides, technicians, social workers, psychologists).

The unit staff and patients form a social structure. Attending physicians, residents, and students become part of this social group whether they wish to or not. Learn how a specific unit is run and who does what when, and participate in some unit activities to help maintain the unit's social process.

The primary goal of unit management is to weld the staff into a cohesive, mutually supportive group. Well-run units establish clear-cut professional roles based on the different skills of each discipline, but also use specific strengths of individual staff regardless of professional identity. Thus, who has what interaction with a given patient may have more to do with the personality of a particular staff member than with that staff member's professional training. Clearly defined professional roles also are important, and the expected contributions of the respective professionals is explicitly stated on well-run units. Optimal unit functioning occurs when everyone interacts with patients, but each discipline is primarily responsible for its own particular area of expertise and where that expertise is intrinsicly valued. A daily patient care and staff activity program and a clearly established treatment philosophy endorsed by all staff members help make an effective acute inpatient unit.

Inpatient Program Structure

The psychiatric inpatient unit is essentially a little community in which most patients are transient members. The experience, as in other communities, is around the clock and can last from days to years. The purposes of acute hospitalization include emergency control of behavior (suicide, violence), supervision of the patient who is unable to function outside the hospital because of severe psychopathology or cognitive impairment, and close monitoring of evaluation or treatment procedures.

Hospitalization also helps structure the patient's daily activities with hourly schedules that help shape his social behaviors. Schedules contain planned activities, each with stated objectives. Frequently, patients are unable to concentrate, plan, or successfully carry out daily tasks. A schedule with appropriate rest periods and free time provides the necessary daily structure until the patient is able to plan for himself. A good schedule is flexible so that as the patient improves he can progressively assume increasing responsibilities for his own activities. This can be done using a "step system" detailing specific behaviors (e.g., no longer hallucinating, complying with treatment) and responsibilities (e.g., doing all self-care, keeping room neat) that patients need to have to obtain privileges (e.g., off-unit activities, passes). The system (like all unit schedules and rules) is simply stated and prominently displayed. Step changes (up or down) are usually decided each morning with input from the entire staff. Part of the step system includes a schedule of daily activities that patients at different steps should or may attend. Some unit activities are helpful in cognitive rehabilitation (see below and Chapter 12) and are truly forms of treatment, not just time fillers.

Psychiatric inpatients are usually fully ambulatory. Once they begin to improve, they need to be occupied. They also need to be educated about their illness and treatments, and they need to deal with illness-related social and occupational disruptions. Some need individualized behavioral programs to alter the frequency of specific behaviors, and all need emotionally supportive interactions with various staff members. A unit daily activity program provides some of these needs. Group meetings for recovering patients educate them about their illness and treatments and can offer practical solutions to interpersonal difficulties they face with family, friends, and employers. Biweekly meetings for all patients and for as many of the staff as can attend are helpful for discussing specific unit problems, activities, and policies.

A daily hourly schedule is also needed for the unit staff. Attending physicians, residents, and students actively participate in this schedule. What staff members are supposed to do, when they are supposed to do it, and why they are doing it are clearly and explicitly stated. A morning report includes as much of the staff (all disciplines) as possible. The charge nurse for the day or the head nurse presents the nursing report from the night shift, briefly summarizes any new admissions to the unit, and reviews any problems from the previous 24 hours. Potential problems for that day, discharges, and last-minute discharge preparations are discussed, and a plan of action for each is devised. A monthly staff meeting for all staff members helps to resolve unit problems, reinforce unit philosophy, and introduce future plans. Evening and night shift staff periodically attend these meetings, which are scheduled close to changes of shift so that little time is lost. To maintain efficiency and enthusiasm, educational activities are a regular part of the staff schedule. The unit structure also takes into account individual staff–patient interactions. What is said to a patient, how it is said, and by whom, are important parts of overall treatment plans.

The hospitalization serves as a period for the patient to get away from a stressful environment, learn some social skills needed for activities of daily living, and get a break from the outside world, whereas treatments resolve psychopathology. By learning to function well in the inpatient community, patients learn skills or their skills are reinforced to better live in the outside world. Social behaviors that get the patient into difficulties on the unit need to be resolved so they will not get the patient into trouble on the outside.

Examples of socially dysfunctional behaviors are monopolizing the phone; lying on the floor in hallways and recreational areas; hoarding common supplies, unit equipment, or another patient's property; exhibiting pseudoseizures; intruding into meetings and conversations; making repeated requests; and standing too close when talking to others. Most of these behaviors are signs of illness and resolve with treatment. Simply stopping the patient from doing the behavior may suffice until the episode of illness is over. Adjunctive behavioral techniques may speed the reduction in the frequency of these behaviors, make the patient feel better, and improve unit functioning. For example, the patient who monopolizes the phone may get some special privilege or treat only if the number of calls or total time on the phone is below a certain level. The patient with pseudoseizures (medically evaluated, moved out of the way, and ignored during each pseudoseizure) is rewarded in some fashion if the number of episodes progressively decreases with time.

Satiation techniques (e.g., giving the patient large amounts of what is being hoarded) may be helpful with the chronic patient who hoards large quantities of primarily useless items: pieces of paper, used paper cups, washcloths, and chalk. Satiation is believed to work because the hoarded items often lose their reinforcing value when the individual has "had his fill" of them. Obviously the condition producing the hoarding also requires treatment.

Some behavioral management of hospitalized patients is almost always needed. Effective behavioral techniques require specific identification of the unwanted behavior and the circumstances in which it occurs (e.g., the target behaviors), determining the frequency of the behavior (i.e., the baseline against which to measure improvement), identification of specific staff responses that are considered reinforcing for the unwanted behavior and then the staff trained not to respond so that with no reinforcement the unwanted behavior eventually stops, and consistent action by all staff members (i.e., the behavioral treatment "dose" must be reasonably consistent to be effective, just like medication blood levels).

Attention is a powerful reinforcer of behavior. Some inappropriate patient interpersonal behavior can be modified or partially extinguishing by ignoring the behavior. Reinforce desirable substitute behaviors to replace the unwanted ones. Reinforcers (i.e., rewards) on an inpatient service include attention and conversation, unit parties, movies and special events, trips to the canteen, trips away from the hospital, visits from friends, and passes. Promotion within the step system can provide the structure for reinforcement. In some centers psychologists develop formal behavior modification systems such as token economies.* These principles can be applied to many behaviors. Examples are as follows.

Pseudosyncopal Episodes

Once morbid causes of fainting or fits are ruled out and the patient is observed not to hurt himself when he falls, pseudosyncopal episodes should be totally ignored. Explain to the other patients why they should do the same. This response is in contrast to the usual experience of such patients that their behavior rapidly mobilizes large numbers of concerned staff. Appropriate behavior is rewarded.

Angry Outbursts

Breaking and throwing things, yelling, slamming doors, and cursing can sometimes be precursors to violence. When further aggressiveness and violence are anticipated, medicate the patient (see below). If the outburst is a temper tantrum, and if a broken article belongs to the patient, be deliberately slow in replacing it. Reward the patient's attempts to mend it. If food is thrown, it should not replaced even if the patient is hungry. Reward periods of normal behavior. To maintain order and quiet on the unit you may need to sedate a patient and place him in a seclusion or quiet room. When the patient has been calm for several hours, he can be released from seclusion and reinforced for normal self-controlled behavior.

---

*A token economy is one in which specific behaviors are rewarded with a specific number of tokens that can then be "cashed in" to purchase items that the patient wants or "tickets" to hospital activities or trips.

Agitation

The patient who is agitated but not assaultive is a management problem. If the patient is not assaultive or irritable, the most likely cause of the agitation is a mood disorder. As the depression improves, the agitation resolves. Until that point, lorazepam 1–2 mg PO or IM (or the equivalent) helps. However, be sparing in using intermediary and long-acting benzodiazepines because several daily doses can lead to a continuously sedated patient who is unable to participate in any unit activities. Symptoms and side effects of other medications may also be masked.

Sexual Behaviors

Most acute treatment inpatient psychiatric units admit men and women. Although "co-ed" admissions increase socialization and normalize patients' behaviors, inappropriate sexual behavior occasionally occurs. Seeing overt sexual behavior in other patients is frightening to some patients, and the sexual behavior, if not stopped, causes other patients to feel that the involved patients are out of control and that the staff is unable to control them. Whereas expressions of warmth and affection can be appropriate, immediately stop specific sexual behaviors (e.g., passionate kissing, embracing, and fondling), and treat them as any other behavior that is inappropriate in a hospital or public setting. Liaisons occurring in patients' bedrooms, although showing some discretion, must also be prevented from recurring, because these too indicate that the participants may have lost control or that one of the participants (with diminished judgment or volition or with hypersexuality) is being taken advantage of by a patient with a less severe illness.

Separation and close monitoring of the patients involved and a reevaluation of their diagnoses and treatments should be your minimal responses. Continued attempts at sexual liaisons by a patient may require seclusion of that patient until a specific treatment (e.g., lithium, neuroleptics) becomes effective. If the patient is voluntarily hospitalized and not a danger to himself, discharge may be necessary. Never ignore overt sexual behavior. Calm but firm discussions with the participants and other patients on the unit helps reduce anxieties. Failing to stop such behavior, in addition to potentially harming a patient, can lead to successful malpractice suits.

Insomnia

Most psychiatric inpatients have difficulty sleeping, particularly during the first few nights of hospitalization. Hypnotics and short-acting benzodiazepines administered on an as-needed basis can help. However, when a patient simply cannot sleep (he is not upset, agitated, or manipulating) and the full hypnotic dose has been administered, do not make an issue of it. Instruct the night staff to allow the patient to sit up in a day area where he can read, watch TV, or talk with a staff member. The insomnia usually improves with resolution of the illness.

Substance Abuse

Patients who are substance abusers are difficult to treat in an acute treatment, general inpatient psychiatric unit. Patients in acute alcohol withdrawal states are at increased risk for seizures and death, may require prolonged intravenous fluid and electrolyte replacement, and are generally best treated on specialized detoxification or medical units.

Occasionally, however, a patient addicted to opiates or barbiturates is admitted to a general psychiatric unit. These patients can cause havoc because they frequently have antisocial traits. They manipulate staff and other patients, abuse other patients, demand and often receive unwarranted medication, and even may give illicit drugs to the unit's other patients. Discharge as quickly as possible all patients who are primarily substance abusers and have no psychosis or major illness such as depression, or who have antisocial personalities.

Medical Professionals and "VIPs"

Patients who are physicians or mental health professionals cause a particular management problem. They often assume a staff-like manner and may actually be of help to other patients. Nevertheless, if they have been appropriately hospitalized (i.e., if they have a major psychiatric disorder), they require the same treatment as anyone else. They may "help out" during the recovery phase of their illness, but do not take for granted their knowledge of their illness and treatments, their response to the illness and family, and their personal concerns. These patients deserve "full service." Patients who are famous or exotic in some way also tempt staff members to respond to reputation or status rather than to personal qualities and to the treatment requirements of their illness. Do not fall into this trap.

Violence

Violence, although relatively infrequent, is the most serious unit problem. The demographics and biology of violence are described in Chapter 16. This section deals with the management of the acutely assaultive patient. Chapters describing specific syndromes increasing the risk for violence (e.g., traumatic brain injury, dementia) detail treatments to prevent or control chronic or periodic violence.

Uncooperative Patients

On inpatient units, the assaultive patient is less common than the agitated and irritable patient who refuses to cooperate with basic unit policies, such as keeping his room and body clean and permitting a physical examination and diagnostic evaluation. The first decision you must make in this situation is whether the patient is suffering from an illness that is causing his uncooperativeness, agitation, and irritability or whether the patient is simply manipulating the hospital system. If you strongly suspect the latter, tell the patient he must either cooperate or be discharged immediately. If he fails to cooperate, discharge him. Always document these and all other significant management decisions.

If you think the patient is ill, then the lack of a physical examination and basic diagnostic tests (e.g., blood work) might be life threatening because a serious illness might progress undiscovered. The question now is whether the patient is capable of participating fully in decisions concerning his treatment. If you think he is capable, explain again the reasons for the examination, diagnostic evaluation, personal hygiene, or other procedures or activities. Tell him that he cannot be helped unless he allows the staff to help him and that he has a choice of cooperating or seeking help elsewhere. If he chooses the latter, notify his family or friends. If they are unable to persuade him, discharged him with a referral to another hospital or physician. Never, however, simply abandon him.

If you think the patient is not capable of making decisions about his treatment or is dangerous to himself or others and is not already in the hospital as an involuntary patient, inform his family of your assessment. If they agree, convert the patient to involuntary status, restrain him, and sedate him if necessary. Then examine him and get blood samples. If x-rays and other tests are needed, do these while the patient is sedated. If the family refuses to support these procedures, which are emergency measures in that a life-threatening illness may be prevented, identified, or treated, ask them to transfer the patient to another hospital. Most families are relieved to know that firm action is being taken to find out what is wrong with the patient and will usually agree to the necessary procedures. Under no circumstances should you permit a hospitalized patient to go over 24 hours without a physical examination and necessary laboratory work.

The agitated, uncooperative patient should be in pajamas. He may need to be sedated and possibly placed in seclusion for varying periods. The overriding issue when a patient is uncooperative because of illness is to ensure that he does not harm himself or others. He must also be prevented from undermining his own treatments and from disrupting the unit's functioning and disturbing other patients. The degree to which you deny the patient's rights are directly related to the degree of need to protect both the patient and the unit. However, once a patient is hospitalized because of illness, he has the right to treatment. If the patient's behavior is dangerous, you are legally permitted to restrain and treat for a limited time. Further involuntary treatment requires court approval. If the patient is not dangerous, but is clearly psychotic or severely ill, decide whether the patient is capable to judge his own condition and follow the prescribed treatments. If he is capable, he should make the decision to be treated. If the patient is not capable, he should be treated. Court approval (declaring the patient incompetent) must be obtained before definitive nonemergency involuntary treatment can be legally administered. Other than for ECT, for which you may not have a legal choice, do not wait and leave the patient in the hospital, untreated until a court decides. In most instances, consultation with the patient's family helps obtain the patient's consent to treatment and reduces the risk of being sued for treating the patient while court approval is being obtained. In the vast majority of instances lawsuits result from nontreatment rather than from treatment.

The use of intramuscular medication, restraints, and seclusion usually does not upset or anger patients if it is clear that these methods are used as treatments and not as punishments and that the staff involved truly cares about the patient's well being. Integral to these responses to deviant behaviors are warm, caring, and concerned supportive responses to the patient's other symptoms and interpersonal needs.

Restraints and Seclusion

Established rules for restraints and seclusion must be clearly understood by each staff member. Physical restraints are used only as a therapeutic measure to protect the patient from injuring himself or others. Restraints are never used to punish or discipline a patient or for staff convenience.

Restraints require a physician's written order. Always examine the patient before applying restraints. Orders for restraints are usually valid for 8–12 hours. Then the patient is reexamined to see if further restraints are needed. In addition, a staff member evaluates the restrained patient every 15–30 minutes, paying special attention to the patient's temperature and fluid intake to avoid dehydration and hyperthermia. When ordering restraints, specify the duration of their application and, in an accompanying progress note, indicate the events leading to the need for restraint and the purpose of the restraint. In emergencies, orders for restraint may be given to a nurse by telephone, or the nurse or other qualified examiner may order restraint, but you need to confirm this in writing within 1 hour and with appropriate documentation.

When a specific seclusion room is not available, use a patient bedroom provided that there is one-to-one staff observation with the room unlocked and free from furniture. All the rules applying to the ordering and monitoring of restraints also apply to the use of the seclusion room.

Suicidal Patient

Occasionally a depressed patient will commit suicide while hospitalized. Placing a suicidal patient on "suicide precautions," although legally necessary, is often insufficient to prevent such deaths. Patients have killed themselves by hanging (using ceiling and shower fixtures), ramming their heads into a wall, jumping off high furniture or a wall molding head first onto the floor, and cutting their wrists with eating utensils or broken window glass. The suicidal patient must be placed in pajamas and be continuously observed by a specifically assigned staff member. The patient may require seclusion and restraints. These patients are never allowed off the unit unescorted. If a patient on suicidal precautions attempts suicide on the unit, emergency ECT is the treatment of choice.

CONSULTATION

Neuropsychiatric consultations assist other physicians and, occasionally, other mental health professionals in the care of *their* patients. Speak with the primary physician. Find out the reason for the consultation. Specify when you will arrive. See hospitalized patients within 24 hours for routine consultations and within minutes or hours for an emergency, depending on circumstances. Recommend temporary measures until then. Have the primary physician tell the patient you will be coming to visit and why.

The principles and techniques of interviewing and diagnosis when consulting are identical to those used for your patients. What differs is the frequency of the conditions observed. Common diagnoses of general medical patients referred for psychiatric consultation include situational reactions and capacity issues, alcohol and substance abuse syndromes, delirium, and depression.

When you finish your examination, tell the patient your general conclusions and recommendations and that the primary doctor will carry these out unless you and he have previously agreed otherwise. Do not write orders unless you are requested to do so by the referring physician. In your recommendations state (1) your diagnosis, or additional information needed to establish a diagnosis (e.g., old records, history from family members, laboratory tests); (2) your thoughts about the patient's present treatments, how they are contributing to the patient's behavioral problem, and what changes, if any, should be made; (3) your specific recommendation about each problem you have identified, including medications, behavioral interventions you think would help, and social supports; (4) any non-invasive interventions you think would help (e.g., visitors, supportive conversations by nurses, visits by a social worker, night light, behavior modification tactics); (5) any follow-up visits on the ward or outpatient clinic or a transfer to a psychiatry service; and (6) your thoughts about the referring physician's other concerns (e.g., whether the patient can tolerate surgery, or can be discharged).

PSYCHOTHERAPY

All good doctors do psychotherapy; most just call it something else. Interacting with patients in specific ways enhances medical care and increases rates of improvement. The most important aspects of this interaction are understanding, developing, and maintaining a good doctor–patient relationship. Some of the tactics for doing this are detailed above and in Table 5.2. Think of psychotherapy as an ongoing process and that the development of the doctor–patient relationship begins at first contact with the patient. By extrapolation, it begins when the patient first calls the answering service or speaks to a secretary, clerk, or nurse in the office or at the clinic. If the patient thinks that person at the other end of the line is respectful, concerned, and helpful, then the doctor–patient relationship is off to a good start.

In every good psychotherapeutic interaction you *always* try to do the following:

> *Be an active listener* by paying attention, reinforcing the patient's statements, asking for clarification and more details, and letting him know you understand and are interested in what is being said. Always ask how the patient felt about the situation being related, or, if you empathically

know how the patient felt, express that empathy (e.g., "that was upsetting"). Encourage the patient to do most of the talking—an 80–20 split is often about right.

Be empathic by letting the patient know that you (and by extrapolation most people) would feel the same way under the same circumstances.

Be respectful. Address all adult patients with their title, Ms., Mrs. Mr., unless otherwise agreed to. A 26-year-old first-year resident or a 23-year-old third-year medical student greeting a 70-year-old recently retired school teacher for the first time with "Hi Chuck" is not respectful; a nurse saying to an 80-year-old arthritic wheelchair-bound woman "How are we today? Here's some goodies for your tummy" is not respectful. Act toward your patients the way you act toward a valued colleague.

Educate, clarify, and accentuate the positive. Psychotherapy implies that the patient is telling you important things. Your job is to educate the patient about the implications of those important things, to help clarify those things for the patient, and, whenever possible, to point out what is good or potentially positive about what the patient is saying. Look for the silver lining in every interpersonal cloud.

Summarize the session at its end. Whenever possible, end on a positive note. Even a chance meeting in a public place can end with "Well, it sounds like things went well. You look better. I'm glad that worked out." Even a more neutral "We should talk about that when we meet tomorrow" offers the hope that something will be done to help the situation.

There is no evidence that all good psychotherapeutic interactions must take place in your office and must last for some specified period of time. What counts is not the place or duration, but the quality of the interaction. A chance meeting or a kindness you do for the patient may have a more positive impact on the patient's perception of your relationship with him than several 50-minute sessions.

The Rehabilitation Model of Psychotherapy

A model of psychotherapy that works well in a medical setting is the rehabilitation model. This model is not particularly designed to determine the "why" of the patient's dysfunctional behavior. Psychodynamic psychotherapy, for example, tries to find out the intrapsychic why: how past interpersonal events shaped the present intrapsychic problem and how that intrapsychic problem now adversely configurates the patient's behavior. The rehabilitation model focuses on the patient's present interpersonal, social, and cognitive strengths and weaknesses. If a person is having trouble getting along in bureaucratic systems in which circumstances require him to work, the focus is not on how he got to be that way but rather on what *exactly* does he do to get into difficulties and then on what interpersonal skills he has that can help him change some of those behaviors. Goals are established (you and patient mutually identify the strengths and weaknesses and then establish the goals) and then worked on. You explore, encourage, and reinforce ways of using the patient's strengths in problem situations and ways of stopping or modifying problem behaviors. The better the doctor–patient relationship, the more powerful the effects of your advice, encouragement, and statements of approval. Understanding the patient's personality helps you to guide treatment; personality is discussed in Chapter 6.

The rehabilitation model of psychotherapy begins with assessment (see Table 5.1). All the areas are assessed so that you can establish treatment goals and start comprehensive management. As part of the rehabilitation model of psychotherapy, the assessment itself becomes an early goal: "We need to find out the following because . . . ." Thus, even obtaining laboratory tests becomes an early goal, and ideally the patient should want the tests done as much as you do. The assessment can educate and clarify problems for the patient as much as it can reveal the diagnosis. Once assessment is complete, long-term goals are established and worked on. Figure 5.1 displays the longitudinal phases of psychotherapy.

Like all treatment, psychotherapy is finite: Inpatients get better and are discharged, outpatients no longer need continuing treatment, and patients and physicians move to different towns. The last phase of psychotherapy is saying good-bye. Next to a good doctor–patient relationship, a good good-bye is the most important phase because it establishes closure on the condition and problems being treated, ends the therapeutic relationship positively so that what has been achieved is not tarnished by bad feelings, and sets a good foundation for any future treatment. Saying good-bye to the patient takes time and should not come as a surprise to the patient.

The biggest goal of treatment is to end it: The patient gets better. At the outset of treatment some sense of how long it will take is almost always a patient concern. "How long will I be in the hospital?" "How long will I have to take this medicine?" These are reasonable questions, and once assessment is complete the patient needs to know the time frame. Specific time frames are discussed in the chapters on syndromes.

Just as each session ends with a summary statement, summaries of how things are going, what has been accomplished, and what is left to do are spaced throughout the treatment period to keep the patient aware that the end of treatment is approaching. As the end point nears, increase the time spent reviewing and reinforcing accomplishments and decrease your involvement (less frequent sessions,

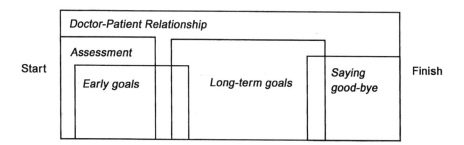

Figure 5.1. Phases of the rehabilitation model of psychotherapy.

offering less advice, encouraging the patient to take more responsibility for treatments). This is tricky because you do not want the patient to take these changes as a rejection. Good preparation helps in setting mutual goals so that the patient looks forward to the day he no longer needs to see you. However, let the patient know he can call you or see you if future problems arise.

If treatment is incomplete, or the patient has a chronic or recurrent illness that will require continuing care, but either you or the patient is moving, it is your obligation to refer to another physician. Good referrals are never made to clinics, programs, or hospitals, they are made to people. Identify the person who the patient will be seeing, and speak with that person. Get the names of appropriate physicians from a state medical or psychiatric society or from colleagues. If a patient is going to a clinic, speak with the clinic doctor. If the clinic is associated with your hospital, have the patient visit it and briefly meet the people there. These strategies greatly increase compliance. Residents should refer to residents and not simply rotate off service leaving the patient to start without any preparation all over again with another trainee. Once the patient is settled in with the new doctor, call the patient to make sure the referral went well. This extra phone call reinforces that you really cared about the patient, and it also guides you about future referrals to that physician.

Rehabilitation psychotherapy has specific goals and limitations. It is designed for patients who have axis I conditions (i.e., states of illness). Although many of its principles and techniques can be used to help persons with personality problems or problems of living, the goals, duration of treatment, and treatment strategies are different for those persons.

PHARMACOTHERAPY GUIDELINES

Diagnose before you treat. Know your treatments well. Individualize treatments to increase compliance by reducing the risks of side effects while maximizing therapeutic response. There are three basic rules to facilitate the effectiveness of your pharmacotherapy:

> 1. *Whenever possible, observe the patient in a drug-free condition.* Any length of time is better than none at all. There are several advantages for doing this. Drug-free observation periods allow for spontaneous remission of psychopathology of recent, acute onset. For nonmelancholic depressions, for example, 25% resolve with placebo. This is also true for patients over 65 years whose behavioral syndromes often result from multiple medications. For may elderly patients, simply stopping these medications can resolve the behavioral syndrome. Some drug-induced states (e.g., the depressive-like syndrome of cocaine withdrawal) and short-lived attacks of mania or hypomania can resolve on their own. Knowing that the remission was spontaneous is important for prognosis and in deciding on long-term treatment and prevention.
>
> A drug-free period allows for observation of symptoms that are

critical to diagnosis (e.g., are the tremors due to illness or are they drug related, is the reduced arousal due to medication or is the patient delirious or suffering from a stroke?). The hesitancy to immediately give psychotropics to a head injury patient should be generalized to most psychiatric patients. Know what is going on first. Only emergencies in which the patient is in immediate danger to himself or others requires immediate psychopharmacologic treatment.

A drug-free period also allows for uncontaminated laboratory investigations such as EEG and neuropsychological testing both of which can be distorted or even rendered uninterpretable by the effects of psychoactive drugs. Do medication-sensitive tests first, if possible, so that if pharmacotherapy is needed those tests get done without unduly delaying treatment.

2. *Know the use of a few drugs thoroughly rather than a large number superficially.* Learn well one or two drugs from each class of drugs. Using too many different drugs in the same class encourages bad polypharmacy (e.g., giving two neuroleptics simultaneously) and can lead to not knowing the rare but important side effects of a drug and what to do to prevent or treat them.

3. *Be sensitive to patients with special pharmacologic needs* (pregnant or breast-feeding women, the elderly, individuals with disease in other systems) and to the life situations and daily habits (e.g., special diets) that may affect their compliance with treatment.

Guidelines for Inpatient Pharmacotherapy

1. Do not treat target symptoms if you can treat the disease process. To identify the disease process, diagnosis always precedes definitive treatment. Treating target symptoms (e.g., hallucinations and delusions, anxiety, despondency) typically leads to bad polypharmacy. For example, depressed patient A is anxious, is having trouble sleeping, and has vague olfactory hallucinations (a bad odor emanating from her mouth and vagina). She is given fluoxetine for her depression, lorazepam for her anxiety and insomnia, and haloperidol for her hallucinations. She becomes lethargic and unsteady. She has a syncopal episode, falls, and hits her head, sustaining a subdural hematoma. The hematoma resolves without surgery, her depression finally resolves after 3 months, and she is discharged on fluoxetine and haloperidol. Both drugs are stopped a year later when it is noticed that slight involuntary choreoathetoid movements have begun in her right hand. Depressed patient B with the same symptoms is given venlafaxine alone and gets better in 6 weeks. Depressed patient C gets ECT and gets better in 3 weeks.

~2. Drugs with half-lives of greater than 18 hours can, and often should, be given once daily: either in the morning if insomnia is a problem or at night if sleep is enhanced or if side effects can be dulled by sleep. You can also give lithium (up to 1,200 mg) once daily after remission is achieved.

3. Once begun and tolerated, do not change or add medications until an adequate therapeutic trial is given, that is, you have given the drug in the proper form, by the proper route, in adequate doses, and for an adequate period of time in steady state (usually two times the steady state period for the decision to continue, add, or change treatments).

4. Get all medications to their steady-state therapeutic levels as fast as can be tolerated by the patient. The steady-state blood level of a given daily dose is achieved at approximately four or five times the drug's half-life.

5. If a drug can be given in a loading dose (e.g., lithium, valproic acid) and is likely to be tolerated by the patient, that is the preferred inpatient strategy.

6. Make only one pharmacologic change at a time. That way, if the change works you know likely cause and effect. If the change leads to side effects you also know cause and effect. Also, if you do two things simultaneously (a drug dose is increased and a second drug simultaneously added) future treatment flexibility is reduced—you have to keep the two changes if the patient gets better (even though only one of them really worked), or you may have to stop both changes if an intolerable side effect develops.

7. When there is a partial response to a drug at its maximum dose, potentiate. When there is no response, switch. When switching medications because of nonresponse, use a different class of drug. For example, if a manic patient partially responds to valproic acid, a next step might be adding lithium rather than carbamazepine. However, if the manic patient did not respond at all to valproic acid, it is highly unlikely that he will respond to carbamazepine, and a next step might be switching to lithium or ECT.

8. Drug–drug interactions are common; always consider them when prescribing. Some interactions are good, but many are not. See specific syndrome chapters for details.

9. The more psychotropics given simultaneously, the less the response and the greater the number and severity of side effects; monotherapy rules.

10. Until the few days prior to discharge, use the oral concentrate or the suspension form of medication. Pills are too easily "cheeked" or regurgitated, are less well absorbed, and do not result in consistent blood levels.

11. When you use medications to treat a hospitalized patient with mood disorder, ECT becomes the best second-line treatment if the first medication strategy is not satisfactory. The reason is that the first drug choice was the one you thought best. Second best sometimes works,

but for mood disorder it rarely works faster, better, or more safely than ECT. ECT is a first-line treatment in many circumstances (see Chapter 7 for details about ECT).

12. Antipsychotics are for psychosis; sedatives or benzodiazepines are to temporarily control agitation or aggression. As-needed sedation is only justified as preparatory to definitive treatment and is rarely justified for any reason beyond 48 hours. Oral or intramuscular lorazepam 1–2 mg is commonly used to control agitation of inpatients without other neurologic disease.

13. Neuroleptics should not be given as needed except perhaps when titrating dosage. Neuroleptics are a definitive treatment, and give them in a set schedule, once a day for oral, two or three times a day for intramuscular. For example, if the patient receives an additional one or two as-needed doses on days 1 and 2 of neuroleptic treatment, the regularly prescribed dose is probably too low and needs to be increased by an amount equivalent to the as-needed doses. Review all as-needed medications every 1–2 days to determine need and efficacy for continuing the order.

14. If, because of severe agitation or assaultiveness, more than one intramuscular neuroleptic dose is needed in a 24–36 hour period, a set intramuscular schedule should be instituted. Switching from intramuscular to oral requires several days of overlap of administration by both routes. This overlap is necessary because the intramuscular dose bypasses the liver, whereas the oral dose does not, so blood levels are initially higher and are achieved more rapidly with intramuscular dosing.

15. Long-acting antipsychotic preparations are never appropriate to treat acutely ill patients. Long-acting neuroleptic preparations (fluphenazine and haloperidol) offer no flexibility and thus are dangerous when treating a patient with an acute psychosis. They are difficult to dose. (How much is enough? When does it become too much?) Once injected the half-life is weeks regardless of side effects or further information that would make you want to stop the drug (e.g., the patient is pregnant, the diagnosis is not schizophrenia but epilepsy). Reserve the use of long-acting neuroleptics for chronically ill, noncompliant outpatients who have failed all other forms of treatment (including ECT). Long-acting neuroleptic use substantially increases the patient's risk for tardive dyskinesia.

16. Risperidone and other "atypical" neuroleptics with "minimum" extrapyramidal side effects are best saved for outpatients or inpatients over age 65, as their side effect advantages are lost on acute psychotics, manics, and other agitated patients for whom high daily doses are needed (e.g., above 8 mg for risperidone). Atypical drugs also do not come in intramuscular form, further limiting their use in acute psychosis. If you must give a neuroleptic to a psychotic depressive, use risperidone or olanzapine to reduce the risks for tardive dyskinesia and neuroleptic malignant syndrome.

Guidelines for Outpatient Pharmacotherapy

1. Other than using pills rather than concentrate and knowing that long-acting neuroleptics have a role in the treatment of noncomplying chronically ill psychotic outpatients, all the guidelines for inpatient pharmacotherapy apply to outpatients.
2. Physiologically stable, otherwise generally healthy patients and young adult outpatients tolerate psychotropics well and can be brought to steady-state therapeutic levels almost as fast as inpatients.
3. Compliance is the biggest challenge in outpatient pharmacotherapy. Compliance can be enhanced. (a) Establish a good doctor–patient relationship. (b) during the few days after the first visit in which medication is started, and periodically until the second visit, make "phone rounds." Tell patients you will be calling them and why and then religiously do it. A 5-minute phone conversation can allay fears, nip a side effect in the bud, and improve confidence and trust in you and the treatment. (c) Uncomfortable side effects are the most common reasons given for noncompliance. Compliance is enhanced by good prevention and treatment of side effects. Educating the patient about the illness and the treatments also improves compliance. (d) Keep appointments and do not keep patients waiting. There is no evidence that your time is more valuable than the patient's. (e) Work with family members. At their best, they are extensions of your eyes, ears, and hands in caring for, monitoring, and supporting the patient.

THERAPEUTICS

Choice of Drug

The principles of pharmacotherapy are the same as those for other classes of drugs. Your choice of a drug within a class is usually determined by differences in preparation route, side effects, physical factors (e.g., color, taste), and the drug's pharmacokinetics (e.g., absorption, distribution, metabolism, and excretion). Specific medications are discussed with each syndrome. In general, however, consider the following:

1. Be a therapeutic optimist. Pick the drug likely to give the patient the best possible response, and, if there is no obvious harm by doing so, always make the diagnosis with the best prognosis.
2. Think in the long-run. Will the drug be best for that patient for acute, maintenance, and prophylactic treatment? For example, even though phenytoin is an effective anticonvulsant, it is rarely given to young persons in part because of gum hyperplasia. Neuroleptics given to

young persons for longer than 3–6 months puts them at great risk for tardive dyskinesia; thus other acute treatment strategies are best for a young patient, not because they are necessarily better than a neuroleptic, but because they are less risky in the long run.

3. The drug with the less disturbing side effects for the specific patient is often the best choice. For example, for a bipolar mood disorder patient who needs fine motor hand function (e.g., a jeweler, a graphic designer), valproic acid may be a better choice than lithium, which is more likely to cause a hand tremor.

4. It is a mistake to think that one class of drug is "safer" or has "fewer" side effects than another. All medications have side effects. Tap water drunk in excess has side effects. Antidepressant drugs are a good example. Serotonin reuptake-inhibiting antidepressants are commonly characterized as having less side effects than the older antidepressants such as desipramine or nortriptyline. In fact, the dropout rates for patients on these different types of antidepressants is about the same; patients just drop out for different reasons.

5. In general, psychotropics are classified by their *pharmacodynamic properties* (i.e., the effects of the drug on the body) and are used based on their *pharmacokinetics* (i.e., the effects of the body on the drug). Pharmacodynamics are discussed for each drug in various chapters throughout the book. Pharmacokinetics are discussed below.

Drug Dosage

Most psychotropic drugs are more effective when administered at the upper rather than the lower end of their dosage range, and inadequate dosing is the most frequent cause of unsuccessful drug treatment. At full therapeutic effect some side effects typically occur. If you think side effects might be a problem, and rapid dose increases are not necessary, slow increases often lead to tolerance developing to many side effects. When not disturbing to the patient, think of mild side effects as indicators that the drug has been adequately absorbed and distributed.

The dose you give mostly depends on the drug's pharmacokinetics, because these factors determine the drug's bioavailability, that is, its availability to the brain. Thus, you need to know the best strategies for maximizing the drug's absorption (e.g., lithium taken on a full stomach), its degree of metabolism in the liver (e.g., carbamazepine is metabolized, gabapentin, another anticonvulsant, is not), and what influences that metabolism (e.g., nicotine increases liver metabolism and lowers some drug levels). Protein binding reduces bioavailability (lithium is not bound, valproate is). The fat solubility of a drug determines its distribution in the body (the more lipophilic, the more it gets distributed in fatty tissue, including brain). You also need to know how each drug is excreted (via kidneys, gut). Table 5.3 displays some drugs and clinical situations that influence drug pharmacokinetics and thus blood levels.

TABLE 5.3. Clinical Situations Affecting Psychotropic Drug Blood Levels

Situations	Drug Blood Level Effect	Mechanism of Action
DRUG–DRUG INTERACTIONS		
Barbiturates	Lower antidepressant levels	Increased liver enzyme activity
Anticonvulsants	Decreased antidepressant, neuroleptic, and other anticonvulsant levels	Lowered protein binding; increased renal clearance; increased liver enzyme activity
Theophylline	Decreased lithium and anticonvulsant levels	Increased renal excretion and liver enzyme activity, respectively
Salicylates	Increased free valproic acid levels	Reduced protein binding
Anti-inflammatory drugs	Variable increases in lithium levels	Increased renal reabsorption
Antibiotics	Increased carbamazepine levels	Reduced renal clearance
Calcium channel blockers (verapamil)	Increased carbamazepine levels	Reduced renal clearance
Methylphenidate and other stimulants, including caffeine	Increased antidepressant levels	Decreased liver enzyme activity
Chlorpromazine	Increased antidepressant levels	Decreased liver enzyme activity
Progestational agents and oral contraceptives	Increased antidepressant and neuroleptic levels	Decreased liver enzyme activity
Alcohol	Decreased antidepressant and neuroleptic levels	Increased liver enzyme activity
Nicotine (tobacco)	Decreased antidepressant and neuroleptic levels	Increased liver enzyme activity
PATIENT CONDITIONS		
Low salt diet	Markedly increased lithium levels	Increased renal reabsorption
Diabetes	Decreased antidepressant, neuroleptic, and anticonvulsant levels	Lowered albumin and, thus, binding
Pregnancy	Increased levels of antidepressant and neuroleptics; lower lithium levels	Decreased liver enzyme activity and increased renal clearance, respectively
Elderly	Increased levels of antidepressants, neuroleptics, and lithium	Reduced liver enzyme activity, first-pass effect, and reduced renal clearance, respectively
Chronic inflammatory disease; recent trauma or surgery	Less available protein-free drug for antidepressants, neuroleptics, and anticonvulsants, although levels remain the same	Increased protein binding

Drug Metabolism

Most psychotropic drugs are metabolized in the liver. Intestinal microflora also metabolize drugs excreted in the feces, and conditions affecting liver and intestinal function affect drug metabolism. Orally administered neuroleptic and nonspecific and partially specific monoamine reuptake-inhibiting antidepressants undergo modification first in the intestinal mucosa and then in the liver via the portal circulation. This *first-pass* effect ensures that when these drugs are orally administered only their metabolites enter the systemic circulation or the brain. Metabolites have degrees of effectiveness different from those of the unmetabolized drug entering the circulation directly from an intramuscular site.

First-pass metabolism primarily involves microsomal cytochrome enzyme systems (e.g., the P450 system) that particularly affect lipophilic drugs such as neuroleptics and most monoamine reuptake-inhibiting antidepressants. These enzymes oxidize lipophilic to less active hydrophilic forms, so they can enter the bloodstream. In this process (termed *biotransformation*) some drug metabolites are excreted in bile, and many are reabsorbed via the enterohepatic circulation and further metabolized. Demethylation resulting in more active substances also occurs during the first pass.

In the second phase of metabolism *(second pass)*, cytoplasmic enzyme systems are primarily involved, and the primary means of biotransformation is conjugation, which further transforms drug metabolites into hydrophilic forms for easier excretion (bile and urine). Thus, liver metabolism of drugs is a prolonged process, and the first several days of treatment with a first-pass, liver-metabolized psychotropic is mostly dosing the liver.

Most monoamine reuptake-inhibiting antidepressants and all neuroleptics are first-pass dependent. Some benzodiazepines (lorazepam) are second-pass dependent. Thus, factors primarily affecting first-pass metabolism (aging, blood flow, intestinal microflora) will have a greater influence on the clinical use of antidepressants and neuroleptics, whereas factors primarily affecting second-pass metabolism (liver damage) will have more of an influence on the use of second-pass dependent compounds.

Figure 5.2 displays the pharmacokinetic steps of many psychotropic drugs. Ninety percent of the dose of most psychotropics gets absorbed because of their high lipophilic properties. Only 40%, however, makes it through the first pass unmetabolized. The more lipophilic the drug, the faster it gets absorbed, but also the faster it will be distributed throughout the body and thus the faster the blood level will drop. This can affect *half-life,* that is, the time it takes for the plasma concentration from a single dose to drop 50%. Obese patients will have greater distribution of high lipophilic drugs than thin patients and thus may need higher doses to get the same plasma level. Elderly patients will also have greater lipophilic drug distribution because, compared with younger persons, their proportion of fatty tissue to body weight is increased. It is the opposite for children, who have less fatty tissue to body weight than do adults.

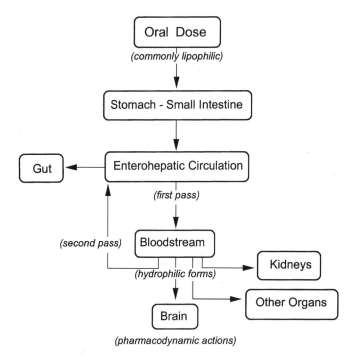

Figure 5.2. Pharmacokinetics of many psychotropic drugs.

Drug Absorption

The choice of preparation and route of administration is determined by factors affecting drug absorption and the clinical needs regarding onset of drug action. For example, intramuscular injection of a soluble salt produces a fast onset of action with neuroleptics. Most benzodiazepines, on the other hand, are highly lipophilic, are poorly absorbed intramuscularly, and are given orally or intravenously if a rapid effect is needed (lorazepam is an exception and is absorbed well intramuscularly). Lithium carbonate can cause more gastric irritation than other forms of lithium. Rapid peak blood levels are needed for sedatives and hypnotics. The rapidity of reaching peak blood level is less a concern for definitive treatments.

For neuroleptics and most monoamine reuptake-inhibiting antidepressants, a single daily dose is safe and clinically effective in part because of the long half-lives of these drugs. The advantages of a single daily dose are (1) if given at bedtime, many side effects may dissipate during sleep, and the quality of sleep may itself be improved by the sedative effect of the drug; (2) nurses have to prepare and distribute medications only once a day; (3) patients at home find it easier to remember to take a single nighttime dose of medication than multiple doses throughout the day, thus missing fewer doses; and (4) taking medication at bedtime is socially acceptable and avoids the potential embarrassment of having to take pills at work or in other public places.

Drug Combinations

There is no hard evidence of true synergism between any two psychopharmacologic agents, although additive effects occur. Certain combinations are frequently used: haloperidol and lithium or an anticonvulsant and lithium for acute mania, and some monoamine reuptake-inhibiting antidepressant and a monoamine oxidase inhibitor for some dysthymias. Specific combinations are discussed in the chapters on syndromes.

Drug Interactions

Many drugs inhibit or induce hepatic enzymes and will raise or lower blood levels of other drugs. Barbiturates induce enzymes and may lower antidepressant blood levels. Benzodiazepines, which have little or no enzyme induction, are a better choice for sedation/sleep in depressed patients. Methylphenidate inhibits enzymes and can raise blood levels of nonspecific and partially specific monoamine reuptake-inhibiting antidepressants by reducing their rate of metabolism. Carbamazepine stimulates liver enzymes that metabolize imipramine and phenytoin, reducing the effectiveness of these drugs. Chlorpromazine reduces liver metabolism of imipramine.

Tobacco (nicotine) and alcohol induce liver enzymes so that larger doses of psychotropic drugs are needed to obtain the usual therapeutic blood level. Steroids, particularly progestational agents (as in oral contraceptives), and pregnancy, with its high progesterone blood levels, all reduce drug metabolism. Under these circumstances more of the dose may get into the blood, and lower oral doses may be needed to avoid toxicity. Once pregnancy is over (or the oral contraceptive stopped) progesterone levels will drop, liver metabolism will become more effective, and dosage may need to be increased. In contrast, lithium is not metabolized in the liver, but is excreted more rapidly by the kidney during pregnancy, when higher doses may be needed.

Bioavailability and Blood Levels

In addition to absorption, metabolism, and solubility in body fat, bioavailability reflects the drug's protein binding and excretion. Although drug blood levels are a gross measure of bioavailability, there is enormous variability in blood levels among patients, and within any given patient over time. Interpretation of drug levels differs across drugs. For example, the variability is small in serum lithium levels if the patient is in normal health and blood levels are measured at a standardized time interval following dose administration, because lithium excretion is mostly a function of renal plasma flow. Thus, big changes in lithium levels are clinically important (e.g., suggesting noncompliance [drop], increasing risk of toxicity [rise]). Because of individual differences in liver and intestinal metabolism, first-pass drugs have extremely variable blood levels after oral doses, and several measurements may be needed to establish a trend.

Drugs have two different types of dose–response curves. Most psychotropics have a linear or sigmoid curve in which increasing blood levels have increasing therapeutic effects until a plateau is reached beyond which no further improvement occurs regardless of blood level. Drugs of this type (e.g., carbamazepine, valproate) can be pushed to their upper dosage range, limited only by their side effects. Drugs with a nonlinear (or inverted U) dose–response curve are characterized by diminishing clinical improvement at higher blood levels, even in the absence of disabling side effects. Thus, if a patient is unimproved on this type of drug (e.g., nortriptyline), the dose may be either too low or too high, and proper treatment cannot be provided in the absence of blood level monitoring.

Finally, bioavailability is in part determined by the amount of the drug that freely circulates in the blood. Most drugs (lithium and the newest anticonvulsants are exceptions) are primarily bound to plasma albumin, leaving only 10%–20% freely dissolved in the plasma water and thus pharmacologically active. Laboratory reports of drug blood levels usually sum both free and protein-bound drug and can give a false impression of active drug available. For example, in liver disease, plasma albumin will be low and total blood levels of a given dose will seem low, although the amount of free drug could be the same as that if the albumin level were normal. The ability of albumin to bind a drug can change: Anticonvulsants and diabetes lower binding, and chronic inflammatory disease, trauma, and surgery increase binding.

Although specific plasma levels for several drugs are used as targets to get within a therapeutic range, the best means of evaluating a drug's effectiveness is by assessing behavioral change and side effects. Blood levels are most important for indicating a patient's compliance rather than if the drug is at a therapeutic dose. Thus, for any patient who is on a psychotropic and then relapses, get a blood level of that drug as soon as possible. If you know the dose the patient is supposedly taking, that blood level will tell you if the patient is a noncomplier or has relapsed while taking adequate amounts of medication. This information is important. In the first instance you might put the patient back on the correct dose of the same medication and try to enhance compliance. In the second instance you might consider a new treatment. The blood level also helps to prevent giving too much of the drug. For example, if a patient is supposedly taking 1,600 mg of carbamazepine daily and becomes ill and is hospitalized, the tendency is again to put him on 1,600 mg daily. But, if he is a noncomplier and his blood level is very low, then 1,600 mg may be an overdose at that point in time. On the other hand, the low blood level will also heighten concerns about withdrawal seizures, ensuring that some carbamazepine will be given.

Duration of Treatment

There are three decisions to make regarding duration of treatment: (1) during acute treatment, how long to continue a drug before you increase its dose, change to another drug, or add a second drug; (2) how long to continue successful maintenance treatment; and (3) when to start and how long to continue prophylactic treatment. Each of these decisions is influenced by the disease being treated, patient variables such as age and general medical health, and the treatment being used and its side effects. These decisions are discussed in detail in the chapters on syndromes. There are three guidelines:

1. Most successful treatments for mood disorders and psychoses requiring hospitalization, and for depressions of all kinds, typically produce *some* response within 7–10 days. If you observe *some* response, continue acute treatment to maximal response (see below). If there is *no response* whatsoever by 10 days (e.g., some improvement in sleep, reduction in anxiety, or no further weight loss), there is little likelihood that continuing that drug will lead to a remission, and some treatment change is probably needed.
2. If acute treatment is successful, maintenance treatment will be necessary through the period of likely relapse. This period varies depending on the diagnosis.
3. Prophylactic treatment is begun only if the patient's illness history is worse than the typical symptom-free period achieved by the prophylaxis. Thus, if a bipolar mood disorder patient had an episode every 8–10 years, prophylaxis may not be warranted because no prophylaxis can do better than that*.

Evaluation of Treatment

Determining when to discontinue or change treatment should be done logically. Both situations are dependent on your assessment of treatment results. For example, the decision to discontinue maintenance medication after a year is based on your conclusion that the patient has achieved the maximum benefit from treatment, and treatment should stop unless symptoms return. Your decision to change treatment is based on your conclusion that the patient has not achieved maximum benefit from treatment, and additional or new treatments are needed. "Maximum benefit" ideally means symptom-free and full return to premorbid function. This standard should be your goal for every patient, but you need to recognize that this standard will not always be met.

In practice, "maximum benefit" for an acute episode is achieved when there is a balance between (1) no additional symptom reduction or functional return over a period of time equivalent to about the typical acute-treatment duration (e.g., 4–6 weeks for antidepressants and neuroleptics, 3–4 weeks for lithium, 6–8 ECTs); and (2) physiological and psychological tolerance to treatment side effects.

Thus, if a patient has not noticeably improved further during the time-frame usually considered adequate for acute treatment with a given treatment regimen and the patient is tolerating the side effects of treatment, he has probably achieved maximum symptom reduction and functional return *with that treatment* at that dose. Further improvement will be unlikely with the same treatment regimen (lithium prophylaxis is one exception to this rule, with the longer the treatment the better the response).

*Some clinicians will automatically prescribe prophylactic treatment for patients following a second episode. Which patients benefit from this strategy, however, is unclear.

If you think the maximum benefit is good (definition will differ for each patient), no changes in treatment need be made until that treatment's typical maintenance phase is completed. If you think maximum benefit is inadequate, then consider the reason(s) for the inadequate response. Focus on (1) misdiagnosis, (2)
incorrect first treatment choice, (3) incorrect dose (almost always too little), (4) incorrect duration of treatment, (5) side effects, (6) noncompliance, and (7) other
physiological factors that can adversely influence treatment (e.g., age, pregnancy,
drug interactions, general medical illness affecting pharmacokinetics). If one of
these possibilities appears causally related to the inadequate response, correct it,
if possible. If none of the above possibilities appears to explain the patient's inadequate response, then choose a new treatment regimen based on the same factors
that determined the original choice.

PRINCIPLES OF REHABILITATION

It is standard practice that following stroke, head injury, or broken bones, the patient undergoes rehabilitation. This rehabilitation is specific: (1) the degree of
strengths and disabilities are assessed; (2) realistic goals for recovery are set; (3)
strengths are maintained and disabilities are repetitively worked on in the rehabilitation laboratory; (4) once in the range of reasonable function, rehabilitation
switches to real-life (in vivo) situations; and (5) follow-up rehabilitation sessions
focus to maintain improvements and offer new skills training if improvement goes
beyond initial expectations. Each step is carefully measured and has gradations of
difficulty designed to keep the patient progressing without discouragement.

Almost all psychotic patients, and many patients with nonpsychotic mood
disorders, even if totally remitted of their symptoms, have suffered a form of
brain trauma and may need some rehabilitation. Thus, you should assess these
patients for their cognitive strengths and social skills, and provide rehabilitation if
needed *as if the problems had been caused by a head injury.*

The brain functions under the guiding principle of "use it or lose it," and
many psychiatric patients who do not get adequate rehabilitation are likely to become chronically less functional than prior to their illness. Examples of the "use it
or lose it" principle are that among healthy persons over age 60 years, those who
regularly play video games, compared with engaging in passive activities (movie
viewing), are substantially improved in their reaction times and performance on
other cognitive tests. Aerobic fitness also improves cognitive performance in the
healthy elderly. Among persons with mild to moderate traumatic brain injury,
cognitive rehabilitation also improves performance on neuropsychological tests.
Neural plasticity does not end with puberty. It lasts a lifetime.

The first step in rehabilitation is assessment. Whenever you think the acute
episode is over, and your patient is ready to enter the maintenance phase of treatment, reassess his cognitive and social skills. This assessment should minimally
include

1. *Level of self-sufficiency in activities of daily living.* Can the patient live on
   his own? Does he have adequate hygiene? Will he be able to prepare

his meals, keep his home reasonably clean and organized, do his shopping, and deal with all the agencies and people needed to maintain a home? If he cannot do all these things, how bad are the deficits? Good frontal lobe function is required to live independently. Match his strengths with placement.

2. *Level of social skills.* How well does the patient interact with others? Does he stand too close when he speaks to others? Does he speak to loudly, have adequate emotional expression, speech and language function? Does he express odd ideas that will put people off? Does he look clean and neat? Good self-monitoring is needed to govern oneself in social situations.

3. *Level of motor behavior.* Is he motorically normal? If he has motor problems, what are their nature and severity?

4. *Level of cognition.* Test attention, abstract thinking, new learning, and visuospatial function. Based on this assessment decide if more elaborate neuropsychological testing is needed.

Thus, neuropsychological testing is done early on to aid with diagnosis and at the end of acute treatment to aid rehabilitation planning. Neuropsychological testing is also used to help determine if the patient can go back to his original work or to plan a rehabilitation program for him.

Good prognostic features include the following:

1. No loss of emotional expression or volition
2. No formal thought disorder during the acute episode
3. Normal motor behavior
4. Good premorbid function, the higher the better (thus, always determine level of education and vocabulary, (gross measures of premorbid IQ)
5. When recovered from the acute episode, good attention, low distractibility, and good serial verbal learning (learning a list of unrelated words [see Chapter 4, Fig. 4.13]).

As for other disorders, rehabilitation for behavioral disorders is done by an expert. If such a person is not directly available to your practice or service, try to refer to rehabilitation specialists in physical medicine, neurology, or a traumatic brain injury program.

Rehabilitation always occurs in incremental steps. For each step the task is broken down into smaller steps. Teaching, learning, and repetition of several tasks within each step covers each function being worked on in several different ways. This provides variety. When a rehabilitation expert is not available, rehabilitation can still be accomplished to some extent through inpatient, clinic, and related hospital activities and through occupational and recreational training sessions. Board and party games requiring some new learning, video games requiring visuoperceptual processing and motor-perceptual coordination, practicing job-related tasks, and role-playing social situations can all help. Failure to adequately rehabilitate seriously ill psychiatric patients after their first episode is a major cause of chronicity. Consider rehabilitation a necessity just as you do medications. This is secondary prevention and cost effective in the long run.

ADDITIONAL READINGS

Ashley MJ, Krych DK (eds): Traumatic Brain Injury Rehabilitation. CRC Press, Boca Raton, 1995.

Caudill W: *The Psychiatric Hospital as a Small Society*. Harvard University Press, Cambridge, 1958.

Guze SB: *Why Psychiatry Is a Branch of Medicine*. Oxford University Press, New York, 1987.

Guze SB: Psychotherapy and the etiology of psychiatric disorders. *Psychiatry Dev* 3:183–193, 1988.

Schwatzberg AF, Nemeroff CB (eds): *Textbook of Psychopharmacology*. American Psychiatric Press, Washington DC, 1995.

Shay KA, Roth DL: Association between aerobic fitness and visuospatial performance in healthy older adults. *Psychol Aging* 7:15–24, 1992.

6

Personality and Personality Disorders

THE TRAIT CONCEPT OF PERSONALITY

Personality represents a combination of stable, habitual patterns of behavior that are characteristic of a person and that develop over the first two decades of life and then change little. Personality patterns are termed *traits* because they are longstanding and consistent, just like other traits such as eye color, hair texture, and height. *State* behavior refers to behaviors that come and go, such as a mood state and many DSM axis I conditions. Abnormal behavioral states are assumed to represent illness and underlying brain dysfunction or disease. Abnormal behavioral traits are assumed not to reflect brain dysfunction or disease, but rather a deviance that has developed during a person's formative years.

There are several reasons why a neuropsychiatrist needs to understand personality:

1. Personality trait behaviors are subserved by brain systems, and so understanding personality teaches us about brain organization
2. Personality disorders are often co-morbid with axis I conditions, and to successfully care for patients it is important to understand the interactions between axes I and II and how to respond to deviant personality behaviors
3. Knowing about personality traits can help shape pharmacotherapy
4. Disorders of the action brain commonly alter personality, and recognizing these changes and being able to manage them are important.

Figure 6.1 illustrates the idea of personality and personality disorders using the analogy of height. Most traits, like height, appear in the general population in a normal distribution. Most persons are in the middle of the distribution, but some are at the extremes. Statistically, persons in the middle are closer to the mean (the norm), whereas persons at the extremes are statistically abnormal (or deviant). For example, if you were to measure the height of all 20-year-old U.S. men you would find their heights to be normally distributed, with the mean (average

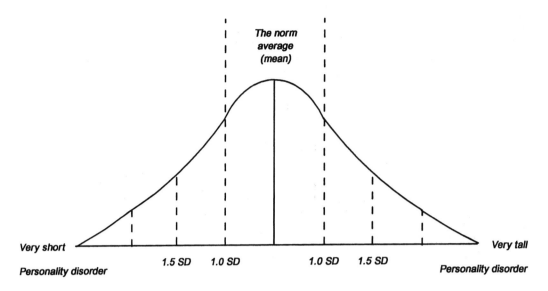

Figure 6.1. Normal distribution of traits: height and personality.

height) about 5 foot 10 inches and a standard deviation of plus or minus 2 inches. All males between 5′ 8″ and 6′ would be close enough to the mean to be considered "normal." The more abnormal or deviant a person is in height, the farther away he is 5′ 10″. A 6′ 7″ professional basketball player is abnormal and deviant in height, but this deviance is clearly not due to disease but rather to a large dose of whatever are the determinants of height (e.g., genes, nutrition, hormonal factors). Being abnormal is not necessarily a bad thing. The average IQ is between 90 and 110. An IQ of 150 is abnormal and deviant, but a good thing. Like other traits, there are multiple determinants of personality, and, based on the interactions of those determining factors, your personality will be somewhere along the normal distribution. The closer to the mean, the more normal your personality. The farther from the mean, the more abnormal your personality.

Persons who are different from the norm often have difficulties because of their deviance. We have designed our society and its expectations of us to reflect the norm. Thus, the 6′ 7″ basketball player will have difficulties finding clothes that fit him and a bed long enough to sleep in comfortably. Because of his body mechanics, he will be prone to lower back problems, particularly as he lifts heavy objects away from his center of gravity. He will have difficulties getting in and out of small vehicles and must be careful not to hit his head on door frames or low light fixtures. His abnormal height, not due to disease, makes him more vulnerable to specific personal difficulties (getting clothes) and to specific disease (back problems, head bruises). Deviant personality also makes a person more vulnerable to specific personal difficulties (e.g., not getting along with people, constantly being taken advantage of) and to specific disease (several conditions in axis I such as anxiety disorder, drug abuse). The DSM axis II classification of personality disorders assumes these conditions to be deviations without disease. However, some of them (see below) may actually reflect disease and conceptually should be in axis I, not axis II. This has happened before, when DSM I and II included cyclothymia as a personality disorder.

Traits, however, can be abnormal because of disease or dysfunction (e.g., short stature in Down syndrome, tall stature in Marfan syndrome), injury (e.g., a leg is shortened), or aging (osteoporosis leads to vertebral compression fractures). Simply measuring a person's height will not distinguish the deviation due to disease from deviation reflecting maturational variability. Personality also may be deviant from brain disease or dysfunction, as well as maturational factors. Table 6.1 displays some of the neuropsychiatric conditions that can dramatically alter normal personality. When a person's personality changes from disease into one of the DSM patterns described below they are said to have *secondary personality disorder* to that disease. Other than a clear change in trait behavior after maturation and after the onset of the brain-changing condition, there are few specific differences between primary and secondary personality disorders. The DSM also does not yet incorporate some of the secondary personality types recognized by the neuropsychaitrist (see Table 6.1).

The Neurobiology of Personality

Like all behavior, personality traits are expressions of brain systems. The basic structure (floor plan) of human personality, its determinants, and underlying brain systems have been partially worked out.

Table 6.1. Conditions That Can Alter Personality

Condition	Common Associations	Typical Personality Change
Epilepsy	Temporal lobe foci	Viscous/adhesive or paranoid (like DSM Cluster A subtype) (see Chapter 10 for details)
Head injury	Large right hemisphere or frontal injuries	Irritable and coarsening, respectively
Stroke	Large or multiple anterior strokes	Avolitional or disinhibited frontal lobe syndromes
Drug abuse	Chronic use of cannabis, inhalants, cocaine	Avolitional, irritable/paranoid, viscous/adhesive, respectively
Bipolar mood disorder	Chronic form	Viscous/adhesive
Degenerative brain disease	White matter dementias, Pick's disease, basal ganglia dementias, chronic metabolic disorders	Avolitional or disinhibited frontal lobe syndromes

Human Personality Structure

Measurements of trait behaviors in thousands of persons in dozens of countries and from all walks of life (rich, poor, urban, rural), religion, race, and ethnicity reveal that

1. *There appears to be a basic human personality structure,* or floor plan, shared by all persons, just as all persons share the same basic floor plan for the human hand and other basic human characteristics. Every person (without developmental anomaly, disease, or injury) has a hand recognizable as the standard four-fingered, oppositional thumbed hand. This hand format comes with all humans, but each person also has a uniqueness about his or her hands. Thus, there is much individual variability within the basic floor plan. The same seems true for personality.

2. *Once fully developed (around age 20–25 years), personality does not dramatically change over the course of one's life unless affected by disease or injury.* For example, the pattern of personality traits does not dramatically change in the same person over many decades, although there is some decrease in impulsivity and curiosity and some increase in cautiousness. The distribution of personality trait scores is similar in persons of different ages (e.g., young adults versus middle age versus elderly persons despite their widely differing experiences).

3. *Personality is composed of several big patterns termed "higher order dimensions."* The number of higher order dimensions and what each is called varies among groups of researchers who, nevertheless, agree on the overall concept.

4. *Each personality higher order dimension is normally distributed in the general population;* thus, most persons are in the mid-range of each dimension, but some are at the opposite extremes (very low or very high).

5. *Each higher order dimension is a continuum* so that any cut-off (high or low) is somewhat arbitrary.

6. *Each higher order dimension is independently determined* so that being high on one does not mean a person must be low on another.

7. *Each higher order dimension is composed of smaller groups of behavioral patterns termed "lower order traits."* Each lower order trait is also a continuum of behavior that can be characterized as high, low, or mid-range.

8. *The combinations of lower order traits determines the "strength" of the higher order dimension that they represent.*

There are several versions of the floor plan of human personality. Figure 6.2 illustrates the basic structure. The differences among versions are substantially less than their agreements. A popular model among psychologists doing personality research is The Five Factor Model. Each factor (or higher order dimension) has a range of scores from low to high. Another model described below is Cloninger's The Temperament/Character Model.

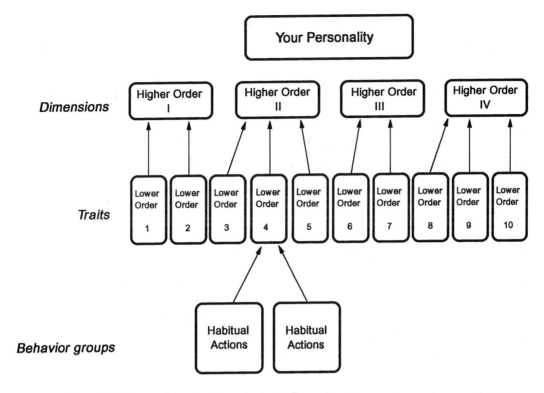

Figure 6.2. Personality structure: the basic floor plan. The number and names for higher order traits, or dimensions, depend on the particular slant of the investigators. Continuous refinement has led to some changes in these details, but the big picture has remained remarkably constant for several decades.

Human Personality and Evolution

Personality structure (the basic floor plan) has evolved just like our other behavioral systems (e.g., memory, language, emotion). Most social mammals (e.g., canines, horses, nonhuman primates) have some evidence of differences in temperament, which is an important aspect of personality. In the small hominid groups of our ancestors, personality, like intelligence and language, provided great survival advantage. Because personality traits once formed are stable, a person's temperament and tendencies to act or not act in certain ways under certain circumstances is predictable. In a small hominid group accurately predicting who you can count on for what has obvious advantages. However, if every person in the group were alike, there would be little group behavioral flexibility; that is, everyone would act the same way, like herd animals that all scatter from danger and run away as fast as they can, sacrificing a few individuals, saving the many. In a small group the loss of a few individuals can be catastrophic, particularly if it repeatedly happens when a predator attacks. However, individuals each with somewhat different tendencies provide flexibility along with predictability. Some individuals will be more aggressive than others. Some will take more chances. Some will be more compliant. Variability also has obvious advantages.

The Genetics of Human Personality

Our understanding of personality derives in part from behavioral genetics. Table 6.2 lists the strategies that behavioral geneticists use. Figure 6.3 displays the determinants of personality and the approximate strengths of each factor's contribution to personality individual differences. Human personality is a complex phenotype, and its structure results from interactions between genetic and environmental factors. Behavioral geneticists want to know how alike are persons based on the degree to which they share the same genes or the same environment, and how different are persons based on these factors, plus their own unique experiences (nonshared environment). For example, two sisters are reared together, receive the same parenting, and are exposed to the same family culture and mores. That represents shared environment. However, because they are 2 years apart in age, they go to different high schools because of redistricting. That represents their nonshared environment. If one sister also had a head injury, influenza, or toxin exposure, that too would be nonshared environment.

Genes can be either one big gene (nonadditive as in Huntington's disease) or a larger number of small genes with an additive effect (as in diabetes and some cancers). Genes are either monomorphic (only one normal form of the gene) or polymorphic (two normal forms like the classic Aa learned in a basic genetics course). Monomorphic genes account for 80% of the human genome. We all share them, and that is why we are all human. We are all much more alike in a fundamental biological way than we are different. Polymorphic genes (20% of the human genome) determine individual differences. Our monomorphic genes determine that we are all mammals, primates, hominids, bipedal, with the basic floor plan for a hand, a brain, and personality structure. Our polymorphic genes account for individual differences in these areas, including personality. Table 6.3 outlines present understanding of the genetics of personality. Table 6.4 lists behavioral traits with high (>40%) heritability.* Note that most of these traits reflect temperament.

Environmental Influences on Personality Development

Most of the nongenetic influences explaining personality differences are from nonshared, not shared, environmental experiences. Evidence for this is that (1) genetically unrelated children reared in the same family do not become more alike in personality than genetically unrelated children reared apart (i.e., there is no shared family environment effect); (2) biologic parents and their adopted away children are no more different in personality than biologic parents and the children living together; (3) dizygotic (DZ) twins reared together are no more similar in personality than DZ twins reared apart; and (4) monozygotic (MZ) twins reared together are no more similar in personality than MZ twins reared apart.

Experiences that are harmful to neural development (e.g., poor maternal nutrition or other gestational problems, ineffectual parenting or neglect, childhood exposure to toxins like lead, disease, head trauma, street drugs) can affect the neural

*Heritability refers to the contribution of genes to the character or behavior of interest; zero means no genetic influence, and 100% means all individual differences are due to genes.

TABLE 6.2. Behavioral Genetic Strategies

Strategy	Purpose
Studying large samples*	Permits analyses of small but meaningful differences, complex multiple interactions, clarification of patterns and subpatterns
Studying large or special pedigrees (a family tree of 200–1,000 individuals, or a family tree with sets of monozygotic [MZ] twins)	Helped identify the Huntington's gene; permits analyses of pattern of genetic transmission (e.g., dominant, recessive, mendelian, nonmendelian)
Assessing MZ and dizygotic (DZ) twins reared together and apart	To look for similarities and differences in personality based on degree of shared genes (100% MZ, 50% DZ) and what effect similar and different rearing has on this, e.g., does being reared together make twins more alike; does being reared apart make them more different?
Adoption studies	To see if adopted children's personalities are more like the personalities of the persons who reared them or more like their biologic relatives who have had no or little contact with them since birth
Cross-fostering studies	To see if the biologic children or the foster children living together and being reared by the same persons become more alike; or if the foster children become more like the rearing parents or their biologic parents
Model fitting	Tests types of genetic transmission, e.g., does the real family and pedigree data match (fit) hypothetical data based on a hypothesized mode of transmission (e.g., major gene, polygenic)
Gene mapping	To find the section(s) on specific chromosome(s) linked with the behavioral trait

*For example, the Virginia family study includes over 30,000 participants, the Colorado adoption study includes close to 500 families, and the Swedish twin registry has close to 13,000 twin pairs.

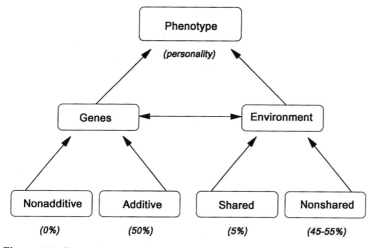

Figure 6.3. Determinants of personality.

TABLE 6.3. The Genetics of Human Personality

Conclusion	Some Evidence
Polygenic transmission is most likely	1. Model fitting and other analyses reject mendelian transmission
	2. Gene mapping has failed to identify a big gene
	3. In nonhumans, temperament breeding takes generations, indicating additive rather than just a few or one gene effect
	4. Most complex phenotypes like personality (e.g., insect eyes and mouth parts) are polygenic
	5. Most neuropsychiatric disorders with substantial heritability appear to be polygenic
Oligogenetic factors likely (i.e., genetic contribution from several sites, probably on different chromosomes, interacting or modifying each other)	1. Survivors of duplications (trisomy 21) and deletions (XO) do not differ much from normals in the big picture format of temperament dimensions
	2. Alzheimer's disease is an example of oligogenesis: at least four different chromosomes are involved in its expression
Monomorphic gene transmission likely	Similarities in personality structure and scores in populations across the planet

TABLE 6.4. Behavioral Traits With High Heritability

Aggressiveness

Altruism

Assertiveness

Constraint

Empathy

Harm avoidance

Impulsivity

Leadership

Nurturance

Persistence

Physicality

Reward dependence

Social closeness

Sociability

Traditionalism

Well-being

substrates of personality. Bad events in one's early life (e.g., parental divorce or death, abuse, chronic family-disrupting illness) are also likely to influence personality development. Bad events and disease may also contribute to deviant personality, but these factors do not explain individual differences among persons within the normal range of personality traits. Whereas bad parenting probably affects personality, adequate or good parenting does not substantially influence normal variations in personality development because differences are small in the way normal parents treat their different normal children. Surveys of parents and children suggest that normal parents treat their normal children similarly. The way siblings and peers treat each other, however, is typically perceived by them as substantially different and is likely to play a role in personality differences.

The above suggest the following:

1. Whatever shared environment contributes to individual differences in personality development, it does so early on (preschool) and it is minimal. The genetic contribution is much more important at this time, assuming normal family life.
2. Nonshared environmental influences (other than intrauterine and illness-related childhood factors) begin to play an increasingly important role as the child has more and more unique experiences (e.g., with playground and school peers, going to school).
3. Once past age 20–25 years, as the number and intensity of new unique experiences diminish (as we settle into life), nonshared environment plays less of a role and neural development is substantially complete.

Thus, after 20–25 years a person's basic personality is unlikely to dramatically change. Clinically this is important. What it means is that any dramatic change in personality after age 30–35 years is likely due to disease or injury. If you have a patient with such a change, always consider it a secondary condition until proven otherwise (see Table 6.1). It also means that if you want to make dramatic changes in a person's personality, you need to do so early on, certainly before age 30 and most likely in childhood or in the teens. Thus childhood, teenage, and young adult treatment programs have a better chance of altering a patient's personality than adult treatment programs. The goals for these programs should be different.

Other Influences on Personality

The neural systems for *emotion* and personality partially overlap (e.g., some personality dimensions relate directly to the limbic system's emotion-generating structures, but some personality dimensions do not). Normal mood states are experienced by persons with very different personalities. For example, you can be a very nasty person or a very nice person and still experience all the mood states. Personality, however, does interact with emotional systems, and temperament traits will influence emotional expression. For example, a person who is high on agreeableness and cooperation and who is outgoing will have a tendency to more often express positive emotions. A person who is low on these traits is more likely to express negative emotions.

Men and women have the same basic personality structure floor plan, and personality traits are normally contributed in both men and women. There are, however, modest gender differences, women tending to score higher on cooperativeness, and in the tendency to maintain behaviors that have resulted in external reinforcement (reward dependence).

There is also a modest interaction between intelligence and personality. The higher a person's intelligence, the lower his scores on personality measures of social conformity. Note, however, that smart people and not so smart people can both be nice or not so nice, outgoing or shy.

DSM PERSONALITY DISORDER

Table 6.5 displays the overall pattern of a DSM personality disorder.

Cluster A

Odd eccentric personality disorders are described in Table 6.6. *Paranoid personality disorder* may be a low-grade variant of delusional disorder and may occur with greater than expected frequency in the families of patients with delusional disorder. Evaluate these patients first for more specific neurologic disease. These include seizure disorder, small vascular malformations, and head injury. Evaluate for drug abuse next (particularly cocaine and inhalants). Treatments for these conditions are more specific and covered elsewhere in this text. If you cannot find these causes, consider a treatment trial with an anticonvulsant and, if that fails, an atypical neuroleptic. Interpersonally, be as nonjudgmental and nonthreatening in words and manner as possible, be nondirective and have limited goals (e.g., a place for the person to live, some funds, and job he is willing to take), and be careful. These patients can be dangerous.

Schizoid personality disorder is the classically described premorbid personality

TABLE 6.5. DSM General Criteria for a Personality Disorder

1. Long-lasting pattern of maladaptive behavior (beginning before age 20 years and ever present since then)
2. Maladaptive behavior in a broad range of personal and social areas
3. Specific areas involved include *cognition* (e.g., poor self-esteem), *affectivity* (e.g., moodiness, emotional outbursts), *interpersonal* (e.g., stormy relationships), and *impulse control* (e.g., suddenly quitting a job)
4. Maladaptive behaviors cause significant impairment in functioning, mating, the expectations of the person's sociocultural background, or subjective distress
5. Maladaptive behaviors cannot be attributed to some other psychiatric disorder (e.g., the person's emotional outbursts and low self-esteem are not due to mood disorder)

TABLE 6.6. Cluster A Personality Disorders: Odd-Eccentric Types

Personality Type	Description	Associated Findings
Paranoid	Distrustful and suspicious, unforgiving and bearing grudges, perceives threats where none exist, vengeful, emotionally aloof or irritable	1. < 1% lifetime population risk 2. Associated with delusional disorder, can be dangerous 3. Stereotype of militia, hate group member, isolated bomber or killer
Schizoid	Emotionally detached and aloof, decreased emotional expression, restricted interests, paucity of activities, sedentary, few friends	1. < 1% lifetime population risk 2. May be low-grade variant or prepsychotic stage of schizophrenia 3. Stereotype of socially awkward, isolated computer hacker
Schizotypal	Schizoid behaviors plus mild perceptual and thinking disturbances and odd ideas	1. 2%–3% lifetime population risk 2. Chronic low grade form of psychosis 3. Their perceptual disturbances, restricted emotional expression, and odd ideas make them like an avolitional version of the FBI agent in "The X-Files"

of schizophrenics. Persons with this rare condition are more likely to become psychotic if their reduced emotional expression is evident from childhood and is associated with the neuromotor and cognitive problems seen in the prepsychotic stage of schizophrenia (see Chapter 9). Schizoid persons who do not become psychotic may function well in situations where there is minimal intense interpersonal interactions and controlled sensory input (a similar need for some adults with mild to moderate autism or Asperger's syndrome). Children with schizoid personality disorder and other associated features benefit from cognitive and neuromotor rehabilitation and minimizing expressed emotion in their environment (also see Chapter 9). Adults with schizoid personality disorder who are concerned about their difficulties will benefit from education, counseling, and attention to their need for low-emotion job and living conditions. Emotionally intense psychological treatment may make these patients worse.

Schizotypal personality disorder is characterized by problems with *emotion* (decreased volition and expression, aloofness and poor interpersonal rapport, or irritability and hypervigilance); *perception* (illusions, dysmorphopsia and dysmegalopsia, depersonalization); *cognition* (missing the point of statements and questions and focusing on details); *ideation* (obsessive concerns with magic, paranormal phenomena, idiosyncratic religious notions, suspiciousness, and ideas of reference); and *behavior* (socially isolative and awkward, make suicidal threats). Persons with this condition may have abnormal eye pursuit, nonspecific EEG and evoked potential abnormalities, and magnetic resonance imaging and cognitive impairments similar to those seen in schizophrenics. They rarely become acutely psychotic. Compared with population rates (2%–3%, males and females equally affected), the morbid risk for schizotypal personality disorder is much higher (10%–15%) in the first-degree relatives of schizophrenics. It may also be higher in the families of some patients with psychotic bipolar mood disorder.

The differential diagnosis of schizotypal personality disorder includes drug abuse (hallucinogens), epilepsy, head injury, vascular malformations, and mood disorder. Look for these first. If not present, some schizoptypal patients will still respond to anticonvulsants or atypical antipsychotics. Focus your interactions with them on correcting misperceptions and odd ideas. Be straightforward, and do not argue if the patient persists in his odd beliefs.

Cluster B

Dramatic-emotional personality disorders are described in Table 6.7. *Antisocial personality disorder* occurs mostly in men. Eighty percent of male felons have antisocial personality disorder and provide the fodder for the stereotyped picture of the tattooed, cold, raspy-voiced psychopath. However, persons with antisocial personality disorder also wear three-piece suits and have traditional jobs. Their weapons are pens, calculators, computers, and administrative and business decisions. Sometimes they too get caught and go to jail. "Style" is less helpful in diagnosing these patients than is behavior. Antisocial persons are cold, callous, deceitful, and remorseless, and they disregard the rights of others. Look for a lifelong pattern of poor behavioral control, impulsivity, irresponsibility, a need for stimulation, and a proneness to boredom. Focus also on aggressive, nondrug-related antisocial childhood behavior and conduct disorder. One third of children with conduct disorder grow up to have antisocial personality disorder. Look for a history of truancy, school failure, and infidelity. Persons with antisocial personality disorder are also more likely as children to bed wet, set and play with fire, and torture animals.

Antisocial personality disorder is familial. Children of such persons who are adopted from birth still have a high risk for developing the condition. Children adopted by persons with antisocial traits, however, do not have a significant increase in their expression of antisocial traits unless their biologic parents also have antisocial traits. Children whose biologic *and* rearing parents both have antisocial traits are *most* likely to also express these traits. Thus, environment and genetic background act synergistically in the expression of antisocial behaviors.

It is rare to find a person over age 55 years who fully meets criteria for antisocial personality disorder. The explanations for this are that as persons age, drive and impulsivity lessen, and so these persons are less likely to get into trouble and thus no longer meet criteria for the disorder; and that the risk for death from violence and drugs and alcohol is high in antisocial persons, so many have not survived to age 55.

Antisocial personality disorder is co-morbid with *histrionic personality disorder* (and perhaps also *narcissistic personality disorder*). These behavior patterns may represent the same personality deviation expressed differently by gender. The evidence for this is (1) 25% of antisocial persons also meet criteria for histrionic personality disorder, and 25% of persons with histrionic personality meet criteria for

TABLE 6.7. Cluster B Personality Disorders: Dramatic-Emotional Types

Personality Type	Description	Associated Findings
Antisocial	Disregard for and the violation of the rights of others; nonconforming to social and legal norms; deceitful, impulsive, aggressive; reckless, irresponsible, remorseless craving for activity and excitement; irrational angry outbursts and tantrums; self-indulgent, vain	1. Lifetime risk 3% of males, 1% of females, but 90% of patients male 2. Associated with drug and alcohol abuse, criminality, violence, and the use of a weapon in fights; spouse and child abuse; sexual crime; somatization disorder; conversion disorder; ADHD; conduct disorder; IQ in 70–90 range; and histrionic personality disorder 3. The cold and callus criminal, lawyer, investment banker, doctor
Histrionic	Excessive emotionality and attention seeking; seductive, dramatic, suggestible; unstable, shallow emotions, and vague speech; exaggerated emotional expressions, self-dramatization and theatrical, craving for activity and excitement; irrational angry outbursts and tantrums; self-indulgent	1. 2%–3% lifetime population risk 2. Associated with somatization disorder, drug abuse, conversion disorder, non-melancholic depression often with dysphoria, and antisocial personality disorder 3. Stereotype of overly dramatic seductive actress/actor
Narcissistic	Grandiose sense of self-importance, sense of entitlement and need for excessive admiration, interpersonally exploitative, takes advantage of others, lacks empathy, has unstable relationships, is self-centered and self-absorbed	1. < 1% lifetime population risk, some overlap with histrionic personality disorder 2. Stereotype of "the Queen Bee"
Borderline	Unstable relationships; distorted self-image; unstable, overly reactive, and intense moods; impulsive, suicidal, self-mutilating, irritabile; lives life like a daytime soap opera	1. 2% lifetime population risk; 2. Associated with mood disorder 3. Other etiologies include drug abuse, head injury, epilepsy, other Cluster B personality disorders 4. Several soap-opera femme fetales rolled into one

antisocial personality disorder; (2) both personality disorders are associated with the same co-morbidities: drug and alcohol abuse, criminality, somatization disorder, conversion disorder, adjustment disorders, intermittent explosive disorder, and sexually transmitted disease; and (3) both personality disorders are familial and have the same family illness pattern: increased risk for antisocial personality and alcohol and drug abuse in males and histrionic personality disorder in females.

Unlike cluster A personality disorders, antisocial/histrionic/narcissistic disorders appear to be non-ill deviations. Other than diagnosis, education about the condition, and general supportive measures for histrionic and narcissistic persons, there are no treatments of demonstrated benefit. If the patient has a co-morbid condition, treat it. If the personality pattern develops after age 35 years, consider it secondary until proven otherwise, and look for head injury, substance abuse, traumatic brain injury, and seizure disorder as likely explanations.

Persons with antisocial or histrionic personality disorder are at greater risk to develop *somatoform disorders*. The DSM includes somatization (encompassing the concept of hysteria), conversion, hypochondriasis, pain disorder, body dysmorphic disorder, undifferentiated somatoform disorder, and somatoform disorder, not otherwise specified. Conversion, pain disorder, and body dysmorphic disorder are described in other chapters. Somatization disorder is described here because it does not appear to be a state of illness, but a consequence of having a Cluster B personality disorder.

Somatization disorder affects about 1%–2% of women and is uncommon in men unless they are seeking or receiving disability compensation. Ninety percent of patients are female. It is characterized by multiple, medically unexplained symptoms in multiple organ systems. Onset is usually in the early teens, or even in childhood, and virtually never begins after age 30. Symptoms fluctuate in intensity and content, but the syndrome appears permanent. The patient with a classic somatization disorder has a long history of medically unexplained complaints and multiple hospitalizations. Symptoms have to be severe enough to require seeing a physician, getting medicine (other than aspirin), or altering life style. Past physicians have typically dismissed complaints as "due to nerves" and have labeled the patient a "crank" or "hypochondriac." The patient is typically dramatic, suggestible, and impulsive. The initial physical examination and laboratory tests reveal no clear abnormalities.

Focus screening questions on vomiting (other than during pregnancy), amnesia, difficulty swallowing, painful menstruation, burning sensations in genitals, shortness of breath without exertion, and extremity pain. Two or more symptoms in men and three or more symptoms in women suggest somatization disorder.

Other complaints include unexplained *malaise* (e.g., feeling weak, easily fatigued); *conversion or pseudoneurologic features* (e.g., difficulty swallowing, loss of voice, deafness, fainting, trouble walking); *gastrointestinal problems* (e.g., abdominal pain, nausea, vomiting spells, diarrhea); *female reproductive difficulties* (e.g., painful or irregular menstruation, excessive bleeding); *psychosexual problems* (lifelong indifference, painful or lack of pleasurable intercourse, impotence, burning sensations in or around genitals); *chronic pain*; and *cardiopulmonary features* (e.g., shortness of breath, palpitations, chest pain, dizziness).

Somatization disorder is familial, occurring in 20% of first-degree relatives (mostly females) of somatization patients. These families also have increased risks for antisocial personality and alcoholism among male relatives. Persons with somatization disorder are more likely than others to marry people with antisocial personality or who abuse alcohol or street drugs. Adoptees whose biologic parents had antisocial personality have a greater than expected frequency of somatization. Somatization disorder is also associated with increased rates of conversion disorders, hospitalization, unnecessary surgery, and receiving polypharmacy. It is common among female felons (about 40%), particularly those with antisocial personality. Although persons with somatization disorder may express suicidal thoughts and make suicidal attempts, they rarely kill themselves.

There is no specific treatment for somatization disorder. Once you make the diagnosis, the following may help:

1. Education that somatization is a medical condition that may lower pain and other sensory thresholds, but the etiology is unknown (i.e., the symptoms are real and partially explainable)
2. Education that there is no specific medical treatment, but there are medical risks to avoid (e.g., seeing too many doctors, getting too many medications, having too many procedures), so one physician should become the primary care front door to medical treatments
3. Regular scheduled visits monitoring symptoms and focusing on the effects of symptoms on social and job functioning are better than as-needed visits, which reinforce symptom development
4. Assessing new symptoms because somatizers get sick too
5. Educating family members about the condition so they can help in limiting unneeded medical interventions while taking a more empathic attitude about the patient's complaints

Although part of Cluster B, *borderline personality disorder* appears to be distinct from the other types in this category. "Borderline" has always been the waste basket for psychiatric diagnosis, first for psychoses and now for persons who have stormy, emotional, disrupted lives and who are impulsive and self-destructive. Assume every patient with a borderline personality disorder diagnosis (even if you made it) to have something else until proven otherwise. An analogy is dementia. You make the syndromal diagnosis "dementia," and then you try to find out which one (e.g., Alzheimer's, vascular). So too for borderline. You make the syndromal diagnosis borderline, and then you try to find out which one. The differential diagnosis includes mood disorder, repeated acute drug-induced states, personality disorder secondary to drug abuse, head injury, epilepsy, vascular malformations, slow-growing anterior brain tumors (typically in the frontal poles or impinging on them), or one of the other Cluster B personality disorders. Borderline personality as a variant of mood disorder is further discussed in Chapter 8. Treat the primary condition. All patients also require respectful firmness, limit setting, and the patience of Job.

Cluster C

Anxious-fearful personality disorders are described in Table 6.8.

The subtyping of anxious-fearful personality disorder is unproven. A common theme for avoidant and dependent personality disorders is the person's tendency to inhibit behavior in novel or stressful situations. They are shy, tense, often dependent, worriers. Persons with obsessive compulsive personality disorder are also worriers, and may be shy, but they tend to over-control situations that are novel or stressful. For example, the shy anxious Cluster C person offered a skiing

TABLE 6.8. Cluster C Personality Disorders: Anxious-Fearful Types

Personality Type	Description	Associated Findings
Avoidant	Socially inhibited, feels inadequate, hypersensitive to criticism; avoids interpersonal contact and risks; views self as inept, inferior, and unappealing	1. 1% lifetime population risk 2. Associated with anxiety disorders, eating disorders, dissociative disorders, benzodiazepine abuse, nonmelancholic depression 3. The wall flower afraid to blossom
Dependent	Submissive, clinging, fearful of separation; indecisive, unassertive; low self-confidence, follower	1. < 1% lifetime population risk 2. Associated with same conditions as avoidant 3. The clinging vine that eventually is cut off or destroys the tree
Obsessive compulsive	Preoccupied with orderliness, perfectionism, and mental and interpersonal control; rigid, not open to new ideas, stubborn; miserly, hoarding; cannot delegate; overly conscientious; ethically scrupulous to the point of unreasonableness; workaholic, efficient	1. 1% lifetime population risk 2. Associated with anxiety disorders, nonmelancholic depression 3. Felix Unger in the "Odd Couple"

trip might avoid going by making excuses or procrastinating until it is too late. The obsessive compulsive personality person might try to over-plan the trip and prepare for any emergency no matter how improbable until no one, including the person, has a good time.

Cluster C personality disorder is familial, but only for the overall category, not for specific subtypes. Thus, a person with an avoidant personality disorder might have relatives with any of the other Cluster C subtypes, but not necessarily avoidant. Persons with Cluster C personality disorders often develop anxiety disorder and nonmelancholic depression. Some develop eating disorders, adjustment disorders, and obsessive compulsive disorder. They may self-medicate with alcohol and sedative-hypnotic drugs. Focus treatment on co-morbidities. Education and general support are helpful. Cognitive behavior therapy may help, but major changes in their pattern of behavior usually requires intervention during the teens or early adult life.

CLONINGER'S TEMPERAMENT AND CHARACTER DIMENSION MODEL OF PERSONALITY

The DSM personality disorder classification has obvious problems that complicate clinical care:

1. Although the personality disorders are supposed to represent non-disease deviations from normal personality, all of Cluster A and many persons in the borderline personality disorder category have brain dysfunction and thus have forms of illness, not deviations. Like cyclothymia before them, these disorders are in the wrong axis.

2. Forty to 60% of persons who meet criteria for one DSM personality disorder also meet criteria for others. Non-illness deviations tend to be in one direction (you are very tall or very short, you cannot be both), suggesting that the subgroups within each DSM cluster do not adequately delineate patients (i.e., the boundaries are behaviorally unclear).

3. Personality disorders, like normal personalities, are supposed to be stable over time (i.e., the personality disorder should not exacerbate and remit like a disease). Some patients in Cluster B, and some schizotypal persons, however, have unstable "personality disorders." That is, one year they meet DSM criteria and the next year they do not. This instability likely reflects an illness.

4. Persons who are clearly different on standard personality tests can, nevertheless, meet DSM criteria for the same personality disorder. For example, some impulsive persons who abuse drugs can meet criteria for antisocial personality disorder, but so too can cold, callous killers.

5. Other than some predictable co-morbidities and the disruptive behaviors for the specific personality disorder, the DSM personality disorder diagnosis does not predict other behavior or likely response to specific interventions, and it is unhelpful in giving you guidance for how to interact with the patient.

Because of these limitations, an alternative dimensional approach that has clinical applications is worth knowing and using. There are several different models of personality that use a dimensional approach (e.g., The Five Factor Model). Some centers assess personality dimensions using extroversion–introversion-related behaviors. The Minnesota Multiphasic Personality Inventory (MMPI) mixes state and trait behavior, but to some extent also measures dimensional behavior. The Temperament/Character Inventory (TCI system) is only one approach, but it fits well in a medical setting. Which dimensional approach you use is less important than using some dimensional measure of personality.

The Cloninger model uses a personality test with 240 true/false questions. Answers can be directly entered (by you or the patient) into a computer, which then gives you a printout of the patient's scores on each higher and lower order trait. It can also be scored by hand. The personality test is the TCI.

The TCI model is by no means thoroughly validated, but it has some practical advantages:

1. Scores on TCI character dimensions predict whether a person has a personality disorder. For example, very high on cooperativeness and very low on self-directedness (both character dimensions) indicate maladaptive dependency.

2. Scores on TCI temperament dimensions can be used to make DSM personality disorder diagnoses, so you do not lose anything by using the TCI system (see below)
3. Scores on TCI temperament dimensions can be used to predict other behaviors (e.g., drug and alcohol use, smoking, and other high risk behaviors). For example, high novelty seeking correlates with use of addicting drugs, including nicotine and caffeine. High harm avoidance predicts difficulty withdrawing from addicting drugs and in staying abstinent.
4. Scores on TCI temperament dimensions can be used to fine-tune the selection of antidepressant medication for the treatment of nonmelancholic major depression (see below).
5. Temperament and character scores can be used to guide treatment: maximizing compliance, aiding drug and alcohol abuse rehabilitation, shaping psychotherapy strategies (see below).

TABLE 6.9. High and Low Temperament Descriptions

Temperament Dimension	High Scores	Low Scores
Harm avoidance	Anxious and Worried	Uninhibited and Optimistic
	Worrying, cautious, inhibited, restrained, pessimistic, fatigable, easily dismayed and disgusted	Confident, uninhibited, risk-taking, optimistic, carefree, energetic
	Shy and Asthenic	Bold and Vigorous
	Fearful, doubtful, timid, easily fatigued, shy	Relaxed, self-assured, bold, daring, dauntless, vigorous
Novelty seeking	Impulsive	Orderly and Reflective
	Impulsive, exploratory, fickle, impressionistic, disorderly, extravagant	Indifferent, reflective, rigid, loyal, particular, orderly, frugal, and regimented
	Excitable	Stoic and Reserved
	Quick-tempered, excitable, curious, exuberant, enthusiastic, easily bored	Slow-tempered, stoical, uninquiring, inexuberant, unenthusiastic, tolerant
Reward dependence	Warm and Good Hearted	Cold and detached
	Loving, sensitive, warm, dedicated, sad if separated, attached,	Unfriendly, insensitive, cool, irresolute, indifferent
	Dependent	Independent
	Sad if separated, attached, dependent	Content if alone, practical, detached, independent
Persistence	Industrious	Lazy
	Industrious and diligent, hard-working, ambitious and overachieving, perseverative and perfectionistic	Inactive and indolent, gives up easily, modest and underachieving, quiting and pragmatic

The TCI system describes four temperament and three character dimensions. Each dimension is independently inherited, with about 60% of individual differences in temperament dimensions and 40% of individual differences in character dimensions due to genes. The interactions among these dimensions result in your personality.

Harm avoidance is the tendency to inhibit behavior when faced with novelty, punishment, or nonreward. Persons with high harm avoidance worry about the risks of contemplated action and so take no action. *Novelty seeking* is the tendency to initiate exploratory behavior, be curious about novel stimuli, and actively avoid punishment and frustrating nonreward. Persons with high novelty seeking are impulsive and engage in high risk behaviors like taking drugs. *Reward dependence* is the tendency to be conditioned and to maintain behaviors associated with reward and nonpunishment. Persons with high reward dependence spend a lot of time and energy pursuing social recognition, wealth, power, and fame. *Persistence* is the tendency to maintain behaviors despite no reward (e.g., stubbornness).

Self-directedness is the tendency to perceive reinforcement as the result of your own actions and to adapt your behavior to fit your goals. Persons with high self-directedness feel autonomous. *Cooperativeness* is the tendency to perceive reinforcement as the result of the responses of others and to identify with and accept other persons (i.e., to be part of "the group"). *Self-transcendence* is the tendency to perceive reinforcement as the result of forces outside your control (e.g., chance, fate, God), to have a belief system (e.g., God, religion, science, a chaotic universe), and to feel part of the natural order of things.

TABLE 6.10. High and Low Character Descriptions

Character Dimension	High Scores	Low Scores
Self-directedness	Reliable and resourceful	Immature
	Mature, strong, responsible, reliable, purposeful, resourceful, effective	Immature and fragile, habits incongruent with long-term goals
	Self-accepted	Unreliable
	Self-accepting, habits congruent with long-term goals	Uneliable, purposeless, inert and ineffective, self-striving
Cooperativeness	Empathic and Tolerant	Intolerant and Critical
	Socially tolerant, empathic, helpful, compassionate and constructive, ethical and principled	Socially intolerant, critical, unhelpful, revengeful and destructive, opportunistic
Self-transcendence	Unconventional	Conventional
	Wise and patient, creative, self-forgetful, united with universe, absentminded, unconventional	Impatient, unimaginative and self-conscious, prideful and lacking humility, conventional, prosaic

TABLE 6.11. Screening for Personality Temperament and Character Dimensions

HARM AVOIDANCE

Do you think of yourself as a nervous person?

Are you the kind of person who worries a lot? Who always sees the possible dangers in doing something, even when other people think everything will be just fine?

Are you a very cautious person?

Do you or others think of you as a timid or very shy person?

Do you or others think of you as a calm, confident person?

Are you a risk-taker?

NOVELTY SEEKING

Are you someone who likes to do new and exciting things, even if there is a modest amount of risk in it? (Examples: white water rafting, rock climbing, traveling to unusual places)

Do you generally think things through before acting, or are you more likely to just do it?

Are you an enthusiastic, energetic person?

Are you quick tempered and excitable?

Are you a neat person?

Are you the kind of person who saves money, or do you spend it when you can?

REWARD DEPENDENCE

Do people think of you as a friendly, sensitive person?

Do you prefer being with friends or family rather than being alone?

Tables 6.9 and 6.10 display the behavioral descriptors of the temperament and character dimensions, respectively. The subheadings in Tables 6.9 and 6.10 reflect "lower order" traits that may eventually help characterize personality subgroups.

In assessing a patient's personality, you could administer the TCI (takes about 30 minutes) or put the descriptors in Tables 6.9 and 6.10 into questions, such as "Are you the kind of person who . . . ?" Table 6.11 lists some questions you might incorporate into your clinical examination for assessing personality. You could formulate additional questions if needed. Questions for self-transcendence are not included because this dimension is clinically useful only within the overall formal TCI analysis. As with all measures of personality, the patient's present behavioral state can influence self-report. For the TCI, harm avoidance is moderately elevated during depressions, whereas the other higher order dimensions are minimally affected.

The TCI system is also based on our present understanding of the brain's behavioral systems. Table 6.12 displays these systems and their association with the TCI temperament dimensions of harm avoidance, novelty seeking, and reward

TABLE 6.11. (*continued*)

Are you a sentimental person?

Do you like to be independent, work on your own, etc., or do you prefer to do things with a group of friends or co-workers?

PERSISTENCE

Do you or others think of you as a perfectionist?

Are you the kind of person who gives up easily?

When things get tough, are you likely to work harder or do you try to do something else?

Do people think of you as stubborn?

Are you a hard worker?

SELF-DIRECTEDNESS

Do you think people count on you a lot to solve problems for them?

Are you the kind of person who "gets the job done," who is very resourceful and can figure out ways to solve problems?

Do you think of yourself, or do people think of you, as a reliable person?

COOPERATIVENESS

Do you get upset with people who have different political or religious opinions than you?

When you hear about natural disasters or accidents with injuries, do you feel almost physically bad for the victims?

If people do you a bad turn, will you go out of your way to get even?

Do you prefer spending your free time helping other people, like doing community service or charity work, or do you think that kind of stuff is overrated?

dependence. High novelty seeking is associated with low baseline dopamine activity within the brain's hedonistic reward system, which partially explains why persons with this trait tend to use dopamine-enhancing drugs. High harm avoidance is associated with high baseline serotonin turnover in the brain's flight/fight system, which partially explains why these persons are anxious-fearful and self-medicate with antianxiety medications. High reward dependence is associated with low baseline norepinephrine activity in the brain's homeostasis system, leading to resistance to extinguish behavior.

HOW TO USE THE TCI SYSTEM

Assessment

You need to assess personality because trait behavior substantially influences long-term management. If you choose to use the TCI system to do this, first con-

TABLE 6.12. Neural Systems Subserving Personality Temperament Dimensions

	Behavioral Activation (Novelty Seeking)	Behavioral Inhibition (Harm Avoidance)	Behavioral Maintenance (Reward Dependence)
Principle monoamine neuromodulator	Dopamine	Serotonin	Norepinephrine
Neural networks	Reward/Pleasure system	Flight/Fight system	Homeostasis system
	Premotor and anterior cingulate	Neocortex	Neocortex
	Amygdala/hippocampus	Basal nucleus of Meynert	Ventral tegmental area
	Nucleus accumbens and ventral striatum	Nigrostriatal nucleus Septal-hippocampal system and habenula	Pontine locus ceruleus
	Ventral tegmental area	Ventral tegmental area	Hypothalamus, limbic system
	Reticular activating system	Brain stem raphe nuclei	
Relevant stimuli	Novelty	Conditioned signals for punishment, novelty, or frustrative nonreward	Conditioned signals for reward or relief of punishment
	Potential reward		
	Potential relief of monotony or punishment		
Behavioral response	Exploratory pursuit	Passive avoidance, extinction	Resistance to extinction
	Appetitive approach		
	Active avoidance, escape		
Physiologic response	Increased heart rate	Increased baseline, physiologic arousal	Reduced habituation (responds to tenth stimulus as if it were the first one)
	Decreased sensation threshold, increased pain perception		
Drug stimuli	Agonists: amphetamine, and cocaine	Benzodiazepines and other GABA-related agents	Blocker: Alpha$_2$ presynaptic agonists (clonidine)
	Facilitators: Alcohol, opiates, opioid neuropeptides	Serotonin reuptake inhibitors	
	Blockers: Neuroleptics		

sider the patient's cooperativeness and self-directedness. Extremes on these dimensions make it highly probable that the patient has a personality disorder. If you use the formal TCI computer version it will tell you the probability in a percentage (e.g., this person has 87% probability of having a personality disorder). Once you decide a patient is likely to have a personality disorder, focus on the temperament dimensions. The patterns listed in Table 6.13 correlate with the DSM system. The TCI also provides information about how the patient answers questions, particularly consistency of answers, thus identifying lying or the patient's "blind spots" about his behavior.

Predictive Co-morbidities

Predictive co-morbidities can help explain why some axis I and II conditions co-occur. The TCI pattern for Cluster B tells us that the primary reason persons get

TABLE 6.13. TCI Temperament Patterns and DSM Axis II

	TCI Temperament Pattern		
DSM Diagnosis	Novelty Seeking	Harm Avoidance	Reward Dependence
CLUSTER A			
Schizoid	Low	Low	Low
Schizotypal*	?	?	?
Paranoid*	?	?	?
CLUSTER B			
Antisocial	High	Low	Low
Histrionic	High	Low	High
Narcissistic	High	Low	Low or average
Borderline	High	High	Average
Borderline†	Low	High	Low
CLUSTER C			
Dependent	Low	High	High
Avoidant	Low	High	High
Obsessive	Low	High	Low

*Never been studied because most investigators assume these to be low-grade forms of illness.

†Because borderline is a mixed group, different TCI patterns are likely. One study found two patterns, the first associated with dysphoric explosive behavior and drug abuse and the second with anxiety or nonmelancholic depression.

these diagnoses is because of their high novelty-seeking behaviors. Low reward dependence in both narcissistic and antisocial persons explains why they often disregard social conventions and cues and violate the rights of others. Their high novelty seeking explains why they are prone to using stimulant drugs, including caffeine and nicotine. High novelty seeking and high harm avoidance, two incompatible behavioral patterns, explains why the lives of some borderlines are in such turmoil.

The TCI pattern in Cluster C tells us that the primary reasons persons get these diagnoses is because of their high harm avoidance coupled with low novelty seeking. Their untempered high harm avoidance makes them prone to anxiety disorders and obsessive compulsive disorder syndromes.

Management of Comorbid Drug and Alcohol Abuse

Drug and alcohol abuse have several determinants (see Chapter 13). Among factors to consider when treating these patients is their personality. For example, the likelihood of smoking increases with increasing novelty seeking. Remaining addicted to nicotine increases with increasing harm avoidance. Low reward dependence and persistence make continued smoking more likely.

The High Novelty-Seeking Drug Abuser

More specifically, a person with high novelty seeking and low or normal harm avoidance is likely to try and perhaps continue to use dopaminergic drugs. Treatment of high novelty-seeking drug abusers includes treating craving with dopaminergic drugs (e.g., bupropion [see Chapter 13 for details]); and modifying the patient's environment to minimize drug-related high risk situations (which stimulate high novelty-seeking persons), minimizing routine (perceived as frustrating nonreward and leading to active avoidance such as drug taking), and maximizing nondrug-related novelty (e.g., giving the patient a socially acceptable outlet).

High novelty-seeking drug abusers who also have low harm avoidance and low reward dependence are likely to be impulsive noncompliers and relapse. Persons with high harm avoidance will be fearful of withdrawal or the social difficulties without the drug for "support," and a serotonin reuptake-inhibiting antidepressant may ameliorate this tendency during the 2–4-month withdrawal period. Drug abusers with normal or high reward dependence have a better prognosis because they are more likely to establish a good doctor–patient relationship with you.

Character traits also affect treatment for drug abuse: Normal or high cooperativeness and normal or low self-directedness help the doctor–patient relationship in the short run because the patient will likely become dependent on you rather than on the drug. Low cooperativeness and high self-directedness are bad prognostic signs because such a person is likely to be a noncomplier.

The relationships among the temperament and character traits in the high novelty-seeking drug abuser apply whether the drug is cocaine, alcohol, or nicotine or caffeine.

The High Harm Avoidance Drug Abuser

High harm avoidance is associated with chronic anxiety and worry. Such persons are at risk for self-medicating with alcohol or anxiety-reducing drugs. When in an abusive relationship with a drug or alcohol abuser, they are prone to join in the drug use to forestall physical abuse (i.e., accepting the lesser of two evils). If the patient is self-medicating, look for anxiety disorder (see Chapter 15) or depression (see Chapter 7) and treat for these. Detoxification may also require a serotonin reuptake-inhibiting antidepressant. Craving should be minimal if novelty seeking is normal or low. If novelty seeking is high, the person is likely to meet criteria for borderline personality, and the strategies described above may help.

If the person with high harm avoidance is in an abusive relationship and is also abusing drugs, physical removal from the abusive environment and establishing an initially dependent relationship with a nurturing caregiver are essential for the treatment of the drug abuse. The person's degree of cooperativeness and self-directedness will also affect outcome.

The High Reward Dependence Drug Abuser

Drug and alcohol abuse in persons with high reward dependence is uncommon unless the person lives in a substance abusing subculture, like a gang. Removal from the drug-related environment at an early age provides the best chance for these persons.

Management of Co-morbid Depression

There is modest evidence that you may increase the number of persons with non-melancholic depression responding well to antidepressants if you choose antidepressants not only because of their side effect profile but also for their interaction with personality. Table 6.14 lists your choices based on the TCI system modified by empirical studies evaluating the efficacy of this approach (see Additional Readings).

Management of Psychotherapy

The most important factor in psychotherapy is the doctor–patient relationship. Table 6.15 displays some patterns of personality and how they may influence your interactions with a patient. All the possible combinations of temperament patterns and how they influence each other cannot be listed here. Think of Table 6.15 as a diagram for guidance only.

TABLE 6.14. Temperament and Antidepressant Response

Temperament Pattern	Suggested Choices
DEPENDENT/AVOIDANT	
High harm avoidance and high reward dependence; novelty seeking low	Venlafaxine first choice (working on both norepinephrine and serotonin), desipramine second choice
High reward dependence only	Desipramine or venlafaxine; clomipramine second choice in women
OBSESSIONAL	
High harm avoidance only; other temperaments normal to low	An SSRI*
BORDERLINE	
High harm avoidance and high novelty seeking, normal reward dependence (irritable/explosive)	Desipramine (in women), bupropion, a combination of bupropion and an SSRI
High harm avoidance only	An SSRI
HISTRIONIC	
High novelty seeking, low harm avoidance, average to high reward dependence	Bupropion, desipramine second choice
NARCISSISTIC	
High novelty seeking, low harm avoidance, average or low reward dependence	Bupropion, desipramine
ANTISOCIAL	
High novelty seeking only	Bupropion, desipramine
NORMAL PERSONALITY	
All dimensions average	Choice based on other factors such as side effects, previous response, and co-morbidities

*SSRI, specific serotonin reuptake-inhibiting antidepressants.

TABLE 6.15. Personality Dimensions and Psychotherapy

Personality Pattern	Effect	Suggested Approach
Self-directedness high, co-operativeness low, reward dependence low	The continuous noncomplier	Any success depends on your ability to get the patient to think treatment goals were his ideas, not yours
High novelty seeking	The impulsive noncomplier	Success depends on other temperament and character dimensions
Low self-directedness, high cooperativeness and high reward dependence	The dependent patient	Use these maladaptive extremes to get the patient dependent on you and to comply with all treatments needed for axis I and any general medical problems; then try to wean the patient using the rehabilitation model where you are the crutch and habitual, adaptive, independent behavior the walking without the crutch; slowly expose the patient to increasing doses of decision making (start with little things like what to wear) strongly reinforce successes and minimize failures
High harm avoidance	Noncomplier when drug side effects occur	Choose drug wisely
		Go slow with doses
		Use other dimensions to keep patient on medication
		Response best reliever of anxiety about side effects
High novelty seeking and high harm avoidance	Irritable/explosive	Refuse to fight
		Do not miss appointments or be late or give any other signs of rejection or abandonment
		Use other personality strengths

ADDITIONAL READINGS

Andrews G, Neilson M, Hunt C, Stewart G, Kiloh LG: Diagnosis, personality and the long-term outcome of depression. *Br J Psychiatry* 157:13–18, 1990.

Bagby RM, Parker JDA, Joffe RT: Confirmatory factor analysis of the Tridimensional Factor Analysis of the Tridimensional Personality Questionnaire. *Pers Indiv Differ* 13:1245–1246, 1992.

Barash D: *The Whisperings Within: Evolution and the Origin of Human Nature.* Harper and Row, New York, 1979.

Benjamin J, Li L, Patterson C, Greenberg BD, Murphy DL, Hamer DH: Population and familial association between the D4 dopamine receptor gene and measures of novelty seeking. *Nat Genet* 12:81–84, 1996.

Berns GS, Cohen JD, Mintun MA: Brain regions responsive to novelty in the absence of awareness. *Science 276*:1272–1275, 1997.

Brown SL, Svrakic DM, Przybeck TR, Cloninger CR: The relationship of personality to mood and anxiety state: A dimensional approach. *J Psychiatr Res 26*:197–211, 1992.

Cadoret RJ: Psychopathology in adopted-away offspring of biological parents with antisocial behavior. *Arch Gen Psychiatry 35*:176–184, 1978.

Cadoret RJ, Troughton E, Bagford J, Woodworth G: Genetic and environmental factors in adoptee antisocial personality. *Eur Arch Psychiatry Neurol Sci 239*:231–240, 1990.

Cadoret RJ, Yates WR, Troughton E, Woodworth G, Stewart MA: Genetic–environmental interaction in the genesis of aggressivity and conduct disorders. *Arch Gen Psychiatry 52*:916–924, 1995.

Cloninger CR: A unified biosocial theory of personality and its role in the development of anxiety states. *Psychiatr Dev 3*:167–226, 1986.

Cloninger CR: A systematic method for clinical description and classification of personality variants: A proposal. *Arch Gen Psychiatry 44*:573–588, 1987.

Cloninger CR: Brain networks underlying personality development. In Carroll BJ, Barett JE (eds): *Psychopathology and the Brain*. American Psychopathological Association Series. Raven Press, New York, 1991, pp 183–208.

Cloninger CR, Bohman M, Sigvardsson S: Inheritance of alcohol abuse. Cross-fostering analysis of adopted men. *Arch Gen Psychiatry 38*:861–868, 1981.

Cloninger CR, Przybeck TR, Svrakic DM, Wetzel RD: TCI: *The temperament* and *Character Inventory (TCI): A Guide To Its Development and Use*. Washington University Center for Psychobiology of Personality, St. Louis, 1994.

Cloninger CR, Svrakic DM, Przybeck TR: A psychobiological model of temperament and character. *Arch Gen Psychiatry 50*:975–990, 1993.

Coccaro EF, Bergeman CJ, McClearn GE: Heritability of heritable impulsiveness: A study of twins reared together and apart. *Psychiatr Res 48*:229–242, 1993.

Condray R, Steinhauer SR: Schizotypal personality disorder in individuals with and without schizophrenic relatives: Similarities and contrasts in neurocognitive and clinical functioning. *Schizophr Res 7*:33–41, 1992.

Costa PT Jr, McCrae RR: *The NEO Personality Inventory Manual*. Psychological Assessment Resources, Odessa, FL, 1985.

Costa PT Jr, McCrae RR: Personality in adulthood: A six-year longitudinal study of self-reports and spouse ratings on the NEO Personality Inventory. *J Pers Soc Psychol 54*:853–863, 1988.

Costa PT Jr, McCrae RR: *NEO-PI/NEO-FFI Manual Supplement*. Psychological Assessment Resources, Odessa, FL, 1989.

Costa PT, Widiger TA (eds): *Personality Disorders and the Five-Factor Model of Personality*. American Psychological Association, Washington, DC, 1994.

Earleywine M, Finn PR, Peterson JB, Pihl RO: Factor structure and correlates of the Tridimensional Personality Questionnaire. *J Stud Alcohol 53*:233–238, 1992.

Ebstein RP, Novick O, Umansky R, Priel B, Osher Y, Blaine D, Bennet ER, Nemanov L, Katz M: Dopamine D4 receptor (D4DR) exon III polymorphism associated with the human personality trait of novelty seeking. *Nat Genet 12*:78–80, 1996.

Eysenck HJ: *The Biological Basis of Personality*. Charles C Thomas, Springfield, IL, 1967.

Eysenck HJ, Eysenck SBG: *Manual of the Eysenck Personality Questionnaire*. University of London Press, London, 1975.

Gunderson JG, Elliot GR: The interface between borderline personality disorder and affective illness. *Am J Psychiatry 142*:277–288, 1985.

Gunderson JG, Silver LJ: Relatedness of schizotypal to schizophrenic disorders. Editor's Introduction. *Schizophr Bull 11*:532–537, 1985.

Guze SB: Genetics of Briquet's syndrome and somatization disorder: A review of family, adoption and twin studies. *Ann Clin Psychiatry 5*:225–230, 1993.

Hellman DS, Blackman N: Enuresis, firesetting and cruelty to animals: A triad predictive of adult crime. *Am J Psychiatry* 123:1431–1435, 1966.

Heinz A, Dufeu P, Kuhn S, Dettling M, Graf K, Kurten I, Rommelspacher H, Schmidt LG: Psychological and behavioral correlates of dopaminergic sensitivity in alcohol-dependent patients. *Arch Gen Psychiatry* 53:1123–1128, 1996.

Hesselbrock MN, Hesselbrock VM: Relationship of family history, antisocial personality disorder and personality traits in young men at risk for alcoholism. *J Stud Alcohol* 53:619–625, 1992.

Joyce PR, Mulder RT, Cloninger KR: Temperament predicts clomipramine and desipramine response in major depression. *J Affect Disord* 30:35–46, 1994.

Kendler KS, Gruenberg AM: Genetic relationship between paranoid personality disorder and the "schizophrenic spectrum" disorders. *Am J Psychiatry* 135:1185–1186, 1982.

Kendler KS, McGuire M, Gruenberg AM, Walsh D: Schizotypal symptoms and signs in the Roscommon family study: Their factor structure and familial relationship with psychotic and affective disorders. *Arch Gen Psychiatry* 52:296–303, 1995.

Kilbey MM, Breslau N, Andreski P: Cocaine use and dependence in young adults: Associated psychiatric disorders and personality traits. *Drug Alcohol Depend* 29:283–290, 1992.

Kinzey W (ed): *The Evolution of Human Behavior: Primate Models.* State University of New York Press, Albany, 1987.

Knutson B, Wolkowitz OM, Cole SW, Chan T, Moore EA, Johnson RC, Terpstra J, Turner RA, Reus VI: Selective alteration of personality and social behavior by serotonergic intervention. *Am J Psychiatry* 155:373–379, 1998.

Lilienfeld SO, Van Valkenburg C, Larntz K, Akiskal HS: The relationship of histrionic personality disorder to antisocial personality and somatization disorders. *Am J Psychiatry* 143:718–722, 1986.

Livesley WJ, Jang KL, Jackson DN, Vernon PA: Genetic and environmental contributions to dimensions of personality disorder. *Am J Psychiatry* 150:1826–1831, 1993.

Livesley WJ, Jang KL, Vernon PA: Phenotypic and genetic structure of traits delineating personality disorder. *Arch Gen Psychiatry* 55:941–948, 1998.

Lyons MJ, True WR, Eisen SA, Goldberg J, Meyer MJ, Faraone SV, Eaves LJ, Tsuang MT: Differential heritability of adult and juvenile antisocial traits. *Arch Gen Psychiatry* 52:906–915, 1995.

Meszaros K, Willinger U, Fischer G, Schonbeck G, Aschauer HN: On behalf of the European Fluroxamine in Alcoholism Study Group, The Tridimensional Personality Model: Influencing variables in a sample of detoxified alcohol dependents. *Comp Psychiatry* 37:109–114, 1996.

Mulder R: The biology of personality. *Austr NZ J Psychiatry* 26:364–376, 1992.

Nixon SJ, Parsons OA: Cloninger's Tridimensional Theory of Personality: Construct validity in a sample of college students. *Pers Indiv Differ* 12:1261–1267, 1989.

Nixon SJ, Parsons OA: Application of the Tridimensional Personality Questionnaire to a population of alcoholics and other substance abusers. *Alcoholism Clin Exp Res* 14:513–517, 1990.

Pervin LA (ed): *Handbook of Personality: Theory and Research.* Guilford Press, New York, 1990.

Pfohl B, Black D, Noyes R Jr, Kelley M, Blum N: A test of the Tridimensional Personality Theory: Association with diagnosis and platelet imipramine binding in obsessive-compulsive disorder. *Biol Psychiatry* 28:41–46, 1990.

Ploman R, Bergeman CS: The nature of nurture: Genetic influence on "environmental" measures. *Behav Brain Sci* 14:373–427, 1991.

Pomerleau CS, Pomerleau OF, Flessland KA, Basson SM: Relationship of Tridimensional Personality Questionnaire scores and smoking variables in female and male smokers. *J Substance Abuse* 4:143–154, 1992.

Reich J, Yates W, Nguaguba M: Prevalence of DSM-III personality disorders in the community. *Soc Psychiatry Psychiatr Epidemiol* 24:12–16, 1989.

Roitman SEL, Cornblatt BA, Bergman A, Obuchowski M, Mitropoulou V, Keefe RSE, Silverman JM, Siever LJ: Attentional functioning in schizotypal personality disorder. *Am J Psychiatry 154:*655–660, 1997.

Ruchkin VV, Eisemann M, Hagglof B, Cloninger CR: Interrelations between temperament, character, and parental rearing in male delinquent adolescents in northern Russia. *Compr Psychiatry 39:*225–230, 1998.

Rutherford MJ, Alterman AI, Cacciola JS, Snider EC: Gender differences in diagnosing anti-social personality disorder in methadone patients. *Am J Psychiatry 152:*1309–1316, 1995.

Scarr S, McCartney K: How people make their own environments: A theory of geno-type–environment effects. *Child Dev 54:*424–435, 1983.

Schuckit MA, Klein J, Twitchell G, Smith T: Personality test scores as predictors of alco-holism almost a decade later. *Am J Psychiatry 151:*1038–1042, 1994.

Siever LJ: Biological markers in schizotypal personality disorder. *Schizophr Bull 11:*564–574, 1985.

Strakowski SM, Dunayevich E, Keck PE, McElroy SL: Affective state dependence of the Tridimensional Personality Questionnaire. *Psychiatr Res 57:*209–214, 1995.

Strakowski SM, Faedda GL, Tohen M, Goodwin DC, Stoll AL: Possible affective-state de-pendence of the Tridimensional Personality Questionnaire in first-episode psychosis. *Psychiatry Res 41:*215–226, 1997.

Svrakic DM, Przybeck TR, Cloninger CR: Mood states and personality traits. *J Affect Disord 24:*217–226, 1992.

Svrakic DM, Whitehead C, Przybeck TR, Cloninger CR: Differential diagnosis of personal-ity disorders by the seven-factor model of temperament and character. *Arch Gen Psychi-atry 50:*991–999, 1993.

Swanson MCJ, Bland RC, Newman SC: Antisocial personality disorders. *Acta Psychiatr Scand (Suppl 376):*63–70, 1994.

Torgersen S: Relationship of schizotypal personality disorder to schizophrenia: Genetics. *Schizophr Bull 11:*554–563, 1985.

Tyrer P, Seivewritht, Ferguson B, Tyrer J: The general neurotic syndrome: A coaxial diagno-sis of anxiety, depression, and personality disorder. *Acta Psychiatr Scand 85:*201–206, 1992.

Western D, Arkowitz-Western L: Limitations of axis II in diagnosing personality pathology in clinical practice. *Am J Psychiatry 155:*1767–1771, 1998.

7

Depression

Depression is common, affecting about 10% of adults in any one year. About 8% of women and 4% men are at lifetime risk for severe depression, and an additional 10% (about 15% overall) are at risk for less severe forms (e.g., adjustment disorders). Depression affects all social classes and all ethnic groups and Western and non-Western societies. Most first depressions occur after puberty and before age 60 years, although childhood depression occurs and is of major clinical concern. The incidence (new cases) of depression increases in persons born more recently (period effect). The age of onset of the first depression is also getting younger (cohort effect). Thus, depression is more common in persons born in the last several decades than in persons born before World War II, and these depressions are occurring for the first time when people are younger. The explanations for these effects are unclear. About 15%–20% of private psychiatric hospital patients and about 10% of public psychiatric hospital patients are admitted for depression. Melancholia affects about 2% of the general population and represents about 20% of all depressions.

Depression is familial with modest heritability when unipolar and with substantial heritability when bipolar. Unipolar patients only have depressions. Bipolar disorders are characterized by a past or present manic or hypomanic episode or long-standing problems with fluctuating moods some of which are elation, excitement, or irritability. Even if a patient experiences only manias and never a depression, the diagnosis is still bipolar. Ninety percent of depressions are unipolar. No longer an official term, *unipolar disorder* is still widely used by clinicians, and it is less cumbersome than the DSM term *major recurrent depression.*

Whenever you suspect depression—the patient looks or acts sad or gloomy, says he is feeling blue or pessimistic about life—your most important clinical question is, "Is this patient suffering from a clinical depression (as opposed to worry or demoralization), and if so, is this clinical depression melancholia or one of the other depressive syndromes?" All treatments and management, all predictions about co-morbid (co-occurring) illnesses or conditions, and all prognostic speculations about depression depend on the answers to these questions because patients with clinical depressions need medical treatment, whereas there are no pills for demoralization and worry.

Symptoms of depression occur in healthy persons in sad circumstances. Many depressed persons have stormy lives during the year of a depression, and stressful events can trigger the depression just as they can trigger, exacerbate, or make a person more prone to many general medical conditions (e.g., stroke, diabetes, infection). Sometimes, however, the moody, irritable early stages of depression lead to interpersonal or job difficulties and a stormy life, and, when the depression unfolds fully, it appears to be precipitated by the stressful events when in fact it caused those events. Only the quality and intensity of the mood state itself helps discriminate depressive illness from worry, demoralization, or bereavement. Determine the mood state using the following clinical rule: The patient has a clinical depression that requires medical treatment if he perceives his mood state to be out of the ordinary, or different from normal sadness or worry *and* he has problems with mood (tearfulness, apprehension, irritability, gloominess), *sleep*, and *cognitive* or *interpersonal functioning* (problems concentrating, loss of interest, feeling pessimistic or helpless, declining function at work, and trouble with family, friends, or employers because of the mood state).

If the patient does not have a clinical depression, but is upset, then brief counseling (clarifying issues, helping setting goals, permitting the patient to "get it off his chest," offering limited advice) may be helpful. If the patient is clinically depressed he requires more specific treatment, and then your clinical concern becomes "Is this clinical depression melancholia or one of the other types of depression?" These "other" choices are major depression without melancholic features, dysthymia, abnormal bereavement, adjustment disorder depressed type, and atypical depression. Although the DSM lists all these nonmelancholic depressions separately, as if distinct illnesses, they have many clinical features in common, and they respond to similar treatments.

CLINICAL PRESENTATION OF DEPRESSIONS

Two clinical features discriminate the two depression groupings: the quality and variability of mood and vegetative signs. Both groupings of depression are associated with feelings of hopelessness, worthlessness, pessimism, and loss of interest, although these tend to be more severe and are sometimes delusional in melancholics. Sometimes the clinical picture is unclear, and it is difficult to decide which type of depression the patient has. Melancholic features take precedent. Thus, no matter how many features of nonmelancholic depression a patient has, if he also has the mood or vegetative signs of melancholia, make that diagnosis and treat for melancholia.

MELANCHOLIA

Mood

The cardinal feature of melancholia is an unremitting, often profound relentless feeling of unnatural gloominess, apprehension, or despair that pervades all mental activity and colors all mental content. When associated with irritability, this mood combination is termed *dysphoria*. The melancholic mood is autonomous from environmental stimuli. It will not "lift" under cheery or lively circumstances, although it may have a rhythmicity of its own (diurnal mood), becoming less intense in the late afternoon or early evening and worse in the early morning. Melancholics do not have "good days." They are anhedonic, that is, they cannot enjoy those things that usually gave them pleasure (e.g., sex, food, hobbies, interests). They appear worried or overwhelmed and mentally "confused" (i.e., unable to think, remember, concentrate). They say they feel different from normal sadness. Even the most minor of daily tasks becomes an unsurmountable burden.

Intense apprehension and self-doubt cause agitation: hand-wringing, pacing, rocking, perseverative rubbing away of skin of the forehead or fingers, or constant questioning and asking for reassurance. Melancholics look worried, apprehensive, frightened, unsure, and lost. Reduced physiologic arousal (psychomotor retardation) can become stupor.

Melancholics rarely complain of "depression." Typical chief complaints include loss of energy, fatigue and disinterest, insomnia, problems concentrating or thinking, problems with sexual performance (males), and problems functioning at work. Patients also complain of ruminations (unrealistic worries about their health, finances, how bad they are, how they might hurt loved ones). Family members may complain that the sufferer is "not himself," is preoccupied, moody, slowed down, no longer animated or with good humor, is not eating, not sleeping, and is talking about death. Complaints about crying are uncommon. Most melancholics have lost their tears. Table 7.1 displays a simplified version of DSM-IV criteria for major depression with melancholic features.

Vegetative Signs

"Vegetative" signs reflect dysfunction in the autonomic and neuroendocrine systems controlled by the hypothalamus. They include alterations in circadian (diur-

TABLE 7.1. Diagnostic Criteria for Primary Melancholia*

A. Profound, unremitting, autonomous mood change characterized by unnatural sadness, apprehension, or dysphoria and a pervasive loss of pleasure

B. Three of the following:
1. Anorexia with a loss of more than 5% of body weight in 3 weeks
2. Insomnia with early morning waking (at least 2 hours before usual time of awakening)
3. Distinct quality of mood different from sadness due to everyday events
4. Diurnal mood swing, worse in the morning.
5. Psychomotor retardation or agitation
6. Feelings of guilt, hopelessness, or worthlessness

C. Not explained by other neurologic or general medical condition and not due to drug or alcohol use

*All criteria must be met.

nal) rhythms that affect the sleep–wake cycle (loss of stage IV sleep and difficulty staying asleep), body temperature (high rather than low in early morning, associated with morning sweats), the menstrual cycle (oligo- and amenorrhea), and libido (reduced). Appetite is decreased, and weight loss is typical. Gastrointestinal secretions and motility are impaired. Resting heart rate is increased. Twenty-four hour cortisol levels are elevated, cortisol peak shifting to the early morning nighttime hours (about 1–2 AM) rather than 1-2 hours after awakening (about 8 AM). Cortisol fails to suppress with dexamethasone challenge (50%–60% of patients). Growth hormone response to amphetamine is blunted, and thyroid response to TSH is reduced. The hypothalamic pituitary axis is in "overdrive."

Associated Features

About 20% of melancholic episodes are associated with delusions or hallucinations (more so with bipolars). Voices are typically accusatory. Some melancholics hallucinate bad odors from their body or in the air They believe they are evil and have done bad things for which they should be punished. They think they are diseased and deserve to die.

Some melancholics drink heavily, and alcoholism is a co-occurring condition (more so with bipolars and male patients). Compared with nonmelancholic depressives, melancholics are more likely to be bipolar. Melancholics may also be at greater risk than nondepressed persons for migraine (women patients), diabetes, and infection.

Depressive Pseudodementia

Melancholia in older patients may present as dementia, exhibiting diffuse cognitive impairment, particularly in attention, concentration, and memory. They may be misdiagnosed as having Alzheimer's disease because their age and cognitive complaints are mistakenly given greater diagnostic weight than the presence of insomnia, weight loss, retardation, and other features of melancholia. Sadness or despondency may be absent, and the patient may appear perplexed, bewildered, or frightened. Scores on the Mini-Mental State Examination average around 20 points (range, 15–25), in the demented range. These patients may live alone and in their confusion neglect to feed and clothe themselves properly. EEG and magnetic resonance imaging (MRI) are unhelpful in differentiating depressive pseudodementia from other dementias in persons over 75 years as both patient groups have nonspecific EEG slowing, and cortical atrophy and ventricular enlargement on MRI. In persons under 75 years, when brain changes due to aging are less confounding, the younger the patient, the more likely MRI will help distinguish pseudodementia from dementias such as Alzheimer's disease.

Table 7.2 displays different characteristics of depressive pseudodementia and Alzheimer's disease. The distinction is important, as patients with pseudodementia respond well to treatment, particularly electroconvulsive therapy (ECT). When in doubt, remember that in persons aged 65–75, depression is four times as common as dementia. However, some Alzheimer's patients become depressed early

TABLE 7.2. Differences Between Depressive Pseudodementia and Alzheimer's Disease

Distinguishing Feature	Depressive Pseudodementia	Alzheimer's Disease
Insight	Exaggerate symptoms and problems	Minimize symptoms and problems and deny illness
Depressive symptoms	More symptoms and more melancholic features; anxiety and agitation	Less symptoms, more apathy and avolition than sadness
Personal history	Previous mood disorder more likely	May have no previous psychiatric illness
Family history	Often mood disorder	Often Alzheimer's disease, Down syndrome, or myeloproliferative disorders
Laboratory tests	1. Some decreased metabolism frontally (hypofrontality) on SPECT	1. Decreased temporoparietal metabolism on SPECT
	2. Bilateral frontal nondominant hemisphere impairment pattern on cognitive testing	2. Bilateral temporoparietal impairment pattern on cognitive testing
	3. EP* shows delay in waves with normal amplitudes;	3. EP shows delay in waves with reduced amplitudes
	4. Normal ventricular enlargement and cortical atrophy	4. MRI most helpful in patients less than 75 years, with Alzheimer's patients showing reduced temporal lobe volume bilaterally and those over 75 showing substantial ventricular and cortical atrophy

*EP, evoked potential.

in the course of their illness. Many of these patients will have a family history of mood disorder. Nondepressed Alzheimer's disease patients rarely do. These depressions will also respond to antidepressant treatment.

Postpartum Mood Disorder

Postpartum mood disorder is rare (1/1,000 births), but during the first several weeks after childbirth women are most at risk (10 times) for severe psychiatric illness. Depression is the most frequent postpartum disorder. Mania accounts for 10%–15% of episodes. The incidence of other DSM disorders does not increase during parturition. Most postpartum mood disorders begin within the first 7–10 days following childbirth. A second, smaller peak occurs 6–8 weeks later with the first postpartum menses.

Although the risk for psychopathology among women is lowest during pregnancy, women who will have a postpartum psychosis usually exhibit some symptoms late in pregnancy, and the presence of psychopathology, however mild, during the third trimester increases the likelihood of a postpartum illness. Except for prior depression, there are no long-term predictors. Two-thirds of patients are primigravid. There is no clear association between postpartum mood disorder and premenstrual syndromes.

Postpartum mood disorder is not a distinct disease. Clinical features, family illness patterns, and treatment response are essentially the same as for major depression occurring at other times. Postpartum depressives, however, are younger than other mood disorder patients (an artifact of being in the child-bearing years), and postpartum manics are more often disoriented, are unable to concentrate, and complain that "things are going too fast," whereas postpartum depressives are more likely to be delusional and to experience hallucinations. Depression also increases the risks for malnutrition and poor prenatal care and is associated with neonatal irritability. Depression that continues after delivery adversely affects maternal–child relationships.

Postpartum mood disorder is extremely responsive to treatment. However, postpartum manics often have cognitive impairment that worsens with neuroleptic or lithium treatment, and postpartum depressives are often delusional and thus less likely to respond to antidepressant drugs alone. ECT is the treatment of choice. It is the safest and most rapid antidepressant for pregnant and breast-feeding mothers who are melancholic (see discussion of ECT, below).

If ECT cannot be given, avoid drugs if possible during the first trimester, and prior to delivery taper medications to avoid newborn withdrawal phenomena (jitteriness, tremor, clonus, seizures, cyanosis on feeding, low birth weight, tachycardia, diaphoresis, premature delivery, and respiratory difficulty). With these qualifications, the use of antidepressants during pregnancy is a minimal risk factor for birth defects and does not affect global IQ, language, or behavioral development in exposed children followed to preschool age. Specific serotonin reuptake-inhibiting antidepressant (SSRI) use, however, may be associated with prematurity, low birth weight, colic, and excessive bleeding at delivery. Avoid neuroleptic use during pregnancy because the long-term risks to the child's brain are unknown. Control agitation with sedative-hypnotics and psychosis with ECT. If a neuroleptic must be given, use an atypical agent (see Chapter 9).

In choosing an antidepressant, follow the management guidelines for melancholia. Anticholinergic properties of the nonspecific reuptake inhibitors can affect the newborn, causing tachyarrhythmias and urinary retention, so the partially specific agents (e.g., desipramine, nortriptyline) are better. Monoamine oxidase inhibitors (MOAIs) require too many dietary restrictions during pregnancy. If you give an SSRI, combine it with vitamin C (1,000 mg daily) to minimize bleeding. Other medications used in mood disorder also have their drawbacks during pregnancy. For example, lithium can produce fetal heart defects and neonatal lithium toxicity, although the mother's blood levels are below toxic concentrations (look for newborn flaccidity, lethargy, arrhythmias and poor myocardial contractibility, poor suck reflex, and cyanosis). Neonatal transient hypothyroidism and nephrogenic diabetes insipidus may occur. Carbamazepine can cause neonatal hemorrhage (vitamin K deficiency), liver damage (vitamin D deficiency), and teratogenesis. Valproic acid can cause teratogenesis, liver failure, and poor clotting (fibrinogen depletion).

Although, long-term outcome for persons with postpartum mood disorder is good, 35%–60% of patients will have subsequent postpartum depressions. If there are no thrombotic problems, the risk for future depressions can be reduced to less than 10% with postpartum estrogen therapy. Heparin 5,000 U BID subcutaneously is given for the first week postpartum. Estrogen (Premarin) is also given orally in a decreasing schedule: 5 mg BID 3 days, 2.5 mg TID 4 days, 2.5 mg BID 5 days, 1.25 mg BID 3 days, 0.9 mg OD 6 days. Noncompliant patients can receive 2.5 mg IV q8h for 2 days and then the oral schedule, if possible.

Stuporous Depression and Catatonia

Some melancholics develop profound psychomotor retardation and become stuporous. They appear sedated despite not receiving medication, and they will sit or lie in bed for hours staring into space and barely responding to stimuli. They may be analgesic to modestly painful stimuli. Some melancholics become catatonic and remain mute and immobile, and posture. The stupor or catatonia may be so striking that observable depressive features are masked, and the patient is unable to express his depressed, hopeless, and suicidal feelings.

Stuporous and catatonic patients typically stop eating and drinking and, when suffering from a co-morbid general medical condition (e.g., diabetes, heart disease) stop taking their medications. Rapid diagnosis and treatment are necessary to avoid a medical emergency or the long-term consequences of a starving, dehydrated, immobile patient.

First, rule out traditional neurologic and general medical causes. In addition to examination and laboratory data, look for a past personal or family history of mood disorder. A highly diluted slowly administered intravenous dose of sodium amobarbital or 1–2 mg IM lorazepam may disinhibit the stuporous or catatonic patient, who will then reveal his depressive thoughts and feelings. A 16–20 mg daily or equivalent dose of a long- or intermediate-acting benzodiazepine may be needed for several days for catatonia. ECT is the definitive treatment for catatonia or depressive stupor (see discussion of ECT, below).

Course

Depressive illness usually begins in the teens or twenties for nonmelancholic depression and 5–10 years later for melancholia. Prepubertal depression is characterized by more general medical complaints but is otherwise indistinguishable from adult-onset depression. Although depressive illness is familial, this is particularly true for prepubertal depression where the family illness risks for mood disorder and alcoholism are two to three times that of controls and two times that of adult-onset depressions. Paternal alcoholism substantially increases a child's risk for depression. Maternal alcoholism, although damaging to the fetus, appears to be etiologically independent of childhood depression.

The earlier the onset of the first depression (<25 years), the more likely the patient will be bipolar (particularly if onset is before puberty, when 33% become bipolar). Bipolar depressions are also more likely to be frequent, severe, psychotic, and ultimately associated with some deterioration in cognitive functioning (particularly in sustained attention, frontal executive functions, and new learning). Ten to 15% of unipolar depressives become chronically ill. The risk for chronicity increases if co-morbidities are present (e.g., alcoholism, drug abuse, head injury, personality disorder). Although frequent or chronic childhood depression may affect personality development, adult-onset unipolar depression does not. Most depressed patients, however, respond well to good treatment. The elderly depressive responds equally well as the young.

Nonmelancholic Depressions

Nonmelancholic depression (about 80% of depressions) is characterized by a mood that is reactive to social situations, is varying (sometimes sad, sometimes anxious or angry), and is associated with a tendency to weep. Nonmelancholic depressives expect not to enjoy themselves (anticipatory anhedonia), but can to some extent do so in pleasurable situations. They complain of fatigue, listlessness, being easily fatigued, loss of interest, tearfulness, and being short tempered. Nonmelancholic depressions often seem to be moody exaggerations of the patient's basic personality, and more than half of such patients have a diagnosable DSM personality disorder (most commonly anxious-fearful, shy and introverted). Unlike melancholics, they can have "good days." At their worst, they feel helpless, blame others or outside circumstances for their troubles, are hypochondriacal, and are filled with self-pity.

Nonmelancholic depressives do not have typical vegetative signs. Although their sleep is often disturbed, they may sleep too much rather than too little. When they have insomnia it is typically falling asleep rather than staying asleep. Nonmelancholic depressives may eat too much and gain rather than lose weight. They are rarely agitated, psychotic, or profoundly slow. When not depressed, these persons tend to feel anxious and have physiologic signs of anxiety, increased muscle tension, and feelings of fatigue and being easily tired.

Major depression without melancholic features and *Dysthymia* are probably variants of the same pathophysiology. Family illness patterns are similar. Major depression without melanchonic features is the more severe episodic form; dysthymia is the milder, chronic form that lasts years. Dysthymia is the most common mood disorder of adolescence. Both forms can occur in the same patient, and these are sometimes referred to as *double depression*. Treatments are similar (see below). Co-morbidities are common (most patients), similar, and include alcohol and drug abuse (particularly marijuana) (30%), cigarette smoking, personality disorder (anxious fearful, 50%), anxiety disorders (all types, 40%–50%), and obsessive compulsive disorders. The combination of a childhood nonmelancholic depression, anxiety disorder (often specific phobia, separation anxiety, or social phobia), and conduct or somatization disorder predicts a poor response to antidepressants (in some studies no better than placebo), and a stormy lifetime course with associated drug and alcohol abuse.

Adjustment disorder with depressive features is in the DSM Adjustment Disorder category and is defined in the DSM as (1) a nonmelancholic depression that does not meet criteria for major depression and that follows a modest stressor (e.g., moving to a new town) in a person who is somehow more sensitive to stress (e.g., because of a premorbid anxious-fearful personality disorder); and (2) the depression resolves within 6 months even without treatment. Evaluate these patients as you would any patient for whom you were considering depression and ask yourself the basic question, "Is it a clinical depression, and, if so, is it melancholic or nonmelancholic?" Treat accordingly.

Bereavement is characterized by many symptoms of depression, including some symptoms of melancholia (e.g., decreased appetite, insomnia). However, bereaved persons do not feel "ill" and usually do not seek psychiatric care. Intense mourning typically lasts about 3–4 months, with lingering feelings for up to a year. Typical bereavement is best resolved within the family. If the bereaved person has no family or friends, a brief period of counseling or joining a support group can help.

Abnormal bereavement is a clinical depression with the loss of a loved one the trigger pushing the person over some threshold into illness. As a clinical depression, abnormal bereavement requires medical treatment, and the big question is still, "Is it melancholia or a nonmelancholic major depression or dysthymia?" Consider the person clinically depressed (i.e., abnormal bereavement) and treat if (1) the intense bereavement lasts longer than 6 months (with the person unable to resume his daily responsibilities), (2) melancholia develops, (3) psychotic symptoms appear, or (4) the person becomes suicidal. The clinical picture is what counts, not whether there is a precipitating event, even one as stressful as the death of a loved one.

Atypical Depressions

Atypical is often a misnomer because the conditions in this group are well defined. They just do not fit the present DSM system.

Dysphoric depression is characterized by gloominess and irritability, oversensitivity to rejection, hyperphagia (for sweets and chocolate), weight gain, hypersomnia (more than 10 hours), feeling "heavy" as if "weighted down" (leaden paralysis), and being easily fatigued. These patients often have co-occurring anxious-fearful personality traits. In the DSM this condition is included under major depression. Another term for it is *hysteroid dysphoria*. These patients are particularly sensitive to medication side effects, so start low, and go slow.

Recurrent brief depression lasts less than 2 weeks, but occurs frequently throughout the year. Symptoms are those of a nonmelancholic major depression. Look for the co-morbid condition and treat these depressions as secondary to it. They include generalized anxiety disorder, panic disorder, dysthymia, major depression, soft bipolar spectrum, and various neurologic and general medical disorders (see below).

Premenstrual dysphoria (i.e., anxiety, irritability, sadness) is rarely confused with other mood disorders. It can be debilitating. It is part of a syndrome that includes *water retention* (breast pain or swelling, weight gain, puffiness and edema, reduced urinary output), *general discomfort* (headaches, backaches, joint or muscle pain, abdominal discomfort), *impulsivity* (irritability, aggressive or violent out-bursts), *impaired social functioning* (staying home from work, concentration diffi-culties, poor judgment, family problems), and brief recurrent *nonmelancholic de-pression* (as described above).

Premenstrual dysphoria is clinically important if symptoms substantially in-terfere with work or interpersonal relationships or if symptoms are severe enough that a clinical depression can be diagnosed.

Women with premenstrual dysphoria have cyclic hormonal changes similar to women without the syndrome, suggesting that the behavioral and emotional symptoms they experience are central in origin with hormonal changes the trig-ger. They have an increased lifetime risk for other mood disorders and are more likely to have phobias and obsessive compulsive disorder. Treatment consists of diuretics, nonsteroidal anti-inflammatory analgesics, and, if the depression war-rants, antidepressants. Fluoxetine at about 20 mg daily helps, as do a high trypto-phan diet (tryptophan is the amino acid precursor of Serotonin), exercise, and re-laxation training (see Chapter 15). Nefazodone 200–500 mg daily has also been reported helpful, as has venlafaxine 25 mg BID increased by 25–37.5 mg/daily with each cycle until remission.

Withdrawal depression ("the crash") is common when a user of high doses of a stimulant stops using the drug. Cocaine withdrawal is best known, but the syndrome also occurs in smokers trying to withdraw from nicotine and to a lesser extent in persons trying to withdraw from caffeine. About 50% of smokers having difficulty withdrawing are dysphoric, with hypersomnia, hyperphagia, and weight gain. Bupropion is the antidepressant of choice if the syndrome interferes with functioning or jeopardizes the withdrawal program. Carbamazepine also is effective.

Chronic fatigue syndrome (CFS) is a debilitating disorder characterized by chronic fatigue and other symptoms, including low-grade fever, sore throat, ten-der and periodically enlarged lymph nodes, muscle and joint pain, headaches, in-somnia and hypersomnia, anxiety, nonmelancholic (usually atypical) depressions, and cognitive impairment (particularly of attention and new learning). Identifi-able pathology sufficient to explain the syndrome is absent, but patients with the condition are not "cranks," "neurotic," "hypochondriacs," or malingerers. They are commonly diagnosed as depressed and given antidepressants.

CFS commonly begins after a viral illness (about 50% of patients); symptoms wax and wane and are aggravated by stress, exertion, and new viral infections. The degree of disability is variable. Epstein-Barr and other herpes and enterovirus infection are the most commonly accepted etiology, and many patients with CFS have persistently high antibody titers to these agents. However, non-ill controls also can have high titers, suggesting that additional factors are needed to cause symptoms. Some patients have immunoglobulin deficiencies and impaired T-cell functions, suggesting immune dysregulation as one of these factors. Other abnor-malities reported in CFS patients include exercise intolerance with an early acido-sis in muscle tissue, electromyography findings suggesting muscle cell membrane dysfunction, low red blood cell magnesium, and hypotension. This last finding is particularly important as this neurally mediated hypotension can be treated by increasing mineral corticoid intake or with beta blockers relieving many of the symptoms of fatigue.

Diagnosis requires

1. Symptom duration of greater than 6 months
2. Fatigue unrelieved by rest
3. A definite onset as opposed to life-long "fatigue"
4. Four or more other symptoms (detailed above)
5. No identifiable explanation for the symptoms other than CFS.

Differential diagnosis of chronic fatigue includes chronic infection, metabolic and nutritional disorders including severe obesity, immune and inflammatory diseases, neuromuscular disorders, malignancy, sedative-hypnotic drug abuse, sleep disorders, Lyme disease, cardiopulmonary disorders, chronic allergies, non-melancholic depression, and generalized anxiety disorder.

Treatment of CFS is nonspecific except for those patients with neurally mediated hypotension. Education about the disorder, counseling, stress management, and gradual aerobic conditioning with flexibility training can help. Low dose, partially specific monoamine reuptake inhibitors (e.g., desipramine, nortriptyline) can also benefit some patients. Outcome is highly variable. Some patients eventually fully recover, although this can take several years.

Suicide

Suicide is common. Over 30,000 suicides are reported in the United States annually, and 70% of these are Euroamerican males. Euroamerican women (20% of the total) make up the next largest group. There may be twice as many unreported suicides, and other ethnic groups may comprise a larger proportion of these persons. In parts of western Europe and in Japan rates exceed 25/100,000 per year.

Suicide rates are higher in the elderly than in persons under age 30, but the rates in the elderly are declining, whereas they are rising in the young due to increased drug use, availability of guns, and cohort and period effects. Rates among persons 30–60 have not changed in decades. Adolescent suicide (2,000/year in the United States) is the second or third leading cause of death in that age group (auto accidents and homicide are higher). Males use guns and hanging more than do females, whereas females use over-the-counter drugs and wrist cutting. Ten to 20% of teenagers say they have thought about suicide, and 5%–10% say they have attempted it. Among those who do, some psychiatric disorder is almost always present (mood disorder, alcohol or drugs, personality disorder). Teenage problems alone are not a risk factor.

Two-thirds of the patients who commit suicide visit their family doctor in the month before their death, and 40% do so in the prior week. More than half receive care for psychiatric illness in the year before committing suicide, and one third receive psychiatric care in the final month. High suicide risk factors are (1) suicidal ideation and intent; (2) diagnosis of melancholia or major depression; (3) alcoholism; (4) serious general medical illness (particularly those that are chronic or painful, including arthritis, emphysema, renal failure, AIDS); (5) middle age or elderly for Euroamericans and younger for other ethnic groups; (6) male gender (one exception is a higher rate among Chinese-American women); (7) single, widowed, divorced, or separated; (8) unemployed or in financial difficulty; and (9) prior suicide attempt or a family history of suicide (associated with a higher risk because it makes it more likely that the patient has a major depression, the real risk factor).

The suicide risk is less when the depressed patient denies intent or ideation, their mood improves as the examination progresses and is reactive to environmental stimuli, and they are in good general health, a child, or are pregnant.

The presence of suicidal intent in a melancholic is the most important factor. Anxious, apprehensive, or agitated depressives and depressives who are bipolar are at the greatest risk. Being male and a heavy drinker are next in importance. Among suicides, about 50% had a major depression. The remaining 50% were persons who were psychotic (drugs most likely), alcoholic, who had a dramatic-emotional personality disorder (DSM Cluster B), or who were facing a difficult life situation. Long-term prediction of suicide is correlated best with severe dysphoria, past alcoholism, and chronic general medical illness.

Most suicidal patients convey their suicidal thoughts to others, and you must always ask a depressed patient if he is contemplating suicide (e.g., "Would you like to go to sleep and never wake up? Would you like to end it all? Are you thinking of harming yourself, of suicide?"). Find out the details about any specific suicidal plan. Suicidal patients are often reassured when your questioning demonstrates an awareness of their desperation and a willingness to stop them from killing themselves. There is no evidence that questions about suicide stimulate suicidal patients to commit suicide.

About 15% of melancholics eventually commit suicide. About 60% do so during the year of the depressive episode, so maintenance treatment for at least a year is important. The risk is highest during the first month after discharge from a psychiatric hospital (sevenfold for men, threefold for women). The risk of suicide in dysthymic disorder is somewhat elevated.

Alcoholism is also highly correlated with suicide. The disinhibiting effects of alcohol associated with depression is deadly. Try to convince all patients with a major depression to *completely* abstain from alcohol for the duration of antidepressant treatment because of its drug–drug interaction with antidepressants, and for a depressed patient any drinking substantially increases suicide risk during the depression and maintenance treatment period. The safest policy is for a person with a previous depression never again to regularly drink alcohol to avoid a recurrence of depression while still using alcohol, but before receiving antidepressant treatment. Alcoholism unaccompanied by mood change or psychosis, however, is rarely an immediate and direct cause of suicide.

DIFFERENTIAL DIAGNOSIS

The first diagnostic question remains, "Is the patient suffering from a clinical depression or something else?" Features that distinguish a clinical depression from demoralization and worry are detailed above. Persons with clinical depressions are also more likely to have prior episodes, prior suicide attempts, and a family history of mood disorder.

Classic, nonpsychotic melancholia is not difficult to diagnose. Diagnosis is harder when a patient (1) does not exhibit all the symptoms needed to meet diagnostic criteria, (2) has many psychotic features traditionally associated with schizophrenia (e.g., persecutory delusions, auditory hallucinations), (3) has ruminations and anxiety that suggest obsessive compulsive disorder (OCD), (4) has a depression associated with diffuse cognitive impairment suggesting dementia, or (5) has an atypical pattern of symptoms (e.g., apathy or avolition rather than gloominess).

Where there is no certainty, probability rules. In the case of an ambiguous mood state, the more mood features the better. If a depression due to a knowable neurologic or general medical condition can be ruled out, or if suspected and there is no obvious contraindication to biologic treatment, diagnose the patient as depressed.

About 20% of melancholics are psychotic, and about 10% have a chronic course. During early episodes, particularly the first episode, the diagnosis may be difficult. First, look for bipolarity (family illness, past behavior patterns consistent with soft bipolar spectrum, discussed in Chapter 8). Second, look for chronic stimulant abuse (stereotyped, awkward, or other motor signs are helpful here). Treat accordingly (see Chapters 8 and 13).

More difficult still is the young male patient whose melancholia is characterized by an oneiroid (daydream-like) state and a delusional mood or vague persecutory delusions. The diagnostic question here is, "do these patients have a severe mood disorder, or are they schizoaffective or schizophrenic?" Some schizophrenics, for example, experience an atypical psychotic depression as their first psychosis, the depression gradually disappearing, leaving the patient in a chronic state. Unlike the schizophrenic, the depressed patient is likely to have a more intense mood. Facial, vocal, and gestural expressions may be absent in both, but in schizophrenics with emotional blunting the subjective experience of emotion is also reduced or absent. Although an important research question (the jury is still out), the clinical issue is simple: If no harm is likely, treat the patient for the illness with the best prognosis. Thus, regardless of the number, severity, and strangeness of psychotic features, if a patient meets other criteria for depression consider them as having a mood disorder and treated for that. More patients will have better, longer, and more productive recoveries with this approach than by being diagnosed schizophrenic and getting neuroleptics and thus probably tardive dyskinesia.

About 50% of melancholics often ruminate about the "bad" things (exaggerated or imagined) they have done or are likely to do. They can appear to have severe OCD when these thoughts are not delusional, and the patients understand their "foolishness" but "can't help thinking about it" and are frightened that they will act on their thoughts. Again, depressive features take precedent and, if sufficient to meet criteria for depression, consider the obsessive thoughts as depressive ruminations and treat for depression. This distinction and diagnosis favoring depression rather than OCD, is critical because both conditions can respond to antidepressants. However, the antidepressants that work best for OCD are limited compared with those that work best for melancholia: clomipramine and other SSRIs for OCD; partially specific and other specific reuptake inhibitors for melancholia (e.g., desipramine, nortriptyline, venlafaxine and perhaps nefazodone). Most importantly the diagnosis of melancholia alerts all to the risk of suicide, whereas the diagnosis of OCD is less likely to focus attention on this life-threatening behavior.

Another difficult decision is when anxiety disorder and depression co-occur, and you need to decide which condition is primary. If the depression is associated with melancholic features, always consider it primary no matter how many anxiety disorder features are present. The reasoning for this is the same as that for OCD versus depression.

Depressions secondary to anxiety disorder are typically nonmelancholic and are characterized by dysphoria, feelings of fatigue, easy fatigability, complaints of breathing problems and being weak, and having palpitations. Patients may be phobic and obsessive and describe themselves as "insomniacs" because their sleep patterns are chronically disrupted in contrast to the primary depressive whose sleep is disturbed only during the depressive episode. These patients describe themselves as being chronically unhappy and dissatisfied. Many have an anxious-fearful personality disorder and physiologic signs of generalized anxiety disorder when not depressed. Some are anxious, orderly, overly conscientious, overly routinized, suspicious individuals and may meet criteria for paranoid personality disorder. These patients, particularly if young and male, do poorly with any treatment.

Distinguishing depression from dementing conditions is another diagnostic challenge. The distinguishing features between pseudodementia and Alzheimer's dementia are described above. This problem relates to the broad difficult question of whether the depression is primary or secondary. Factors to consider in identifying secondary psychiatric disorder and when considering the etiology of any behavioral syndrome are

1. Atypical present episode (e.g., a depression marked by apathy rather than apprehension or gloominess; hallucinations that last only a few minutes or occur at the same time each day)
2. Atypical course (e.g., a depression that lasts hours or days rather than weeks and months; an anxiety disorder that begins for the first time after age 40)
3. Physical examination evidence of another disorder that could account for the behavioral syndrome (e.g., enlarged thyroid)
4. Historical evidence of another disorder that predates the behavioral syndrome and that could account for the behavioral syndrome (e.g., previous stroke)
5. Laboratory evidence of a general medical or neurologic condition that could account for the behavioral syndrome (e.g., HIV-positive blood test, epileptic-like EEG [spikes and sharp waves, bursts of slow waves]
6. A family history of illness consistent with another disease that affects the brain (e.g., no family history of mood disorder, but several first-degree relatives ill with Huntington's disease)

Although secondary depressions can be severe, they rarely are typically melancholic, particularly in mood, which is often more anergic and avolitional than apprehensive or dysphoric. Think of secondary depression when you hear the words (sleep problems, loss of interest, pessimistic), but not the music (pervasive gloom apprehension) of melancholia. Secondary depressions due to discrete lesions (stroke, injury) can also have other discriminating features. For example, patients with depressions from posterior nondominant hemisphere lesions look depressed, but often deny it. Patients with dominant anterior depressions say they are depressed but look or act more apathetic. Many medications can cause a depressive-like syndrome (Table 7.3). Drug-induced depressions vary in pattern: atypical lethargic (sedative-hypnotics, anticonvulsants), apathetic (all others), melancholic (reserpine), pseudodementia-like (antihypertensives, H_2 blockers). Assume any medication listed in Table 7.3 guilty until proven otherwise, particularly in a person over age 65. If the cause, reduce or stop. If the depression persists *without any symptom reduction* five times the drug's half-life (the time to reach steady state), treat as if a primary depression. This will rarely be needed, and if so, the patient will most likely have a co-morbid mood disorder.

The severity of secondary depressions, however, is not correlated with the severity of the disability resulting from the underlying cause. For example, persons with mild Parkinson's disease can have severe depressions. These secondary depressions reflect the fact that brain systems involved in mood generation and regulation are also involved in the pathophysiology of the neurologic condition.

Depressions from *head trauma* (25% of brain injury patients) typically begin several years after closed head injuries (as scaring develops), whereas they can start within days of an open head injury or an injury with a skull fracture or intrahemispheric bleed. Depression-producing sites include dominant frontal and orbitomedial areas and the nondominant hemisphere, the last producing a dysphoric depression with irritability. If the lesion appears excitatory (lots of emotion and psychotic features), treat as you would for depression with epilepsy (see

TABLE 7.3. Medications That Often Cause Secondary Depression

Class	Examples
Antihypertensives	Reserpine, propranolol, methyldopa, hydralazine, nifedipine
Antiarrhythmics	Quinidine, procainamide, lidocaine
Anticonvulsants	Phenytoin, barbiturates, ethosuximide
Antibiotics	Penicillins, mycins
Antineoplastics	Vincristine, mycins
Hormonal agents	Corticosteroids, progestational agents (particularly oral contraceptives), estrogens
H_2 blockers	Cimetidine, ranitidine
Sedative-hypnotics	Benzodiazepines, chloral hydrate, alcohol
Others	Baclofen, cyproheptadine, disulfiram, methysergide

below and Chapter 10). If the lesion is ablating (more avolition than strong mood), treat as you would for depression with stroke (see below and Chapter 11).

The *postconcussion syndrome* is also associated with depression. Patients complain of headaches, dizziness, problems with concentration and new learning, anxiety, and atypical depressive features. Abnormal evoked potential (slowed) and vestibular caloric testing are helpful laboratory tests. Treat with buspirone (Buspar) if anxiety features or irritability predominate. Treat with a stimulant or bupropion if concentration and atypical depressive features predominant. Treat with an SSRI if a major depression is present. *Cluster* and *migraine* headaches can also produce depression, so you have to distinguish these conditions from postconcussion headache. If present, treating them usually resolves the depression (see Chapters 10 and 16).

Depression from *stroke* (10%–30% of stroke patients) is typically late onset, nonpsychotic, and avolitional and apathetic. Behavioral, cognitive, and motor signs of dominant frontal lobe dysfunction (lesion in the head of the caudate or frontal lobe) or dysphoria and agitation (posterior nondominant temporoparietal areas) are two patterns. Magnetic resonance imaging (MRI) findings and single photon emission computed tomography (SPECT) hypometabolism can identify these lesions. EEG is usually normal. If stroke involves frontal circuits, dopamine agonists with antidepressant properties are the first choices: bupropion (Wellbutrin), nortriptyline (Pamelor), desipramine (Norpramin), and ECT. If the depression is apathetic, methylphenidate (Ritalin) helps. If the nondominant hemisphere is involved, any appropriate antidepressant drug or ECT can work (also see Chapter 11).

Forty percent of *epileptics* (particularly those with complex partial fits) develop depression. When associated in or around the seizure, the depression is brief (hours or days to a week or two), frequent, and nonmelancholic with anxiety, panic attacks, psychosensory features, problems with olfaction, avolition, and fatigue rather than profound gloom. EEG evaluation requires frequent tracings with sleep deprivation, 24-hour telemetry, and other specialized techniques. SPECT hypermetabolism during fits and hypometabolism interictally combined with MRI (decreased temporal lobe or frontotemporal volume or showing a specific lesion [e.g., vascular malformations]) are helpful diagnostic tests. ECT is the best choice if the patient has a psychotic depression. Carbamazepine (Tegratol) has both anticonvulsant and antidepressant properties. If the depressions are associated with bipolar features (see Chapter 8), valproic acid (Depakote) is the drug of choice. Neuroleptics can worsen symptoms, as can combining anticonvulsants (also see Chapter 10).

Basal ganglia disease typically produces depression. For Parkinson's disease (50%–70% of patients become depressed) look for a late onset depression with slight bilateral resting hand tremor, muscle stiffness, and bradykinesia. MRI and EEG tests are normal in early stages. SPECT may show bilateral basal ganglia hypometabolism. Treatments are the same as for depression with stroke. If apathy and loss of energy are main features of the depression, bromocriptine (Parlodel) helps the depression and motor features. Huntington's disease begins with depression in about one third of patients. Look for dysarthria, awkward movements, chorea, and a family history of movement disorder and dementia. MRI shows "butterfly" ventricles, and SPECT shows hypometabolism in the basal ganglia and orbitofrontal regions. Dopamine agonists (including ECT) can worsen motor symptoms, but methylphenidate is least likely to do this. SSRIs help. (See also Chapter 12.)

Dementia can also produce depression (25%–30% of dementia patients). Alzheimer's disease often begins with a mild depression, and dopamine agonists, bupropion, or sertraline work best. *White matter degenerative disease* such as multiple sclerosis produces a depression (30% of patients) associated with anxiety and weakness. Look for other neurologic signs. Treatment is the same as for primary depression. HIV can also produce a white matter dementia with an apathetic depression and bradyphrenia. AIDS is already present. Stimulants and other dopamine agonistic-like drugs (e.g., bupropion) can help.

Endocrinopathies often cause depression. Thyroid disease (30% of patients) must be corrected before antidepressant treatment is likely to work. This is also true for patients with primary depression and co-morbid thyroid disease. Hyperthyroidism produces a nonmelancholic depression with striking anxiety features, panic attacks, and irritability. Hypothyroidism (sometimes associated with arthritis and hypercholesterolemia) produces a nonmelancholic depression with lethargy and weakness. Once the patient is euthyroid, treat as for primary depression if needed.

Hyperparathyroidism (15% of patients) also causes a nonmelancholic depression with lethargy, easy fatigability, and weakness. Look for a history of calcium renal stones and hypercalcemia. You must correct the parathyroid dysfunction to successfully treat the depression.

Cushing's disease (30% of patients) can produce an agitated, anxious depression with suspiciousness and other psychotic features. Look for classic signs of steroid overproduction, but remember that primary melancholics have abnormal 24-hour cortisol and abnormal dexamethasone suppression tests (DSTs). Correcting the Cushing's disease often resolves the depression. *Lupus erythematosis* (look for skin, kidney, joint, and other organ disease) can produce depression, as can its treatments. If the depression is due to lupus, treat as if it were primary.

Cancer can cause depression. Lung cancers can produce neurotoxins that damage white matter. Carcinoma of the head of the pancreas can produce a melancholia months before this deadly cancer is obvious. Radiation and chemotherapy can cause avolitional depressions. If the depression requires, treatment, use lower doses and increase more slowly to avoid side effects because cancer patients are more at risk for many of these.

Viral illness can result in depression. Mononucleosis can produce an atypical depression with lethargy, fatigue, lymph adenopathy, and hepatomegaly. Look for a depression that quickly follows a flu-like syndrome. Avoid drugs that are metabolized by the liver. Low dose stimulants may help. Encephalopathies associated with herpes, Epstein-Barr, and similar viruses produce atypical avolitional nonmelancholic depressions. If associated with an attention deficit syndrome or visuospatial problems, use stimulants. If depressive features are prominent, treat as if the depression was primary nonmelancholic.

TABLE 7.4. Laboratory Profile of Primary Depression

Measurement	Findings
Brain Metabolism	
Cerebral blood flow (CBF)	1. Reduced CBF in some depressives; left anterior cingulate and left dorsolateral prefrontal cortex; increased cerebellar vermal CBF
	2. Patients with cognitive impairment also have left medial frontal gyrus hypometabolism
	3. Perhaps greater activation in left anterior and right posterior regions during cognitive tasks seen with EEG.
PET/SPECT	1. Diffuse low metabolic rate, most marked in frontal regions, particularly anterior cingulate gyrus, in bipolar more so than unipolar melancholics
	2. Left dorsal anterolateral prefrontal pattern in melancholics; low caudate metabolism, low amygdala metabolism, increased cerebellar vermal activity
	3. Some studies find increased metabolism in the left medial thalamus ventrolateral prefrontal cortex, and amygdala
Brain structure: CT/MRI	1. Many delusional melancholics (50%–80%) show modest ventricular enlargement and cortical atrophy with frontotemporal accentuation (may be reversible as it is associated with high cortisol levels). This reversibility is also seen in patients receiving steroids or who have Cushing's disease

CFS produces apathetic, brief depressions. Look for persistent or waxing and waning fatigue with a definite onset over a minimum of 6 months associated with impaired short-term memory, concentration, headaches, anorexia and nausea, postexertional malaise lasting more than 24 hours, tender lymph nodes, and a sore throat. If associated with postural hypotension, treat with salt tablets or fludrocortisone. If not, use stimulants or bupropion.

Fibromyalgia (chronic fatigue immunodeficiency syndrome) also can cause brief apathetic depressions characterized by fatigue, myalgia, night sweats, insomnia or hypersomnia, generalized aches and stiffness with points of tenderness affected by weather and stress, headache, joint swelling, irritable bowel syndrome, hepatomegaly, pharyngitis with painful lymph nodes, abnormal Romberg sign, limb numbness, sluggish accommodation, and visual blurring and photophobia. MRI is normal. SPECT shows hypometabolism frontally and in the midbrain. Bupropion, nortriptyline, nefazodone, and venlafaxine can help.

Laboratory findings are of limited help in differentiating primary from secondary mood disorders because many laboratory findings are abnormal in both groups. Secondary mood disorders are more often associated with focal or circum-

TABLE 7.4. *(continued)*

Measurement	Findings
	2. On MRI also greater T_1 relaxation time in frontotemporal areas (indicating more water or cell loss) and white matter hyperintensities.
	3. Diminished caudate volumes in some depressives. These findings are related to melancholia and severity, not to family history or years of illness
Information Processing	
Resting EEG	25%–30% of patients have mild, diffuse theta, a choppy EEG with transient small sharp waves, and, on computerized or topographic EEG, increased alpha power in dominant frontal and nondominant posterior regions, all suggesting decreased activation
Evoked potential	In delusional melancholics, delay between stimulus and wave forms (i.e., increased latency) and variable amplitude changes
Sleep EEG	Disturbed sleep architecture, reduced REM latency, loss of stage 4 (deep) sleep, frequent awakenings
Cognition	Significant proportion of patients have mild to moderate impairment in attention and new learning and other findings reflecting bifrontal and nondominant hemisphere dysfunction
Hypothalamic–pituitary axis	1. High 24-hour cortisol levels or phase-shifted diurnal cortisol curve
	2. DST nonsuppression, reduced growth hormone response to amphetamine, blunted thyroid-stimulating hormone response to thyrotropin-releasing hormone

scribed findings. The DST, abnormal in 50%–70% of melancholics (they are cortisol nonsuppressors to dexamethasone challenge), is unhelpful because many causes of depression can lead to nonsuppression (e.g., dementia, alcohol-related conditions). Table 7.4 displays the laboratory findings in patients with primary depression.

The depressed patient with a chronic general medical illness is a particular diagnostic problem because you have to consider if the condition is demoralization and worry or a clinical depression and if the depression is primary (i.e., co-occurring but unrelated to the general medical problem) or secondary to the general medical condition or its treatments. The above guidelines to resolve these issues especially pertain to these patients. In addition, vegetative signs are less helpful because many general medical patients, particularly those hospitalized, will have sleep and appetite problems. The quality of the mood state thus becomes the most important depressive feature to consider. Also consider the onset of the mood changes, because in 25% of depressed general medical patients the depression antedates the general medical condition (i.e., the depression is co-occurring but unrelated).

Depression in general medical patients is common (8%–30%), and treating the depression is important because, all other things being equal, compared with nondepressed patients, depressed general medical patients have more morbidity and mortality from their general medical condition.

THE NEUROLOGY OF DEPRESSION

Primary emotions (anger, sadness, happiness, anxiety) are observed in social mammals (e.g., canines, primates, hominids). Depressive-like states are also observed in these species (e.g., a dog who pines away for his dead master; a young chimpanzee that stops eating, drinking, and interacting following the death of his mother or who socially isolates himself after the death of a play or preening companion; human depressions) From a phylogenic perspective, the neurology of emotion and depression should and does include subcortical systems: brain stem and midbrain arousal systems and the limbic system bilaterally.

The differing specializations and information-processing styles of the cerebral hemispheres modify emotional expression. Social emotions, such as shame, nostalgia, guilt, and disgust, and emotions based on the qualities attributed to an object, person, or situation (e.g., a used condom, Hitler, a funeral) are strongly linked to language and are altered by dominant hemisphere, particularly prefrontal cortical circuit, lesions. Bereavement (from loss of a person, possession, or status) and dominant anterior brain lesions thus produce depressions that have many of the verbal characteristics of primary depression (e.g., being pessimistic, thinking the situation is out of one's control) but that also differ in important clinical features (more apathy or avolition rather than a melancholic mood, few vegetative signs, plus a self-awareness in the bereaved that the quality of their mood state is not abnormal).

The nondominant hemisphere processes low frequency information and processes information in a more diffuse pattern than does the dominant hemisphere. It is more responsive to changes in arousal and mood (a low frequency internal stimulus). Right hemisphere lesions typically produce mood-related symptoms. Anterior nondominant hemisphere lesions produce loss of emotional expression, and posterior lesions result in the inability to recognize the emotions of others. Depressive-like syndromes with dysphoric moods and irritability and violent behavior can result from nondominant temporoparietal lesions.

Patients with primary depression, particularly melancholia, have action brain dysfunction (see Table 7.4). Anterior cingulate gyrus, prefrontal cortex, caudate, amygdala, and cerebellum (the vermis modulates the limbic system) all seem to be involved with reducing metabolism in this system. Action brain structural changes are also seen. EEG slowing and delayed information processing seen with evoked potentials are consistent with reduced metabolism in this system. Cognitive impairments in depressed patients also suggests action brain dysfunction.

Although the dysfunction cannot be further circumscribed, intrinsic problems in the anterior limbic system are likely. Mood expression recruits arousal systems in the midbrain and brain stem, and disturbances in these systems are involved in mood disorders. Mood expression also influences anterior brain systems through limbic connections to the basal ganglia and directly into the anterior cingulate frontal circuit. The limbic disturbance likely produces the subjective mood state,* while the disruption of anterior brain systems produces the social behaviors and other symptoms of depression (bradyphrenia [slow thinking] and bradykinesia [slow movement]) and mania (the frontal lobe disinhibited syndrome). Limbic mood disturbances also affect hypothalamic function, causing disruptions in circadian rhythms and pituitary end-organ axes.

Persons with mood disorder have a genetic vulnerability. The vulnerability may be expressed in unstable or intense mood responses, particularly to stress. The exact nature of this vulnerability, however, is unknown. States of mood disorder (e.g., episodes of depression) may then further sensitize the limbic system, leading to more episodes (even without stress) and shorter well intervals. Mood-stabilizing drugs work directly on the limbic system, whereas dopamine agonists improve the arousal disruption in the frontal circuits.

TREATMENT AND MANAGEMENT

As discussed in Chapter 5, consider treatment in three stages: treatment of the acute episode, maintenance of the maximum response to acute treatment, and prophylaxis to prevent future episodes and minimize functional decline.

Treatment of Acute Depression

Melancholics and nonmelancholic depressives respond differently to treatments and require different management strategies. Both patient groups, however, require the help of family members in treatment. Minimally, and with the patient's concurrence and understanding of the importance of family involvement, you need to educate close family members about the patient's illness and treatments. They need to understand that the patient is not just "lazy" or "weak willed" and the folly of the idea that "if he only tried harder, he'd overcome it." They need to know that the patient is suffering from a medical condition of the brain, that his role as a patient is legitimate, and that biologic treatment and family support and understanding are essential for recovery. Sometimes family support groups and mood disorder organizations are helpful in reinforcing these treatment needs.

Melancholia

Melancholics often require hospitalization because of suicide risk, profound anorexia and weight loss, retardation or stupor with dehydration, or psychosis. These patients are treated in a locked unit under close observation, and ECT is

---

*This is one explanation why many secondary depressions are characterized by avolition (anterior brain underarousal) rather than the typical depressed mood.

often the treatment of choice. Even in the absence of specific suicidal thoughts or behavior, melancholics are at risk for suicide, particularly if they are older, have recently lost a spouse or have no social support system, or are in poor general medical health.

Do not engage melancholics in intense interpersonal exchanges or force them into unit activities. Exploratory and interpretive psychotherapy is not indicated. These patients often feel guilty and worthless, and these feelings may intensify with such interactions. Tell them that their illness has a biologic basis that is not under their voluntary control and that they are likely to make a rapid and full recovery. You will need to frequently reassure them because their self-doubts and guilty ruminations quickly return.

Nursing and other professional staff also provide support and reassurance. They observe and record patients' behavior and help in suicide prevention. Acutely suicidal patients may require continuous one-to-one observation because a determined patient can kill himself while hospitalized (e.g., jumping head first off an armoire).

Patients should be weighed daily and their sleep charted to document alterations in these vegetative features and to provide a baseline for assessing improvement. Severely depressed patients do best with short visits with family members until they are significantly improved. Many melancholics are unable to feel any emotion even for their loved ones, and seeing them may increase their guilt and self-reproach.

Nighttime sedation for insomnia is commonly needed. Short-acting benzodiazepines work well, but do not routinely use them to control agitation and anxiety or to enhance sleep past the first few days of hospitalization. Doing so often leads to a stormy course because the sedating effects of benzodiazepines may be mistaken for either improvement or antidepressant oversedation. In the former instance, higher antidepressant doses are mistakenly thought unnecessary, and in the latter instance the antidepressant dose may be mistakenly lowered or the drug discontinued. Prolonged benzodiazepine use over several months also can cause addiction. An alternative or adjunct to benzodiazepines is a transdermal nicotine patch (17.5 mg). This may improve REM sleep for some depressed patients and slightly elevate their mood during the first week of treatment before the antidepressant begins working. Nicotine's induction of liver enzymes is minimal at that dose and short duration of administration.

If the melancholic is receiving outpatient pharmacotherapy, the first several weeks are critical. Daily phone rounds can be life saving during the first week, and phone calls several times weekly during the first month, or until the patient is well on the way to recovery, are also helpful. Outpatient phone rounds and more frequent follow-up visits early on reduce hospitalizations, help prevent suicide, increase compliance, increase patient satisfaction, reduce law suits, and reduce overall costs to the system.

The first follow-up visit should be in 7–10 days unless severity requires an earlier visit. Do not prescribe medication for beyond this point because a 2-week supply of most antidepressants is a lethal dose. The second visit is a crossroad. If some response has occurred (e.g., improved sleep, no further weight loss), continued or augmented treatment is indicated. If *no response whatsoever* by 10 days to your first choice drug, a later good response to it is less likely, and switching treatment is often necessary at this point. Most textbooks accept little or no response for 4 or more weeks before altering treatment. This delay is not warranted, as the longer the depression lasts the greater is the risk for suicide or chronic social and cognitive dysfunction.

If there were only one treatment for melancholia, it should be ECT. For severely ill melancholics it gives the fastest response, thus reducing the length of hospital stays. It is the most efficacious and safest antidepressant treatment. If you can convince a melancholic patient to accept ECT, do so and give it.

If ECT is used and is successful, give all patients a minimum of a 6-month course of maintenance drug treatment to reduce relapse rates (10% rather than 30%–60%). All things being equal, select the drug for maintenance that you would have picked as the best choice for the patient's acute depression. If, however, the patient has already not responded to your first choice drug, choose a different one. For patients who relapse despite maintenance drug treatment, continued treatment with ECT can be effective (see below).

If you use medication to treat the acute depression, follow the guidelines in Tables 7.5 and 7.6. Although there is no clear evidence for therapeutic differences among antidepressants, most clinicians have their favorites. For melancholia, partially specific reuptake inhibitors seem to work better than the specific reuptake inhibitors. Among the specific reuptake inhibitors, venlafaxine, nefazodone and sertraline affect several neurotransmitter systems (i.e., they are less specific than the other "specific" agents). These three agents would be drugs of choice after the partially specific monoamine reuptake antidepressants for moderate to severe melancholia. In addition, nefazodone with its serotonin autoreceptor antagonism plus its serotonin reuptake inhibition may act as its own "enhancer." It also is good if insomnia is a problem for the patient. Pure SSRIs often cause agitation and an akathesia-like syndrome in melancholics. This is attributed to their serotonin enhancing effect.

There is some anecdotal evidence that dosing by the patient's circadian rhythms (often disrupted in depression) may maximize therapeutic effect. Typically, for depression, the best time to dose is late afternoon, and most antidepressants can be given in a single daily dose. For patients who experience insomnia with the afternoon dose, switch to a morning dose.

Lithium and carbamazepine also have some antidepressant properties and can be added to benefit some bipolar melancholics if the first choice antidepressant is only partially successful and for both unipolar and bipolar melancholics with psychosis. The idea that bupropion compared with other antidepressants reduces the risk for "breakthrough mania" is unproven. If there are no past manic, hypomanic, or soft bipolar behaviors (see Chapter 8) to help you decide polarity, the likelihood that a depressed patient is bipolar (and therefore should not receive an antidepressant only) increases when major depressions (1) begin before age 25 years; (2) are associated with a reversal of vegetative features (e.g., hypersomnia, overeating); (3) are psychotic, postpartum, or seasonal; or (4) the patient has a family history of bipolarity.

TABLE 7.5. Medication Guidelines for Treating Unipolar Melancholia

I. INITIAL MEDICATION CHOICE

A. In an otherwise healthy patient under age 65

Consider first desipramine or nortriptyline (harder to use because of the U-shaped dose-response curve and need for blood levels). Response rate* about 65%, with initial changes seen within 7–10 days and remission in 4–8 weeks

B. In a patient over age 65 or who has modest complicating comorbidities, making risky† the use of partially specific reuptake inhibitors

Consider more specific reuptake inhibitors with relatively broad neurotransmitter spectrums: venlafaxine, sertraline, nefazodone. Response rate about 55%–65% with initial changes seen within 10–14 days and remission in 6–8 weeks

II. SECOND CHOICE MEDICATION

A. If no improvement whatsoever in 10–14 days

1. ECT if consent given, or
2. Switch medications or enhance. Enhancement works best when there is a partial response

III. ENHANCEMENT

A. If the patient is over 75% improved in 4–8 weeks, continue the initial drug for another 4 weeks before enhancing

B. If the patient is less than 50% improved in 4–8 weeks, offer ECT and use it if consent is given

C. If the patient is less than 75% improved and refuses ECT, enhance

D. Women who are *not* extremely anxious, agitated, or suicidal, enhance with L-triiodo-thyronine (cytomel) T$_3$ 25–50 µg daily‡

E. Several other enhancing medications can be used (an additional 10% respond to these)

1. Bromocriptine (7.5–60 mg daily) for both men and women melancholics who are not psychotic or suicidal
2. Methylphenidate (5–60 mg daily) for both men and women melancholics who are not psychotic, suicidal, or agitated; in addition to stimulant effect, it inhibits liver enzymes, resulting in increased antidepressant drug blood levels
3. Pindolol (2.5 mg TID) for both men and women melancholics receiving a specific SSRI
4. Mirtazapine (30–45 mg daily) for both men and women melancholics receiving an SSRI or venlafaxine
5. Lithium (600–1200 mg daily) for both men and women melancholics even if unipolar; 60% of initial partial responders will benefit; because lithium increases serotonin formation and release, it can be used as an enhancer with all antidepressants
6. MAOI (phenelzine 60–120 mg daily) can be added to nonspecific or partially specific reuptake inhibitors. It cannot be added to agents with substantial serotonin reuptake inhibition
7. Other specific reuptake inhibitors as a last medication resort can be added at modest doses (e.g., sertraline, bupropion, or nefazodone); may help some melancholics not responding to other enhancers (data for this are anecdotal)

TABLE 7.5. (*continued*)

IV. FOR PSYCHOTIC MELANCHOLICS WHEN ECT IS NOT AN OPTION

A. Antidepressants alone do not work better than placebo; ECT is the first choice and, if refused, automatic enhancement of an antidepressant is needed

B. Desipramine, venlafaxine, nefazodone, sertraline are the antidepressants to consider first

C. Automatic enhancement is necessary. Consider lithium first and then carbamazepine (each has some antidepressant properties, and a psychotic depressive is more likely to be bipolar)

D. Risperidone is the antipsychotic of choice in doses below 8 mg daily. Wean the patient from this during the maintenance period of 3–6 months. Olanzapine, 15 mg daily, is the next best choice. Clozapine's side effects of salorrhea and syncope and anticholinergic effects are a substantial problem for elderly patients

---

*Response is defined as resolution of the depression, not just symptom reduction. If there is absolutely no response in 2 weeks, the likely response rate by 6–8 weeks is only 35%; if there is no response by 4 weeks, the subsequent likely response rate is less than 20%.

†You must individually judge risk in a patient over age 65 who is otherwise healthy.

‡T_3 is begun at 12.5 μg and increased in 3–5 days to 25 μg and then 50 μg by several weeks; monitor dose with pulse rate and any increase less than 20% above baseline is fine. T_4 (thyroxin or synthroid) can also be used, but its action onset is slower. Thyroid enhancement only works in women, and the reason for this is unknown. If thyroid is used to enhance the antidepressant, once the depression resolves (about 4–8 weeks) taper and then stop the thyroid to avoid any long-term side effects of this treatment.

TABLE 7.6. Medication Guidelines for Treating Bipolar Melancholia

I. INITIAL MEDICAL CHOICE

A. Choose an antidepressant as you initially would for unipolar melancholia

B. Automatically "cover" this with a mood stabilizing drug to avoid inducing mania. Lithium is the first choice, valproate the second choice, and carbamazepine the third choice

II. ENHANCEMENT

A. Decide on the need for enhancement as you would for unipolar melancholia

B. Enhancer choices are lithium or carbamazepine, thyroid, or adding an MAOI

III. FOR PSYCHOTIC BIPOLAR MELANCHOLIC WHEN ECT IS NOT AN OPTION

A. Same as for steps IV A–D for unipolar melancholia

B. Valproate is an additional option for a mood stabilizer

If your original drug choice was a partially specific reuptake inhibitor, and the series of steps outlined in Table 7.5 do not work and ECT still cannot be given, pick a different enhancing combination. For example, if your original choice was venlafaxine, nefazodone, or sertraline, and ECT or the partially specific reuptake inhibitors cannot be used, try bupropion because its therapeutic spectrum and pharmacology are different from those of SSRI-like drugs.

For elderly melancholics, remember that the body fat to body mass ratio may be increased, cardiac output may be decreased (and thus hepatic flow may be decreased), and loss of hepatic cells may have reduced the liver's capacity to metabolize drugs. Half-lives of drugs can be two to three times *longer* than for younger patients, so lower doses or every other day dosing (Monday, Wednesday, Friday) may be sufficient. A guideline for pharmacotherapy in the elderly is to start low and go slow.

Improvement in sleep and a reduction in apprehension are often the first signs of recovery and usually are observed by 7–10 days. However, significant therapeutic effects may not occur for 4 weeks. In melancholics who refuse ECT and are resistant to antidepressant enhancement, look for so-called *subclinical hypothyroidism*. Assess all depressed patients for physical examination and history evidence of thyroid dysfunction (dry thick skin, loss of outer third of eyebrows, coarsening or loss of hair, sluggish ankle jerks, slow heart rate, low blood pressure, overweight, cold intolerance). If not previously assessed, do so for the treatment-resistant patient. Hypothalamic pituitary thyroid dysfunction occurs in some melancholics, so laboratory testing is helpful only when several test results are substantially abnormal. Nevertheless, measure thyroid-stimulating hormone (TSH) levels (elevated), response of TSH to thyroid-releasing hormone (TRH) (enhanced), and antithyroid antibody titers (elevated). Some patients with subclinical thyroid disease have an autoimmune condition that also includes osteoarthritis, rheumatoid arthritis, and hypercholesterolemia. You must correct any thyroid problem first, and then the patient may no longer be treatment resistant. The most important factors in obtaining remission are *accurate diagnosis* (melancholia or not, primary or secondary); *adequate dosing;* and *compliance* (a function of the patient's personality, co-morbidities [e.g., alcoholism], side effects and their management, and the doctor–patient relationship).

Nonmelancholic Depression

Patients with nonmelancholic major depression or dysthymia usually do not require hospitalization. When they are hospitalized, it is usually for a suicide attempt or because they threaten suicide if not admitted. ECT rarely benefits these patients, and there is no advantage in giving them one of the partially specific monoamine reuptake-inhibiting antidepressants. Use of one of the specific reuptake-inhibitors. Choose within this class by the patient's co-morbid conditions, and, as for all medications, risks of side effects. Table 7.7 lists guidelines for use of antidepressants in the treatment of nonmelancholic depression. MAOIs may be particularly good for nonmelancholic depressives who have not responded to your first drug choice or who have a primary atypical depression

TABLE 7.7. Guidelines for the Use of Antidepressants in the Treatment of Nonmelancholic Depression

Co-Morbid Conditions	Suggested Antidepressant
Stimulant drug or alcohol abuse	Bupropion, because drugs with dopamine agonistic-like properties can reduce craving
Obsessive compulsive disorder or its variants	Fluoxetine
Generalized anxiety disorder	Phenelzine or paroxetine (other SSRIs can worsen anxiety); buspirone (15–50 mg daily) can also be effective as an enhancer in 75% of patients
Anorexia nervosa	Paroxitine, because weight loss is less than with other SSRIs
Bulimia nervosa	Sertraline; consider adding lithium if there is a family history of bipolar mood disorder. Because of the potential for fluid and electrolyte problems in bulimics, add lithium while the patient is in the hospital.
Personality deviation (see Chapter 6 for details)	
a. High novelty seeking with other temperament traits normal or low (antisocial; personality pattern with the least favorable outcome)	Bupropion or desipramine
b. High harm avoidance with other temperament traits low or normal	Any SSRI or, for women, desipramine
c. High harm avoidance and high reward dependence (passive-dependent or passive-aggressive)	Venlafaxine or, for women, desipramine
d. Low levels of novelty seeking, harm avoidance, and reward dependence (schizoid)	Good response to any antidepressant chosen by other factors (e.g., side effect considerations)

characterized by a reactive mood, hyperphagia, hypersomnia, easy fatigability, and inertia. Early side effects of concern are insomnia and orthostasis.

Pharmacotherapy for nonmelancholic depressives is enhanced with concurrent psychotherapy that pays close attention to interpersonal and social problems that may exacerbate the depression and to how the patient's habitual ways of dealing with these problems can be altered to reduce stress. Some depressives respond to cognitive therapy. Most likely to do so are those with mild pretreatment depressive features, those who are married, and those who have few or mild dysfunctional attitudes about themselves and their life situation (e.g., perfectionistic standards, concern about approval from others, degree of feeling inadequate).

Stereotactic cingulotomy is also reported to benefit some patients with intractable depression, particularly the nonmelancholic type. Side effects are modest (less than 1%) and are those of any neurosurgical procedure (bleeding, infection, seizures). This treatment is best limited to patients with intact personalities who have failed all other forms of treatment.

Secondary Depressions

Secondary depressions are often responsive to treatment. The same treatment in the same doses that work for primary depression often work for secondary depression. ECT is particularly effective and safe. Consider the treatment suggestions discussed above. Additional guidelines are

1. If the syndrome is characterized by avolition, apathy, and anergia more than gloominess and anxiety, and the patient is not psychotic or suicidal, use a dopamine enhancing agent such as methylphenidate (20 mg up to 0.5 mg/kg body weight) or bromocriptine (20–60 mg).
2. If the depression is associated with several psychosensory features or untypical perceptual experiences (e.g., olfactory hallucinations) or atypical behaviors (e.g., self-injurious but not suicidal behavior), use carbamazepine or ECT.
3. If the depression is associated with ruminations disproportionately more severe than other features, use an SSRI or venlafaxine.

Table 7.8 lists additional psychopharmacologic treatment suggestions for secondary depressions and depressions co-occurring with other conditions. Diabetes, heart disease, and depression are each common disorders and thus occasionally co-occur. Treating the depression is particularly important in these patients because, compared with the nondepressed, depressed diabetics and cardiac patients are at greater risk for morbidity and death from their diabetes or heart disease. Depression, for example, increases the risk for malignant arrhythmias and sudden cardiac death in post-myocardial infarction patients and for thrombosis. Depression also suppresses immune function, making depressed patients more infection prone.

MAOIs and, to a lesser extent, antidepressants that substantially affect noradrenergic or dopamine systems are contraindicated in diabetics. MAOIs produce hypoglycemia by enzyme inhibition blocking of long-chain fatty acid oxidation in glucogenesis. Noradrenergic and dopaminergic antidepressants increase plasma glucose, decrease insulin secretion, and reduce insulin resistance. SSRIs reduce plasma glucose and insulin, reduce insulin resistance, and are the safest antidepressants for diabetics. SSRIs are also safe for cardiac patients, although they may slow the heart rate two to three beats per minute. Nonspecific monoamine reuptake inhibiting antidepressants, contraindicated in ischemic disease, have quinidine-like properties and are thought relatively safe as type 1A antiarrhythmics. However, like quinidine, they increase mortality from drug-induced ischemic changes. Specific and partially specific monoamine reuptake-blocking antidepressants are also contraindicated in persons with heart block (e.g., first degree heart block, bundle branch block) because of their quinidine-like effect.

TABLE 7.8. Psychopharmacologic Treatment Suggestions for Secondary and Other Depressions

Condition	Medication Suggestion
Epilepsy	MAOI (least effect on seizure threshold in therapeutic doses and adherence to MAO diet), fluoxetine, desipramine; do not use bupropion, which lowers seizure thresholds
Dementia (Alzheimer's)	Venlafaxine, bupropion, fluoxetine, sertraline
Parkinson's disease	Bupropion, sertraline, stimulant; fluoxetine may worsen motor symptoms
Tardive dyskinesia	Bupropion, fluoxetine, sertraline
Migraine	Nortriptyline
Chronic pain	Amitriptyline, imipramine, desipramine
Narrow angle glaucoma	Venlafaxine, bupropion, nefazodone
Diabetes	Sertraline, other SSRIs
Ischemic heart disease	SSRIs
Congestive heart failure, coronary artery disease	Bupropion, fluoxetine, sertraline, venlafaxine
Cardiac conduction defect	MAOIs (least effect on the heart), bupropion, SSRIs, venlafaxine
Stroke	SSRIs, stimulants if dominant anterior lesion
Prostatic hypertrophy	SSRIs, MAOIs
Hypertension (if treated with drugs such as prazosin, terazosin, doxazosin, labetalol)	Fluoxetine, paroxetine, bupropion; do not use venlafaxine in high doses; do not use MAOIs with pheochromocytoma as it can cause hypertensive crisis
Hypertension (if treated with drugs such as clonidine, guanabenz, guanfacine, methlydopa)	Bupropion, paroxetine, fluoxetine
Hypertension (if treated with drugs such as guanethidine, guanadrel)	Bupropion, nefazodone, fluoxetine
Hypertension (mild and untreated)	MAOI (when diet is maintained, more likely to lower than raise blood pressure)
Postural hypotension	Venlafaxine, fluoxetine, paroxetine, bupropion, sertraline, desipramine; do not use MAOI

They can cause second- or third-degree block. MAOIs are relatively safe for heart patients and would be a second choice after SSRIs.

Maintenance Treatment

Maintenance treatment is always required after the successful acute treatment of a depression. What is to be maintained is always the best possible acute treatment result, hopefully a remission. If the patient has not fully recovered, he needs different or more treatment to resolve the depression, not maintenance of less than full recovery. Because untreated depressions last 7–14 months, maintenance is usually about 1 year. Maintenance less than 6 months most often results in re-lapse. An abnormal DST after acute treatment predicts early relapse. Even with good acute and maintenance treatment, 20%–30% of depressed patients relapse within 1 year of the depression.

The goal of maintenance treatment is to prevent relapse of the acute episode you successfully treated. Because 60% of depressed patients who kill themselves do so during the year following a depression, good maintenance treatment is also good suicide prevention. Determinants of successful maintenance treatment are the same as those for acute treatment. Guidelines for maintenance medication treatment are:

1. The medications that resolved the acute depression are the medica-tions used in maintenance, usually at the same doses. Reducing the dose for maintenance often leads to relapse.
2. The duration of maintenance treatment for depression is 8–12 months; longer treatment is prophylaxis against future episodes.
3. Taper treatments over a period of several months to avoid rebound withdrawal syndromes.
4. Insist that the patient avoid any alcohol use during the maintenance period to minimize drug–drug interactions and impulsive suicide at-tempts and then avoid heavy drinking thereafter. Co-morbid alco-holism requires aggressive treatment if the depressed patient is to re-main in remission (see Chapter 13).
5. Maintenance and prophylaxis treatments *always* include educating the patient and family about medications, how to take them, and their side effects; and the patient's specific early symptoms of his depression and the need to rapidly abort any impending relapse.
6. Discussions with the patient, and sometimes family members, about recent and future interpersonal and job problems related to the de-pression.

Prophylaxis

Prophylaxis treats the patient over the long haul, sometimes for a lifetime. The goals of prophylaxis are to prevent future episodes, to reduce the severity of future episodes, and to maximize interepisode function. Guidelines to prophy-laxis are

1. *Sometimes you cannot do better than nature.* For example, a patient who gets depressed every 5–10 years may not need prophylactic treatment because there are no treatments that do better than that. Such a patient does, however, need early detection of a new episode so that you can restart treatments rapidly, avoiding undue suffering and hospitaliza-tion. Although 60% of persons with a first depression will have recur-rences, there is no present way of knowing who will, so do not give long-term pharmacotherapy to recovered first episode depressives.

2. *Severity breeds severity.* The more episodes a patient has, the more these episodes interfere with interpersonal and job functioning, the greater the interepisode deficits, and the more the need for prophylaxis. Patients with well intervals of more than 5 years may not benefit from continuous pharmacotherapy. Bipolar patients and patients with comorbidities (particularly alcohol and drug abuse or anxiety disorder) may benefit most from long-term treatment. Also, the more episodes a person has, the more likely they are to have subsequent episodes with shortening well periods. Treatments that worked for the acute episode and during maintenance are also the likely choices for long-term management.

3. *Cognition predicts long-term function.* Always assess the patient's cognitive function (screening for verbal and visual new learning, attention, and cognitive flexibility) after each episode has resolved.* Depression is a brain disease, and 10%–15% of unipolar depressives become chronically dysfunctional with permanent cognitive problems. If the patient shows no decline, good. If your screening suggests some decline, get more extensive neuropsychological testing. If that testing confirms some decline, treat the patient as if he had suffered a head injury and provide cognitive rehabilitation (see discussion of rehabilitation in Chapter 5).

4. *Maximizing patient compliance is the key for both maintenance and prophylactic treatment.* Fifty percent of patients receiving long-term treatment are to some degree noncompliers. The keys to maximizing compliance are a good doctor–patient relationship that is maintained throughout the long-term treatment period, successful treatment of the original episode, and minimizing medication side effects. Despite appropriate prophylaxis, some patients will have breakthrough symptoms that can lead to noncompliance and relapse. For all the treatments for depression there is no evidence that long-term prophylaxis is dangerous or debilitating.

Prophylactic Drugs

Carbamazepine in doses and blood levels therapeutic for epilepsy (5–12 µg/ml) reduces the frequency of both unipolar and bipolar depressions. MAOIs reduce the frequency of unipolar depressions, and MAOIs plus lithium reduce the frequency of bipolar depressions. All antidepressants have some prophylactic benefit for unipolar depression. Use the antidepressant that worked for the acute episode and during maintenance as the prophylactic drug.

Abruptly stopping SSRIs can produce a withdrawal syndrome characterized by dizziness, paresthesias, lethargy, vivid dreams, irritability, and gloominess.

---

*During the acute episode many depressed patients do poorly on cognitive tests because of concentration problems. You want a baseline assessment when the patient is well so you can monitor follow-up and plan rehabilitation.

Taper SSRIs with short half-lives (clomipramine, paroxitine, sertraline) over a period of several months. Fluoxetine, with a half-life of several weeks, should still be tapered, but withdrawal symptoms are very uncommon with abrupt stopping of this drug.

Gradually discontinue antidepressants with anticholinergic properties. Suddenly stopping these drugs may cause a cholinergic rebound with anorexia, nausea, vomiting, abdominal distention or cramps, diarrhea, drooling, headache, muscle pain, drowsiness, agitation, irritability, dizziness, and insomnia and nightmares. Some patients develop akathesia, bradykinesia, and muscle rigidity. This syndrome can be treated with an anticholinergic drug such as benztropine or with diphenhydramine.

"Resistant" Depression

No depressed patient should be labeled treatment resistant until he has failed to respond to a course of bilateral ECT (8–12 generalized seizures of greater than 25 seconds). The most common explanations for depressed patients not responding to treatment are

1. *Inadequate dosing:* More than 70% of "resistant" depressed patients fall into this category.
2. *Incorrect diagnosis:* Most often a secondary depression goes unrecognized, but will respond to alternative treatments.
3. *Noncompliance:* This is most often due to poor side effect management and inadequate education of the patient to his disease and treatments.
4. *Interfering co-morbidities:* Co-morbidities can be deviant personality traits not adequately considered when prescribing an antidepressant for a nonmelancholic depression, alcohol or drug abuse disrupting treatments, or they can be unrecognized (e.g., subclinical thyroid disease) or poorly treated (e.g., giving too many medications, compounding adverse central effects) general medical conditions.

Specific Use of Antidepressants

Antidepressant categories are summarized in Table 7.9. The number of benzene rings each drug has does not predict the drug's efficacy or receptor specificity. Antidepressants are classified by their pharmacodynamics (i.e., what they do at the synaptic/neuronal level [Table 7.10]). Their therapeutics are based on their pharmacokinetics (i.e., how they are absorbed, metabolized, distributed, and excreted [Table 7.11]).

Nonspecific Monoamine Reuptake-Inhibiting Antidepressants

Except for some specific childhood conditions and some chronic pain syndromes, the older drugs (the original "tricyclics") are rarely used because of their anticholinergic and other side effects (e.g., orthostasis, lethargy). They are relatively contraindicated in the elderly (falls with hip fracture, paralytic ileus, subacute anticholinergic delirium), in persons with heart or prostate disease, and in epileptics (the nonspecific reuptake-inhibition antidepressants, like many psychotropics, lower the seizure threshold).

Partially Specific Monoamine Reuptake Inhibiting Antidepressants

Partially specific monoamine reuptake antidepressants are best used in healthy patients under age 65. Their common side effects are anticholinergic (e.g., dry mouth), sedation, and orthostasis. Discontinuation rates are similar to those for SSRIs.

Specific Monoamine Reuptake-Inhibiting Antidepressants

The serotonin specific reuptake inhibiting agents (SSRIs) have similar overall efficacies. Although many patients respond at the recommended starting dose, if there is *no* response in 7–10 days, or if the response is well below expected, increase the dose. Sertraline is the exception where dose increases are done similar to those for partially specific monoamine reuptake-inhibiting antidepressants. Their common side effects are sexual (delayed ejaculation or anorgasmia, male impotence), gastrointestinal (nausea, vomiting), neurologic (headache, tremor, euphoria, anxiety and nervousness with agitation, insomnia, dizziness), and weight loss with anorexia.

Bupropion is also a specific reuptake inhibitor, but it is not an SSRI. It inhibits dopamine reuptake. Venlafaxine inhibits the reuptake of norepinephrine and serotonin. Nefazodone inhibits norepinephrine reuptake and also blocks autoreceptors, making that neurotransmitter more available.

Monoamine Oxidase Inhibitors (MAOIs)

Monoamine oxidase inhibitors work intracellularly in the presynaptic neuron, reducing the metabolism of all monoamine neurotransmitters and thus making them more available for discharge into the synaptic cleft. MAOIs can be used alone or to enhance non-SSRI reuptake-inhibiting antidepressants. Common side effects are excessive weight gain, muscle twitching, ankle edema, and orthostasis hypotension.

Management of Side Effects

Selecting an antidepressant for nonmelancholic depression is initially based on side effects. Table 7.12 summarizes the nature and management of side effects of monoamine reuptake-inhibiting antidepressants. Table 7.13 summarizes the nature and management of MAOI side effects.

TABLE 7.9. Antidepressant Categories and Some of Their Characteristics

Category	Drug	Characteristics	Clinical Issues
Nonselective monoamine reuptake inhibitors	Imipramine (Tofranil) Amitriptyline Elavil, (Endep), Doxepin (Sinequan), Trimipramine, (Surmontil), Protriptyline (Vivactil)	The old "tricyclics" all have substantial anticholinergic side effects, limiting their use	Low doses of imipramine and amitriptyline are still used 1. To minimize the hypertensive risk of MAOIs, 2. In the treatment of ADHD with depression, 3. For chronic pain syndromes
Partially selective monoamine reuptake inhibitors	1. Clomipramine (Anafranil)	1. Has substantial serotonin reuptake inhibition and used for obsessive compulsive disorder; also has norepinephrine reuptake inhibition 2. Half-life 24 hours 3. Daily dose range 200–300 mg, beginning with 75 mg and increasing by 25 mg daily	Sedating with moderately high anticholinergic and postural hypotensive (orthostasis) properties
	2. Desipramine (Norpramin, Pertofrane)	1. Has substantial norepinephrine reuptake inhibition and a 22–70 hour half-life 2. Easy to use with once a day dosing between 150–300 mg, beginning at 75 mg and increasing by 25 mg daily to 150–200. After 14 days, can go higher	1. Sedating with moderately low anticholinergic and orthostasis properties and only moderate cardiac conduction (quinidine-like) effects 2. A good choice for the otherwise healthy melancholic; also a good choice for women with nonmelancholic depressions who have an anxious-fearful personality disorder; slow clearance so remains in body 2 weeks after last dose

3. Nortriptyline (Pamelor, Aventyl)

1. Most difficult to use as it has inverted U-shaped dose–response curve and plasma levels need to be monitored to keep drug in therapeutic range of 50–170 ng/ml usually seen at doses of 75–150 mg daily

2. Given once daily. Start with 50 mg; 24–30 hour half-life

1. Sedating, alpha adrenergic, and orthostasis properties; slow clearance so remains in body 2 weeks after last dose

2. Cardiac effect modest and quinidine-like. If QRS complex and P–R interval prolonged, patient is likely above therapeutic window

Selective monoamine reuptake inhibitors

1. Fluoxetine* (Prozac) (an SSRI)

1. Primarily inhibits serotonin reuptake in doses of 20–60 mg.

2. Has longest half-life, 2–15 days

3. Most nonmelancholic depressives respond to 20 mg, but if improvement not considerable within 3–4 weeks, increase by 10 mg Q3–4 weeks; given once daily

1. Do not use with other antidepressants because it inhibits liver enzymes leading to high blood levels relative to dose given

2. Most troublesome side effect is altered sexual function (decreased libido, anorgasmia, delayed ejaculation); can also cause anxiety, nausea, akathesia

2. Paroxetine (Paxil) (an SSRI)

1. Most potent SSRI†; shortest half-life, 18–24 hours, of SSRIs

2. Most nonmelancholic depressives respond to 20 mg, can increase up to 50 or 60 mg; morning dosing minimizes insomnia and daytime drowsiness

1. Drowsiness and fatigue, nausea and sweating

2. The SSRI with minimal weight loss, so is the SSRI of choice for anorexia and bulimia

3. Nefazodone (Serzone) (an SSRI)

1. An analogue of trazodone and a first-line drug when insomnia is a major concern

2. Has serotonin reuptake and autoreceptor antagonism, so acts as its own enhancer

3. Daily doses 300–600 mg (begin at 200 mg daily); half-life (3 hours)

Side effects (mostly at doses above 300 mg) include chronic fatigue-like syndrome, hypotension, bradycardia, blurred vision, sinus congestion and upper respiratory problems, nausea, dry mouth, edema.

TABLE 7.9. Antidepressant Categories and Some of Their Characteristics (*continued*)

Category	Drug	Characteristics	Clinical Issues
		requires 3–4 doses daily increased by 100 mg/day after 4-5 days and then every 10 days as needed	
	4. Sertraline (Zoloft) (an SSRI plus)	1. Has broadest reuptake inhibition spectrum of "selective" drugs and second-most potent SSRI effect, thus good at doses 50–200 mg for all types of depression	1. Give after evening meal to avoid nausea and maximize absorption; can also cause diarrhea, tremors, insomnia, and dry mouth
		2. Half-life 1–3 days; begin at 50 mg and increase to 100–150 mg after 1 week	2. Tolerated well by the elderly
	5. Bupropion (Wellbutrin)	1. A dopamine reuptake inhibitor with a 12-hour half-life; also has direct dopaminergic agonistic properties	1. Nonsedating; no anticholinergic, antihistamine or orthostatic properties; and no weight gain
		2. Works in doses 150–300 mg daily for nonmelancholic depressions, particularly in patients with high risk taking behaviors, and drug and alcohol problems as it may reduce craving	2. May cause seizures at higher doses, and eating disorder and epileptic patients are at particular risk; do not give with dopamine agonists or antagonists
		3. Some depressed patients require daily doses up to 450 mg	3. More common side effects: restlessness, hyperactivity, tremors, insomnia, and nausea
	6. Venlafaxine (Effexor)	1. Norepinephrine and serotonin reuptake inhibitor with a half-life of 3–13 hours requiring 2–3 doses daily	1. Elevated blood pressure occurs in some patients above 225 mg daily for more than 2 months
		2. Second choice to desipramine for melancholia in daily doses 200–400 mg	2. Below 225 mg can cause nervousness, drowsiness, anorexia, dizziness, insomnia, nausea, dry

| Monoamine oxidase inhibition | Phenelzine (Nardil) | 1. Twice daily or morning-only doses to avoid insomnia; begin at 15 mg and increase by 15 mg every other day to 60 mg; if response not complete in 3 weeks continue increasing to 90 mg
2. Works alone for nonmelancholic depressions and with a nonspecific reuptake-inhibiting antidepressant for melancholia. | mouth, constipation, sweating, headache, impotence, delayed ejaculation, anorgasmia; abrupt withdrawal can cause headache, nausea, abdominal discomfort, fatigue, tinnitus, sinus congestion
3. Useful for obsessive compulsive disorder with depression
1. Diet and drug–drug interactions biggest problems
2. Can also cause hypotension, resulting in syncope |
| | Selegiline (Eldepryl, Atapryl) | 1. MAO-B selective inhibition
2. Antidepressant dose 20–60 mg daily | 1. A second-line MAOI when patient is allergic to sulfur (other MAOIs come in sulfate form) or is treatment resistant
2. Minimal complications from tyramine-containing foods, and mostly occurring with long-term treatment and in doses above 30 mg daily)
3. Side effects include insomnia and occasional episodes of dizziness and light-headedness (from some lowering of blood pressure)
4. Good choice for depressed patient with Alzheimer's or Parkinson's disease |

TABLE 7.9. Antidepressant Categories and Some of Their Characteristics (continued)

Category	Drug	Characteristics	Clinical Issues
Dopamine agonists	Bromocriptine (Parlodel)	1. Poorly absorbed (<30%), liver metabolized, 90% protein bound. Ergot alkaloid with D_2 agonistic activity 2. Higher doses work at postsynaptic receptors, mimicking dopamine 3. Daily doses vary: neuroleptic malignant syndrome (NMS): 7.5–60 mg; Extrapyramidal side effects (EPS)7.5 mg; depressive syndromes, 10–220 mg (average, 40 mg); cocaine withdrawal over 10 mg	1. Useful for neuroleptic malignant syndrome, cocaine withdrawal depression, apathetic syndromes, Parkinson's disease with and without depression 2. Side effects occur early and at doses above 20 mg daily: nausea, abdominal cramps and constipation, headaches and dizziness, psychosis in persons at higher risk for psychosis
	Amantadine (Symmetril)	300 mg once daily	Useful for cocaine withdrawal depression and the avolitional depressive-like syndrome associated with chronic cocaine use
Other agents	Lithium	As an enhancer and prophylactic agent	See Chapter 9 for details
	Carbamazepine (Tegretol)	For bipolar depressions in combination with lithium, but effect is weak	See Chapter 9 for details
	Pindolol (Visken)	1. A 5-HT_1 autoreceptor and beta-adrenergic 1 and 2 antagonist 2. Peak plasma level in 1 hour, 95% absorbed, no first-pass, 60%–65% hydroxylated in liver, 40% protein bound, half-life 8 hours, dose 2.5 mg TID	1. Used with SSRIs to keep serotonin production and release ongoing; combination may bring substantial relief within 4—10 days 2. Contraindicated in heavy smokers and asthmatics (bronchospasm), diabetics (blocks the

		tachycardia warning in hypoglycemia), persons with hypothyroidism, heart block, or heart failure; also used to treat akathesia (5 mg) and childhood aggression
Mirtazapine	1. An alpha$_2$ adrenergic receptor blocker and norepinephrine agonist 2. Also a 5-HT$_2$ and 5-HT$_3$ postsynaptic and 5-HT$_1$ presynaptic receptor blocker 3. Does not inhibit monoamine reuptake 4. Cytochrome P450 metabolized with a 20–40 hour half-life; can be used once daily 5. Begin at 15 mg daily, increase to 30 mg in 3–4 days, and then up to 45 mg if needed; half-life 20–40 hours	1. Early sedation and weight gain at doses below 15 mg 2. Minimal sexual dysfunction, some dry mouth 3. Best as an enhancer of SSRIs and perhaps venlafaxine and nefazodone 4. Has some antianxiety properties

*Fluvoxamine is a similar drug, but with a shorter half-life (about 20 hours) and no clinical advantages over other SSRIs.

†SSRI potency and therapeutic efficacy not highly correlated.

TABLE 7.10. Pharmacodynamic Profiles of Commonly Used Monoamine Reuptake-Inhibiting Antidepressants

*Neurotransmitter and Receptor Relative Potencies**

Drug	Norepinephrine (NE)	Serotonin (5-HT)	Dopamine (DA)	Histamine (H1)	Adrenergic receptor (Alpha1)	Dopamine presynaptic receptor (D2)	Anticholinergic (Muscarinic)
Desipramine	High	<1	–	Low	Low	<1	Low
Nortriptyline	Modest	<1	–	Low/Modest	Low	–	<1
Clomipramine	Low/Modest	Modest	–	Low	Low/Modest	<1	Low
Fluoxetine	<1	Modest	–	–	–	–	–
Fluvoxamine	<1	Modest	–	–	–	–	–
Sertraline	<1	Modest/High	<1	–	<1	–	<1
Paroxetine	Low	High	–	–	–	–	<1
Bupropion	–	–	<1	–	–	–	–
Venlafaxine	Modest	Modest	–	–	‡	–	–
Nefazodone	<1	<1†	–	–	Low	<1	–

* <1, Meaningful, but small effect; – clinically meaningless effect

† Also 5-HT$_2$

‡ Also beta-adrenoreceptor downregulation.

TABLE 7.11. Pharmacokinetic Profiles of Commonly Used Antidepressants

Drug	Starting Dose (mg)	Dose Range (mg)	Gastrointestinal Absorption	Metabolism* (First-Pass, Liver, P450)	Plasma Protein Binding (percent)	Half-Life (hr)
Desipramine	50	100–300	Slow, 4–8 hr to peak	Oxidation and conjugation	90	12–30
Nortriptyline	20	75–150	Slow, 4–8 hr to peak	Oxidation and conjugation	93	
Clomipramine	75	200–300	Fairly slow, 2–6 hr to peak	Demethylation and conjugation	97	14–79
Fluoxetine	20	20–80	Slow, 4–8 hr to peak	Oxidation and conjugation	94	26–220
Fluvoxamine	100	100–300	Slow, 4–8 hr to peak	Oxidation and conjugation	77	22
Sertraline	25–50	50–200	Slow, 4–8 hr to peak	Oxidation and conjugation	98	24
Paroxetine	10	20–50	Rapid, 2 hr to peak	Oxidation and conjugation	93	4–65 (20 average)
Bupropion	200	200–450	Rapid, 1–3 hr to peak	Hydroxylation	88	4–24 (average 12)
Venlafaxine	75	200–375		Demethylation		2–7†
Nefazodone	200	200–600	Rapid, 1 hr to peak; food delays it	Hydroxylation 20% higher in older people and women	99	2–4†

*Paroxetine is nonlinear inhibiting its own metabolism; thus, as drug concentrations increase, clearance is prolonged.
†Despite short half-life, steady state is still 4–5 days as metabolites accumulate.

TABLE 7.12. Management of Monoamine Reuptake-Inhibiting Antidepressant Side Effects

Side Effect	Management
ANTICHOLINERGIC EFFECTS (ESPECIALLY THE NONSELECTIVE AND PARTIALLY SELECTIVE MONOAMINE REUPTAKE INHIBITORS)	
Dry mouth (melancholia also causes dry mouth)	1. Sugar-free fluids or hard candy (sugar causes weight gain and predisposes to oral candidiasis), commercial saliva substitutes such as Moi-Stir or Orex twice daily or as needed 2. If above fails: pilocarpine 5 mg PO or a 1% oral rinse TID, or bethanechol 10–50 mg PO TID or QID (but can cause abdominal cramps, nausea, diarrhea)
Constipation (melancholia can lead to constipation)	1. High fiber diet, exercise, hydration, bulk laxative (e.g., psyllium) or stool softener 2. If above fail, pilocarpine or bethanechol as above 3. Do not use Milk of Magnesia, as it reduces gastric absorption of most drugs.
Delirium (restlessness, mydriasis, myoclonic jerking, and choreo-athetoid movements can occur without peripheral signs of dry skin and mucosa, tachycardia, and hot flushed skin)	Physostigmine 2 mg IV or SC up to 8 mg daily for 1–3 days
Sexual dysfunctions (melancholia often reduces libido)	1. When due to anticholinergic effect, bethanechol 10–50 mg PO 1–2 hours before coitus, or Neostigmine 7.5–15.0 mg 30 minutes before coitus 2. Sexual dysfunction can also be caused by serotonergic or alpha-adrenergic effects
Blurred vision	1. Caused by a combination of anticholinergic (mydriasis) and sympathomimetic effect (meiosis) 2. Pilocarpine 1% ophthalmic solution, one drop in each eye BID
SEROTONIN SYNDROME (MOST COMMON WHEN SSRI PRESCRIBED SIMULTANEOUSLY WITH OTHER SEROTONERGIC DRUGS)	
1. May be fatal when an SSRI or meperidine is combined with an MAOI; resembles neuroleptic malignant syndrome with gastrointestinal symptoms 2. Manifestations include restlessness, lethargy, insomnia, delerium, skin flushing, sweating, tremor, hyperreflexia, nausea, diarrhea, abdominal	1. If mild, lower dose and prescribe cyproheptidine 4–8 mg/day 2. If severe, discontinue serotonergic drugs, provide supportive measures (e.g., cooling for hyperthermia), and prescribe cyproheptidine plus dantrolene (mg/kg/day in 4 divided doses). Propranolol (20 mg Q8h) or methysergide (2 mg BID) are adjunct treatments

TABLE 7.12. *(continued)*

Side Effect	Management
cramps, and, when more severe, hyperthermia, ataxia, shivering, rigidity, hypertension, rhabdomyolysis, and myoglobinuria. Distinguished from carcinoid syndrome (a serotonin-secreting bowel or lung tumor), which is similar but with cyanosis with flushing, and hypotension	3. ECT can also resolve the syndrome

NEUROLOGIC EFFECTS (PARTICULARLY THE NONSELECTIVE AND PARTIALLY SELECTIVE DRUGS)

Side Effect	Management
Postural tremor	1. Usually due to sympathomimetic effect 2. Propranolol 20–60 mg/day (propranolol can raise blood levels of other psychotropic medications)
Lowered seizure threshold	Maprotiline and bupropion both contraindicated in epileptics, and bupropion also contraindicated in anorexia and bulimia nervosa
Myoclonus	Clonazepam 0.25 mg TID
Stimulation and insomnia (particularly SSRIs with fluoxetine the most likely)	1. For antidepressants with long half-lives and proneness to stimulation and insomnia, prescribe entire dose in morning 2. During worst of depression, short half-life benzodiazepine at night 3. If symptom remains troublesome, change antidepressant 4. Nefazodone least likely of newer drugs to cause insomnia

EXTRAPYRAMIDAL SIDE EFFECTS

Side Effect	Management
Akathesia	1. Can occur with fluoxetine or amoxapine; Amoxapine should not be first-line treatment for depression 2. Propranolol 20–80 mg per day
Parkinsonism, neuroleptic malignant syndrome, tardive dyskinesia	1. Can occur with amoxapine, which is not a recommended antidepressant 2. Treat as described for neuroleptics (see Chapter 9)

CARDIOVASCULAR EFFECTS

Side Effect	Management
Postural hypotension	1. Education about gradual position change; increase salt in diet or give salt tablets 600–1,800 mg; use

TABLE 7.12. Management of Monoamine Reuptake-Inhibiting Antidepressant Side Effects (*continued*)

Side Effect	Management
	support hose, abdominal binder; one cup brewed caffeinated coffee in morning or when symptoms most pronounced
	2. Can add methylphenidate (5 mg), triiodothyronine (25 µg), thyroxine (100–200 µg daily), or 9-alpha-fluorohydrocortisone (0.025–0.05 mg BID)
	3. Because thyroid is an antidepressant enhancer, it should be tried before other agents
Sinus tachycardia (without other antidepressant side effects)	Benign and requires no treatment
Conduction disturbances (non-specific and partially specific monoamine reuptake inhibitors)	1. Quinidine effect (prolonged cardiac repolarization with prolonged QT intervals), predispose to ventricular tachycardia
	2. Switch to another antidepressant

AGRANULOCYTOSIS

Side Effect	Management
Rare; most common among older women in second month of antidepressant treatment	1. Check white blood cell (WBC) counts stat in patients on antidepressants who become febrile
	2. Stop drug if WBCs below 2,000

WEIGHT GAIN

Side Effect	Management
Nonspecific and partially specific monoamine reuptake antidepressants and MAOIs cause weight gain; SSRIs cause weight loss	Prevent and treat as for weight gain of any cause: low calorie diet, medically directed exercise regimen, stimulus control

SEXUAL DYSFUNCTION

Side Effect	Management
Reduced libido, reduced erection or lubrication, delayed or absent orgasm (any antidepressant can cause these, but bupropion least likely to do so)	1. Instead of stopping or switching antidepressant, "allow" antidepressant to alleviate depression; improved mood or tolerance to sexual side effects may restore function
	2. If dysfunction persists despite improved mood, treat as follows: If antidepressant's anticholinergic effect is the likely cause (erectile and ejaculatory dysfunction with preserved libido), treat with bethanechol (a cholinergic agonist) 10–40 mg 30–60 minutes before coitus; if antidepressant's serotonergic effect is the likely cause, cyproheptidine (a serotonin antagonist) 4–12 mg PO 1–2 hours before coitus; for erectile or arousal dysfunction unresponsive to above, yohimbine (alpha$_2$-autoreceptor antagonist) 10 mg PO 1–2 hours before coitus; some patients will have substantially

TABLE 7.12. *(continued)*

Side Effect	Management
	improved sexual function with the addition of 50–75 mg of bupropion or 100–200 mg of amantadine
Priapism	1. Caused only by trazodone (at doses around 150 mg daily) due probably to alpha$_1$-adrenergic receptor blockade
	2. Do not prescribe trazodone to men
	3. If priapism occurs, discontinue, and refer for prompt urologic surgery
Spontaneous ejaculation	1. Rare; occurs most often with SSRIs
	2. Treat with cyproheptidine as described above

Drug–Drug Interactions

In addition to avoiding the use of stimulant-containing drugs and narcotics, persons taking MAOIs must avoid tyramine-containing foods. Table 7.14 lists foods to avoid. Patients taking an MAOI should also carry a 10 mg nifedipine gelatin capsule in case they unwittingly ingest a high tyramine-containing food or develop hypertensive symptoms. Should either occur, the patient bites open and swallows the capsule and immediately seeks medical attention.

After discontinuing an MAOI, avoid prescribing any antidepressant drug for 14 days. ECT, however, can be given immediately but not with barbiturate anesthesia. After discontinuing an SSRI, avoid prescribing an MAOI for 2–6 weeks, depending on the half-life of the SSRI (fluoxetine has the longest half-life [36 hours to several weeks], and paroxitine the shortest [18 hours]). After stopping clomipramine, let 3 weeks elapse. After sertraline, paroxetine, or fluvoxamine, let 2 weeks elapse, and after venlafaxine, 1 week.

You can start an MAOI after giving a partially specific reuptake antidepressant (e.g., desipramine, nortriptyline) or start an MAOI and the partially specific reuptake antidepressant together. This combination actually reduces the risk for an MAOI hypertensive crisis. The combination strategy is done when treating refractory depressions.

Antidepressants are metabolized by the liver, so drugs inducing hepatic enzymes decrease antidepressant blood levels, requiring slightly higher antidepressant doses. Enzyme inducers include alcohol, nicotine, many anticonvulsants, (gabapentine is an exception), barbiturates, chloral hydrate, glutethamide, and oral contraceptives. Antidepressants and alcohol have additive effects in causing drowsiness. Antidepressants can be used in persons with mild but not severe liver disease.

Phenothiazines and butyrophenones inhibit metabolism of antidepressants, increasing antidepressant blood levels. SSRIs also inhibit metabolism of other antidepressants and of benzodiazepines, elevating blood levels of these drugs. In decreasing order, potency of hepatic enzyme inhibition by drug is fluoxetine, flu-

TABLE 7.13. Side Effects of MAOIs

Side Effect	Manifestations	Treatment
Hypertensive crisis	1. From ingesting high tyramine foods or sympathomimetic agents 2. Throbbing headache that often affects occiput, sore neck, nausea, sweating, photophobia	1. Give 50 mg amitriptyline daily to prevent 2. Give 10 mg capsule of nifedipine to bite on if it occurs, followed by emergency room control of blood pressure with phentolamine (an alpha-blocker) 5 mg IV, then 0.25–0.50 mg IV Q4–6h 3. The patient should be in a seated, not lying down, position to reduce gravity effect and its cerebrovascular accident risk
Postural hypotension	1. Syncope after taking several steps immediately upon getting up from a seated or lying down position 2. After nonspecific monoamine reuptake-inhibiting antidepressants, MAOIs most likely type of antidepressant to cause this	Education about gradual position change; increase salt in diet or give salt tablets 600–1800 mg; support hose, abdominal binder; one cup brewed caffeinated coffee in morning or when symptoms are most pronounced
Tremor	Sympathomimetic effect	Propranolol 20–60 mg/day
Weight gain	1. Can be substantial and may lead to noncompliance in weight-conscious patients 2. Most likely antidepressant to cause this	Diet, exercise, dose reduction
Sexual dysfunction	Increased or decreased libido, male erectile disorder or female arousal disorder, delayed orgasm	1. For erectile problem, yohimbine (alpha$_2$- autoreceptor antagonist) 10 mg PO 1 hour before coitus 2. For reduced libido, wait until depression has resolved; if libido has not improved, dose reduction; for other problems, dose reduction
Anticholinergic effects	1. In organs with dual adrenergic and cholinergic innervation 2. Mydriasis with blurred vision, dry mouth, constipation (anticholinergic effects)	Usually mild, requiring no treatment. If not tolerated, follow treatments for anticholinergic problems from other antidepressants and neuroleptics
Psychosis	Amphetamine-like psychosis (especially with tranylcypromine)	1. Rarely seen with phenelzine 2. When it occurs it is mania-like and consider the patient bipolar and give lithium
Neurologic signs	Pyridoxine deficiency: paresthesias, ataxia, hyperreflexia, (harbinger of carpal tunnel syndrome), insomnia, myoclonus, seizures	Pyridoxine 150–300 mg PO daily

TABLE 7.14. The MAOI Diet

Foods To Avoid	Drugs To Avoid
Most cheese and cheese-containing foods (some safe cheeses are ricotta cheese, cottage cheese, cream cheese)	Cold medications (Dristan, Contac) and other over-the-counter sympathomimetic drugs
Fermented or aged foods (e.g., corned beef, salami, pepperoni, sausage; but pickled herring [brine is unsafe], smoked salmon, smoked whitefish are safe)	Nasal decongestants and sinus medications (allergy and hay fever medication)
Liverwurst	Stimulants (meperidine, cocaine, amphetamines, methylphenidate, appetite suppressants)
Broad pea pods	Direct-acting sympathomimetic amines (epinephrine, isoproterenol, methoxamine, levarterenol [norepinephrine])
Meat or yeast extracts (bovril and marmite, though baked goods containing yeast are safe, as is fresh yogurt)	Indirect-acting sympathomimetic amines (phenylpropranolamine, ephedrine, cyclopentamine, pseudoephedrine, tyramine)
Overripe or spoiled fruits	Direct- and indirect-acting sympathomimetic amines (metaraminol, phenylephrine, local anesthetics with epinephrine, levo-dopa for parkinsonism, dopamine)
Soy sauce, fermented bean curd	
Sauerkraut	
Shrimp paste	Narcotics of all types
Beer and ale	
Vermouth, sherry, cognac, full-bodied red wines	

voxamine, paroxetine, sertraline, and venlafaxine. Propranolol can increase the blood levels of other psychotropic drugs. Caffeine and nicotine induce liver enzymes and reduce blood levels of most psychotropics metabolized in the liver. Table 7.15 lists some drug–drug interactions of particular concern.

ELECTROCONVULSIVE THERAPY (ECT)

ECT is used throughout the world. In the United States, 2% of psychiatric admissions to public hospitals, about 10% of admissions to teaching hospitals, and 20% of admissions to private hospitals receive ECT.

ECT is a medical procedure performed in a special suite by a treatment team, including a psychiatrist, anesthetist/anesthesiologist, nurse, and nursing assistant. EKG and EEG monitoring are routine, vital signs are measured and recorded at regular intervals, and, following treatment, the patient is observed by trained personnel in a separate recovery area until fully alert and ambulatory. Patient apprehension is reduced or eliminated by premedication and by fast-acting barbiturates inducing general anesthesia. Muscle relaxants minimize seizure induced muscle contractions, and the patient is ventilated with pure oxygen.

Table 7.15. Drug–Drug Interactions of Particular Concern

Antidepressant	Concerns
Nefazodone	Do not give with over-the-counter antihistamines, as combination may cause cardiac conduction problems (prolonged QT interval) and ventricular tachycardia and death
SSRI	MAOI–SSRI combination may cause lethal serotonin syndrome
MAOI	Cold and cough over-the-counter mixtures with sympathomimetic or narcotic properties can cause a lethal hypertensive crisis
Nonspecific and partially specific monoamine reuptake	Adding an MAOI is okay; adding these to a person already taking an MAOI can cause a lethal hypertensive crisis
Bupropion	Fluoxetine will inhibit liver metabolism of bupropion, leading to higher plasma levels and increased seizure risk

Some transient memory impairment occurs in most patients, but most find their memory fully restored by 30 days following ECT. Some experience a longer lasting but finite period of dysfunction, and a few assert that the treatment permanently impaired their memory. There is no clear evidence for permanent post-ECT memory disturbance as measured by mean memory-test scores in patients versus control groups. When persons who claim such impairment are tested, they function normally on standard memory test batteries. Many high functioning individuals have been successfully treated during their careers without any loss in ability.

Three possibilities may account for the persistent subjective feeling in some patients that their memory long after ECT is not as good as it was before ECT:

1. There is no ECT-related long-term memory deficit, but patients who have received ECT have been sensitized to that possibility and so overinterpret normal aging changes in memory. Education and counseling is the best treatment for this possibility.
2. There is a real ECT-related long-term memory deficit, but it is too small or subtle to be detected by present cognitive tests. If there is some loss of memory, it is a small price to pay for successful treatment and suicide prevention.
3. Depression is a brain disease, and some depressed patients appear to have a limbic sensitization pattern that in bipolar disorder is associated with memory problems independent of ECT (see Chapter 8). Thus, the long-term memory problems that exist in some depressed patients may result from their disease, not their treatment. Rapid and effective treatment of episodes and good maintenance and prophylaxis

offer the best safeguard against this sensitization, and, ironically, ECT may be the best treatment to do this.

Indications

The primary indication for ECT is depression (melancholia and major depression respond best). The more symptoms of depression a patient has, the better the response to ECT. Six to eight induced seizures work for most melancholic episodes (85%–95% response rate). For delusional depression, for the melancholic who is a serious suicide risk, and when the choices are ECT or an antidepressant plus neuroleptic or some combination of other drugs (e.g., lithium, carbamazepine, MAOI), ECT is the most rapid, definitive, and safest treatment. ECT is also the first-line, most effective, rapid, and safest treatment for the depressed patient who is stuporous. Depressed patients who have not done well with the first-line medication choice, usually respond well to ECT. Response is better for those patients who have failed to respond to a specific rather than to a partially specific reuptake inhibitor, but no depressed patient should be thought treatment resistant until he has failed to respond to medications and ECT. Mania is also extremely responsive to ECT (8–15 treatments).

Catatonia (often part of a melancholia) is also extremely ECT responsive, and almost all patients respond fully to two to four seizures. The eventual outcome is determined by the prognosis of the underlying condition. The neuroleptic malignant syndrome and lethal catatonia, variants of the typical catatonic syndrome, are also successfully treated with ECT. Other conditions that respond to ECT are drug-induced psychosis (the more excitement or mood disturbance the better), epileptic psychoses, and most secondary mood disorders. The more acute the episode, and the more episodic the lifetime course of illness, the more likely the patient will respond to ECT. For the depressed patient who has a co-occurring general medical problem, who is pregnant or breast feeding, or who is over age 65, ECT is the most effective and safest antidepressant treatment.

Pretreatment Evaluation

The ECT work-up is the same as for any procedure under general anesthesia: medical history and physical examination, EKG, complete blood count, urinalysis, fasting blood sugar, and blood urea nitrogen. Skull x-rays and an EEG are not useful pretreatment screening tests. Almost one-third of melancholics exhibit pretreatment nonspecific EEG abnormalities that do not predict an unfavorable outcome. If you suspect a brain lesion, get an MRI, but the only absolute contraindication to ECT is increased intracranial pressure. A brain tumor without increased intracranial pressure is not an absolute contraindication (Table 7.16). Chest x-rays are needed only if you suspect the patient has pulmonary disease. Patients with a specific general medical or classic neurologic condition may need additional tests. Pre-ECT spine films are unnecessary with modern techniques. You may need a consultation for the high risk patient (see below) to help stabilize or resolve a problem prior to treatment. Consultants, however, do not approve patients for ECT. The decision to treat is the psychiatrist's.

TABLE 7.16. High Risk ECT Problems and Their Management

Problem	Possible Consequence if Given ECT	Management
Pre-ECT severe hypertension	Can result in post-ECT hypotension and bradyrhythmia	Pretreatment with propranolol (Inderal) 0.5 mg IV and keep blood pressure below 150/100; 0.25 mg atropine IV post-treatment to resolve
Pre-ECT premature ventricular contractions (PVCs)	Ventricular fibrillation	ECT given with lidocaine drip ready should PVCs increase post-ECT; pre-ECT control with propranolol or libidolol
Degenerative joint disease/severe osteoporosis	Fractures	Older women most at risk; increase calculated succinylcholine dose by 40% or more
Prosthetic heart valve	Embolus	Maintain prothrombin time at about 1.5 times, control with maintenance warfarin therapy
Demented patient	More severe and prolonged ECT-induced cognitive impairment	Use unilateral ECT or reduce bilateral treatments to twice weekly or three biweekly
Brain tumor that causes increased intracranial pressure	Further increase in pressure, causing cell damage	A tumor without increased pressure is not a contraindication, and controlling ECT-induced hypertension will control cerebrospinal fluid pressure. Use nitroglycerine sublingually or libidolol to keep blood pressure below 150/100; then treat and have a benzodiazepine ready should an emergence delirium occur. When a patient needing ECT has a tumor causing increased cerebrospinal fluid pressure, a surgical shunt procedure needs to be done

Review all the patient's medications before giving ECT. Benzodiazepines, most other sedative-hypnotics, anticonvulsants, and lidocaine and its analogs all block or reduce seizure length and can be reduced rapidly (1 week) to doses low enough to permit an ECT-induced seizure without causing withdrawal seizures. The most likely problem will be with benzodiazepines. This can be resolved with flumazenil, a benzodiazepine antagonist given 0.2–0.5 mg IV at the time of treatment. Once the seizure has ended, 5 mg diazepam IV will cover the withdrawal period until the next ECT. Antidepressants are unnecessary and increase the risk of emergence delirium. Taper these and then stop them, if possible. Barbiturate anesthesia cannot be given with an MAOI. Lithium (in levels above 0.7 mg/L) exacerbates cognitive side effects and postseizure delirium, and it may cause post-ECT spontaneous seizures. Theophylline in blood levels above 30 µg/dl can lower seizure threshold and cause prolonged seizures. Mycin antibiotics can pro-

TABLE 7.16. (*continued*)

Problem	Possible Consequence if Given ECT	Management
		first; when pressure reduced, treat as above
Pheochromocytoma	Hypertensive crisis	Same as for patient with brain tumor
Unstable cardiac function	Heart failure, fibrillation	Stabilize if possible before ECT, pacemaker; severe hypertension can be controlled by sublingual nitroglycerine
Recent myocardial infarction	Can extend infarction	Wait 6 weeks and treat; if treatment essential before that, best done by ECT expert
Recent stroke	Intracranial hemorrhage	Delay treatment, reduce hypertension as above
Demand pacemaker	May respond to ECT-induced muscle potentials, resulting in severe bradycardia	Convert to fixed mode operation during seizure by placing ring magnet over the pacemaker's pulse generator
Aortic aneurysm or surgical graft	Rupture (although no reported cases)	Increase muscle relaxation
Pulmonary disease	Patients with chronic obstructive pulmonary disease or asthma may be taking theophylline which can cause prolonged seizures and posttreatment spontaneous seizures	Theophylline blood levels below 30 μg/dl safe

long post-ECT apnea. Reserpine can cause fatal hypotension with ECT and should be stopped. Higher doses of *low potency* neuroleptics can lead to severe post-ECT hypotension, cardiovascular collapse, or death. If a neuroleptic is needed during the early part of the ECT treatment course, use a high potency typical or an atypical agent.

Written informed consent for ECT is necessary, unless ordered by a court. The degree to which patients agree to ECT depends greatly on your enthusiasm and knowledge of the treatment and on how much time you are willing to devote to educating and convincing the patient. Ask family members to help.

In some states, the patient who suddenly and unexpectedly becomes acutely suicidal and is in immediate danger of killing himself may be given emergency ECT. Convert the patient to involuntary commitment, often (but not always) first obtaining the family's consent and that of the hospital director or service chief.

Many states now also insist that informed consent for ECT be obtained from involuntary patients as well. If you are thoroughly convinced that the potential benefits of ECT justify involuntary treatment, petition the court to direct that ECT be given against the patient's will. In addition to state requirements, the American Psychiatric Association recommends that informed consent be specific, including the number of treatments (give a range, not a single number) and whether ECT will be continued as maintenance, and that consent may be withdrawn at any time.

Preanesthesia and Anesthesia

The written order to give ECT includes (1) treatment days and starting times, (2) the patient not eating or drinking the day of treatment to avoid vomiting and aspiration, and (3) giving atropine 0.6–1.0 mg IV (preferred in persons under 60 years who are otherwise healthy) or glycopyrarolate 0.2–0.4 mg IV in the ECT waiting area or treatment room immediately before treatment to minimize the risk of vagally-mediated bradyrhythmias or asystole and to reduce bronchial secretions.

Remove and safely store the patient's dentures and eyeglasses. Have patients urinate before going for treatment to avoid incontinence. Make sure the patient's hair and scalp are thoroughly clean to maximize good electrode–scalp contact (see discussion of impedance below).

The ultra-short-acting barbiturate methohexital is the anesthetic of choice. It is the same anesthetic used in minor oral surgery, and it has low risk of EKG abnormalities. Start an intravenous drip with a 250-cc container of glucose and water, using a 19–21 gauge, thin-walled butterfly needle assembly.* After recording vital signs, give a bolus of 60–80 mg of methohexital (1 mg/kg) rapidly into the intravenous tubing. When the patient is asleep, inject 40–50 mg succinylcholine (0.5–1 mg/kg) into the tubing and run it in. You may have to modify subsequent succinylcholine dosage according to the strength of the first seizure. If the patient has substantial osteoporosis, increase the highest range calculated succinylcholine dose by 30%–40%. If the patient has low muscle mass for his body weight, use the lower range of the calculated dose. Watch the patient for muscle fasciculations, representing the depolarization phase of succinylcholine activity. These start in the face, chest, and arms and progress to the legs over 10–20 seconds. When the fasciculations begin to fade in the calves and small muscles of the feet (watch the toes and arches), the patient is ready to be treated. A peroneal nerve stimulator can also be used to determine full muscle relaxation.

Oxygenate with 100% oxygen at a flow rate of at least 5 L /min and a respiration rate of 15–20 breaths/min from the onset of anesthesia until resumption of spontaneous respirations, except during the brief period of the application of the stimulus and the subsequent muscular spasm before the actual seizure begins.

---

*If the patient is a chronic alcoholic, pretreat with intramuscular thiamine and give 400 mg IV thiamine with the intravenous glucose to prevent a Wernicke's encephalopathy (see also Chapter 13).

Use a flexible mouth bite to protect teeth and mouth from damage. For patients with special dental problems, a dentist may have to customize the mouth bite or pull isolated teeth. Extend the patient's head and neck slightly to help maintain an airway. Hold the patient's chin during the passage of the current to keep the jaws tightly closed to avoid injury. The anesthesiologist usually does these procedures. Touching or holding the patient will not lead to injury as with cardiac defibrillation. Voltage is less, and, unless you are in direct contact with the electrode surface or some conducting gel, you feel nothing.

Treatment Electrode Application

Bilateral ECT, the original method, is administered through bifrontotemporal electrodes, one on each side of the head, placed an inch above the midpoint of an imaginary line joining the outer canthus of the eye and the external auditory meatus (Fig. 7.1). Unilateral ECT, a modification introduced in 1958, is administered through electrodes placed over the nondominant hemisphere only. The lower (temporal) electrode is placed as for bilateral ECT, and the upper electrode is placed above this, as far up to the vertex and midline as possible. Right-sided unilateral ECT is given initially even to left handers. If a left hander exhibits verbal memory impairment after the first treatment, move treatment electrodes to the left hemisphere for further treatments.

Unilateral electrode placement

Bilateral electrode placement

Placement of EEG electrodes

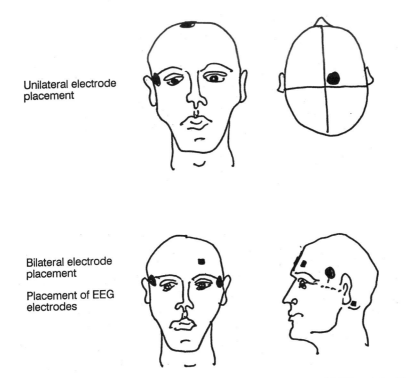

Figure 7.1. Electrode placements for unilateral and bilateral ECT and for EEG monitoring.

For patients treated for depression, which electrode placement to use remains controversial. Bilateral ECT is recommended here because less treatments are needed and the response to unilateral is more variable. If you begin with unilateral, however, change to bilateral if you do not observe significant improvement after three to four treatments. When you need a rapid response, as in suicidal, psychotic, agitated, or stuporous depressives, give bilateral ECT. Manics, catatonics, and other psychotic patients should always get bilateral ECT.

Treatment Current and Dosing

Modern ECT uses only brief pulse current. It is more efficient in inducing a seizure and uses less electricity than the old sinusoidal wave machines, thus causing less memory problems.

Most pulse-wave ECT machines deliver about the same amount of energy, and settings are based on manufacturer specification. In general, the primary consideration is to deliver an adequate amount of energy to induce a grand mal seizure. Some considerations are

1. Seizure thresholds are higher (and therefore more energy is needed for a seizure) in the elderly and in men.
2. Seizure thresholds increase over the course of treatment in about 30%–40% of patients, so energy doses may need to be increased after three to four treatments.
3. With unilateral ECT, stimuli marginally above the seizure threshold are less therapeutic than those delivered at a higher intensity (about 50% above threshold), but grossly suprathreshold stimuli lead to more cognitive impairment without an equivalent increase in therapeutic effect (an inverted U-shaped dose–response curve analogous to that of nortriptyline).

Because the amount of energy delivered to a large extent determines if a patient has a seizure and how much memory problems he will have, you need to determine the proper level for each patient. For bilateral ECT, take half the patient's age as a percentage of the maximum energy the machine can deliver, and use that energy level for the first treatment (e.g., a 60-year-old person gets 30% of the maximum). For most patients this will be adequate to induce a seizure. If not, immediately restimulate (up to four total stimulations during that first session), raising the energy level by increments of 20% of maximum until a seizure is induced. Then use that level for the remaining treatments. For unilateral ECT you have two methods: One, start with 80% or 100% of maximum for patients under and over age 60, respectively, whereas for adolescents and young adults, start with 40% of maximum. Two, be prepared to stimulate several times beginning at a low energy and going up by 50%–100% until you find the threshold and then treating at 50% above that. For example, if you started with 10% and got a seizure at 40%, you would treat at 60%.

Always check each patient's scalp to electrode to machine hook-up for impedance (the resistance to the energy you want to deliver). Too low an impedance (<100 ohms) indicates a short circuiting of the current flow (e.g., conductive gel that spread between electrodes, hair oils not thoroughly washed out). Too high an impedance (>2,700 ohms) indicates an inadequate circuit (e.g., poor electrode contact with the skin, skin not properly cleaned, defective wires or cables), and you will not get a therapeutic seizure. Impedance of about 1,000 ohms is a good medium.

The Seizure

Inducing a fully developed grand mal *brain* seizure is necessary to have a therapeutic effect. The motor part of the seizure is irrelevant. Missed, abortive, or partial seizures occasionally occur, most often with unilateral ECT. Even with extreme degrees of muscle relaxation, you can see the tonic seizure phase and its pronounced plantarflexion lasting for 5–10 seconds. If you do not see this, repeat the electrical stimulation immediately to take advantage of the temporarily lowered seizure threshold from the initial stimulus. Additional evidence that you induced a seizure is sudden tachycardia. You can also indirectly monitor brain seizure activity throughout the procedure by inflating a blood pressure cuff beyond systolic blood pressure over one arm or leg before you give the succinylcholine. You can then observe the unmodified muscle seizure in the occluded limb. Use the ipsilateral limb when you give unilateral ECT so you can see if the seizure generalized to the opposite hemisphere.

EEG monitoring is the best way to determine adequate seizures. If total seizure time is less than 25 seconds (18–20 seconds in the elderly) or is otherwise inadequate, restimulate at a higher intensity after waiting about 1 minute for the refractory period to pass. It is almost never necessary to give additional succinylcholine in this event, as an adequate degree of muscle relaxation for ECT continues for several minutes after the peak effect has been reached. The above does not mean that the longer the seizure the better, but rather that seizures of longer than 25 seconds are more likely to be full grand mal seizures. The length of the grand mal seizure beyond 25 seconds is not correlated with therapeutic outcome. A minimum of a single-channel EEG recording is standard procedure for all ECT (one lead on the left forehead 1 inch above the eyebrow mid-pupil and the other behind the left ear over the mastoid bone as close to the hairline as possible). This frontomastoid, two-lead set-up monitors EEG over the left hemisphere so you can see if the seizure really generalized when giving right unilateral ECT. Two-channel EEG monitoring is better (eliminate any EMG leads to do this) because then you can see left and right hemisphere activities and any symmetry of EEG.

The characteristics of an adequate EEG seizure are

1. Duration of 30–40 seconds or more except for patients over age 70, when 18–25 seconds is acceptable.
2. Both hemispheres become synchronous in their electrical discharges (i.e., the tracings of the two channels look similar).
3. There is a pattern of a slow build up followed by 30-40 seconds of high

amplitude slow waves with spikes or spikes on top of the slow waves followed by a breaking up of the high amplitude discharge.

4. There is a relatively sharp end point followed by low amplitude waves.

Some machines provide an analysis of the EEG, giving you the amount of seizure energy produced. Total seizure energy below 800 is inadequate. Total seizure energy of 1,500 or above is good.

Missed or inadequate seizures usually result from poor electrode contact, premature termination of the stimulus, or disconnected cables. Occasionally, despite maximum energy doses and proper equipment, some patients will still not have a seizure. At the next session reduce somewhat the dose of anesthetic, hyperventilate prior to stimulation, and give 200–1,500 mg caffeine IV over a 1-minute period 2–3 minutes prior to anesthesia or a 500-mg theophylline suppository the night before treatment to lower the seizure threshold sufficiently to permit seizure induction. Caffeine augmentation at higher doses may raise pre-ECT blood pressure beyond 150/100 in some hypertensive patients and cause arrhythmias in some cardiac patients. Use theophylline for these patients.

After the seizure ends, ventilate for several minutes until spontaneous respirations return. Then remove the intravenous tubing, turn the patient on his side, and wheel him to a nearby recovery area where he is observed until he awakens. During the recovery phase, an airway and adequate exchange of air are maintained. Suction and oxygen equipment, although rarely required, should be immediately available.

ECT stresses the cardiovascular system directly through an initial Valsalva effect and then from seizure-induced generalized autonomic and motor discharges. Heart rate and blood pressure initially increase. Pulse rates typically rise to 130–150 beats/min with accompanying systolic blood pressure around 200 mmHg. A sharp drop in heart rate correlates with the end of the seizure (usually less than 1 minute), and both heart rate and blood pressure return to baseline by 1 minute or so after the seizure ends. Cerebral blood flow increases after an initial brief reduction during the electrical stimulus, and this is accompanied by doubling of cerebral oxygen consumption and glucose utilization during the induced seizure. However, there is no cerebral anoxia during succinylcholine-modified ECT because of the high blood oxygen saturation during ventilation and the very small amounts of oxygen used peripherally by the paralyzed muscles.

Complications and Side Effects

Emergence delirium from anesthesia affects about 5%–10% of patients. Reassurance or firm persuasion does not help. Restrain the patient and give the short-acting benzodiazepine midazolam 2 mg IV to terminate the episode. Repeat episodes usually occur with each subsequent treatment and can be prevented by giving midazolam immediately after the seizure. Untreated, emergence delirium rarely lasts longer than 15–20 minutes.

Prolonged apnea is an extremely rare complication of ECT muscle relaxation and results from a relative deficiency of pseudocholinesterase, the enzyme that degrades succinylcholine. If spontaneous respirations do not return by 5 minutes after the seizure has ended, prepare to intubate; if assisted respiration is still required after 10 minutes, intubate. Most patients with this complication will breathe spontaneously within 30 minutes and the remainder within 60–90 minutes.

Occasionally, a seizure will persist for more than 120 seconds. *Prolonged seizures* are not beneficial, so terminate with 10 mg diazepam IV any seizure that lasts longer than 120 seconds.

The main side effect of ECT is *temporary disorientation and memory loss,* mostly seen after several bilateral ECT. This side effect may be exaggerated in patients over age 60. The memory loss consists of a fully recoverable retrograde amnesia for events preceding the first treatment, with amnesia more pronounced for recent than remote events, and a permanent anterograde amnesia from failure to consolidate new memories during several post-ictal hours. Once treatments have ended, the retrograde amnesia resolves over several weeks and usually disappears by 30–60 days. Because of the anterograde amnesia, however, patients often complain of memory gaps for parts of their hospital stay. As depression also impairs cognitive function, memory may also be incomplete for events prior to treatment when the depression was at its worst. Memory impairment from depression improves with remission whether the treatment is medication or ECT.

Memory changes following unilateral ECT administered to the nondominant hemisphere are much less than those with bilateral ECT. Immediately following a seizure, personal orientation returns more rapidly with unilateral than with bilateral ECT, as does recall of items learned immediately prior to the seizure. Both retrograde and anterograde amnesia are reduced, as well as the cumulative memory impairment following a course of treatment. By 1 year post-ECT, patients' memory functions are similar to those of controls. When memory and cognition concerns during the 6 weeks post-ECT are of paramount importance, use unilateral ECT. For most patients, bilateral will be more therapeutic.

Induced convulsions are characterized not only by the electrical discharge of the seizure but by *EEG changes* that persist into the interseizure period. These changes include increased amplitude, slowing, and increased rhythmicity. They appear all over the scalp, the degree of slowing directly related to the number and frequency of seizures and the location of the treatment electrodes. Consider these EEG changes a transient side effect indicating that you gave adequate treatments.

Other problems that can arise from ECT are: *jaw and tooth fractures* (dental consults when needed and special mouth bites can eliminate these), *vertebrae fractures* (almost always due to not allowing enough time for the succinylcholine to work and only in elderly women patients; when in doubt use a muscle stimulator to tell when paralysis complete), and, most commonly, *headache* (40% of patients on the day of treatment, most analgesics work). The *death* rate associated with ECT is 10% that from natural childbirth, and all documented ECT induced deaths were due to error, not to the procedure itself.

High Risk Patients

There are no contraindications to ECT, although several conditions increase the risk for side effects and complications. Although many of these conditions occur in the elderly, if left untreated, the mortality rate of the depressed elderly is increased. The risks from pharmacotherapy, however, are also greater in the elderly than in younger patients, as elderly patients are more likely to have co-occurring chronic general medical illness and are physiologically more sensitive than are younger patients to the anticholinergic, cardiotoxic, and hypotensive effects of medications. If appropriate precautions are taken, the risks from ECT in these patients are substantially less than those from medications. The elderly may also respond to ECT better than younger patients.

ECT complications are more likely when a patient has cardiovascular disease (arrhythmias, hypertension, recent myocardial infarction, occlusive vascular disease, aneurysms and their surgical repair, recent stroke), chronic obstructive pulmonary disease, degenerative joint disease, severe osteoporosis, dementia, brain tumor, or pheochromocytoma. Table 7.16 lists some high risk problems and techniques to resolve them or minimize risks.

Although ECT is the safest antidepressant treatment for the severely ill depressed pregnant woman, pregnancy requires special attention in ECT technique. Consider the following guidelines:

1. There is a greater than typical risk for *aspiration* because of prolonged gastric emptying time or from gastric reflux. Treat as if the stomach were full, even though the patient has had nothing by mouth. During the third trimester, this may require preventative intubation to protect the airway. Use small instruments to minimize damage. Also use sodium citrate (30 cc of 0.3 M sodium citrate 15–20 minutes before ECT), a nonparticulate antacid, to minimize gastric acidity and thus any aspiration pneumonitis.

2. *Maternal aortocaval compression* can occur after 20 weeks gestation when lying prone. Elevate one hip to shift the uterus, and hydrate with normal saline prior to treating to minimize this.

3. Use *glycopyrrolate* rather than atropine. The latter crosses the placenta and causes fetal tachycardia. Glycopyrrolate minimally crosses the placenta.

4. Prior to ECT, obtain an *obstetrical consultation* and, if needed, have the obstetrician available during treatment. If possible, discontinue all anticholinergic medications; after ECT recheck for vaginal bleeding, uterine contraindications, and fetal arrhythmias (fetal heart rate typically remains unchanged during ECT).

Continuation ECT Treatment

Without some maintenance treatment the post-treatment 6-month relapse rate with ECT ranges from 30%–60% (peaking during the first 10 days and over the first 6 weeks post-ECT). Follow-up treatment with antidepressants (for unipolar melancholia) or lithium or an anticonvulsant (for bipolar disorder) after a successful course of ECT reduces the relapse rate to about 10%–15%. Maintenance drug doses are the same as those used in acute treatment of depression. For patients who relapse despite continuation pharmacotherapy, consider continuation of ECT. With continuation ECT, patients return at regular intervals for additional treatments even in the absence of any recurrence of symptoms.

Although there is no broad consensus on how to prescribe continuation ECT, several factors are known: The largest number of relapses occur in the first 10 days after a successful course of ECT, with the majority of the remaining relapses occurring during the next 5 weeks; and relapses while receiving continuation ECT tend to occur when treatments are spaced beyond every 2 weeks. To maximize the efficacy of the continuation period consider doing the following:

1. Carefully monitor symptoms and follow with periodic DSTs to pick up relapse early on.
2. Begin continuation treatments the first week after the successful course.
3. Give weekly ECT for the next 6 weeks.
4. Give biweekly treatments for the next 4–6 months.
5. If symptoms begin to recur or DST reverts from suppression to non-suppression, give a treatment as soon as possible and temporarily increase the frequency back to once weekly until the DST reverts back to suppression.

The above regimen adds up to 14–19 treatments or more if relapse begins. At this point reevaluate. If you think more ECT is necessary, continue at 1 every 2 weeks and reevaluate again in 3 months (another six to seven treatments). If more is still needed, continue at 1 every 2 weeks (another six to seven treatments), with a continuation period now of 1 year with a total of about 33 treatments.

If after 6, 9, or 12 months you decide to switch from continuation ECT to medications, do the following:

1. Keep the patient in the hospital after the last ECT. The patient does not have to be on a locked psychiatric ward for this admission.
2. The day of the last ECT, following recovery, give an evening loading dose if the drug of choice is lithium or valproate.
3. The following day, if the drug is tolerated, give the full therapeutic dose; if this is tolerated, discharge the patient on that dose. Steady state should be achieved in 4–5 days.

The patient will then be at steady state with the therapeutic dose of your first choice maintenance drug for 9–10 days before what would be the next ECT. This period permits some patients to continue a successful maintenance period without continuing ECT. If you cannot hospitalize or use the loading dose strategy, overlap the ECT with the drug by 1–3 weeks, depending, on the half-life of the drug. If, however, the patient relapses on the drug, and previous medication trials (single or in combination) have not worked, then continuation ECT may be needed for a prolonged period. The alternative is rehospitalization and an attempt to stabilize the patient on a combination of medications. Patients usually given continuation ECT are those with multiple hospitalizations and who have failed to respond to multiple drug regimens. Although studies are few, rehospitalization for these patients can drop by two-thirds with continuation ECT. Some patients will need a treatment every 2–4 weeks for an indefinite period of time.

ADDITIONAL READINGS

Abrams R: *Electroconvulsive Therapy,* 2nd ed. Oxford University Press, New York, 1992.

APA Task Force on Electroconvulsive Therapy: *The Practice of Electroconvulsive Therapy.* The American Psychiatric Association, Washington, DC, 1990.

Bancroft J: The premenstrual syndrome. A reappraisal of the concept and the evidence. *Psychological Medicine Monograph Supplement 24,* Cambridge University Press, Cambridge, England, 1993.

Barchas JD, Bunney WE Jr (eds): Neuroscience of depression: Part A: Diagnostic, epidemiologic, and physiologic aspects. *Clin Neurosci* 1:69–112, 1993.

Barchas JD, Bunney WE Jr (eds): Neuroscience of depression: Part B: Neurobiological, genetic, and molecular aspects. *Clin Neurosci* 1:115–121, 1993.

Barraclough B, Bunch J, Nelson B, Sainsbury P: A hundred cases of suicide: Clinical aspects. *Br J Psychiatry* 125:335–373, 1974.

Berner P, Musalek M, Welter H: Psychopathological concepts of dysphoria. *Psychopathology* 20:93–100, 1987.

Blier P, Bergeron R, de Montigny C: Selective activation of postsynaptic 5-HT$_{1A}$ receptors induces rapid antidepressant response. *Neuropsychopharmacology* 16:333–338, 1997.

Borson S, Claypoole K, McDonald GJ: Depression and chronic obstructive pulmonary disease: Treatment trials. *Semin Clin Neuropsychiatry* 3:115–130, 1998.

Bouckoms AJ: The role of stereotactic cingulotomy in the treatment of intractable depression. In Amsterdam JD (ed): *Advances in Neuropsychiatry and Psychopharmacology, vol 2, Refractory Depression,* Raven Press, New York, 1991, pp 233–242.

Brumback RA: Is depression a neurologic disease? In Brumback RA (ed): *Behavioral Neurology, Neurologic Clinics, vol 11.* WB Saunders, Philadelphia, 1993, pp 79–104.

Burton SW, Akiskal HS (eds): *Dysthymic Disorder.* The Royal College of Psychiatrists, Gaskell, 1990.

Calev A, Nigal D, Shipira B, Tubi N, Chazan S, Ben-Yehuda Y, Kugelmass S, Lerer B: Early and long-term effects of electroconvulsive therapy and depression on memory and other cognitive functions. *J Nerv Ment Dis* 179:526–533, 1991.

Casey P, Meagher D, Butler E: Personality, functioning, and recovery from major depression. *J Nerv Ment Dis* 184:240–245, 1996.

Clauw DJ: The pathogenesis of chronic pain and fatigue syndromes, with special reference to fibromyalgia. *Med Hypoth* 44:369–378, 1995.

Devanand DP, Dwork AJ, Hutchinson ER, Bolwig TG, Sackeim HA: Does ECT alter brain structure? *Am J Psychiatry* 151:957–970, 1994.

Duggan CF, Sham P, Lee AS, Murray RM: Can future suicidal behavior in depressed patients be predicted. *J Affect Disord* 22:111–118, 1991.

Fink M: Response to commentaries on "How does convulsive therapy work?" *Neuropsychopharmacology* 3:97–99, 1990.

Fink M: Impact of the antipsychiatry movement on the revival of electroconvulsive therapy in the United States. *Psychiatr Clin North Am Electroconvulsive Ther* 14:793–801, 1991.

Fink M: What is an adequate treatment in convulsive therapy? *Acta Psychiatr Scand* 84:424–427, 1991.

Fink M: Optimizing ECT. *L'Encephale* pp 297–302, 1994.

Fink M: Combining electroconvulsive therapy and drugs. A review of safety and efficacy. *CNS Drugs* 1:370–376, 1994.

Fink M: The decision to use ECT: For whom? When? In Rush AG (ed): *Mood Disorders, Sys-*

tematic Medication Management. Modern Problems in Pharmacopsychiatry, vol 25. Karger, Basel, 1997, pp 203–214.

Fink M, Sackeim HA: Convulsive therapy in schizophrenia. *Schizophr Bull* 22:27–39, 1996.

George MS, Ketter TA, Post RM: SPECT and PET imaging in mood disorders. *J Clin Psychiatry* 54(suppl 11): 6–13, 1993.

Gitlin MJ: Psychotropic medications and their effects on sexual function: Diagnosis, biology, and treatment approaches. *J Clin Psychiatry* 55:406–413, 1994.

Glassman AH, Bigger JT Jr: Cardiovascular effects of therapeutic doses of tricyclic antidepressants: A review. *Arch Gen Psychiatry* 38:815–820, 1981.

Greenberg L, Fink M: The use of electroconvulsive therapy in geriatric patients. *Clin Geriatr Med Psychiatr Disord Late Life* 8:349–354, 1992.

Heilman KM, Satz P (eds): *Neuropsychology of Human Emotion.* Guilford Press, New York, 1983.

Henriques JB, Davidson RJ: Regional brain electrical asymmetries discriminate between previously depressed and healthy control subjects. *J Abnorm Psychol* 99:22–31, 1990.

Herrmann N, Shulman Kl (eds): Mood disorders in old age. *Clin Neurosci* 4, 1997.

Jablinsky A: Prediction of the course and outcome on depression. *Psychol Med* 17:1–9, 1987.

Kato T, Inubushi T, Kato N: Magnetic resonance spectroscopy in affective disorders. *J Neuropsychiatry Clin Neurosci* 10:133–147, 1998.

Katon W: The effect of major depression on chronic medical illness. *Semin Clin Neuropsychiatry* 3:82–86, 1998.

Kellner CH, Pritchett JT, Beale MD, Coffey CE: *Handbook of ECT.* American Psychiatric Press, Washington, DC, 1997.

Klein DN, Riso LP, Donaldson SK, Schwartz JE, Anderson RL, Ouimette PC, Lizardi H, Aronson FA: Family study of early-onset dysthymia. *Arch Gen Psychiatry* 52:487–496, 1995.

Kocsis JH, Zisook S, Davidson J, Shelton R, Yonkers K, Hellerstein DJ, Rosenbaum J, Halbreich U: Double-blind comparison of sertraline, imipramine, and placebo in the treatment of dysthymia: Psychosocial outcomes. *Am J Psychiatry* 154:390–395, 1997.

Koren G, Pastuszak A, Ito S: Drugs in pregnancy. *N Engl J Med* 338:1128–1137, 1998.

Krishnan KRR, Hays JC, Blazer DG: MRI-defined vascular depression. *Am J Psychiatry* 154:497–501, 1997.

Krystal AD, Coffey CE, Weiner RD, Holsinger T: Changes in seizure threshold over the course of electroconvulsive therapy affect therapeutic response and are detected by ictal EEG ratings. *J Neuropsychiatry Clin Neurosci* 10:178–186, 1998.

Krystal AD, Weiner RD, Coffey CE: The ictal EEG as a marker of adequate stimulus intensity with unilateral ECT. *J Neuropsychiatry Clin Neurosci* 7:295–303, 1995.

Kulin NA, Pastuszak A, Sage SR, Schick-Boschetto B, Spivey G, Feldkamp M, Ormond K, Matsui D, Stein-Scheckman AK, Cook L, Brochu J, Rieder M, Koren G: Pregnancy outcome following maternal use of the new selective serotonin reuptake inhibitors: A prospective controlled multicenter study. *JAMA* 279:609–610, 1998.

Lejoyeux M, Ades J: Antidepressant discontinuation: A review of the literature. *J Clin Psychiatry* 58(suppl 7):11–16, 1997.

Leonard BE: Pharmacological effects of serotonin reuptake inhibitors. *J Clin Psychiatry* 49(suppl):12–17, 1988.

Liu B, Anderson G, Mittmann N, To T, Axcell T, Shear N: Use of selective serotonin-reuptake inhibitors or tricyclic antidepressants and risk of hip fractures in elderly people. *Lancet* 351:1303–1307, 1998.

Lustman PJ, Clouse RE, Freedland KE: Management of major depression in adults with diabetes: Implications of recent clinical trials. *Semin Clin Neuropsychiatry* 3:102–114, 1998.

Maes M, Cosyns P, Maes L, D'Hondt P, Schotte C: Clinical subtypes of unipolar depression. Part I. A validation of the vital and nonvital clusters. *Psychiatry Res* 34:29–41, 1990.

Maes M, Maes L, Schotte C, Vanderwoude M, Martin M, D'Hondt P, Blockx P, Scharpe S,

Cosyns P: Clinical subtypes of unipolar depression: Part III. Quantitative differences in various biological markers between the cluster analytically generated nonvital and vital depression classes. *Psychiatry Res 34:*59–75, 1990.

Maes M, Schotte C, Maes L, Cosyns P: Clinical subtypes of unipolar depression: Part II. Quantitative and qualitative clinical differences between the vital and nonvital depressive groups. *Psychiatry Res 34:*43–57, 1990.

Mann SC, Caroff SN, Bleier HR, Antelo E, Un H: Electroconvulsive therapy of the lethal catatonia syndrome. *Convulsive Ther 6:*239–247, 1990.

Maser JD, Cloninger CR (eds): *Comorbidity of Mood and Anxiety Disorders.* American Psychiatric Press, Washington, DC, 1990.

Mayberg HS: Frontal lobe dysfunction in secondary depression. *J Neuropsychiatry Clin Neurosci 6:*428–442, 1994.

Moellentine C, Rummans T, Ahlskog JE, Harmsen WS, Suman VJ, O'Connor MK, Black JL, Pileggi T: Effectiveness of ECT in patients with parkinsonism. *J Neuropsychiatry Clin Neurosci 10:*187–193, 1998.

Moldin SO, Scheftner WA, Price JP, Nelson E, Knesevich MA, Akiskal H: Association between major depressive disorder and physical illness. *Psychol Med 23:*755–761, 1993.

Murphy GE: The physician's responsibility for suicide: I. An error of commission. *Ann Intern Med 82:*301–304, 1975.

Nasrallah HA, Coffman JA, Olson SC: Structured brain imaging findings in affective disorders: An overview. *J Neuropsychiatry 1:*21–26, 1989.

Nemeroff CB: The neurobiology of depression. *Sci Am 278:*42–49, 1998.

Nobler MS, Roose SP: Differential response to antidepressants in melancholic and severe depression. *Psychiatr Ann 28:*84–88, 1998.

Nulman I, Rovet J, Stewart DE, Wolpin J, Gardner HA, Theis, JGW, Kulin N, Koren G: Neurodevelopment of children exposed in utero to antidepressant drugs. *N Engl J Med 336:*258–262, 1997.

Nutt D: Not only but also? Comments on "How does convulsive therapy work?" *Neuropsychopharmacology 3:*93–95, 1990.

O'Brien JT, Desmond P, Ames D, Schweitzer I, Tuckwell V, Tress B: The differentiation of depression from dementia by temporal lobe magnetic resonance imaging. *Psychol Med 24:*633–640, 1994.

Parker G, Ray K, Hadzi-Pavlovic D, Pedic F: Psychotic (delusional) depression: A meta-analysis of physical treatments. *J Affect Disord 24:*17–24, 1992.

Philibert RA, Richards L, Lynch CF, Winokur G: Effect of ECT on mortality and clinical outcome in geriatric unipolar depression. *J Clin Psychiatry 56:*390–394, 1995.

Preskorn SH: Comparison of the tolerability of nefazodone, imipramine, fluoxetine, sertraline, paroxetine, and venlafaxine. *J Clin Psychiatry 56* (suppl 6):17–25, 1995.

Rabheru K, Persad E: A review of continuation and maintenance electroconvulsive therapy. *Can J Psychiatry 42:*476–484, 1997.

Ross ED, Rush AJ: Diagnosis and neuroanatomical correlates of depression in brain damaged patients. Implications for a neurology of depression. *Arch Gen Psychiatry 38:*1344–1354, 1981.

Rush AJ, Weissenburger JE: Melancholic symptom features and DSM-IV. *Am J Psychiatry 151:*489–498, 1994.

Sackeim, HA, Decina P, Kanzler M, Kerr B, Malitz S: Effects of electrode placement on the efficacy of titrated low-dose ECT. *Am J Psychiatry 144:*1449–1455, 1987.

Schatzberg AF, Haddad P, Kaplan EM, Lejoyeux M, Rosenbaum JF, Young AH, Zajecka J: Possible biological mechanisms of the serotonin reuptake inhibitor discontinuation syndrome. *J Clin Psychiatry 58* (suppl 7):23–27, 1997.

Schatzberg AF, Nemeroff CB (eds): *Textbook of Psychopharmacology.* American Psychiatric Press, Washington, DC, 1995.

Shores MM, Pascualy M, Veith RC: Major depression and heart disease: Treatment trials. *Semin Clin Psychiatry 3:*87–101, 1998.

Squire LR, Chace PM: Classics in ECT research: Memory functions six to nine months after electroconvulsive therapy. *Convulsive Ther 12:*239–256, 1997.

Stoudemire A: Recurrence and relapse in geriatric depression: A review of risk factors and prophylactic treatment strategies. *J Neuropsychiatry Clin Neurosci 9:*208–221, 1997.

Sturm R, Wells KB: How can care for depression become more cost-effective? *JAMA 273:*51–58, 1995.

Sunderland T, Cohen RM, Molchan S, Lawlor BA, Mellow AM, Newhouse PA, Tariot PN, Mueller EA, Murphy DL: High-dose selegiline in treatment-resistant older depressive patients. *Arch Gen Psychiatry 51:*607–615, 1994.

Suominen KH, Isometsa ET, Henriksson MM, Ostamo AL, Lonnqvist JK: Inadequate treatment for major depression both before and after attempted suicide. *Am J Psychiatry 155:*1778–1780, 1998.

Terman M, Amira L, Terman JS, Ross DC: Predictors of response and nonresponse to light treatment for winter depression. *Am J Psychiatry 153:*1423–1429, 1996.

Tollefson GD: Adverse drug reactions/interactions in maintenance therapy. *J Clin Psychiatry 54*(suppl):48–58, 1993.

Tsuang MT, Faraone SV: *The Genetics of Mood Disorders.* The Johns Hopkins University Press, Baltimore, 1990.

Warner P, Bancroft J, Dixon A, Hampson M: The relationship between perimenstrual depressive mood and depressive illness. *J Affect Disorder 23:*9–23, 1991.

Wessely S: The neuropsychiatry of chronic fatigue syndrome. *Ciba Found Symp 173:*212–237, 1993.

8

Bipolar Mood Disorders

Bipolar mood disorder is defined as the presence sometime during a person's life of mania, hypomania, or variants of these intense mood states. The number and severity of depressions are irrelevant to the category. A patient with only recurrent mania is bipolar. A patient with many recurrent depressions and only one mania is bipolar. Table 8.1 displays the bipolar disorders and their definitions.

About 1%–2% of the general population is at lifetime risk for bipolar disorder, and another 2%–3% may have milder forms (the soft bipolar spectrum). Bipolar disorder is familial, with age-corrected prevalences of 5%–10% for bipolar disorder *and* 10%–15% for unipolar in the first-degree relatives of bipolar patients. Adopted children with an ill biologic parent are also at greater risk for mood disorder. A person's risk increases 3-fold if one parent is ill and 10-fold if both parents are ill. The relatives of bipolar patients are also at greater risk for some eating disorders.

Concordance rates (both twins having it) among monozygotic and dizygotic twins are about 65% and 25%, respectively, and the rate is higher for bipolar than for unipolar twin pairs. In about 20% of concordant twins one member is bipolar and one unipolar. Some common (but unknown) genotype obviously exists for some bipolar and unipolar patients. Genes on the long arm of chromosome 18 may play a role in some families. Genes in this area relate to G-protein (part of the postsynaptic intracellular second-messenger system associated with some dopamine receptors). Most likely other genes on other chromosomes are also involved.

The risk for suicide is also high among bipolar patients. Among teenagers, bipolar patients are twice as likely to kill themselves as are unipolar patients. The risk for teenage suicide is directly related to drug use, access to guns, and lack of treatment for the mood disorder. For persons aged 25–60 years, suicide rates are similar for unipolar and bipolar patients. Among persons over 60 years, the rate for suicide is slightly higher for unipolar patients.

TABLE 8.1. Bipolar Disorders

Disorder	Definition	Clinical Issues
Bipolar I	Episodes of mania and depression, both requiring treatment	1. Rapid cyclers, mixed syndrome; schizoaffectives, substance abusers; chronic patients in this group are difficult to treat
		2. ECT is sometimes most effective, and can avoid polypharmacy.
some	Bipolar II 1. Unlike recurrent unipolar depression, these depressions are hypomanias or soft bipolar spectrum behaviors that usually do not get treated	Episodes of depression that require treatment, plus more likely to respond to lithium and anticonvulsants
		2. Treating these depressions with antidepressants alone can precipitate a more serious mania (30% of patients)
Mixed mood state	Signs and symptoms of mania and depression occur in the same episode, usually in sequence, but occasionally simultaneously	Harder to treat than pure episode; Not a distinct subgroup
Schizoaffective mania	A mania with psychosis in a more chronic patient	Treat as a mood disorder
Hypomania	A mild mania	1. Treat if it interferes adversely with functioning or a subjective feeling of well being
		2. Follow untreated patients and do periodic assessments for cognitive and sensitization problems (see text) and then treat to prevent further decline
Cyclothymia	A low-grade chronic mood disorder of gradual shifts from abnormal energetic optimism to mild depression	Manage like patients with hypomanias
Soft bipolar spectrum	Mild to moderate disturbances in temperament and mood that begin in early adulthood and remain fairly constant	Manage like patients with hypomanias and cyclothymia

CLINICAL PRESENTATION

Mania

The classic features of mania are disturbances in mood (euphoric, irritable, labile), motor behavior (hyperactivity), and speech (rapid, pressured, and distractible). A lot of intense emotion, actions and movements, and speech are the hallmarks of mania.

Ten to 20% of manic patients have mixed states of rapidly shifting manic and depressive symptoms. Mixed states are difficult to treat. They more often produce psychotic features. Another 10%–20% of bipolar patients only have manias. About one third of bipolar patients experience a significant number of psychosensory symptoms. These patients, however, have no clinical or EEG evidence of seizure disorder. Psychosensory features are consistent with temporolimbic disease and are one indication that anticonvulsants might be helpful for that patient.

Psychosensory features in mania include *memory problems:* deja vu (as if it has all happened before), jamais vu (suddenly everything is unfamiliar); *perceptual disturbances:* dysmegalopsia (objects seem to change in size), dysmorphopsia (objects seem to change in shape); and *alterations in sense of reality:* depersonalization (sudden feeling of being detached from oneself, as if floating, watching oneself "go through the motions"), derealization (sudden feeling as if the world is no longer real, like a dream or cartoon).

About 20% of manics have catatonic features during their manic episodes. Manics with catatonia do not have a different illness. They are just more severely ill, but they still respond well to treatment. Rarely, some bipolar patients have a sudden onset of intense excitement (a mixed state of mania and delirium), develop catatonic features, and become febrile, although apparently in previously good health. This syndrome, "lethal catatonia," was first described in the 19th century. Without treatment, death resulted in about 50% of cases. When a specific cause can be ruled out (most often infections), electroconvulsive therapy (ECT) can be life saving, often leading to remission. Lethal catatonia is often indistinguishable for neuroleptic malignant syndrome (NMS). One difference is that the fever in lethal catatonia develops as the patient becomes catatonic, whereas the fever in NMS develops after the patient has become catatonic. Patients with NMS also rarely have echophenomena, ambitendency, or bizarre postures. Their postures are more mundane as in the bradykinetic positions of Parkinson's disease. NMS also responds to ECT.

Manics are dramatic and changeable. Their moods can shift in seconds, and in mixed states the shifts can be from a stuporous melancholia to extreme manic excitement bordering on delirium. Shifts from morning depression to afternoon mania is most typical and can partially be controlled by restricting the depressed patient's activity and light exposure and by encouraging sleep. Manic behaviors can dominate a psychiatry unit. Manics rush to greet persons entering the inpatient unit. They salute staff and comment on their clothes or hair, disrupt meetings, bother other patients, are demanding, impulsive, and perseverative, can be sexually provocative, and occasionally get into fights with other patients because of their intrusiveness. They can be loud, vulgar, obscene, verbally abusive, aggressive, and violent. Most hospitalized manics are irritable rather than euphoric. When euphoric they sing, dance, laugh, and talk nonstop. They have flight-of-ideas and racing thoughts dominated by themes of religion, grandiosity, persecution, and sex. They may speak in rhymes, with accents in made up languages. They often wear bright-colored clothing and may decorate themselves with buttons, ribbons, signs, and strange haircuts. Among hospitalized manics, 20% are catatonic, 15% have first-rank symptoms, 20% hallucinate, and 40%–50% are delusional.

Outside the hospital manics disrupt their households and neighborhoods. They may throw objects out of windows, use make-up or profanity out of keeping with their socioeconomic background, create disturbances at airports, and upset traffic at busy intersections. They require little sleep, have intense appetitive behaviors (eating, hypersexual) and are impulsive and may go on sudden trips, buy unnecessary gifts, give away money or belongings, gamble, and drive recklessly. The likelihood of a psychotic patient being manic increases with the more noise he makes, the more questions he asks, the more jokes he tells, the more words he utters, the more biblical or religious references he makes, and the more often he is observed on the inpatient unit. Manics live in excess. They can take off all their clothes or walk around in multiple layers. Table 8.2 lists diagnostic criteria for mania. DSM criteria also include other manic features, but these additional requirements do not improve discrimination. However, manics with avolition or formal thought disorder (about 5%–10% of patients) do not respond well to treatment and are often chronically ill.

Manic patients are often psychotic, and they do strange things. Some examples of odd behavior seen in manics who responded to treatment for mood disorder are wearing a pile of ashes on the top of her head, like a hat, to ward of gamma rays; using household furniture as stepping stones to avoid touching the floor and thus endangering her children; dressing in black leather pants and jacket and attacking skyscrapers with a large kitchen knife; shaving half of his head and beard; dressing as "Robin Hood" and holding up a convenience store with a bow and arrow; carrying her feces around in the palm of her hand to demonstrate her good health; wearing self-made and decorated paper clothes; walking around the house in only panties even in the presence of her children and other adult relatives; and wearing many layers of clothes in summer.

TABLE 8.2. Diagnostic Criteria for Mania (All Must Be Met)

1. An altered mood characterized by sustained euphoria or irritability or lability with periods of euphoria and irritability
2. No avolition or loss of emotional expression
3. Hyperactivity
4. Rapid or pressured speech
5. No evidence of other neurologic disease, medication use, substance or alcohol abuse, or general medical condition that better explains the mood state

Because one third or more of manics become chronically ill, the combination of psychosis and mood disorder and chronicity has led to the concept of *schizoaffective disorder*. Schizoaffective disorder has been divided into schizoaffective manic and schizoaffective depressed. It is unclear whether schizoaffective disorder represents a variation of schizophrenia or mood disorder, is the middle ground of a psychosis continuum with schizophrenia at one end and psychotic mood disorder at the other, or is a disorder distinct from both schizophrenia and mood disorder. Think of these patients clinically as (1) severely ill with both mood and psychotic features; (2) more likely to be frequently hospitalized and poorly functioning between episodes; (3) more likely to have a family history of schizoaffective disorder, mood disorder, *and* schizophrenia; and (4) responsive to treatments for mood disorder, but less so than nonpsychotic mood disorder patients. Ten to 30% of acutely hospitalized psychotic patients are diagnosed schizoaffective.

There is a relationship between bipolar mood disorder and creativity. Among writers, artists, and musicians, for example, there is a high prevalence of bipolar mood disorder and alcoholism. The other side of the coin is consistent, as there is also a greater than expected degree of creativity among bipolar II mood disorder patients. The reasons for this co-occurrence are unclear. Bipolar patients who are creative artists are often productive during their hypomanic episodes or cyclothymic highs and unproductive during their manias, depressions and drinking bouts. They do not want to lose their highs and thus are often noncompliant with treatment .

Soft Bipolar Spectrum

Mild forms of bipolar disorder rarely lead to hospitalization or even medical treatment, but nevertheless can cause social and job disruptions. These forms typically begin in the teenage years or earlier and are ongoing more than episodic, although episodes of mood disorder can also occur. Thus, they appear to be personality patterns rather than the expressions of illness that will respond to medication.

Cyclothymia is analogous to dysthymia. It is a mild prolonged form of a mood disorder. The cyclothymic person has gradual mood swings lasting weeks or months. When "up," they are extroverted, outgoing, cheerful, optimistic, impulsive, restless, talkative, and uninhibited. They need less sleep and have increased appetitive behaviors. When "down," they are moody, irritable and short-tempered, lethargic, hypersomnic, taciturn, inactive, shy, unsure, pessimistic, and slow in thinking.

Hyperthymic temperament is characterized by being overtalkative, extroverted, uninhibited, overly optimistic, restless, meddlesome, vigorous, needing less sleep, bombastic, cheerful, irritable, and, at times, mildly hypomanic. *Dysthymic* temperament is characterized by being hypersomnolent, brooding, anhedonic, self-blaming, passive, and indecisive. *Irritable* temperament is characterized by being brooding, hypercritical and complaining, dysphoric and restless, sarcastic, irritable, and choleric.

The importance of the soft bipolar spectrum is that these behaviors can cause social and job dysfunction and, if identified, will respond to mood stabilizing medications. Also, a substantial proportion of patients with atypical depression (e.g., reversed vegetative signs, atypical mood; co-morbid anxiety disorders) have these behaviors, and they do best when treated for bipolar rather than unipolar disorder. The risk of suicide is also high among soft bipolar patients, so recognizing their illness can be lifesaving.

Borderline Personality Disorder

Borderline personality disorder is included in the DSM axis II Cluster B category. However, it represents several different conditions. The pattern of borderline personality disorder is long-standing stormy interpersonal experiences, much emotionality, and a difficult treatment course with poor doctor–patient relationships. If you have a patient with this diagnosis (made by you or someone else), consider it only the first step. You have characterized the syndrome; now you must determine cause. A significant proportion of borderline patients have a form of bipolar mood disorder. Many of the diagnostic criteria for borderline require mood changes, and symptoms are consistent with a variant of bipolar affective disorder (e.g., *impulsivity* that is self-damaging, like spending to much money, having risky sex, abusing drugs, shoplifting, driving recklessly, binge eating; *affective instability*, such as marked reactivity of mood with intense episodic dysphoria, irritability, or anxiety usually lasting a few hours and only rarely more than a few days; *angry mood*, with inappropriate, intense anger or a lack of control of anger; and recurrent *suicidal* threats, gestures, or behavior or self-mutilating behavior.) Most of the other criteria for borderline reflect the consequences of these mood disturbances. Among the associated borderline features in the DSM are "psychotic-like symptoms," including hallucinations and ideas of reference.

Some of the other indications that borderline personality disorder represents a mild state of illness rather than a pattern of deviant nonpathological traits include (1) a large proportion of borderline patients (25%–50%) meet criteria for bipolar II or cyclothymia, and bipolar disorder and borderline disorder co-occur in the same individuals; (2) the relatives of borderline patients have an increased risk for mood disorder and alcoholism; (3) a large proportion of borderline patients (about 50%–60%) fail to suppress with dexamethasone; (4) some (25%–30%) have other laboratory findings similar to those seen in more typical mood disorders (e.g., abnormal EEGs, evoked potentials, and neurologic soft signs, although computed tomography [CT] findings are normal); and (5) some respond to monoamine oxidase inhibitors (MAOIs), anticonvulsants, and lithium.

Brief Psychotic Disorder

This DSM syndrome is said to resolve within a month. It is similar to the European tradition of reactive psychosis and to the concept of combat neurosis. Criteria basically include

1. A precipitating stressful event
2. A rapid-onset psychosis developing soon after the stressful event
3. Significant affective lability and mood intensity

4. Symptom content congruent with the stress event
5. Rapid resolution once the stressful circumstances are ameliorated.

Some predisposing vulnerability is implied but has never been established. The validity of this disorder is also unclear. However, brief psychotic disorder tends to occur early in the course of illness, followed by classic episodes of mania and depression. Among ill families, the younger relatives are more likely to have brief psychotic disorder while older relatives have classic mood disorders. You should treat episodes of brief psychotic disorder as a mood disorder because doing so provides the best short- and long-term recovery for these patients.

Seasonal Affective Disorder

Seasonal mood disorder refers to recurrent winter depressions. Other mood disorders also have seasonal variability: Manias are more common in the spring and summer, and depressions are more common in the fall and winter. For most patients, however, episodes do not occur like clockwork (e.g., every May a mania). An uncommon exception are patients who develop a depression every winter (usually beginning in November and lasting through February) that seems related to the reduced amount of winter daylight.* These depressions are nonmelancholic and are characterized by lethargy and hypersomnia, fatigue and apathy, overeating with a craving for carbohydrates, and weight gain. This depression is treated with antidepressants, mood stabilizers, and 30 minutes of high intensity light exposure (a 10,000 Lux light box) every morning during winter months. The therapeutic effect of bright light is modest and is not mediated through changes in melatonin circadian secretion, which is normal in these patients. However, the frontal, anterior cingulate, and thalamic hypometabolism seen in these patients improves with successful treatment.

Seasonal mood disorder may be more common in male patients. Over the years, some patients become less sensitive to seasonal changes, and the timing of their depressions and hypomanias become unpredictable. Seasonable mood disorder is also more common in persons living at higher latitudes where seasonal light changes are more dramatic.

Seasonal depressives with melancholic features or Cluster C personality disorders with high harm avoidance behaviors do not respond well to light therapy. Patients with some eye diseases (e.g., retinal disease, glaucoma, cataracts, optic nerve disease, inflammatory disease) should be approved for light treatment by an ophthalmologist. Because the light used is fluorescent with low ultraviolet (radiation) and infrared (heat) properties, light therapy has no clear side effects (headache and vague visual complaints are most common).

Because seasonal depression is symptomatically similar to the cocaine withdrawal "depression" or "crash," stimulant drugs such as methylphenidate may also be effective if light therapy is unavailable. Among the antidepressants,

*Severity of episode correlates with length of daylight, but not to cloud cover, rainfall, or atmospheric pressure.

bupropion is the best choice. Morning propranolol may help symptoms of anxiety. Because of the sleep disturbances in these patients, good sleep hygiene is also important in obtaining and maintaining remission. Going to bed at a set time is important. Using melatonin (only the extended release form has demonstrated efficacy) and maintaining a tryptophan-rich diet (experimentally lowered tryptophan levels cause relapse) may also help. Treat melancholic depression in the wintertime as suggested in Chapter 7 for melancholia. If the patient with winter depressions has a bipolar II pattern, add lithium to the antidepressant or light therapy. If the depression is typical of other mood disorders, treat as you would for any bipolar II patient.

CO-OCCURRENCE OF MOOD DISORDERS, ALCOHOLISM, AND DRUG ABUSE

Thirty to 50% of bipolar patients abuse alcohol, and 20%–40% abuse street drugs. Half of those who abuse these substances are also dependent on them.

Alcoholism and mood disorder are both familial, and mood disorder and alcoholism co-occur in the same families. It is unclear if this familial co-occurrence represents the same pathophysiology, mood disorder patients self-medicating with alcohol, or some other unknown relationship. There appears to be no significant familial relationship between street drug abuse and mood disorder.

Mood disorder patients with co-occurring alcoholism or drug abuse (referred to as "dual diagnosis" patients) are difficult to treat. Programs designed to treat patients with mood disorders are rarely equipped to handle the alcohol- or drug-dependent patient, and many alcohol and drug rehabilitation programs adopt an antimedical and antimedicine model; thus, many mood disorder patients on maintenance medication are not eligible for treatment. Specialized dual diagnosis programs have been developed for these patients, but combining strategies for treating bipolar patients described below with the treatments for alcohol and substance abuse described in Chapter 13 also works for many patients.

COURSE

Illness onset of mania is usually acute (within a 3-month period), with the first episode appearing in the late teens (25%–30%) or early twenties. Thirty percent are hospitalized by age 25. Females are slightly at greater risk than are males. Half the time a stressful event precedes an early episode. Depression as the first episode of bipolar disorder occurs in only 5%–10% of patients. Suspect a first episode depressed patient as bipolar when the patient

1. Is under 25
2. Has a family history of bipolar disorder or mood disorder of any type in several first-degree relatives

3. Has a depression with hypersomnia or stupor or other atypical features or has a postpartum depression
4. Complains of racing thoughts while depressed and elaborates on answers and comments rather than having reduced slow speech
5. Has a predepression personality consistent with one of the soft bipolar spectrum conditions
6. Has winter-only depressions

About 85% of first-episode bipolar patients will have subsequent episodes. About one third will never have a depressive episode, but these "unipolar manics" are similar to patients who have both manic and depressive episodes.

Typical episodes of mania are rare before puberty. Children at risk for bipolar disorder, however, usually have (1) a family history of bipolar mood disorder, (2) a temperament pattern consistent with a soft bipolar spectrum disorder, (3) a history of aggressiveness or hyperactivity and related school problems, and (4) IQ testing (WISC) results in which there is a discrepancy between verbal (normal) and performance (low) IQ.

Bipolar children rarely have clearcut manic episodes. Instead, these children have long-standing patterns of emotional lability or a low grade long-standing mania-like syndrome. Children with emotional lability (5% prepubescent, 10% of teens) are school and family challenges. They are anxious and silly, they sleep less, they are hyperactive, reckless, explosive, irritable, and overtalkative, and they have periods of mood elevation. Most have co-morbidities, including major depression (60%), phobias (50%; animal and blood most common), episodic conduct disorder or ADHD (40%), oppositional defiant disorder, and drug abuse. They are also more likely than their peers to be enuretic and have migraine symptoms, Raynaud's phenomena, learning disorders, and severe fingernail biting. Teens with emotional lability typically abuse drugs. Drug use, however, is not the cause of their emotional lability, nor is it an attempt at self-medication.

Teens and children with these "soft" bipolar behaviors and co-morbidities are extremely difficult to treat (lithium does not appear to work well), and anticonvulsants offer the best hope. As adults, these patients have a clearer form of bipolar disorder, but continue to have all the co-morbidities and their associated problems. Almost one third have a family history of mood disorder and substance abuse. In ruling out other causes, look for head injury, developmental disorders, and epilepsy.

In adults, the course of bipolar disorder is rarely cyclical. Episode frequency varies with periods of quiescence interspersed with periods of sporadic episodes and periods of episode clusters. During these paroxysms rapid cycling can occur (four or more episodes in a year). Rapid cyclers are not a distinct subgroup.

The *likelihood of relapse* from a given manic episode increases with the following *episode characteristics*: psychosis, psychosensory features, formal thought disorder, multiple psychosocial stressors, a family or post-episode environment with high expressed emotion (intense emotions, many negative emotions, and criticism), and low socioeconomic status.

Among the 30%–50% of bipolar patients who become chronic there is a progressive increase in episode numbers and length with a concomitant decrease in interepisode duration and functioning. For example, the typical interval between the first and second episode is 2–4 years, whereas the typical interval between episodes five and above is about 1 year. As patients become chronic they become increasingly resistant to lithium and then to other drugs. The likelihood of a bipolar patient eventually becoming *resistant to standard treatments* increases with (1) illness onset age at or before puberty; (2) co-morbid alcohol or substance abuse, particularly cocaine; (3) history of head injury or other neurologic disease; (4) the presence of formal thought disorder and avolition during episodes; (5) the presence of psychosensory features between episodes; (6) episodes with mixed features, rapid onsets, and psychosis; (7) periods of rapid cycling; (8) low premorbid cognitive and intellectual functioning (e.g., low IQ, failure to complete high school); and (9) structural brain changes (e.g., enlarged ventricles, small temporal lobe volume). Patients who relapse often and have treatment-resistant episodes develop interepisode cognitive impairment with interepisode avolition and are likely to be chronically dysfunctional.

Chronicity includes social and job problems and cognitive impairment affecting new learning. A temporolimbic sensitization process has been hypothesized to explain this pattern (see below) whereby early episodes, triggered by environmental stress, adversely and permanently sensitize temporolimbic systems leading to more frequent, prolonged, and severe future episodes that can occur without stress. This vicious circle continues to chronicity and affects treatment and management considerations.

The sensitization pattern of episodes suggests that to reduce chronicity the treatment of early episodes should be aggressive and rapid and should be followed by equally aggressive, multidimensional maintenance strategies, including biological treatments that have direct effects on kindling and sensitization and behavioral interventions that focus on stress reduction and the development of adaptive behaviors to stress. Furthermore, faced with a patient in the midst of multiple, closely spaced episodes, do not become pessimistic, as these episodes may reflect a paroxysm that if aggressively treated could lead to a period (sometimes years) of relative quiescence.

DIFFERENTIAL DIAGNOSIS

The differential diagnosis of bipolar disorder falls into three groups: classic bipolar disorders; primary disorders not presently classified as bipolar but that, when treated as bipolar, offer the patient the best prognosis; and secondary bipolar disorder.

The duck principle always rules when you suspect a patient has primary bipolar disorder. If arousal is increased with an intense mood, and speech and other motor behaviors are increased, the likelihood is great that the patient has what you suspect. This is also true for patients whose illness develops outside the expected age of a first episode (20–40 years, typically around 25). The tendency is to reject the likelihood of a first mania in the very young (<15) and the elderly (>60).

However, although content may differ (particularly in children), the form of the illness is the same at all age groups.

A more difficult decision is when the patient is psychotic or chronically ill. The DSM offers categories such as schizoaffective and not otherwise specified (NOS), but these choices do not suggest how to treat such patients. A simple rule is, if the patient meets the basic criteria for mania in Table 8.2 and there is no evidence of a secondary syndrome, consider him bipolar regardless of the number or intensity of psychotic features or the patient's chronicity. Many bipolar patients become chronically ill, but this does not mean that they do not have bipolar disorder. It means that they have the most severe form of it. Chronic bipolars are avolitional, but have adequate emotional expression. They may experience more psychosensory features during and between episodes, their course of illness may suggest sensitization, and they are likely to be lithium nonresponders. Even when asymptomatic they are likely to have substantial cognitive problems, particularly with new learning.

Identifying secondary bipolar disorder is a challenge. As with all syndromes, the more atypical the episode or course of illness, the more likely it will be secondary. Laboratory findings are helpful if they are specific to another condition or suggest localized brain dysfunction. Primary bipolar patients, however, also have brain disease and have abnormalities on many measures of brain function and structure (Table 8.3). For example, deep white matter hyperintensities on T_2 weighted MRI scans are seen in 40% of primary bipolar patients. Hyperintensities cluster in frontal and frontoparietal regions near the corona radiata, which connects the cerebral cortex to the limbic system and basal ganglia. The clinical sig-

TABLE 8.3. Laboratory Abnormalities in Bipolar Patients

Assessment Method	Findings
Brain structure (CT, MRI)	Lateral and third ventricle enlargement (10%–30%), cerebral cortical atrophy (15%), cerebellar vermal atrophy (25%), deep white matter hyperintensities (40%)
Brain metabolism (SPECT/PET)	Decreased perfusion in right basal temporal cortex; diminished frontal and anterior cingulate blood flow and glucose metabolism
Brain information processing (EEG, EP)	Mild diffuse slowing or "choppy" waveforms more in right posterior leads (EEG); augmentation on EP (repeated stimuli produce waves with greater amplitude)
Cognition	Bifrontal nondominant hemisphere impairment pattern during acute episodes; problems with new learning (verbal and visual) in chronic patients
Neuroendocrine	High nighttime cortisol levels (most patients), nonsuppression of cortisol to dexamethasone (50%), blunting of thyroid-stimulating hormone response to thyroid-releasing hormone (some patients)

PET, positron emission tomography; EP, evoked potential.

nificance of these abnormalities is unclear (less than 5% of controls have them), but they are also seen in patients with demyelinating disease and after brain infections and post-traumatic anoxia. On many neuropsychological tests chronically poor functioning, but asymptomatic bipolar patients under age 55 years perform at levels similar to those found in older persons.

Bipolar patients (particularly those who develop psychoses) also have a greater likelihood of having a history of mild developmental delays (walking and talking), neonatal and infant neurologic problems (lower Apgar scores, low birth blood oxygen levels, neonatal convulsions, postnatal viral infection). A bipolar patient with a history of such events, but with an otherwise normal developmental and neurologic history is most likely primary. These perinatal findings are also seen in more severe forms in children who become schizophrenic (see Chapter 9).

Many conditions can produce bipolar symptoms. The most common error is to diagnose secondary bipolar disorder in a patient who has periods of irritability and agitation from a head injury or drug abuse. Those patients do not have clear episodes of mania (with euphoria, multiple plans, flight-of-ideas), rarely if ever have a major depression, and are avolitional without a temporolimbic sensitization pattern. They often are psychotic with complete auditory hallucinations, other first-rank symptoms, and persecutory delusions. They can be violent. True secondary mania responds either to specific treatment (e.g., an anticonvulsant for epilepsy or stopping or reducing the dose of the drug that is inducing the mania, as can happen with levodopa treatment for Parkinson's disease) or to standard treatment for bipolar disorder (e.g., lithium, valproic acid, ECT). True secondary mania is characterized by (1) rapid syndrome onset, (2) marked sleeplessness, (3) hyperactivity, and (4) classic features such as euphoria, high risk financial or physical activities, press of speech, and flight-of-ideas.

Many prescription and over-the-counter preparations can also induce a manic-like episode. It is unclear whether these states are intoxications (as seen with mania secondary to cocaine) or whether the agents are triggering a mania in a potentially bipolar person. The more abrupt the onset following ingestion of the agent and the shorter the episode of mania, the more likely it is due to the drug. Some drugs of particular concern are baclofen (after sudden withdrawal), captopril, dextromethorphan, cyclobenzaprine, and sympathomimetics. Bromocriptine-induced mania is typically associated with severe hyperactivity and stereotypes. Corticosteroids and ACTH (in higher doses), levodopa (more in older patients with prolonged use), digitalis (at higher doses), and antidepressants (10% of patients) can also cause mania. If the drug can be withdrawn rapidly, do so, and control the mania with sedative-hypnotics for 48 hours, or taper withdrawal if indicated by the drug's pharmacology (e.g., steroids). If the patient improves, wait and full improvement may occur without further treatment. If no improvement *whatsoever* occurs in 48 hours, treat as if it were a primary mania. However, some drug-induced manias may continue after the drug is fully withdrawn. Once remission is achieved (the usual result), treat for 6 weeks to avoid relapse and then withdraw the antimanic drug. Avoid neuroleptics unless you have no other choice. Recurrences are less likely than in primary mania, and prophylactic treatment other than avoiding mania-causing agents is unwarranted.

Some street drugs can also induce mania (also see Chapter 13). *Phencyclidine* (PCP) causes an extreme psychotic excitement state with violence and periods of catatonia. Hypertension, other sympathetic arousal signs, vestibular-cerebellar signs (dizziness, rotary nystagmus, ataxia), and generalized analgesia distinguish PCP mania from primary mania. A history of drug use and a drug screen can confirm the diagnosis. In most cases the patient will need to be hospitalized, and restraints may also be needed. Use lorazepam or diazepam for agitation. Acidify the urine with ammonium chloride 4–8 g daily and 40 mg IV furosemide to increase PCP excretion. Give propranolol or another beta-blocker if sympathetic symptoms are severe. Loading dose strategy with valproic acid may also be needed (see Table 8.4). If this does not break the mania, use intramuscular or intravenous haloperidol, and, if successful, follow with oral haloperidol for 3–6 weeks, overlapped with mood stabilizers for 3–6 months of maintenance. If haloperidol does not rapidly break the mania, a course of bilateral ECT usually does and is the recommended first-line treatment to avoid polypharmacy and delayed improvement.

Stimulant drugs, particularly cocaine, also can induce mania. Cocaine-induced mania is characterized by a hyperkinetic, hyperarousal state with suspiciousness and irritability. Hallucinations of geometric shapes and bugs crawling under the skin are classic. The patient may have stereotypies and other perseverative behaviors (palalalia, stock words) and typically moves in a jerky bird-like manner. Treatment is the same as for PCP, but neuroleptics and ECT are only needed in the severest psychotic states.

Hallucinogens can cause secondary mania with sudden euphoria, hyperactivity, and sleeplessness. Hallucinations in multiple sensory modalities are common. Formal thought disorder combined with flight-of-ideas, avolition, and personality deterioration are associated with chronicity. Control agitation with lorazepam or diazepam. ECT is the recommended treatment. A loading dose strategy of lithium

TABLE 8.4. Loading Dose Strategies for Acute Manics

	Lithium	*Valproate*
Day 1, PM dose	600–900 mg	20–30 mg/Kg body weight, so that for a 70 kg person, dose will be 1400–2100 mg
Day 2, AM dose	Same as Day 1, PM dose	Same as Day 1, PM dose
Day 2, PM dose	Same as AM dose or 50% of that dose, depending on tolerance, so that day 2 total dose will be 900–1800 mg	Same as AM dose or 50% of that dose depending on tolerance, so that day 2 total dose will be 2100–4200
Day 3	Continue the Day 2 total dose or double the day 1 dose, whichever is best tolerated	Continue the Day 2 dose or double the day 1 dose whichever is best toelerated
Day 7–8	Steady state	Steady state

or valproic acid, an anticonvulsant mood stabilizer, works moderately well for patients without signs of chronicity. Neuroleptics are the last resort. Relapse following street drug–induced mania depends on the degree of (1) initial response to rapid interventions (the faster the better), (2) cognitive deficits once the manic symptoms have resolved (the more deficits, the worse the prognosis), and (3) continued drug use.

Some *strokes* (<1%) can cause sudden euphoria, hyperactivity, sleeplessness, and risk-taking manic-like behaviors. Those behaviors usually develop within days or weeks of the stroke, but there can be a 3–6 month delay. Strokes most likely to cause mania affect large areas of nondominant hemisphere (frontotemporal) or the nondominant thalamus or caudate. When nondominent basal ganglia structures are involved, obsessive compulsive disorder (OCD) features are often seen with the mania. OCD and mania due to stroke often are associated with hypoperfusion on single photon emission computed tomography (SPECT), whereas primary OCD is one of the few neuropsychiatric conditions with orbitofrontal hyperperfusion. Magnetic resonance imaging (MRI) also helps distinguish primary from secondary mania due to stroke. Patients who develop post-stroke mania are also more likely to have a family history of bipolar mood disorder. Treat post-stroke mania as you would acute primary mania, but integrate this management with stroke rehabilitation and prevention strategies. Relapse following stroke-induced mania depends on (1) the size and location of the stroke; (2) the degree of initial response to treatment; and (3) the degree of long-term cognitive, motor, and sensory impairment.

Traumatic brain injuries to orbitofrontal and nondominant basotemporal cortex, nondominant anterior limb of the internal capsule, head of the caudate, and thalamus can cause mania. In children, birth or early head trauma can result in irritability, distractibility, hyperactivity, and social disinhibition that mimics mania but that responds to stimulants as does ADHD. If mood stabilizers do not work for secondary mania from head trauma, low doses of stimulants may help, but do not prescribe these to psychotic patients who can be made worse by them. Relapse factors are the same as those for stroke.

Epilepsy can also lead to mood disorder. Partial complex epilepsy with a mesial temporal or frontal lobe focus (nondominant > dominant) and an onset around puberty is the most likely to cause mania. Psychotic features and mood changes may be brief (minutes or hours), prominent at particular times of the day (upon awakening or when fatigued), or, in women, premenstrually. The mania is usually associated with irritability or delirium, and psychosensory features often occur. Look for frontal or temporal lobe auras and identifiable fits. SPECT and MRI are the most helpful distinguishing tests after EEG (see Chapter 10 for details). ECT or valproic acid works best for acute episodes.

Demyelinating disease can also produce hypomania and atypical mood states associated with emotional dysregulation, pseudobulbar affect with sudden laughter or weeping without emotional stimulation, and modest euphoria without grandiosity or flight-of-ideas. Multiple sclerosis (MS) and AIDS are the most likely etiologies. For MS look for fluctuating scattered neurologic findings and optic nerve neuritis when the onset is in a young adult or cerebellar signs when onset is closer to middle age. Oligoclonal IgG bands and elevated IgG turnover in cerebrospinal fluid, abnormal evoked potentials, and white matter lesions seen on MRI help to diagnose MS.

Hypomania or mania occurs late in the course of AIDS, so the etiology is rarely in question. In both MS and AIDS, the more frontotemporal lesions the patient has, the more likely he is to develop a mania-like syndrome. Although Mini-Mental State scores can be in the high 20s, these patients have other cognitive problems that are worse than expected from their relatively modest manic-like or hypomanic features. Look for deficits in sustained attention (A test), cognitive flexibility (poor Trail Making) and other frontal lobe features. Many patients will have features of the lateral orbitofrontal disinhibited syndrome, and AIDS patients may have a personal or family history of bipolar mood disorder. Treat these patients as you would for primary bipolar disorder after eliminating demyelinating disease treatments (e.g., steroids) as a cause.

Basal ganglia disease can also cause secondary mood states: depressions with dominant lesions, manic-like syndromes with bilateral or nondominant lesions. Ten percent of Huntington's disease patients develop shallow euphoric frontal lobe disinhibited syndromes with mood changes predating the most striking motor features. Thus, no matter how mild, any frontobasal ganglia motor features in atypical manics need further evaluation. Patients will often have a family history of Huntington's and sometimes also mood disorder. Dopaminergic agonistic-like treatments (e.g. ECT, bupropion) can worsen the motor features. Lithium and valproic acid are first-line treatments.

About 2% of Parkinson's disease patients also develop hypomania. Ten percent of patients taking levodopa become euphoric or hypomanic, and some become psychotic. Bromocriptine and pergolide may also cause hypomania. When the Parkinson's syndrome is postencephalitic, midbrain and hypothalamic lesions are likely (get an MRI). ECT treats both the mood disorder and the parkinsonian motor features.

Some patients with Wilson's disease, because of its putamen and thalamic lesions, will develop hypomania. These patients will be teenagers or young adults. Look for upper limb motor abnormalities, liver involvement, and abnormal copper metabolism. Lithium is the drug of choice if liver involvement is severe.

Focal cerebellar lesions (trauma, MS, stroke, tumor) can result in a rapid cycling mania with abnormal eye movements (jerky, poor pursuit), dystonias or ataxia, and compulsive behavior without obsessions (stereotyped checking of locks, turning light switches on and off, and other utilization behaviors akin to what you can observe in some autistic patients). Lithium and valproic acid are first-line treatments.

Midline *brain tumors* anywhere from the frontal poles to the subcortical forebrain, diencephalon and brain stem, or third ventricle can cause hyperkinetic episodes with euphoria and sleeplessness. Treatment is the same as for primary bipolar disorder, and ECT can be used if there is no increased intracranial pressure.

General paresis was the most common cause of psychosis in the 19th century. Lesions in the frontal lobes can produce a frontal avolitional syndrome with

Witzelsucht, or disinhibition with grandiosity. In addition to treating the syphilis, treat as for primary bipolar disorder.

Endocrinopathies may cause secondary mania or hypomania. Patients may become frenetic and delirious. Hyperthyroidism, hyperparathyroidism, and Cushing's disease are the likely etiologies. You must correct the endocrinopathy if the bipolar disorder is to be resolved. Then treat as for primary bipolar disorder.

Finally, 40% of patients with the *fragile-X syndrome*, particularly women carriers, develop a chronic mood disorder. Five percent become psychotic. Flight-of-ideas with palalalia is a common feature in these patients. In addition to learning difficulties since birth, delayed speech, infantile hypotonia, and low IQ, look for triangular-shaped face (long with decreased head circumference), large protruding ears, macrognathia with speech difficulties and high-arched palate, loose joints, soft velvety skin, and large gonads (96% of male patients). Treat as for primary bipolar disorder.

THE NEUROLOGY OF BIPOLAR DISORDER: KINDLING AND SENSITIZATION

Limbic sensitization and kindling have been proposed as potential analogues to the pathophysiology of bipolar mood disorder. *Electrophysiological kindling* refers to the propensity of some neurons to become sensitized to repeated low-level electrical stimulation so that eventually a previously subconvulsive stimulus induces an electrical seizure. Continued stimulation further lowers the seizure threshold so that spontaneous seizures without stimulation eventually occur. *Behavioral sensitization* is similar to kindling. In this model neurons become increasingly responsive (as measured by behavioral activity) to repeated administrations of the same dose of a stimulant drug (e.g., cocaine): Behaviors become more severe, onset is more rapid, changes are more prolonged, and behaviors are more likely to be triggered by stress without the offending drug being a necessary inducer. The propensity of neurons to be sensitized (and to kindle) involves a significant genetic component, raising the possibility that the proposed genetic liability in mood disorders is to such a process. Furthermore, in nonhuman studies, younger animals are more vulnerable, akin to the early-onset pattern of bipolar disorder.

The hippocampus and amygdala are particularly prone to kindling and sensitization. This provides a useful model for mood disorders because (1) MRI and CT abnormalities have been observed in the frontotemporal regions of these patients, (2) secondary mood disorder syndromes have been clinicopathologically associated with frontolimbic disease, (3) about 30% of patients with mood disorder exhibit psychosensory features (e.g., deja vu, dysmegalopsia), (4) the course of mood disorders with increasing episode frequency over time is a kindling-like pattern, (5) chronic asymptomatic bipolar patients have cognitive problems consistent with temporal lobe disease, and (6) treatment modalities (ECT, anticonvulsants) that raise the seizure threshold and modifying kindling are efficacious in mood disorder. Furthermore, lithium, effective early in the course of illness, becomes less so, and, as the proposed sensitization develops, anticonvulsants must be used.

Early in temporolimbic sensitization mood responses to stress are unstable and inappropriately intense and prolonged. When severe, this mood response could account for the psychotic, psychosensory, and emotional disturbances seen in bipolar patients. First, the limbic system influences frontal lobes via limbic participation in frontosubcortical circuits (the mesial circuit to the anterior cingulate cortex) and limbic connections to the thalamus and basal ganglia. Second, the effects of emotion on arousal with temporolimbic disorders often produce "frontal lobe symptoms" (e.g., the disinhibited syndrome, stuporous and catatonic states, poor executive function, increased motor [including speech] behavior), which are also characteristic of mania. Third, thalamic dysfunction, linking action and perceptual-integrating brain systems, could account for many of the psychotic features seen in some manics.

Early illness episodes may act as further sensitizing agents and may affect (along with stress) gene transcription (hypothesized in third meninger C-fos m-RNA systems) that may lead to long-lasting changes in neural synaptic plasticity affecting short- and long-term memory. Kindling also leads to synaptogenesis and cell death. Thus, stress and then multiple mood disordered episodes can cause permanent temporolimbic dysfunction and chronicity.

MANAGEMENT OF ACUTE MANIA

The treatment of acute mania is a challenge, always requires urgent intervention, and is often a medical emergency. Excitement, overactivity, and elation may be rapidly replaced by irritability and assaultive behavior. Intrusive, importunate, and demanding patients may become extremely angry at only slight provocation. When persecutory delusional ideas are present, the risk of violent attack is increased. Do not interview potentially assaultive and extremely uncooperative patients alone in a closed office. Restraints and seclusion may be necessary. If so, sedate with an intravenous benzodiazepine (e.g., 2–4 mg IV lorazepam) or 250–500 mg IV sodium amobarbital. If the patient requires restraints do not initially use oral medication because the delay in drug action onset by this route can lead to an uncontrollable patient injuring himself or others.

First, try to avoid the use of neuroleptics by a loading dose strategy with lithium or valproate. Table 8.4 lists the steps in this procedure. Excitement should be controlled within 36–48 hours with either drug, although the mania may not resolve for several weeks. If the excitement is not controlled with lithium, add or substitute valproate loading. If neither drug nor their combination controls the excitement, then use a neuroleptic.

If the acute excited manic is psychotic, a neuroleptic may initially be needed. In choosing a neuroleptic consider the following. Among the atypicals (see Chapter 9 for details) risperidone rarely controls acute mania at below 8 mg the maximum dose to avoid extrapyramidal side effects, and it presently has no intramuscular or intravenous form. Olanzapine also is an oral preparation, and may excite patients with a history of excitement. Clozapine has more severe side effects (anti-cholinergic, agranulocytosis, sudden death) than haloperidol, is expensive, and cannot be given with a benzodiazepine often used to sedate manics and treat associated catatonia. Haloperidol and fluphenazine, in contrast, can be used orally, muscularly, and intravenously. They also come in a long-acting form for chronic noncompliers. They are safe and have been widely used with lithium and anti-convulsants. Like all typical high potency neuroleptics, their biggest drawback is short-term extrapyramidal side effects and, in the long-term, tardive dyskinesia. Use one if there is no alternative, and then for the shortest duration. Haloperidol is the more widely used and is recommended for otherwise healthy patients of average or above body weight between ages 16 and 60 years. Initially give haloperidol 20–30 mg.* The large volume of solution (4–6 ml) may require the dose to be split into two injections, one in each buttock. Nurses prepare the necessary syringes and paraphernalia in advance of any confrontation. Lower hourly dosages (e.g., 2–5 mg haloperidol) until the desired effect is achieved (termed *neuroleptization*) only delays the process and increases the risk of injury to patients and staff.

The typical order is for 20 mg haloperidol IM "stat and BID." Continue this for at least 48 hours even if there is a dramatic response to the first injection, as too hasty a switch from intramuscular to oral administration often leads to rapid relapse. Most acutely ill manics respond well, although some patients may need 20 mg IM TID or 30 mg IM BID. Do not give a "stat" dose of a neuroleptic and then injections on an as-need basis. This method increases the likelihood that patients will develop acute symptoms again between doses. Once you decide to treat, carry it out systematically to provide continuous relief.

When you change to oral medication, briefly overlap it with intramuscular treatment. For most patients start with a single nighttime oral dose 30%–50% greater than the daily intramuscular one. Give this dose for two to three nights before discontinuing the intramuscular dosage. The increase in dosage is to counter the reduced efficacy of the oral versus the intramuscular dose.

If the intramuscular neuroleptic is insufficient to resolve a patient's excitement state, use intravenous haloperidol. The patient should be physiologically stable and unresponsive to total daily intramuscular doses up to 80 mg. Then (1) after discontinuing all other psychotropics, administer an IV bolus of 10 mg of haloperidol diluted into 1 cc of saline; (2) immediately follow the haloperidol bolus with 1 mg of lorazepam diluted into 1 cc of saline administered IV over 1 minute to sedate and prevent delirium as the patient awakens; and (3) monitor blood pressure and pulse every 15 minutes for 1 hour. This procedure can be repeated daily for up to 5 days at the same dose or for up to 3 days at 20 mg of haloperidol. Dramatic reduction in psychosis and excitement can occur with this procedure. Once the manic excitement is controlled, use more typical neuroleptic administration or other appropriate medication.

---

*Intramuscular doses below 10 mg often produce acute dystonias. Intramuscular doses above 15 mg rarely produce dystonia and commonly cause sedation. Patients of small body weight do well with 15 mg IM. Elderly acute manics often respond to lower doses (5–10 mg).

Reserve intravenous haloperidol for the most severely ill patients. Monitor temperature and muscle tone several times daily to quickly identify early signs of neuroleptic malignant syndrome (see Chapter 9 for treatment of this rare condition). By the end of the first week of neuroleptic treatment, most manic patients are fully stabilized, and lithium treatment can be started. Combining lithium and a neuroleptic is routine, and once the patient has been in steady state with lithium for several weeks, taper the neuroleptic and then discontinue. This may take 1–3 months.

About 10% of acute manic patients do not respond to even the most intense drug treatments and may progress to a toxic, dehydrated, and febrile state. If loading strategies or 5 days of parenteral, high-dose neuroleptic treatment have not ended the acute phase of the illness, discontinue medications, and give ECT without further delay. Two bilateral ECTs daily for 2–3 consecutive days may be needed to break the excitement. The remainder of the ECT course is given at the usual frequency. Manics require more ECTs than depressives, the average number being 8–12 treatments, and up to 25 treatments may ultimately be needed. However, even if the patient recovers by the fifth or sixth treatment, it is best to continue to at least eight to avoid rapid relapse.

Because medical practice does not occur in a vacuum, what is ideally the best treatment may not always be the treatment that can be given. The semi-official strategy for treating severe manic excitement is (1) loading with either lithium or valproate; (2) combining lithium with valproate, if necessary; (3) using a neuroleptic orally, intramuscularly, or intravenously if lithium and valproate do not work; and (4) using ECT as a last resort. Nevertheless, the least used strategy, but the safest, and possibly the best way of avoiding temporolimbic sensitization from a prolonged manic excitement is to use ECT initially. Response rates of manics to ECT are at least equivalent to those with drugs.

MANAGEMENT OF MANIA AND HYPOMANIA

When the manic patient is not extremely excited, or assaultive, and is willing to take oral medication, lithium is still the drug of choice unless there is a specific contraindication (e.g., poor renal function, severe allergic rash when last exposed to lithium) or (2) there is good reason to believe that the patient is a lithium nonresponder (i.e., an often psychotic manic who as been ill for many years and has previously not done well on lithium). As there is a several-day lag before the onset of substantial antimanic activity with lithium, the staff (and the other patients) must be able to tolerate the frequently annoying and occasionally disruptive behaviors typical of manic patients. In a healthy patient without clinical evidence of renal, thyroid, parathyroid, or cardiac disease, you can start lithium as soon as blood is drawn for the initial laboratory tests without waiting for the results. A dose of 1,200–1,800 mg/day will usually produce a blood level within the upper half of the therapeutic range (1–1.5 mEq/L) by the end of 7–10 days. Measure serum lithium levels twice weekly until steady state.

Because lithium is not bound to protein or metabolized in the liver, the plasma level primarily reflects the last dose and the time since it was given. If adequate levels are not obtained for a given dose, consider (1) the patient is not swallowing all of the medication, (2) polyuria with excessive lithium loss is occurring, or (3) the dose is too low. Some manic patients with grandiose or persecutory delusions hide lithium tablets or capsules in their cheek or under their tongue. They rush to the water fountain or bathroom as soon as they have "swallowed" their pills. Using liquid preparations, or having the patient sit in or near the nursing station for 20 minutes after each dose resolves this problem.

The anti-antidiuretic hormone (anti-ADH) effect of lithium causes some patients to excrete a large volume of dilute urine, carrying with it a considerable amount of lithium, and making it difficult to obtain a therapeutic level. Potassium-sparing diuretics (amiloride [Midamor]) can block the anti-ADH effect, reducing urinary output and increasing serum lithium levels. Watch these patients for signs of lithium overdose, and monitor serum lithium levels more frequently.

A small number of patients require more than 1,800 mg/day of lithium to reach a therapeutic level. These patients typically exhibit no side effects at 1,800 mg/day. Remember, treat the patient, not the blood level or dose.

Treating most acute classic manics is straightforward. Table 8.5 outlines the steps to consider. If the patient is hypomanic or is a manic under reasonable control (20% of patients), try lithium alone first. Patients who ultimately respond show clinical changes quickly, usually within 4 days of an adequate lithium dose.

TABLE 8.5. Treatment of Acute Mania

HYPOMANIC/CONTROLLABLE MANIC

1. Lithium alone for 3–4 weeks
2. If less than 75% improvement, ECT for mania
3. If ECT refused, or if the patient is hypomanic with less than 75% improvement on lithium alone, add valproate to lithium. Use carbamazepine as a second choice anticonvulsant
4. If the patient continues to be resistant to 3 weeks of anticonvulsant–lithium combination, again offer ECT; if the patient refuses, taper original anticonvulsant and introduce the other anticonvulsant, then discontinue the original
5. If the patient continues to be resistant, the only options are ECT or experimental pharmacotherapy (e.g., other anticonvulsants, verapamil)

UNCONTROLLABLE MANIC

1. Control behavior with valproate or lithium loading; use lorazepam sparingly during the first 24–48 hours until loading strategy has its effect
2. If this fails, offer ECT or treat with intramuscular neuroleptic
3. If neuroleptic (including intramuscular and intravenous administration) does not control behavior within 1 week, again offer ECT
4. Once controlled, treat with lithium or combined pharmacotherapy as outlined in treatment steps for controllable mania

---

These subtle changes include increased sleep time, a dusky skin color and loss of skin luster in Euroamericans (in contrast to a rosy cheek, shiny skin appearance during mania), a moderate slowing of speech, and a decrease in activity level. Three weeks of steady-state treatment resolves most, if not all, psychopathology in most moderately ill patients. If after 3 weeks there is less than 75% improvement, consider ECT or adding an anticonvulsant to the lithium regimen.

If your first choice was valproate, and you did not get what you consider a maximum response, add lithium. If the combination does not work, then consider ECT. For the patient with moderate mania, carbamazepine may also work. You cannot load with carbamazepine, however, as headache and dizziness with falling may occur. Carbamazepine also does not seem to work as well as valproate for acutely excited manics, so reserve it for the moderately severe manic who has not responded to lithium, or use it as an adjunct to an antidepressant in bipolar II patients who cannot tolerate lithium.*

As described above, if the patient is manic and assaultive or otherwise uncontrollable, a neuroleptic may be required. Follow the steps outlined above regarding overlapping oral haloperidol or, in rare instances, intravenous haloperidol followed by the oral form. Once the patient is taking an oral neuroleptic, give lithium and taper the neuroleptic.

Carbamazepine and valproate are the drugs of choice for manics who also have Parkinson's disease because lithium can exacerbate this condition by decreasing dopamine synthesis. General medical conditions that aggravate mania (e.g., thyroid disease, low estrogen levels) must be controlled as quickly as possible, as these conditions can cause pseudoresistance to antimanic drugs.

MAINTENANCE AND PROPHYLAXIS MANAGEMENT

The goal of maintenance treatment is to prevent relapse from the resolved acute episode. The goal of prophylaxis is to prevent or ameliorate future illness episodes. Because of potential limbic sensitization, good maintenance and prophylactic treatment minimize interepisode chronicity.

Maintenance pharmacotherapy is relatively uncomplicated if the acute episode is adequately treated. Periodic drug blood levels testing, renal or liver function monitoring, thyroid studies, and other testing in the high functioning physiologically and behaviorally stable patient are mostly needed for medicolegal reasons. Blood drug level testing every 2–4 months and laboratory monitoring of other organ systems likely to be affected by long-term pharmacotherapy every 12 months is usually sufficient. Changes in behavior may occur weeks before full relapse, so educate the patient and his family about the early signs that typify the patient's episodes. Patients with a co-occurring general medical condition or other neurologic illness and those over 65 years of age (renal clearance is reduced) require more frequent and specific testing. Maintenance lithium over a 10-year period reduces the number, intensity, and duration of manic episodes. Mainte-

*Unlike valproate, carbamazepine has a weak antidepressant effect.

nance with anticonvulsants has a somewhat more modest effect. Table 8.6 summarizes maintenance and prophylaxis strategies.

Because mania can be very disruptive to a person's life, bipolar patients need advise, education, and counseling about social and job problems resulting from their illness. Common themes are (1) a disrupted career or a lost job and the need to start again, (2) family members who were frightened, embarrassed, or demoralized by the patient's behavior, (3) a spouse who "has had enough," and (4) the embarrassment the patient now has at having to face friends or colleagues who observed the manic behaviors. Additionally, patients are concerned about (1) losing their minds, (2) getting sick again, (3) becoming dependent on medicine, (4) getting side effects from medicine, and (5) fears that their children will inherit the disease. Assess the patient's situation to see if these concerns apply, and then use the psychotherapy strategies described in Chapter 5.

Never consider a bipolar patient treatment resistant unless he has failed an adequate course of bilateral ECT. If a patient has not responded (remained symptomatic) with adequate trials (loading strategies included) of lithium, valproate, lithium plus valproate, carbamazepine alone or with lithium, or ECT, some will respond to other anticonvulsants alone or in combination (the least desirable choice). Two newer choices are *lamotrigine* (about 200 mg daily: begin with 25 mg BID and increase weekly by 25 mg each dose, drowsiness and skin rash most common side effects) and *gabapentin* (begin 300–900 mg daily with 4,800 mg daily maximum). Gabapentin has the advantage of not being metabolized by the liver

Table 8.6. Maintenance and Prophylaxis Strategies for Bipolar Disorder

1. Maintenance of remission for 8–12 months with the pharmacologic regimen that worked for the acute episode. If a neuroleptic was used, taper and discontinue it over 3–6 months. If ECT was used, either give continuation ECT as detailed in Chapter 7 or prescribe a mood stabilizer that would have been your first choice if ECT had not been given

2. Prophylaxis for future episodes with lithium, valproate, or their combination based on
   a. Frequency (<5 years) and number (> 2) of episodes
   b. Presence of any reduced function after resolution of symptoms
   c. Evidence of sensitization (spontaneous episodes without stress, presence of psychosensory features, increasing numbers of episodes with short well intervals, comorbid cocaine use)

3. Stress reduction, particularly after first episode to minimize development of sensitization

4. Rapid and vigorous treatment of future episodes; use of ECT for mixed states and beginning of a rapid cycling period to prevent prolonged duration of active illness, thus minimizing sensitization

5. If symptom free for 5 years and without other evidence of a continuing chronic process (e.g., cognitive deficits) about 10% of bipolar patients (particularly those over age 65 years) may no longer need single-drug prophylaxis. If you and the patient decide to stop treatment, taper over a 6-month period and follow closely for signs of relapse

or bound to protein so its onset of action is faster and it can be given to patients with liver problems. Either drug can be given with lithium. The combined effect is modest, at best.

Verapamil, a calcium channel blocker, has also been used to treat bipolar patients, but alone it has no clear benefit and with lithium it can cause neurotoxicity.

Some chronic psychotic bipolar patients will require a neuroleptic beyond their acute episodes and may need a neuroleptic indefinitely. Bipolar patients when acutely ill are at greater risk than other psychotic patients for neuroleptic malignant syndrome and when maintained on a neuroleptic at greater risk for tardive dyskinesia. To minimize these risks, whenever possible, offer ECT before a neuroleptic. If you must use a neuroleptic acutely, haloperidol or fluphenazine remain the best choices if the patient is violent or in a state of psychotic excitement. If these concerns are not a factor, risperidone may be the safest choice. Avoid olanzapine because it may make manics more excited and hyperactive. Clozapine would be a last resort. Combining a neuroleptic with ECT can also work for some chronic patients unresponsive to either alone.

LITHIUM

Pharmacokinetics

Lithium is a naturally occurring alkali metal with the atomic weight of 3. With food it is rapidly absorbed from the stomach (time to peak blood level is 1–2 hours). Half-life is 36 hours, and steady state is reached in 5–7 days. It is not metabolized by the liver, and it is not protein bound. Lithium is distributed in all body compartments, is actively transported into red blood cells and neurons, and is excreted unchanged by the kidneys.

Pharmacodynamics

Although the exact mechanism of therapeutic action is unknown, lithium's pharmacodynamics suggest that it works on inositol 1,4,5-triphosphate and diacylglycerol second-messenger systems. Lithium inhibits neurotransmitter–receptor coupled adenylate cyclase activity and cyclic AMP formation by preventing the neurotransmitter receptor linking to G protein. The G protein is not activated, and thus the adenylate cyclase system is not activated, and ion channel permeability is altered. Lithium's thymoleptic long-term (i.e., mood stabilization) effect is explained through this mechanism.

Lithium also decreases beta-adrenoceptor–mediated stimulation of adenylate cyclase, increases alpha$_2$-adrenoceptor downregulation, and increases serotonin turnover in presynaptic neurons, because tryptophan uptake increases (particularly in the hippocampus). This last effect leads to postsynaptic diminished binding of serotonin receptors. These changes are hypothesized to explain lithium's weak antidepressant effect. Dopamine receptor supersensitivity is also blocked, and GABAnergic activity and acetylcholine turnover are increased by lithium. These changes have also been related to lithium's acute antimanic properties.

Therapeutics

Lithium works best in patients with acute episodes of mood disorder with well intervals and with a family history of mood disorder. About 60%–90% of pure manics respond, and less than 30% relapse when blood levels are maintained around 1 mEq/L. Less likely to respond are patients who (1) are rapid cyclers, (2) have brief cycles (multiple shifts over several days or weeks), (3) are drug abusers, (4) have families who often express intense and negative emotions, (5) develop troublesome side effects, and (6) have complicating endocrine problems (particularly thyroid or parathyroid disease). Age at illness onset, number of previous episodes, and age when you see the patient have no predictive value. The presence of a sensitization pattern of illness, social and marital disruption, avolition between episodes, the combination of formal thought disorder and avolition during episodes, abnormal motor behavior, severe tardive dyskinesia, and cognitive impairment between episodes also predict resistance to lithium. In general, the longer a patient stays on lithium, the better he does. Thus, the second year of lithium prophylaxis is better than the first, the third is better than the second, and so on.

The proportion of bipolar patients benefiting from lithium prophylaxis ranges from 40%–80%, depending on the above response factors. Among unipolar patients, lithium is a weak prophylactic agent (antidepressants are better). Prior to lithium's use, assess the patient for heart disease and renal function (dysfunction in these organs is the main contraindication to giving lithium), and get baseline measures of thyroid and parathyroid function (because 3% and 10% of patients, respectively, develop dysfunction in these glands). Tests to perform are EKG, blood urea nitrogen, and urinalysis with specific gravity, serum creatinine, T_3/T_4 levels (some medical centers also test thyroid-stimulating hormone), serum calcium, and electrolytes.

Plasma lithium levels are used to monitor acute treatment. Get blood samples in the morning, 12 hours after the last dose. Levels of 1.0–1.5 mEq/L are optimal, but do not treat blood levels, treat patients. Thus, if a patient goes into remission with a blood level less than 1 mEq/L, he is on the correct dose. If a patient becomes toxic with a blood level of less than 1.5 mEq/L, he is getting too much. If a patient responds well and has only modest side effects with a blood level of 1.7 mEq/L this is the correct level for that patient. Like all psychotropics for which blood levels are readily obtainable, use lithium levels to monitor compliance. Use the patient's behaviors and physical examination findings to monitor treatment response and side effects.

After remission of symptoms, the dose that worked for the acute mania is the dose for maintenance. Blood levels are usually obtained twice weekly until steady state is reached, then weekly levels for inpatients and monthly or bimonthly levels for outpatients during the first year. There is no reason to obtain routine blood levels in patients on long-term lithium prophylaxis. Measure blood levels when the patient's physiologic status has changed (e.g., he develops pneumonia) or is about to change (e.g., he is to have surgery).

Lithium is actively reabsorbed in the proximal tubule by the sodium transport system with which it competes. Thus, in the presence of a reduced renal sodium load (e.g., a low salt diet), more lithium will be reabsorbed, possibly leading to toxicity. This is the likely mechanism for most of the deaths reported when lithium was marketed as a salt substitute in the 1940s.

Lithium diffuses passively across all cell membranes and is actively extruded against a gradient by several mechanisms. It is not significantly stored anywhere in the body, and in steady state the amount circulating in blood reflects a balance between oral dose and urinary excretion. During the first week or so of lithium treatment there is a sodium diuresis, with polyuria, as lithium replaces a portion of intracellular sodium. This is followed by several days of lithium diuresis around the time of substantial clinical improvement. Following lithium diuresis, steady state occurs in which lithium and sodium, as well as water and potassium, reach a stable balance and maintain equilibrium for the remainder of the treatment course.

Lithium has few behavioral effects at nontoxic doses. Normal subjects given lithium report some reduced "mental efficiency" and some motor slowing at blood levels around 1 mEq/L. Most adult bipolar patients receive 1,200–1,800 mg of lithium daily, usually in two divided doses with meals.

Lithium will exacerbate acne and psoriasis, and, when these conditions are severe, consider other treatments first. The risk benefit of lithium is particularly important when considering using it in patients with cataracts (lithium can alter lens electrolyte balance), lupus erythematosus (may exacerbate symptoms), myeloproliferative disorders (relatively contraindicated in patients with myeloid leukemia because of lithium's bone marrow–stimulating effects), low sodium diets, steroid therapy (as in some rheumatoid arthritis patients who then retain too much lithium), myasthenia gravis (lithium may interfere with acetylcholine release and may potentiate effects of myorelaxant drugs), and Parkinson's disease (exacerbates motor symptoms and a neurotoxic syndrome can occur).

Lithium peaks in the blood about 1.5–2 hours after ingestion. For patients with intense side effect "peaks," use the slow release preparation (Lithobid 300 mg or Eskalith CR 450 mg) or lithium in one nightly dose with a snack. Single-dose administration is often preferable because (1) lithium's elimination half-life (24–36 hours) permits 24-hour maintenance of adequate blood levels; (2) patient compliance improves with fewer doses; and (3) once-daily lithium may reduce the risks of renal histologic change. There is no intramuscular or intravenous lithium preparation. Converting from a divided to a single dose schedule raises lithium blood levels 10%–20%.

Side Effects

During the initial week or so of treatment, patients may experience a fine tremor (30%–50% of patients), mild fatigue or drowsiness, nausea, abdominal fullness and anorexia (30% of patients), increased thirst and polyuria (30%–40% of pa-

tients), a metallic taste, mild ankle edema (10%–15% of patients), and mildly reduced accommodation. These symptoms usually do not require lowering the
dose, and they usually remit during steady state. When *tremor* is prolonged (more
likely in males and heavy coffee users), or because interpersonal or job factors
make the tremors problematic, prescribe lithium once daily at bedtime with a
snack, and, if needed, give propranolol (20–120 mg daily) or other beta-blockers
less likely to depress mood (nadolol 20–40 mg or metoprolol 25–50 mg, each twice
daily.) Beta-blockers, however, are contraindicated for pregnant women and for
persons with asthma, diabetes, or hyperthyroidism. Reducing the dose may be
needed for some patients. Give lithium with food or once daily at night to avoid
nausea and vomiting. Side effects usually correlate with high peak blood levels,
and most patients (80%) experience at least one.

Lithium toxicity rarely appears below serum lithium levels of 2.0 mEq/L and is
characterized by profuse vomiting or diarrhea, slurred speech with thick discolored saliva (lithium is secreted in saliva), ataxia, coarse tremor, and lethargy. If untreated, myoclonus, stupor, coma, and death can occur. *Atypical neurologic syndromes* may occur, with unilateral focal signs mimicking a stroke. Treatment of
moderate lithium toxicity is supportive. Stop the drug, force fluids, and give salt
tablets. There is no specific antidote. Renal hemodialysis can actively remove
lithium if toxicity is severe (usually at blood levels above 3.3 mEq/L).

Use lithium with extreme caution for patients with impaired renal function:
low doses (e.g., 150 mg BID or TID) and frequent serum lithium determinations.
This is a last resort for such patients who refuse ECT and have not responded to
other mood stabilizers.

Lithium can also cause *cardiac repolarization abnormalities.* Do not prescribe it
for cardiac patients receiving diuretics or a low sodium diet because severe
lithium poisoning may occur rapidly in salt-depleted patients.

Because it inhibits cyclic-AMP/adenylcyclase, lithium impairs the function of
antidiuretic hormone (ADH) and thyroid hormone (T_3/T_4). The effect on ADH is
to prevent its action on the kidney, producing *secondary nephrogenic diabetes insipidus* (which is ADH resistant). Diabetes insipidus, which occurs in up to 20% of
lithium patients, is characterized by a large output of dilute urine (specific gravity
<1.010) and mild hypernatremia with normal blood sugar levels. With such a
large urine volume (>6–8 L/day) it becomes difficult to maintain adequate serum
lithium levels, and patients may relapse. Give a potassium-sparing diuretic (e.g.,
amiloride) to reduce urine volume and increase serum lithium levels. The response to amiloride, however, is slow (several weeks), and an interim rapid response (hours or days) can be obtained with indomethacin (see below for details).
Monitor blood levels until a new steady state occurs.

Patients with diabetes insipidus or a history of severe lithium toxicity may develop glomerular changes. Long-term lithium use can cause reduced renal function (10%–20% of patients develop reduced glomerular filtration rates and have
elevated serum creatinine), but renal failure is rare (1–2 cases in over 40 years of
worldwide use).

Because lithium blocks the release of T_3/T_4, about 3% of patients receiving
long-term maintenance lithium treatment develop *nontoxic goiters* that shrink

with discontinuation of lithium or with the addition of small doses of thyroid. Onset is usually between 5 and 24 months of treatment. The patients are usually clinically euthyroid, but signs of hypothyroidism and myxedema may occur. T_3/T_4 levels are often reduced, and there is an increased uptake of radioactive iodine (30% of patients). Women and cigarette smokers are more frequently affected than men.

Lithium may also cause *parathyroid hyperplasia* (10% of patients) leading to elevated levels of parathyroid hormone and hypercalcemia. Most of these elevations are mild and require no treatment or change in medication. Some patients, however, develop symptoms of hyperparathyroidism: osteoporosis, fatigue, hypertension, mild or atypical depression. Unlike primary hyperparathyroidism, renal calculi are rare in lithium-induced hyperparathyroidism because it leads to hypo- rather than hypercalciuria. Serum phosphate levels are also normal in lithium-induced hyperparathyroidism rather than low as in primary hyperparathyroidism. Increased serum levels of magnesium are, however, found. If symptoms are substantial, lithium needs to be discontinued. Calcium levels will return to normal within a month. If lithium continuation is essential, treat the hyperparathyroidism with norethindrone (counteracts the effects of elevated parathyroid hormone). Subtotal parathyroidectomy may be needed in some patients (extremely rare). Because of its effect on calcium metabolism, lithium's use in prepubescent children requires careful monitoring of bone growth.

Avoid giving lithium to *pregnant women* during their first trimester. Teratogenic heart problems (Ebstein's tricuspid valve anomaly) may occur. Lithium after the first trimester is acceptable, but it has an insulin-like effect on carbohydrate metabolism, and newborns exposed to lithium tend to have heavier birth weights. Because early signs of lithium toxicity (nausea, vomiting) are similar to complaints seen in pregnancy, developing toxicity can more easily be missed. If a pregnant woman is given lithium, fetal development is followed with level II ultrasound and echocardiography. Lithium is also excreted in mother's milk, and mothers on lithium treatment should bottle feed their babies. Infants exposed to lithium are also reported to be lethargic with decreased muscle tone. ECT is still the safest treatment for the pregnant or breast-feeding bipolar woman.

Excessive weight gain and *acneiform eruptions* are frequent troublesome side effects of lithium. The former frequently occurs in women and is often the primary reason for noncompliance. Other than dose reduction, diet and exercise are the only remedy. Some patients who stop lithium because of rash can restart it without a recurrence. If a patient suffers *hair loss* from lithium treatment, hair will grow back after stopping the drug, but the loss will reoccur with subsequent treatment.

About 50% of manics successfully treated with lithium become mildly depressed. If depression occurs, and is mild, continue lithium. If the depression becomes significant, you may need to add an antidepressant or give ECT.

Lithium affects some laboratory tests. These include elevated thyroid-stimulating hormone, leukocytosis due to increased production of normal neutrophils (no treatment required), flat EKG T waves (no treatment required); sleep EEG showing increased slow wave sleep and reduced REM sleep duration with no

REM rebound or reduced sleep time (no intervention required); and reduced sperm count and motility (effect on fertility unknown).

The elderly, children, and persons who regularly exercise or do strenuous physical activity require special attention. Older patients have lower glomerular filtration rates than do younger persons so that, at a given oral dose, older people are more apt to have side effects. Use lower starting doses for the elderly (300–600 mg/day), and do not give them a loading dose. Use ECT instead. Lithium is not FDA approved for children under 12 years, but it can be prescribed safely and effectively for manic children. Most children have good renal function and can tolerate high lithium doses. Patients in good general medical health who take lithium may exercise and do strenuous physical activity. More lithium than sodium is lost in sweat. Thus, patients taking lithium who exercise or do strenuous physical activity need higher doses of lithium on days they sweat heavily. They should drink fluids amply.

Noncompliance with lithium most commonly is due to (1) unpleasant side effects (e.g., weight gain, cognitive problems, tremor, thirst, fatigue, rash), (2) missing hypomanic highs or feeling less creative, and (3) feeling well and seeing no need to continue treatment. Patients most likely to be noncompliers include the young, males, patients with infrequent episodes, and patients incompletely responding to lithium.

Drug-Drug Interactions

Table 8.7 lists some of the drugs you can prescribe safely with lithium. Drugs to be concerned about are as follows.

1. Hydrochlorothiazide and chlorothiazide cause lithium retention. Patients receiving these agents with lithium need lower doses and more frequent serum lithium monitoring.
2. Theophylline and aminophylline (mild osmotic diuretics) increase

TABLE 8.7. Some Drugs That Can Be Prescribed with Lithium

General Medical Drugs	Psychotropic Drugs
Antineoplastic agents	Benzodiazepines
Amiloride	Carbamazepine
Aspirin	Cyclic antidepressants
Cromolyn	Monoamine oxidase inhibitors
Digitalis	Neuroleptics
Disulfiram (Antabuse)	Selective serotonin reuptake inhibitors
Furosemide	Valproic acid
Pindolol	
Prednisone	
Propranolol	
Sulindac	
Thyroxine	
Topical steroids	

lithium excretion. Large amounts of caffeine can also increase lithium excretion. When these agents are used along with lithium, a higher lithium dose is usually needed. Cromolyn has no effect on serum lithium.

3. Indomethacin, phenylbutazone, naproxen, and ibuprofen cause lithium retention. Of these, the lithium retention is greatest with indomethacin (100% increase in levels), which should not be prescribed with lithium. One exception to this injunction is the patient with lithium-induced diabetes insipidus who is slow to respond to diuretics. Low doses of indomethacin (25–75 mg daily) may reverse the electrolyte loss and reduce urinary output to normal. At this point, using an alternative to lithium may be the safest choice, but if lithium must be used by such patients, prescribe very low doses, get frequent blood levels, and monitor behavioral signs of impending toxicity (thick or discolored saliva, unexplained lethargy or concentration problems, weakness, and fatigue). If phenylbutazone, naproxen, or ibuprofen must be given with lithium, prescribe lower doses of lithium. Always ask patients whether they take any over-the-counter medications, such as Advil or other ibuprofen products. Aspirin causes a clinically insignificant increase in lithium levels.

4. Mazindol, an appetite suppressant, causes lithium retention and should not be prescribed with lithium. Metronidazole, an antiprotozoal, can also do this.

5. Lithium may potentiate neuroleptic dopamine blockade. A lithium-neuroleptic combination can cause a toxic encephalopathy, although this idiosyncratic neuroleptic malignant syndrome-like reaction is extremely rare. Also, the liquid forms of lithium and many neuroleptics are incompatible and when given together result in a precipitate that is not absorbed, leading to underdosing.

6. Clozapine (see Chapter 9) causes a potentially fatal agranulocytosis in 1%–2% of patients. The agranulocytosis usually occurs rapidly without warning, but may be preceded by a neutropenia. Because lithium has a myelostimulatory effect, a clozapine–lithium combination might mask a clozapine neutropenia and its potential to warn against agranulocytosis.

7. Tetracyclines, used to treat acne, should not be used with lithium because the combination may produce a nephrotoxic reaction. Drugs like isotretinoin can be used with lithium, although lithium exacerbates acne.

ANTICONVULSANT MOOD STABILIZERS

Carbamazepine and valproate are widely prescribed for mood disorder patients, particularly those with bipolar disorder. These drugs substantially benefit 25%–50% of patients. They are rapidly metabolized by the liver and must be taken several times daily to maintain effective blood levels. They also induce cytochrome enzymes, thus lowering blood levels of most psychotropics, and reduce the levels of oral contraceptives and other steroids and can cause false-positive pregnancy tests. Thus, drug–drug interaction is a particularly important consideration when prescribing anticonvulsants.

Anticonvulsants should be used by women of childbearing age with caution as they cause fetal neural tube defects (e.g., craniofacial, spina bifida) in 1%–2% of patients. Vigorous birth control, careful monitoring for pregnancy, and prophylactic folic acid minimize the risks if anticonvulsants must be used.

Carbamazepine

Carbamazepine (CBZ) is structurally similar to nonspecific monoamine reuptake-inhibiting antidepressants. CBZ blocks voltage-dependent sodium channels in the cortex and hippocampus. This basic effect results in a variety of other pharmacodynamic changes: reduced synthesis and thus turnover of dopamine, reduced GABA turnover, and increased release of intracellular potassium. GABA regulates gating (opening or closing) of chloride ion channels. The overall result is a decrease in the frequency of sustained repetitive firing of action potentials of hippocampal neurons. High frequency sustained repetitive firing is necessary for seizure generation. Thus, CBZ stabilizes ion channels in an inactive mode and delays recovery from this state. CBZ also acts on peripheral-type benzodiazepine receptors. Although it cannot prevent kindling, CBZ inhibits kindling.

CBZ is fairly rapidly absorbed in the gastrointestinal tract, and peak blood levels occur between 1 and 5 hours. CBZ is metabolized (oxidation) by the liver cytochrome P450 systems, 70%–80% protein bound, and has an initial half-life of 15–30 hours with a 4-day duration to steady state. Because of autoregulation (i.e., it increases its own metabolism), after 1–3 months half-life decreases to 10–15 hours. You may need to increase oral doses at that time to avoid relapses. Therapeutic blood levels for seizure disorders are 4–15 µg/ml, with typical oral doses between 800 and 1,600 mg. A typical starting dose for mood disorder patients is 200 mg BID followed by an increase of 200 mg every 4–7 days. For epileptics, dosing is slower by half. Some patients require as much as 2,400 mg. Asian, some African-American, and elderly patients reach therapeutic blood levels at lower oral doses.

CBZ is effective as an adjunct treatment of bipolar depression and for mania, in the treatment of resistant bipolar states, and in the prevention (modest effect) of manic and depressive episodes. It also is used to treat alcohol withdrawal and, combined with lithium or beta-blockers, to control assaultive behavior in patients with stroke or head injury.

CBZ is combined routinely with lithium and, to a lesser extent, with neuroleptics. The latter combination often involves haloperidol, despite the fact that CBZ decreases haloperidol blood levels.

In addition to lowering the blood levels of most psychotropic medications, CBZ levels are in turn lowered by calcium channel blockers, cimetidine, terfenadine, barbiturates, phenytoin, primidone, erythromycin, and itself. It is unclear if valproate affects overall CBZ levels, but CBZ lowers valproate levels, and the combination (possibly synergistic in mood disorder) can produce more free plasma CBZ (displaced by valproate, making for more bioavailability) and more of the metabolite CBZ-E. Fluoxetine leads to more CBZ being biotransformed to the 11–10 epoxide metabolite, which is neurotoxic. At high levels, CBZ can cause an encephalopathy or a Parkinson's syndrome. CBZ also lowers the blood levels of oral contraceptives and anticoagulants. Furthermore, it should not be used with clozapine because of the potential of both drugs to suppress bone marrow activity. Do not prescribe CBZ for persons who received an MAOI in the previous 2 weeks or have narrow angle glaucoma or a bone marrow–suppressing disorder.

Side Effects of CBZ

Common CBZ side effects involve (1) the *central nervous system:* drowsiness, dizziness, headache (change dosages slowly); (2) *gastrointestinal tract:* nausea (take with food, usually transient); (3) *blood:* leukopenia (benign, no response needed); and (4) *skin:* rash (10%–15% of patients).

Drowsiness and dizziness that are significant or associated with ataxia or diplopia and blurred vision usually result from increasing doses too fast. Nausea, vomiting, and diarrhea can occur. A common error in treating newly hospitalized bipolar patients who are receiving CBZ is to restart them on the drug before measuring blood levels. Always obtain an admission blood level for CBZ and for every drug for which assays are readily available so that you can determine if the patient's hospitalization results from *noncompliance* or *breakthrough relapse*. If noncompliance is the problem and you automatically put the patient back on his "usual" CBZ dose that he is no longer taking, you will likely induce an overdose. Breakthrough relapse suggests that the medication may no longer be working, and enhancing it or changing it may be needed.

Rare adverse CBZ reactions that require stopping the drug include (1) agranulocytosis and aplastic anemia, which develop between months 2 and 6 of treatment (mild depression of white cells is more common and does not require intervention, only careful follow up); and Stevens-Johnson syndrome (mucosal and skin lesions, exfoliative dermatitis, chills, fever).

Other side effects include hepatocellular or cholestatic jaundice, hypnoatremia, water intoxication, and dystonias. A temporary dose reduction usually resolves these difficulties. After several weeks of treatment, liver enzyme-increased metabolism often increases drug tolerance. Because of liver and blood side effects, obtain liver and blood studies prior to treatment and then weekly until steady state. Afterward, assess monthly for 6 months and then semiannually. Cardiac conduction changes are similar to those with other tricyclic compounds (slowing). If you discontinue CBZ, taper it gradually over several weeks because withdrawal seizures may occur, even in nonepileptics.

Valproate

Valproate (VP) is available in four forms: valproic acid (Depakene), sodium valproate syrup, divalproex sodium (Depakote), and a sprinkle form to put on food for children and persons who cannot easily swallow tablets. The divalproex sodium seems to cause less gastrointestinal side effects. VP directly upregulates GABA hippocampal receptors, similar to the effects of diazepam and phenobarbital. Dopamine turnover and GABA turnover are reduced, whereas GABAnergic action increases. It also blocks sodium channels. VP at high doses also acts on peripheral-type benzodiazepine receptors. Thus, VP can prevent as well as inhibit kindling.

VP is sluggishly absorbed from the gastrointestinal tract, with peak blood levels in 3–5 hours. It is metabolized (oxidation and conjugation) by liver cytochrome P450 enzyme systems, is 90%–95% protein bound, and has a half-life of 6–16 hours with a 3–4-day duration to steady state.

When divalproex is used and given after meals, side effects are uncommon. Of these, nausea, diarrhea, sedation, and tremor occur most often. Some VP metabolites (e.g., 2-propyl-4-pentanoic acid) are hepatotoxic. VP will typically produce mild and transient liver transaminase elevations. Severe hepatotoxicity with delirium, ataxia, and dysarthria can, but rarely, occurs (usually in the first 3 months of treatment). This potentially fatal hepatitis is an idiosyncratic reaction seen more in epileptics and persons under age 10 years than in bipolar patients, probably because the former often take several anticonvulsants concurrently. Chronic treatment with VP, however, can cause elevated serum ammonia levels because of VP's inhibitory action on carbamyl phosphate synthase, the first enzyme in the urea cycle. Some patients tolerate the high ammonia levels (other liver enzymes may be in the normal range), but if a patient who has previously tolerated VP develops unexplained lethargy and bradyphrenia (timed cognitive tests are an inexpensive, sensitive way of assessing this) obtain an ammonia level test. *Carnitine* (1 g BID), a nutrient found in meat and dairy products (and health food stores), is a cofactor in oxidative metabolism of long-chain fatty acids. It can specifically reverse the enzyme inhibition, resolve symptoms, and permit the patient to remain on VP.

Blood dyscrasias with VP are very rare, although thrombocytopenia can occur in elderly patients. CBZ reduces VP plasma levels. Aspirin, fluoxetine, and erythromycin increase VP plasma levels.

VP is effective for acute mania and as a prophylaxis for both manic and depressive episodes. It can be used alone or with lithium. VP may be helpful in treating panic disorder and is used in benzodiazepine withdrawal. For outpatients, the usual dose schedule for mood disorders is to begin at 250 mg twice daily and increase slowly by 250 mg every few days to a serum level of 50–100 µg/ml. For acute manic inpatients, give VP in a loading dose as described above. Elderly patients and patients with impaired liver function should receive lower dosing schedules. The daily dosage range is 750 to 4,500 mg. Aspirin displaces VP from protein binding, increasing free drug levels. Thus greater bioavailability can be achieved with a lower oral dose. Salicylates, however, should not be routinely given with VP. When side effects are troublesome and dose reduction necessary, adding aspirin may allow continuation of the drug while lessening side effects.

Discontinuation of VP, as with CBZ, should be done gradually over several weeks. One modification of the rule occurs when you have decided to give ECT to a patient receiving VP or CBZ. Because VP and CBZ raise the seizure threshold, they can make it difficult or impossible to safely induce a therapeutic seizure. Waiting several weeks to taper the drug is often impractical. In this situation reduce the drug by 25% every 2 days until the patient is on 25% of his original dose. Most patients will then be able to successfully undergo ECT (which raises the seizure threshold) without having spontaneous withdrawal seizures. The last 25% of the drug can be stopped after the first or second ECT. The schedule would be— down 25% Friday, down another 25% Monday and again on Wednesday, ECT on Friday and Monday, down the last 25% Wednesday.

Side Effects of VP

Common side effects of VP are tremor (10%; use a beta-blocker if severe), ataxia (slowly reduce dose if severe), increased appetite and weight gain (exercise and diet are the only treatments) Hepatic transaminase elevations are also common and dose dependent. Alone, however, they cause no hepatic toxicity and have no clinical significance. Alopecia can occur, as can lethargy, sedation, dysarthria, and flushing. Side effects can be minimized by gradual dose increases. Serious side effects that require stopping VP are *hepatic toxicity*, with jaundice, malaise, nausea, vomiting, and edema; *pancreatitis* (rare); *hematologic abnormalities*, particularly bleeding; and allergic *rash*. These usually occur within the first 6 months of treatment and are less common in elderly patients. Pretreatment evaluation and serial liver function studies help to identify early signs of toxicity.

Additional Readings

Abou-Saleh MT, Filip V (eds): Prediction in psychopharmacology. *Br J Psychiatry 163*(suppl 21), 1993.

Adams F: Emergency intravenous sedation of the delirious medically ill patient. *J Clin Psychiatry 49*(suppl):22–26, 1988.

Akiskal HS: The prevalent clinical spectrum of bipolar disorders: Beyond DSM-IV. *J Clin Psychopharmacol 16*(suppl 1):4s–14s, 1996.

Akiskal HS, Akiskal K: Cyclothymic, hyperthymic, and depressive temperaments as subaffective variants of mood disorders. In Tassman A, Riba MB (eds): *American Psychiatric Press Review of Psychiatry,* vol 11. American Psychiatric Press, Washington, DC, 1992, pp 43–62.

Akiskal HS, Mallya G: Criteria for the "soft" bipolar spectrum: Treatment implications. *Psychopharm Bull 23*:68–73, 1987.

Akiskal HS, Maser JD, Zeller P, Endicott J, Coryell W, Keller M, Warshaw M, Clayton P, Goodwin FK: Switching from "unipolar" to bipolar II: An 11-year prospective study of clinical and temperamental predictors in 559 patients. *Arch Gen Psychiatry 52*:114–123, 1995.

American Psychiatric Association: Practice guideline for the treatment of patients with bipolar disorder. *Am J Psychiatry 15*:(suppl), 1994.

Andrulonis PA, Glueck BC, Stroebel CF, Vogel NG: Borderline personality subcategories. *J Nerv Ment Dis 170*:670–679, 1982.

Angst J: Switch from depression to mania: A record study over decades 1920–1982. *Psychopathology 18*:140–154, 1985.

Atre-Vaidya N, Taylor MA: The sensitization hypothesis and importance of psychosensory features in mood disorder: A review. *J Neuropsychiatry Clin Neurosci 9*:525–533, 1997.

Carter JG: Intravenous haloperidol in the treatment of acute psychosis (Letter). *Am J Psychiatry 143*:1316–1317, 1986.

Casey DA: Electroconvulsive therapy in the neuroleptic malignant syndrome. *Convuls Ther 3*:278–283, 1987.

Cummings JL, Mendez MF: Secondary mania with focal cerebrovascular lesions. *Am J Psychiatry 141*:1084–1087, 1984.

Davis GC, Akiskal HS: Descriptive, biological and theoretical aspects of borderline personality disorder. *Hosp Commun Psychiatry 37*:685–692, 1986.

Dubovsky SL, Buzan RD: Novel alternatives and supplements to lithium and anticonvulsants for bipolar affective disorder. *J Clin Psychiatry 58*:224–242, 1997.

Eastman CI, Young MA, Fogg LF, Liu L, Meaden PM: Bright light treatment of winter depression. *Arch Gen Psychiatry 55*:883–889, 1998.

Fernandez F, Holmes VF, Adams F, Kavanaugh JJ: Treatment of severe refractory agitation with a haloperidol drip. *J Clin Psychiatry 49*:239–241, 1988.

Fogarty F, Russell JM, Newman SC, Bland RC: Mania. *Acta Psychiatr Scand Suppl 376*:16–23, 1994.

Freeman MP, Stoll AL: Mood stabilizer combinations: A review of safety and efficacy. *Am J Psychiatry 155*:12–21, 1998.

Gershon ES, DeLisi LE, Hamovit J, Nurnberger JI Jr, Maxwell ME, Schreiber J, Dauphinais D, Dingman CW II, Guroff JJ: A controlled family study of chronic psychoses: Schizophrenia and schizoaffective disorder. *Arch Gen Psychiatry 45*:328–336, 1988.

Hare E: The two manias: A study of the evolution of the modern concept of mania. *Br J Psychiatry 138*:89–99, 1981.

Inskip HM, Harris EC, Barraclough B: Lifetime risk of suicide for affective disorder, alcoholism and schizophrenia. *Br J Psychiatry 172*:35–37, 1998.

Johnson FN: *Depression and Mania, Modern Lithium Therapy*, IRL Press, Oxford, England, 1987.

Kahlbaum KL: *Catatonia*. The Johns Hopkins University Press, Baltimore, 1973.

Kasanin J: The acute schizoaffective psychoses. *Am J Psychiatry 13*:97–126, 1933.

Kelsoe JR: The genetics of bipolar disorder. *Psychiatr Ann 27*:285–292, 1997.

Ketter TA, Pazzaglia PJ, Post RM: Synergy of carbamazepine and valproic acid in affective illness: Case report and review of the literature. *J Clin Psychopharm 12*:276–281, 1992.

Kraepelin E: *Manic-Depressive Insanity and Paranoia*. Barclay RM (trans), Robertson GM (ed). E&S Livingstone, Edinburgh, 1921; Arno Press, New York, 1976.

Lauterbach EC: Bipolar disorders, dystonia and compulsion after dysfunction of the cerebellum, dentatorubrothalamic tract, and substantia nigra. *Biol Psychiatry 40*:726–730, 1995.

Manzano J, Salvador A: Antecedents of severe affective (mood) disorders, patients examined as children or adolescents and as adults. *Acta Paedopsychiatrica 56*:11–18, 1993.

McElroy SL, Keck PE, Jr, Stanton SP, Tugrul KC, Bennett JA, Strakowski SM: A randomized comparison of divalproex oral loading versus haloperidol in the initial treatment of acute psychotic mania. *J Clin Psychiatry 57*:142–146, 1996.

Mukheijee S, Sackeim HA, Schnur DB: Electroconvulsive therapy of acute manic episodes: A review of 50 years' experience. *Am J Psychiatry 151*:169–176, 1994.

Mungus D: Interictal behavior abnormality in temporal lobe epilepsy: A specific syndrome or nonspecific psychopathology? *Arch Gen Psychiatry 39*:108–111, 1982.

Perugi G, Akiskal HS, Cecconi LD, Mastrocinque C, Patronelli A, Vignoli S, Bemi E: The high prevalence of "soft" bipolar (II) features in atypical depression. *Compr Psychiatry 39*:63–71, 1998.

Perry PJ, Alexander B: Dosage and serum levels. In Johnson FN (ed): *Depression and Mania, Modern Lithium Therapy*, IRL Press, Oxford, 1987, pp 67–73.

Placid GF, Signoretta S, Liguori A, Gervasi R, Maremmani I, Akiskal HS: The semistructured affective temperament interview (TEMPS-I): Reliability and psychometric properties in 1010 14–26 year old students. *J Affect Disord 47*:1–10, 1998.

Pope HG, Jonas JM, Hudson JI, Cohen BM, Gunderson JG: The validity of DSM-III border-line personality disorder. *Arch Gen Psychiatry 139*:1480–1483, 1982.

Pope HG Jr, Lipinski JF: Diagnosis in schizophrenia and manic-depressive illness: A re-assessment of the specificity of "schizophrenic" symptoms in light of current research. *Arch Gen Psychiatry 35*:811–828, 1978.

Pope HG Jr, Lipinski JF, Cohen BM, Axelrod DT: "Schizoaffective disorder": An invalid di-agnosis? A comparison of schizoaffective disorder, schizophrenia, and affective disor-der. *Am J Psychiatry 137*:921–927, 1980.

Post RM: Transduction of psychosocial stress into the neurobiology of recurrent affective disorder. *Am J Psychiatry 149*:999–1010, 1992.

Post RM, Rubinow DR, Ballenger JC: Conditioning, sensitization, and kindling: Implica-tions for the course of affective illness. In Post RM, Ballenger JC (eds): *The Neurobiology of Mood Disorders*. Williams & Wilkins, Baltimore, 1984, pp 432–466.

Post RM, Weiss SRB: Kindling: Implications for the course and treatment of affective disor-ders. In Modigh K, Robak OH, Vestergaard P (eds): *Anticonvulsants in Psychiatry*. Wrightson Biomedical Publishing Limited, Petersfield, U.K., 1994, pp 113–137.

Post RM, Weiss SRB, Pert A: Cocaine-induced behavioral sensitizations and kindling: Im-plications for the emergence of psychopathology and seizures. *Ann NY Acad Sci 537*: 292–308, 1988.

Price LH, Heninger GR: Lithium in the treatment of mood disorders. *N Engl J Med 331*:591–598, 1994.

Sangiovanni F, Taylor MA, Abrams R, Gaztanaga P: Control of psychotic excitement states with intramuscular haloperidol. *Am J Psychiatry 130*:1155–1160, 1973.

Starkstein SE, Fedoroff P, Berthier ML, Robinson RG: Manic-depressive and pure manic states after brain lesions. *Biol Psychiatry 29*:149–158, 1991.

Starkstein SE, Mayberg HS, Berthier ML, Fedoroff P, Price TB, Dannals RF, Wagner HN, Leiguarda R, Robinson RG: Mania after brain injury: Neuroradiological and metabolic findings. *Ann Neurol 27*:652–659, 1990.

Taylor MA: Catatonia: A review of a behavioral neurologic syndrome. *Neuropsychiatry, Neuropsychol and Behav Neurol 3*:48–72, 1990.

Taylor MA, Abrams R: The phenomenology of mania. A new look at some old patients. *Arch Gen Psychiatry 29*:520–522, 1973.

Turk J: The fragile-X syndrome, on the way to a behavioral phenotype. *Br J Psychiatry 160*:24–35, 1992.

van Gorp WG, Altshuler L, Theberge DC, Wilkins J, Dixon W: Cognitive impairment in euthymic bipolar patients with and without prior alcohol dependence. *Arch Gen Psychi-atry 55*:41–46, 1998.

Van Reekum R, Conway CA, Gansler D, White R, Bachman DL: Neurobehavioral study of borderline personality disorder. *J Psychiatry Neurosci 18*:121–129, 1993.

Winokur G, Clayton PJ, Reich T: *Manic-Depressive Illness*. CV Mosby, St. Louis, 1979.

Zanarini MC, Frankenburg FR, Dubo ED, Sickel AE, Trikha A, Levin A, Reyonlds V: Axis I comorbidity of borderline personality disorder. *Am J Psychiatry 155*:1733–1739, 1998.

9

Psychosis

The DSM separates "psychotic disorders" from "mood disorders," defining psychotic disorders as conditions in which hallucinations, delusions, or related behaviors (e.g., grossly "disorganized" speech, thought, or social behaviors) *must* be present. Depression and mania can be severe enough to produce hallucinations and delusions, but these and related phenomena are not necessary for a diagnosis of mood disorder. This dichotomy is dangerous because it influences you to not diagnose mood disorder when a patient is also psychotic. However, 20% of melancholic and 30%–50% of manic episodes are of psychotic severity, and if you understand the treatment needs of such patients their response to treatment is good.

Nevertheless, psychosis is a severe state of illness that requires specific diagnostic and management decisions. Table 9.1 displays the differential diagnosis of psychosis from the most to the least common. Although psychotic patients often require neuroleptics, think of psychotic features as indicators of severity rather than of specific pathophysiology. Thus, your goal is to identify the syndrome and its cause and then decide the best treatment for that patient, which may (but not necessarily) include a neuroleptic. The diagnosis and treatment of mood disorders are covered in Chapters 7 and 8. The principles and guidelines for treating psychotic patients are covered below with details for different conditions presented in subsequent chapters.

CLINICAL PRESENTATIONS

Delirium

Delirium is caused by many drugs (illicit, over the counter, and prescribed) and has multiple etiologies. Delirium affects 10%–15% of all acute medical–surgical patients, and 30% of elderly medical inpatients will have acute or subacute delirium. Ninety percent of cases go unrecognized, making it one of the most missed diagnoses. Table 9.2 lists criteria with which to assess delirium. The pattern of delirium

TABLE 9.1 The Differential Diagnosis of Psychosis*

Condition	What To Look For and Consider
Mood disorder (40%) (bipolar, unipolar, schizoaffective)	1. The most common (apply Sutton's law) 2. Signs and symptoms of depression or mania should always take precedence over psychotic features (make the diagnosis with the best prognosis, use the duck principle) 3. Past episodes, family history may confirm diagnosis
Drug-induced states (25%)	1. Delirium (decreased arousal due to the direct toxic effects of the drug, as with sedative-hypnotics) 2. Intoxications (arousal may be increased by the direct toxic effects of the drug such as with phencyclidine, reduced from many prescribed drugs, or clear but still associated with hallucinations also with many prescription drugs) 3. Withdrawal states (usually producing altered arousal such as with alcohol delirium tremens) 4. Chronic or recurrent psychosis (due to permanent brain damage from a drug such as LSD) 5. Drug screen, physical examination findings, history of drug abuse may confirm diagnosis
Epilepsy (<5%)	Complex partial fits with temporal or frontal lobe focus most likely to produce psychosis. See Chapter 10 for details
Head Trauma or Stroke (5%)	Frontal and temporal lobe and nondominant hemisphere lesions most likely to produce psychosis. See Chapter 11 for details
Dementia (5%)	Vascular and other subcortical dementias most likely to produce psychosis. See Chapter 12 for details.
DSM "Psychotic Disorders"† (5%)	Schizophrenia, schizophreniform disorder, delusional disorder, and other non-DSM disorders are primary psychoses without past or present mood disorder. See text for details
Basal ganglia disease (<5%)	Huntington's and Wilson's diseases most likely to produce psychosis
Other neurologic disease (5%–10%)	1. Delirium from many causes can result in psychosis when metabolic changes are rapid 2. Tumors, syphilis, vascular malformations, and other masses in frontotemporal regions can result in psychosis. See Chapters 12 and 16 for details
Psychotic disorders not in DSM (5%)	Positive symptom nonaffective psychoses and paraphrenias

*numbers in parentheses are approximate percentages of acute psychotic patients admitted to a general hospital psychiatric service. In some hospitals, drug induced psychotic states are most common.

†Brief psychotic disorder is discussed in Chapter 8; postpartum disorder is discussed in Chapter 7; shared psychotic disorder (Folie a deux) is without validation and is not discussed.

TABLE 9.2. Diagnostic Criteria of Delirium

Criterion	Operational Definition
Diffuse cognitive impairment	Mini-Mental State score of <22
Altered sensorium	Abnormal Letter Cancellation Test or missing the time of day by more than 2 hours; lethargic, dozing off during the examination; or having delayed reaction time
Fluctuating behavior	A rating of "2" or more on the following scale for increasing fluctuation: 0, none; 1, questionable; 2, definite (mild, at least one discrepancy in global behavior during nursing shifts or change in performance on cognitive tests); 3, definite (two or more discrepancies or changes)
Increased motor activity	A rating of "2" or more on the following scale for increased motor activity: 0, none; 1, questionable; 2, restless (fidgets in bed, plays with bedclothes); 3, agitated (needs siderails and restraints)
Altered sleep–wake cycle with insomnia or daytime drowsiness	Less than 5 hours of sleep at night or more than 3 hours of sleep during the day

is (1) diffuse cognitive impairment, (2) altered sensorium (reduced arousal), (3) fluctuating behavior, (4) increased motor activity (restlessness or severe agitation), and (5) altered sleep–wake cycle with insomnia or daytime lethargy.

Acutely delirious patients are perplexed, disoriented, anxious, and agitated. Tremor, tachycardia, sweating, and vasoconstriction with cold, clammy skin and circumoral pallor are common. These patients are "fitful," cannot understand events around them, fear staff and other patients, and may become irritable and assaultive. They are often worse at night (the "sundown" syndrome), when reduced lighting and fewer interactions with staff exacerbate already impaired brain function.

Delirious patients commonly have illusions and visual hallucinations. They often assume conversations among staff or visitors are about themselves, and they may become delusional. Random fragments of nongoal-directed associations are typical (rambling speech). Cognitive impairment is most striking for attention (poor A test performance), immediate recall, and new learning (a form of anterograde amnesia). Disorientation for time of day is almost pathognomonic. Motor coordination also is often impaired. Onset may be gradual or acute. Most deliria resolve with good treatment, although 30% of patients die within a month of the delirium.

Severe delirium is rarely misdiagnosed. Suspect subacute delirium in patients whose general medical condition and treatments do not fully explain their behavior. These patients are unexpectedly lethargic and easily fatigued. They have difficulty feeding, washing, or dressing and cannot understand simple instructions. They appear uncertain, hesitant, or perplexed by simple tasks like going to the bathroom and navigating from the visitor's lounge to their room.

Delirium is a syndrome. You must find the etiology to effectively treat it. For medical or surgical patients, the most likely cause of delirium is medical treatment (particularly drugs) or a metabolic problem due to the disease that led to treatment. Drugs with substantial anticholinergic properties or with a narrow safety margin between therapeutic and toxic doses such as lithium and digitalis are common offenders. Psychotropic drug use is a common cause in the elderly. General medical problems likely to cause delirium are those associated with fluid and electrolyte imbalance, hypoxemia, hypoglycemia, infection, or fever. Other common causes of delirium are drug overdoses, drug withdrawal, seizure disorder, mania, epilepsy, cerebral edema from head trauma, central nervous system infection, urinary tract disease, pulmonary and cardiovascular dysfunction, and systemic infection.

Most often you will find the cause in the order sheet (medications given) or among the commonly ordered laboratory studies. The rate of change is more likely associated with delirium than simply having an abnormal finding For example, end-stage renal disease produces a very high blood urea nitrogen value (>100 mg/ml) but rarely delirium, whereas acute renal failure with lower blood urea nitrogen values usually causes delirium.

The EEG pattern of delirium is diffuse high voltage slowing. A normal tracing is strong evidence *against* delirium. Delirium tremens is the exception; its EEG pattern is increased fast activity. Most deliria do not suggest etiology. Specific symptom patterns that do are anticholinergic delirium, Wernicke's encephalopathy, and delirium tremens (the last two are discussed in Chapter 13).

Anticholinergic drug-induced delirium is common because of the large number of these agents and their overuse and overprescription. Drugs to worry about are nonspecific and partially specific monoamine reuptake-inhibiting antidepressants, antispasmodics, antihistamines, antiparkinsonians, and clozapine and olanzapine. Many over-the-counter preparations have significant anticholinergic properties. These include cold remedies (Allerest, Coricidin, Romilar, Sine-Off, Contac, Sinutab, Dristan), analgesics (Excedrin PM, Cope), and hypnotics and tranquilizers (Compoz, Devarex, Dormirex, Nytol, Sleep-Eze, Sominex).

Patients with anticholinergic deliria have parasympathetic blockade. They have dry, hot, flushed skin; widely dilated pupils; dry mucous membranes; decreased bowel and bladder motility; mild hyperthermia; tachycardia; palpitations; and arrhythmias. They are severely agitated and have a clouded sensorium and diffuse cognitive impairment, rambling speech, and perceptual disturbances (illusions and hallucinations). They may be delusional. When antidepressants are involved, cardiac arrhythmias are common and heart block may occur. The clinical mnemonic is "blind as a bat, dry as a bone, red as a beet, and mad as a hatter."

Phenothiazines and other psychotropics with anticholinergic properties are obviously contraindicated for anticholinergic delirium because they exacerbate and prolong the syndrome. Emergency treatment may require restraints. Primary treatment is physostigmine, which crosses the blood–brain barrier and counters both peripheral and central cholinergic blockade. Initially give 1–2 mg IV or SC and repeat in 30 minutes and again at 30–60-minute intervals, if needed, for a total dose of 6–8 mg. Neostigmine does not enter the central nervous system. You may need to give physostigmine for several days because most anticholinergic drugs have a substantially longer half-life than does physostigmine. If agitation and anxiety continue, look for diarrhea, abdominal cramps, and salarrhea, indicating severe anticholinergic withdrawal from giving too much physostigmine.

Treatment of Delirium

The first step in treating the delirious patient is to achieve behavioral control to prevent self-injury. Then treat the cause. If this is not known, concentrate on conditions that are life threatening or cause permanent brain damage. Hypoglycemia, hyperthermia, and hypoxemia require rapid intervention. Test the blood glucose levels of all patients with deliria of unknown etiology. If there is any question regarding the glucose level, give intravenous dextrose (50 ml of a 50% solution) and immediately examine for hyperthermia, hypotension, myocardial infarction, and cardiac arrhythmia (frequently causing deliria in the elderly), pulmonary disease, and anemia. If the patient is a known or suspected alcoholic, give thiamine 100–400 mg IV if glucose is administered to avoid precipitating a Wernicke's encephalopathy. Thiamine is a cofactor in glucose metabolism, and many alcoholics with already low thiamine levels cannot tolerate a large glucose load.

The delirious patient is best managed in a quiet, calm, structured setting. A softly lit hospital room with constant observation by familiar people and staff who clearly identify themselves and what they are doing reduces the patient's anxiety and agitation, often making pharmacotherapy unnecessary. When sedation is needed, use benzodiazepines in low doses given widely apart to avoid overlapping half-lives and further deterioration in arousal and cognition.

Occasionally standard treatments fail to relieve agitation, assaultiveness, or self-destructive behavior in a patient for whom the treatment of the underlying process (e.g., infection) has not begun to take effect. This is a life-threatening situation in which death can result from cardiovascular collapse (from initial fluid and electrolyte imbalance, compounded by struggling against restraints), the thwarting of primary treatment (e.g., pulling out intravenous tubes, ripping off surgical dressings), or self-injury (e.g., jumping out of the window to escape "the voices"). ECT can be used safely to ameliorate these symptoms of delirium. One or two treatments can resolve agitation and permit treatment of the underlying process.

Psychotic Drug-Induced States

Psychosis due to drug use falls into three categories: intoxications (sometimes delirium), withdrawal states, and recurrent psychosis from permanent drug-caused brain damage (also termed *post-hallucinogen perceptual disorder).*

Intoxications are typically nonspecific, but are usually associated with (1) an acute onset; (2) some alteration in arousal (reduced in delirium, raised in excitement states) that results in poor concentration, attention, or responsivity; (3) an intense mood (particularly anxiety or euphoria); (4) agitation (sedative-hypnotics in high doses and opiates are exceptions); and (5) hallucinations, often in multiple sensory modalities. Table 9.3 displays behavior patterns of some specific intoxications. Many prescription drugs also cause intoxication with psychosis, and the likelihood increases if the patient (1) is elderly, (2) lives in a nursing home, (3) receives more than two medications, (4) has a general medical condition known to affect brain function, or (5) has known neurologic disease. Intoxications in the young are most often from street drugs, whereas intoxications in the middle-aged and in elderly persons are often from prescribed drugs. Prescribed drugs that produce intoxication are described in Chapter 13.

Withdrawals that cause psychosis are uncommon. Only 5% of withdrawals from alcohol result in delirium tremens. These patients are typically physically debilitated from chronic alcohol abuse (e.g., cirrhosis, pancreatitis). Table 9.4 lists some withdrawal syndromes.

Recurrent drug-induced psychoses are treatment resistant, often chronic illnesses that result from permanent brain damage from drug use. Even after years of abstinence a person can have these recurrent psychoses. The characteristics of a drug induce psychosis are (1) acute onset, (2) agitation, (3) irritability and lability of mood (particularly anxiety and euphoria), (4) multiple types of hallucinations, (5) multiple psychosensory features, and (6) substantial cognitive impairment (frontal executive functions, attention, visuospatial, memory) in clear consciousness (very different from intoxications). The presence of avolition and formal thought disorder are particularly poor prognostic signs. The absence

TABLE 9.3. Specific Intoxication Behavior Patterns

Drug	*Pattern*
LSD	Synesthesias,* perceptual distortions (particularly visual, e.g., illusions, dysmorphopsia, dysmegalopsia), anxiety, sympathetic arousal
Peyote/mescaline	Panoramic hallucinations (scenes like a movie), euphoria, flushed skin, catatonia
Phencyclidine (PCP)	Intense manic-like excitement, violence, catatonia, vestibulocerebellar dysfunction (dizziness, rotary nystagmus, poor muscular coordination), analgesia, hypertension, tachycardia
Cocaine	Excitement, lability of mood (euphoria, expansiveness, irritability, suspiciousness), sympathetic hyperarousal, hallucinations of geometric shapes and bugs crawling on or under the skin
Anticholinergics	Delirium, hot flushed skin, dry mucosa, dilated pupils, tachycardia, low-grade fever, myoclonus if severe
Alcohol	Ataxia of speech, gait, and thought; initial excitation followed by reduced arousal

*Stimulus produces a hallucination in a different sensory modality (e.g., seeing colors when hearing music).

TABLE 9.4. Characteristics of Some Withdrawal Syndromes

Cause of Withdrawal	Characteristics
Alcohol	Agitation, coarse tremor, multiple types of hallucinations, reduced arousal and diffuse cognitive impairment, sympathetic hyperarousal, fast activity on EEG (the only delirium to produce this), seizures
Barbiturates and benzodiazepines	Grand mal seizures may be first sign of withdrawal. Early signs include restlessness, anxiety, sense of ill ease. Late signs include obsessive compulsive–like behaviors (with benzodiazepines) and poorly formed hallucinations
Stimulants	An apathetic nonmelancholic "atypical" depression ("the crash"), hypersomnia increased appetite (particularly for carbohydrates and sweets), attention and concentration problems, poorly formed hallucinations irritability, and delusional mood
Opioids/opiates	Restlessness, abdominal cramps and diarrhea, muscle cramps and spasms, tearfulness, rhinorrhea, headache, piloerection, poorly formed hallucinations, and irritability

of these signs, and the more classic manic features a patient has, the better the prognosis.

Patients at greatest risk for recurrent drug-induced psychoses are those (1) who used inhalants or hallucinogens, (2) whose drug use onset began before or during puberty, (3) who used multiple drugs in large doses for long periods of time, (4) who had a "bad trip" or prolonged hallucinosis during an acute intoxication, (5) with co-morbid head injury, (6) with a predrug abnormal personality (e.g., schizotypal) or psychiatric disorder (e.g., depressive illness), and (7) with a family history of mood disorder. Among the relatives of patients with a chronic drug-induced psychosis, the morbid risk for mood disorder is three to four times that of the general population.

Patients who used stimulants heavily and for long periods may also have motor and attentional problems. They are distractible, continuously scan their environment, are fearful, and move in a jerky, bird-like manner. Stereotypes are common (e.g., automatic, repetitive movements such as constantly touching one's face, automatically patting the surface of furniture).

Patients who used heavy doses of cannabis for long periods of time may become apathetic and avolitional. They may have poor pulmonary function from chronic cannabis smoking.

Patients who used hallucinogens are often avolitional and, when psychotic, very emotional (irritable, mania-like). They may express fantastic confabulations and ideas (e.g, machines around the earth, flying in a spaceship) and formal thought disorder superimposed on flight-of-ideas. Delusions are usually persecutory or grandiose. These patients may also be violent.

Epilepsy

Any form of epilepsy can cause psychosis (see Chapter 10 for more details). Those epileptics most likely to become psychotic are those who (1) developed their seizure disorder during puberty, (2) have more than one type of seizure, (3) have complex partial epilepsy, and (4) have a temporal lobe seizure focus. Psychosis can occur during the days or weeks prior to a fit (usually grand mal), several days after a fit (also usually grand mal), during and immediately after a fit and lasting for days or weeks (usually partial complex), and between seizures (all forms, but usually after 5–10 years of seizure disorder).

Epileptic psychosis can be of any type. Acute onset, short duration, great emotionality, multiple perceptual disturbances, and psychosensory features are common threads. When it occurs before the fit, irritability and moodiness are common. When it occurs during the fit and is an extension of it (as in status), some alteration of consciousness or attention (oneiroid or stuporous states), catatonic features, or delirium can occur. When interictal, positive symptom nonaffective psychoses followed in frequency by atypical psychotic mood disorders are most likely.

Head Trauma/Stroke

Psychosis from head trauma is most likely when the lesion is frontal (producing an avolitional or disinhibited syndrome plus hallucinations and delusions) or is to the nondominant cerebral hemisphere, particularly temporoparietal (irritability and violence, or depression plus hallucinations and delusions).

Psychosis from stroke is most likely from multiple small strokes to frontotemporal and frontosubcortical loop circuits. Large strokes cause psychosis when they are parietal (unilateral or bilateral) or temporal (usually bilateral). These psychoses do not neatly fit into DSM categories. Unilateral parietal lobe lesions can cause neglect syndromes and unilateral catatonia contralateral to the lesion.

Dementia/Basal Ganglia and Other Neurologic Disease

There is no characteristic psychosis associated with dementia. Although Alzheimer's disease is the most common dementia, vascular dementias with their multiple focal lesions are more likely to produce psychosis. These psychoses are similar to those seen in patients with individual strokes. Pick's disease, with its frontal, temporal, parietal progression is associated with a psychosis that resembles schizophrenia (see below). Dementias due to basal ganglia disease are associated with mood disorder, and occasionally hallucinations and delusions, so that these dementias are associated with behavior that resembles psychotic mood disorder or schizoaffective disorder.

Syphilis that involves frontal brain structures is associated with a chronic manic-like illness characterized by fantastic and other grandiose delusions, expansiveness, and delusions of persecution.

Space-occupying lesions (tumors, hemorrhage, vascular malformations, cysts) can cause psychosis depending on their location, size, and rapidity of growth.

General medical conditions that can affect the brain (e.g., diabetes, chronic obstructive pulmonary disease) can produce psychosis. Most of these are atypical and do not clearly fit into standard DSM categories.

DSM Psychotic Disorders: Schizophrenia

Although the "flagship" psychiatric disease for decades, schizophrenia is relatively uncommon. Less than 4% of acute admissions to general hospital psychiatric units meet DSM criteria for it. Among chronic patients the numbers are higher, but mood disorder is still more common among chronic patients unless you consider schizoaffective disorder a subtype of schizophrenia. About 0.5% of the general population is at lifetime risk for schizophrenia, and the incidence may be lessening, perhaps due to better prenatal and infant health care. Among first-degree relatives of schizophrenics the risk for schizophrenia is about 5%. Schizophrenia is familial. Twin concordance rates (40%–50% for monozygotic, 5%–10% for dizygotic) and other data indicate that it is highly heritable. Table 9.5 lists the

TABLE 9.5. Classic Features of Schizophrenia*

Perceptual disturbances (100%)	Auditory hallucinations (voices), illusions, perceptual distortions
Delusions (30%–40%)	Usually persecutory, both primary and secondary to perceptual disturbances and first-rank symptoms
First-rank symptoms (65%–75%)	In addition to complete auditory hallucinations, (most common), they include experiences of alienation and control, thought broadcasting, delusional perception
Speech and language disturbances (40%)	Paucity of speech and thought, disorganized speech (formal thought disorder that resembles subcortical aphasia); speech can be manneristic or stilted
Emotional blunting (80%)	Avolition and loss of emotional expression (also seen in milder forms in non-ill first-degree relatives); abnormal social behaviors (collecting garbage, hoarding food, talking to self in public, lying on hospital floor), dirty, disheveled, and unkempt
Motor disturbances (30%–50%)	*Frontal circuit* (adventitious overflow, impersistence, poor sequencing, poor eye tracking, perseveration, motor inertia [difficulty starting and stopping], stereotypies such as rubbing head or twisting hair), and *cerebellar* (dyssynchrony, past-pointing, poor coordination,); *eye tracking problems* (sluggish or jerky persuit) also seen in non-ill first-degree relatives and may be a marker for risk
Cognitive disturbances (80%–100%)	Poor sustained attention and working memory, difficulty changing sets, problems with new learning, problems with word finding, thinking, and executive functions

*Numbers in parentheses are percentages of patients with those features.

classic features of schizophrenia. In the DSM, schizophreniform disorder is linked to schizophrenia, but is defined as being of less severity with less loss of function and of shorter duration (<6 months). In clinical practice, this distinction is meaningless, and the DSM version of schizophreniform is ignored or considered a milder form of schizophrenia.

Subtype schema for schizophrenia have limited clinical usefulness. The DSM subtypes paranoid, catatonic, undifferentiated overlap, making discrimination difficult. The same is true for the positive–negative symptom and the paranoid–nonparanoid dichotomies. For example, patients characterized as nonparanoid often have persecutory delusions (i.e., they are "paranoid"), and patients with negative symptoms often also have positive symptoms (i.e., hallucinations and delusions). Positive symptoms or persecutory delusions are not clinically helpful in predicting prognosis, treatment response, or biological markers, whereas the degree of emotional blunting and mood disorder features do predict these factors. A general clinical rule is, once you decide a patient is psychotic, the more negative features and the fewer mood disorder features, the worse the prognosis. The reverse is also generally true. Patients who satisfy diagnostic criteria for schizophrenia will usually be those with no or minimal mood disorder features. Further dividing schizophrenics into those with and without significant negative features is probably more useful than the present DSM subtyping system.

Schizophrenics have brain disease. Table 9.6 summarizes the evidence for this. In addition, schizophrenics have more "minor" physical anomalies than expected. These are nonlife-threatening, nondysfunctional body abnormalities indicating some developmental insult. They include low-set ears, wide-set eyes, and abnormal hair swirls. Increased visibility of nailfold capillary plexi is also found in some schizophrenics and may also indicate susceptibility to the disorder.

The psychoses of schizophrenia begin in the late teens and early twenties. The disorder, however, is probably present at birth in most patients. As a group, children at risk for schizophrenia (i.e., they have an ill parent) who also have histories of gestational, labor, or delivery problems, maternal exposure to influenza, or other maternal health and pregnancy problems are at great risk for psychosis. Persons who become psychotic have childhood problems with sustained attention and working memory, frontal and cerebellar motor problems, delayed motor landmarks, low IQs, and a tendency to be emotionally aloof and irritable. The more severe the prenatal difficulty the more severe are these childhood problems. The more severe these childhood problems, the more likely the person will become psychotic and the psychosis will be chronic.

Childhood-onset schizophrenia psychosis is rare (modal age around 10 years), and most persons with this diagnosis are found to have other conditions (e.g., mood disorder, Asperger's disorder). Children with schizophrenia are likely to have high rates of family illness (particularly schizotypal [10%], mood disorder [20%–25%], and, in boys, *isolated* features of pervasive developmental disorder [(e.g., stereotypies, odd speech and speech delay, arm flapping, disturbances in social behavior such as poor eye contact and no interest in peers, slow in developmental milestones, and low IQ—30% are in special education programs and 50%

TABLE 9.6. Brain Disease Findings in Schizophrenia

Areas	Findings
Brain structure (CT, MRI)	1. 40%–50% of patients have ventricular enlargement from thinned cortex and subcortical structures (e.g., thalamus); cerebellar vermal atrophy and third ventricle enlargement in 30% of patients; widespread cerebral gray matter volume deficits, basal ganglia sclerosis in some patients, thalamic and surrounding white matter changes
	2. The greater the structural changes, the worse the cognitive dysfunction and likelihood of chronicity
	3. Larger lateral and third ventricle changes seem to be in nonfamilial forms; smaller head size and cerebral areas (bitemporal/cerebellar) seem to occur more commonly in familial forms
Brain metabolism (PET, CBF)*	Frontal hypometabolism at rest and when doing frontal lobe tasks (40%–50% of patients); thalamic, cerebellar, and posterior cingulate hypermetabolism
Brain information processing	
EEG	40%–50% of patients have reduced alpha at rest posteriorly plus increased slow waves centrally and frontally
EP†	Delayed waveforms, particularly P300 (a cortical wave); reduced amplitude and distorted waves in visual, auditory, and somatosensory systems
Cognition	50%–75% of patients have moderate to severe (in the demented range) impairment on standard clinical neuropsychological tests; impairment pattern is bilateral frontotemporal and dominant hemisphere; low IQ scores
Neurotransmitter	D_1 receptors reduced prefrontally related to avolition and poor cognitive performance; reduced cortical glutamate activity and increased midbrain dopaminergic activity

*CBF, cerebral blood flow
†EP, evoked potentials.

repeat grades]). These children may have co-morbid ADHD, but differ from primary ADHD children in the other features described above, plus having abnormal MRI findings (small brain size due to gray matter reduction, increased ventricular size, and small thalamus). The smaller the thalamus, the earlier the onset of schizophrenia and the more chronic the course.

The first episode of psychosis in schizophrenia, however, typically begins within the decade after the beginning of puberty. For the patient who develops a schizophrenia-like psychosis after age 35–40 years, consider other diagnoses first. This so-called "late-onset schizophrenia" is a diagnosis to avoid. These patients are more often women (2:1) with mild cognitive changes (executive functions), no or little emotional blunting, and no clear structural brain changes. They are more likely to commit suicide. Think of mood disorder first and then secondary conditions. If neither of these applies, think of positive symptom nonaffective psychosis (described below) and treat for that.

Also consider other diagnoses than schizophrenia if the patient (1) has been or is married with children (particularly if a man*), (2) has no loss of emotional expression, and (3) has none of the findings listed in Table 9.6. Consider secondary schizophrenia whenever you can identify an event (e.g., head trauma) or condition (e.g., drug abuse, epilepsy) that predates the patient's schizophrenic features and is known to cause brain dysfunction. Schizophrenia is a last resort diagnosis. Giving the patient another diagnosis can (1) lead to specific treatments (e.g., an anticonvulsant for epilepsy), (2) justify not using a neuroleptic (thus preventing tardive dyskinesia), and (3) justify a better prognosis and more specific management strategies (e.g., cognitive rehabilitation for head trauma).

Eighty to 90% of schizophrenics become chronically ill, and all have some permanent decrement in functioning. Most of the loss of function occurs during the 3–5 years after the first psychosis, but many schizophrenics have cognitive difficulties from childhood. Hallucinations and delusions diminish in intensity and frequency over the years and many chronic schizophrenics ill for decades are primarily emotionally blunted and virtually demented (a frontal lobe pattern; see Chapter 12), and have only brief periods when they are acutely psychotic. Men become ill earlier than women, are more chronic, and have more structural brain changes. Women schizophrenics are more likely to be irritable and have a family history of schizophrenia. The lower morbidity risk among the relatives of male schizophrenics is explained by there being more phenocopies among male patients. A phenocopy is a biologic characteristic similar to the characteristic expression of a genotype (termed a *phenotype)* but that is due to environmental (e.g., head trauma, drugs) rather than direct genetic causes (e.g., Huntington's disease).

Think of schizophrenia as a developmental disorder: gestational problems in a genetically vulnerable individual triggering problems in neural development (e.g., abnormal cell migration and pruning). The genes involved seem to be multiple, each with a small additive effect. The vulnerability is probably not for the psychosis but to biological stressors in neural development (e.g., nutrition, exposure to toxins such as alcohol and nicotine, viral infection, mechanical stress, and anoxia during delivery). Because neural development continues for decades (myelinization is not completed until the late twenties or early thirties; cell and dendritic pruning and dendritic and synaptic formation continue throughout life), childhood and adolescent events (head trauma, viral infection, street drug use) can also push a genetically vulnerable person over the threshold of illness. Schizophrenia may also be a disease of the industrial revolution, as descriptions of it are rare before that time, whereas descriptions of other disorders (e.g., mania, depression) are common.

---

*Male schizophrenics have a fertility rate 10% of expected; female schizophrenics have a fertility rate about 20% of expected.

In addition to the classic symptoms and course from childhood to late adult-hood both being consistent with a developmental disorder, other evidence for schizophrenia being a developmental disorder include 1) converging data from brain function studies that suggest that schizophrenics have action brain system dysfunction (most susceptible to developmental and gestational adverse events); (2) the motor signs and minor physical anomalies seen in schizophrenics and children at risk for it; (3) the increased prevalence of gestational and developmental adverse events in persons who become schizophrenic; and (4) cytoarchitectural changes in action brain areas of schizophrenics showing reduced number of cells, ectopic cells, and no gliosis (gliosis is expected after brain injury unless the injury occurs during fetal life). Table 9.7 lists the developmental phases of schizophrenia.

The developmental model of schizophrenia has practical clinical importance. It suggests that prevention and rehabilitation should reduce the incidence of the disorder and the degree and prevalence of its consequences. For example, for pregnant women with a personal or family history of psychosis, make every effort to provide the needed prenatal care to minimize risk situations. That is primary prevention. At birth, an infant at risk should be assessed for the markers of future problems. Young children at risk should also be assessed. If they are free of these, nothing needs to be done. If they have postnatal and childhood markers, they need motor, cognitive, and behavioral rehabilitation, and their parents may need counseling, treatment for expressed emotion (see below), and help with parent-ing skills. When similar programs are provided for children with autism or As-parger's disease, improvement in levels of functioning can be dramatic. This is secondary prevention and may prevent future psychosis. In the decade following puberty it is also important to look for the earliest signs of psychosis so that im-mediate and vigorous treatment can begin. Because the major part of cognitive decline occurs within a few years following the first psychosis, vigorous treat-ment and rehabilitation may minimize long-term dysfunction. This is tertiary prevention.

Psychotic Disorder: Delusional Disorder

Delusional disorder is uncommon (<0.03% of the population). It is character-ized by the patient endorsing an organized delusional story in the absence of other psychopathology. The delusional story is typically mundane, about love, jealousy, corporate or city corruption, rather than strange or fantastic. Patients with delusional disorder have minimal emotional blunting, no speech and lan-guage disorder, and no history of bipolar mood disorder. Nonmelancholic major depression can sometimes occur during an episode, but these depressions are usually mild and of short duration. Delusional disorder appears unrelated to mood disorder or schizophrenia. Onset is usually after age 30 years. Men and women are equally at risk, and more than half are married at the time of onset. Twenty-five to 40% become chronically ill.

Some delusional disorder patients can trace their delusional ideas to experi-ences that turn out to be misperceptions and misidentifications. These patients may have mild to modest visuospatial deficits. Family members may be at greater

TABLE 9.7. Phases of Schizophrenia

Prenatal*	Perinatal*	Childhood	Psychosis	Illness Course
1. Second trimester adverse event, viral infection (influenza, rubella)	1. Low Apgar scores	1. Delayed walking and speech onset	1. Onset within decade of puberty onset	1. Further cognitive decline for several years
2. Gestation <37 weeks	2. Neonatal convulsions	2. Low IQ	2. Atypical, apathetic, psychotic depression may be first episode	2. Slow reduction in frequency and intensity of positive symptoms
3. Bleeding	3. Low blood oxygen	3. Neuromotor frontal or cerebellar signs	3. Typically nonaffective psychosis with loss of emotional expression and avolition a. Avolitional frontal lobe syndrome b. Motor aprosodia c. Perceptual disturbances	3. Negative symptoms predominate
4. Genetic vulnerability to the above	4. Difficult labor and delivery	4. Emotional aloofness, irritability, and sensitivity to criticism		
	5. CNS infection (viral) in infancy	5. Sustained attention and working memory problems		
	6. Birth weight <2,500 g	6. Head injury and drug abuse increase risk		
	7. Premature rupture of membranes	7. Small thalamic volume and ventricular enlargement		
	8. History of incubation or resuscitation			
	9. Genetic vulnerability to the above			

*Placental insufficiency, hypoxic events, and viral or nutritional adverse effects on neural development in a genetically vulnerable person appears to be the big risk pattern.

than expected risk for paranoid personality disorder, but there is no increased family risk for schizophrenia or mood disorder.

(Non-DSM Psychoses (Labeled NOS or Atypical): Positive-Symptom Nonaffective Psychosis

Some patients periodically become psychotic, although they retain emotional expression and have no past or present evidence of a mood disorder. They rarely have speech and language problems, they have only mild cognitive impairment that resolves with the psychosis, and between episodes they seem to function better than schizophrenics. The durations of episodes vary, some less than 6 months (filling the schizophreniform criterion) and some more than 6 months.

Over the decades many terms have been used to try to characterize these patients (e.g., *cycloid psychosis* when associated with anxiety; *reactive psychosis* when preceded by a stressful event that seems connected to the content of the psychotic features; *brief reactive psychosis* when less than 1 month; and *schizophreniform psychosis* [European version] when associated with a normal premorbid personality, substantial emotionality during the psychosis, and a relatively good outcome). The reason for not labeling these patients schizophrenic is to avoid the initial use of neuroleptics. Many of these psychoses are secondary; therefore, carefully hunt for the cause that may respond to more specific treatment. Table 9.8 lists some of the many possibilities to consider.

Non-DSM Psychoses

Kraepelin described paraphrenia as a psychosis that develops after age 30 and more often after age 60, with no emotional blunting, formal thought disorder, or progression to dementia. He considered it unrelated to schizophrenia. It has been subtyped into delusional, depressive, phonemic, and late (after age 60) paraphrenia. Phonemic paraphrenia is a condition in which the patient hears voices, but has little other psychopathology and is aware that the hallucinations are symptoms of illness. Delusional disorder was also considered a paraphrenia before it was incorporated into the DSM. The implications of paraphrenia are the same as those for the positive-symptom nonaffective psychoses.

TREATMENTS AND MANAGEMENT

Acute Treatment

Hospitalization is needed for psychosis if the patient is dangerous, suicidal, unable to function, or doing things that will cause job or family disruption if not stopped. Sometimes these patients are hospitalized because of an inadequate response to treatment and the need to reevaluate therapy or because of a change in treatment that requires close monitoring of side effects.

The acute management of psychotic excitement is discussed in Chapter 8.

TABLE 9.8. Possible Causes of Secondary Positive Symptom Nonaffective Psychoses and the Paraphrenias

---

Many prescribed and some over-the-counter drugs (particular culptrits are disulfiram, cimetidine, digitalis, bromides)

Frontosubcortical circuit neuronal or white matter infarctions

Small frontotemporal vascular malformation

Frontal lobe pole meningioma

Seizure disorder with frontal lobe, parietal lobe, temporal lobe (left > right) focus

Head trauma localized to the tips of the frontal or temporal lobes

Herpes or other viruses with an affinity to the temporal lobes (look for bilateral EEG slowing with sharp waves)

Brain damage from drug abuse (particularly with inhalants)

Thyroid disease (hyperthyroidism, particularly)

Third ventricle cysts

Cerebellar disease

Normal pressure hydrocephalus

Sela tursica masses

Sickle cell disease

Tuberculosis

Syphilis

Metal toxicity (mercury, arsenic, manganese, thallium)

When lives and limbs are not in danger, always diagnose first before treating. Do not automatically prescribe a neuroleptic. Indeed, make neuroleptics your last, not your first, resort.

Steps to consider are

1. If you can identify a specific cause for the psychosis and there is a specific treatment for it, give that treatment (see Table 9.9). See other chapters for more details.
2. If you cannot identify a specific cause or there is no specific treatment, try to match the syndrome to one of the idiopathic or specific secondary syndromes and treat for that. Thus, if the psychosis best fits mania, treat for bipolar disorder. If the psychosis best fits epilepsy, treat for that.
3. If you cannot identify the specific cause or match the syndrome, determine if the patient meets sufficient indicators for ECT (see Chapter 7); if so, give ECT.

4. If none of the above steps pertains, determine if the psychotic features are so disruptive that treatment is still necessary. If so, consider a neuroleptic following the guidelines in Table 9.10. Note that only a few neuroleptics are identified as models. There is no reason to use all of the drugs on the market. Learn a few medications very well rather than many superficially.

Once you have done all assessments and have begun treatment, it is in the patient's best interest not to dwell on his psychotic experiences and symptoms. Respectfully let the patient know you now want to focus your attention not on the illness, but on the patient, on his strengths and weaknesses, his rehabilitation and response to treatment, and his plans when he leaves the hospital. Talking with the patient about his real-life problems and their potential solutions is far more productive than rehashing delusions and hallucinations. A patient who insists on talking about psychotic themes is still actively ill.

Stress that participating in ward activities, going for cognitive and vocational rehabilitation, and repairing any family or job damage are as important as taking medication or ECT.

Consider ECT for a neuroleptic treatment–resistant schizophrenic, particularly if the patient is not emotionally blunted. Treatment resistance is a minimal response after 4 weeks of steady-state, maximum dose treatment of two neuroleptic trials, one with an atypical and one with a high potency typical. The addition of lithium to the neuroleptic will also benefit a small percentage of schizophrenics despite the absence of mood disorder features. However, the use of anticonvulsants has not been found to benefit such patients.

All psychotic patients have brain dysfunction. Consider them analogous to persons who have suffered a traumatic brain injury. When their psychopathology is mostly resolved, assess their cognitive strengths and weaknesses and provide adequate rehabilitation (see below and Chapter 5). Educate both the family and patient about the patient's illness and treatments. Help them plan for discharge and further treatment, rehabilitation, and resolution of family, housing, financial, and job problems. Patient and family support groups are helpful, and ally yourself with these organizations.

Long-Term Management

Maintenance treatment is usually needed following an acute psychotic episode. For patients in full remission, 3–6 months of maintenance pharmacotherapy or ECT are necessary to prevent relapse. For schizophrenics, patients with delusional disorder or paraphrenia, up to 12 months of maintenance therapy is typically needed to prevent relapse. Longer prophylactic treatment, which may be for a lifetime, is usually needed for patients with (1) more than one episode; (2) cognitive impairment following resolution of most or all symptoms; (3) avolition, emotional blunting, or formal thought disorder during the acute episode; and (4) poor premorbid or interepisode social and job functioning but without acute symptoms

TABLE 9.9. Some Treatments for Specific Psychotic Conditions

Condition	Suggested Treatments
LSD intoxication	In the emergency room
	1. Calm, quiet setting; reassuring, nonthreatening staff
	2. intermediate-acting benzodiazepine (lorazepam 1–2 mg) for agitation not controlled by supportive measures
	3. If hallucinosis persists beyond 1–2 hours, or is intense, give a single dose of risperidone 1–2 mg or a single intramusclar dose of a low potency neuroleptic, e.g., chlorpromazine 25–50 mg, to avoid acute dystonia in young men who are typical LSD users
	On admission to hospital
	ECT, VP, or CBZ if hallucinosis persists past 48 hours; if VP or CBZ is used, a neuroleptic may also be needed. With bilateral ECT, no other augmentation is usually needed
Phencyclidine	1. Restraints if violent
	2. ECT, VP, or high potency neuroleptic (low potency would need higher doses and have too many anticholinergic properties)
	3. Acidify urine to aid excretion (ammonium chloride 4–8 g daily)
	4. Beta-blockers or clonidine for sympathetic hyperarousal
Cocaine	In the emergency room
	1. Calm, quite setting, reassuring staff

Haloperidol (50 mg/ml) and fluphenazine (25 mg/ml) are also available in long-acting (depot), intramuscular form. You can give these forms every 2–3 weeks to noncompliant patients who have previously been successfully treated with an oral neuroleptic. The administration of the long-acting intramuscular form should overlap with oral administration, which is then tapered and discontinued, leaving the patient on the maintenance dose (0.5–1 ml of haloperidol or 1–2 ml of fluphenazine or higher). Many patients will develop significant extrapyramidal side effects unless doses for the long-acting forms are gradually increased. The risk for tardive dyskinesia is also greater among patients receiving prolonged treatment with the long-acting preparations. They are the preparations of last resort. Do not use until all other methods have failed for increasing compliance (e.g., using single, bedtime doses; having family members or other caregivers monitor compliance or administer medication; using behavior modification techniques to reward compliance). Long-acting preparations

TABLE 9.9. (*continued*)

Condition	Suggested Treatments
	2. Intermediate-acting benzodiazepine (lorazepam 1–2 mg)
	On admission to hospital
	1. Treat "crash" behaviorally as above, bupropion if antidepressant needed
	2. For psychosis, ECT, CBZ, neuroleptic
	3. Beta-blockers or clonidine for sympathetic hyperarousal
	4. Acidify urine to aid excretion
DTs	1. Long-acting benzodiazepines (diazepam or chlordiazepoxide titrated to produce mild sedation)
	2. Thiamine and multivitamins; if intravenous fluid needed, avoid glucose because thiamine is a cofactor in glucose metabolism and the glucose load will deplete thiamine, perhaps causing a Wernicke's encephalopathy
Epilepsy	ECT, VP, CBZ
Head trauma or stroke	1. Avoid psychotropics if possible during acute phase
	2. Use risperidone for nonaffective positive symptom psychosis if CBZ does not work; use CBZ or VP for mood syndromes
Secondary causes listed in Table 9.6	1. Specific treatments, ECT, VP, CBZ, "atypical" neuroleptic if patient not violent or excited
	2. High potency neuroleptic if patient is violent
Mood disorders	See Chapters 7 and 8

provide no therapeutic flexibility and are inappropriate for the treatment of acute episodes.

Assess all patients at the end of their acute episode for their cognitive strengths and weaknesses and their personality patterns. If cognitive deficits are substantial, cognitive rehabilitation is essential to minimize later chronicity. Rehabilitation typically focus on (1) motor skills, (2) cognitive flexibility, (3) attention, and (4) new learning. Practicing these abilities by doing cognitive or neuropsychological tests, playing video games and motor skills games, and performing specific job-related skills may improve performance to within normal levels and prevent or reduce long-term decline. Avolitional or poorly motivated patients need specific reinforcers to keep them progressing, and all patients need tasks and instructions explained in great detail to help them assimilate the information and use it. Personality assessment is necessary to guide psychotherapy (see Chapters 5 and 6).

Always assess the patient's family or living situation for expressed emotion

TABLE 9.10. Guidelines for Choosing a Neuroleptic as the Last Resort

Situation	Suggested Choice
Excited, violent, severe psychotic state	High potency (haloperidol the model)
Positive symptom nonaffective state	High potency (haloperidol the model)
Schizophrenia	"Atypical" neuroleptic (olanzapine the model) or low potency neuroleptic (chlorpromazine the model)
Tardive dyskinesia with psychosis that is not associated with violence or excitement	"Atypical" neuroleptic (risperidone the model, but in daily doses of < 8 mg)
Dementia with psychosis	"Atypical" neuroleptic (risperidone the model)

(EE). Although described initially as a factor in the relapse rates for schizophrenia, EE affects all seriously ill psychiatric patients. The higher the EE in the patient's environment, the greater the chance for relapse. High EE refers to (1) frequent expressions of hostility, (2) often making critical comments, (3) being overly involved in the patient's daily activities and overcontrolling on large issues, and (4) often and intensely expressing both positive and negative emotions. High EE by hospital, clinic, and office staff also contributes to relapse.

Reducing EE reduces relapse rates by 50%. Education, counseling, and role playing with the patient and significant persons in the patient's hospital and placement environments are needed. Typical family- and crisis-oriented therapies that rely on "getting things out in the open" often result in high EE episodes and are counterproductive for these patients.

NEUROLEPTICS

Pharmacodynamics

Neuroleptics are drugs that in therapeutic doses tranquilize without sedating. The therapeutic effect of traditional neuroleptics is believed due to dopamine (DA) receptor blockade in the mesolimbic system. They also affect DA receptors D_1 to D_5 in the mesolimbic, nigrostriatal, and tuberoinfundibular systems. Neuroleptics also have alpha-adrenergic–blocking, anticholinergic, antihistaminic, and antiemetic properties, and some neuroleptics have calcium channel–blocking properties.

D_2 nigrostriatal and tubolofundibular blockade results in extrapyramidal (increased tone, tremor, bradykinesia) and endocrine (increased prolactin release, galactorrhea, amenorrhea, pseudopregnancy) side effects, respectively. Anticholinergic properties result in dry mouth, mydriasis with sluggish accommodation, reduce gastrointestinal tract motility, and urinary retention (men with benign prostatic hypertrophy)). Alpha-adrenergic effects cause sedation, weight gain, and postural hypotension. All the above neurotransmitter effects play a role in the sexual dysfunction associated with neuroleptic administration.

Pharmacokinetics

Neuroleptics are absorbed well and rapidly from the stomach, with peak plasma levels reached in 1–4 hours; half-lives are 10–30 hours, an once-a-day dosing at night is preferred. Steady state is reached in 3–5 days. All neuroleptics undergo "first-pass" metabolism in the enterohepatic circulation and are further metabolized in the liver through conjugation, hydroxylation, oxidation, demethylation, and sulfuride formation. Metabolites are complex and highly lipophilic. Ninety percent is protein bound, but twice as much drug is stored in skin, fat, lung, and brain. Most of any given dose is excreted in a metabolized form in the feces and urine. Table 9.11 lists the traditional neuroleptics and some of their characteristics.

Haloperidol is an all around neuroleptic and the high potency drug of choice. A second high potency choice is fluphenazine.* Chlorpromazine is the low potency drug of choice, although it is rarely used. There is no advantage in using any of the other agents with the exception of pimozide for several nonpsychotic conditions (e.g., Gilles de la Tourette's syndrome).

There are three widely used atypical neuroleptics: risperidone, clozapine, and olanzapine. These agents are termed *atypical* because at low and moderate doses they have more selective mesolimbic D_2 affinity than the older neuroleptics and they have serotonin receptor affinity (usually greater than their D_2 affinity). Clozapine and olanzapine are benzodiazepine derivatives. The atypical neuroleptics have two advantages: In moderate doses they have little extrapyramidal side effects and thus theoretically less risk for tardive dyskinesia, and clozapine and olanzapine may improve emotional blunting better than other neuroleptics.

Olanzapine (Zyprexa) (10–20 mg daily typical, but you can prescribe up to 40) is recommended† for young, first or second episode schizophrenics because it works as well as the other atypicals (perhaps better than risperidone for acute psychosis because you can prescribe higher doses without causing extrapyramidal side effects), improves negative symptoms, has a low risk for tardive diskinesia and extrapyramidal side effects, has less severe anticholinergic side effects (clozapine has many), and has none of the lethal effects of clozapine (e.g., sudden hypotension and death, agranulocytosis). In addition, benzodiazepines cannot be given with clozapine because of the increased risk for hypotension and death with that combination, so that controlling agitation or irritability during the

---

*About 50% of patients with neuroleptic malignant syndrome (NMS) received haloperidol, and thus some clinicians believe that haloperidol holds a greater NMS risk than other high potency neuroleptics. However, it is more likely that the relationship between the drug and NMS is due to its high frequency of use compared with other neuroleptics for acutely hospitalized excited psychotic patients. Fluphenazine is the only other neuroleptic available in all forms of administration.

†Comparison studies with haloperidol used relatively low doses of haloperidol; thus overall response to olanzapine is probably not better than to haloperidol, but its use has less of a risk for tardive diskinesia.

TABLE 9.11. Traditional Neuroleptics

Class/Subclass	D2 Nigrostriatal Tubulofundibular	Anticholinergic	Alpha-Adrenergic	Daily Dose (mg)	Comments
Phenothiazine					
Aliphatic					
Chlorpromazine (Thorazine)	Modest	Moderate	Substantial	400–800	Low potency drug of choice
Piperazine					
Fluphenazine (Prolixin)	Substantial	Modest	Modest	20–80	High potency depot and intramusclar forms available; depot form has limited role for chronic patients who are noncompliers
Trifluoperazine (Stelazine)	Substantial	Modest	Modest	10–60	High potency; not recommended
Piperidine					
Thioridazine (Mellaril)	Weak	Substantial	Substantial	200–600	Low potency; risk of retinitis pigmentosa at doses >600 mg; not recommended
Thioxanthenes					
Aliphatic					
Chlorprothixene (Taractan)	Modest	Moderate	Substantial	400–600	Low potency; no advantage over chlorpromazine

				Dosage (mg)	Comments
Piperazine					
Thiothixene (Navane)	Substantial	Modest	Modest	20–80	High potency; no advantage over fluphenazine
Butyrophenone					
Haloperidol (Haldol)	Substantial	Modest	Modest	20–80	High potency drug of choice; intramuscular, intravenous, and depot forms best for excitement states
Diphenylbutylpiperidine					
Pimozide (Orap)	Modest	Weak	Weak	10–30	High potency; not good for psychosis except for delusional disorder; also used for Gilles de la Tourette's syndrome, trigeminal neuralgia; has some calcium channel blockade so get EKG before using; has long half-life, 55–150 hours, and can be given every other day
Dihydroindolamine					
Molindone (Moban)	Modest	Modest	Weak	20–200	Less likely to reduce seizure threshold
Dibenzoxazepine					
Loxapine (Loxitane)	Modest	Modest	Modest	60–100	No advantage

first several weeks of treatment with clozapine may require substantial doses of other sedating drugs (e.g., diphenhydramine). A benzodiazepine to control agitation during the first few weeks of olanzapine treatment is safe. Do not, however, prescribe olanzapine for patients with a history of excitement or disinhibition. It will often make them worse. Olanzapine has substantial anticholinergic, moderate alpha-adrenergic, and serotonin receptor affinity. It is a weak D_1 and a modest D_2 blocker. Initial side effects are similar to those with chlorpromazine: dizziness (10%), somnolence (25%), constipation (10%), orthostasis (5%), weight gain (5%–10%), and small liver enzyme changes (common but clinically insignificant).

Because *risperidone* (Risperdal) presently has no intramuscular form and, above 8 mg, similar extrapyramidal side effects as other neuroleptics,* it is recommended at lower doses in conjunction with an antidepressant for psychotic depression and for nonagitated psychoses in elderly patients. Risperidone has substantial alpha-adrenergic and serotonin receptor affinity. It has only weak anticholinergic properties and thus is reasonably tolerated by older patients. Its D_2 mesolimbic blockade is greater than the other atypicals, whereas its D_2 nigrostriatal/tubulofundibular blockade is about the same as other atypicals.

Clozapine (Clozaril) is the drug of last resort. Clozapine has substantial anticholinergic and alpha-adrenergic properties. Its D_2 mesolimbic and serotonin receptor blockade is moderate; its D_2 nigrostriatal/tubulofundibular and D_1 blockade are weak. Its peak plasma level is 1–4 hours after ingestion, first-pass and liver metabolism include demethylation and oxidation, 94% is protein bound, and its half-life is about 16 hours. Dosing usually begins at 25–50 mg on day 1 and is increased by 50–100 every 3–7 days to a maximum of 900 mg. Weekly expensive blood counts are needed to monitor early signs of agranulocytosis. Common side effects are hypotension, dizziness, constipation, fatigue, weight gain, and dose-related seizures. Sialorrhea causing nausea, sedation, and tachycardia can, with care, be treated with a peripheral beta-blocker such as atenolol.

Additional atypical neuroleptics are coming on the market. They will get shelf space, but they are not more effective or safer than presently used neuroleptics. *Quetiapine* (Seroquel) is a dibenzothiazepine with atypical neuroleptic pharmacodynamics. Effective doses are above 250 mg daily (750 mg typical maximum), and common side effects include headache, agitation, and hypotension. Quetiapine has a half-life of only several hours and, thus, must be given three times a day. There is no advantage in using it.

Sertindole, another new atypical neuroleptic, has mesolimbic D_2, 5-HT_2, and alpha-, and noradrenergic receptor selectivity. Therapeutic doses are about 20 mg daily. Its half-life is 1–4 days. Sertindole is a more potent 5-HT_2 antagonist than olanzapine or clozapine. Side effects include hypotension and dizziness, nasal congestion, mild peripheral edema, reduced ejaculatory volume, and perhaps an increased risk for cardiac death. There is no compelling advantage in using it.

---

*Most clinicians prescribing risperidone report that the rare patient will have these side effects even at very low doses.

Management of Side Effects

Most neuroleptic side effects resolve when the drug is discontinued, but some (e.g., tardive dyskinesia) are permanent, and some (e.g., neuroleptic malignant syndrome) [NMS] are life threatening. Prescribe a neuroleptic only when there is no other treatment choice. Compared with low potency neuroleptics, high potency neuroleptics have more frequent and severe extrapyramidal side effects and less frequent and less severe anticholinergic, sedative, and postural hypotensive side effects. Table 9.12 summarizes neuroleptic side effects and their management. Table 9.13 summarizes drugs used to treat neuroleptic extrapyramidal side effects.

Most patients treated with a neuroleptic for an acute psychosis become drowsy with each dose increase until a stable dose and its steady state are reached. Anticholinergic side effects are common with low potency neuroleptics and with clozapine and olanzapine. In younger, otherwise healthy patients, most of these are tolerable and require education and reassurance only. Sometimes they can be specifically managed as described in Table 9.12. In the elderly, or persons with general medical illness (e.g., cardiovascular disease), they can produce delirium and dementia-like syndromes.

Except when prescribing depot neuroleptics, do not prescribe one of the antiparkinsonians until symptoms develop. About 30%–40% of patients (taking high potency more than low, traditional more than atypical neuroleptics) will need one of these agents. After 3–4 months, however, taper and then discontinue the antiparkinsonian over a 6-week period. Only 30%–40% of patients need to be restarted or kept on the drug. Thus, among all patients who receive long-term neuroleptic treatment, only 10%–15% will need an antiparkinsonian longer than 4 months. Continued use of these agents increases the risk for tardive dyskinesia, so try to wean patients off them. Too rapid a reduction of drugs with anticholinergic properties can cause a cholinergic rebound (tearing, watery eyes, cramps and diarrhea, vomiting, sweating, and bradycardia). When discontinuing a neuroleptic, also taper it slowly (6–12 weeks). This is to avoid any anticholinergic rebound and to minimize relapse. If a patient who is being tapered off neuroleptics is also receiving an antiparkinsonian, first taper and discontinue the neuroleptic (longer half-life).

NMS is rare, but life threatening. One theory considers it an idiosyncratic response to dopamine (D_2) blockade. Another idea is that it is a variant of catatonia induced by the neuroleptic. Consistent with this is the impression that bipolar patients, 10%–20% of whom may have catatonic features, are also at particular risk for NMS. NMS also has all the features of lethal catatonia. In lethal catatonia postures may be more extreme and unusual, whereas in NMS the patient looks more parkinsonian. Both conditions are characterized by high fever (occurs early in lethal catatonia and late in NMS). Based on the idea that NMS is an idiosyncratic response to D_2 blockade, standard treatment consists of (1) controlling hyperthermia, (2) giving dantroline as a muscle relaxant, and (3) giving a dopamine agonist (e.g., bromocriptine, amantadine, levodopa, apomorphine). This regimen may take several days to work, and for many patients relief is only partial. Despite this

TABLE 9.12. Neuroleptic Side Effects and Their Management

Side Effect	Characteristics	Management
Extrapyramidal		
Dystonia	Most common in young patients; involuntary spasm or cramp-like contraction: torticollis, tongue contraction, opisthotonos, laryngospasm (rare)	Diphenhydramine 25–50 mg IM or IV or benztropine 2–4 mg IM or IV. IV works immediately; IM takes 20–40 min. Follow-up with antiparkinson agent
Tardive dystonia	Due to months or years of neuroleptic use. Same as for acute dystonia (see above).	Butulinum toxin (see text)
Parkinsonism	Bradykinesia (expressionless face, slow gait with small steps, tremor, cogwheel rigidity), micrographia, greasy skin, drooling, pill-rolling, common in women and in persons >35	1. Amantadine (an antivival dopaminergic antiparkinson agent) 100–300 mg per day 2. Benztropine 1–2 mg BID or TID
Rabbit syndrome	Rhythmic mouth tremor	Same as for parkinsonism
Acute dyskinesia	Choreoathetosis within days or weeks of starting treatment	Same as for parkinsonism
Akinesia	Reduced spontaneity of movement, gestures, and speech; resembles emotional blunting (causing misdiagnosis of schizophrenia); can be misdiagnosed as depression	Same as for parkinsonism
Akathisia	Onset usually within days or weeks: inner-restlessness with pacing or rocking; may lead to noncompliance, elopement, or suicide attempt; distinguishable from agitation in that akathisia patients (1) recently started neuroleptics (2) cannot usually give reason for restlessness, and (3) rock from foot to foot rather than just pace	Propranolol 20–80 mg per day, usually in two divided doses; benzodiazepines are effective, but cause dependence, buspirone (Buspar) in moderate doses
Tardive dyskinesia (TD)	Choreoathetoid movements of mouth, cheeks, tongue, extremities (especially fingers and initially in preferred hand); ballistic arm movements; lordosis; rocking or swaying; pelvic thrusting; chest dyskinesia with secondary cyanosis or stridor; dysphagia; and cognitive dysfunction. Many patients unaware of their TD. TD variants: tar-	Prevention: Do not use neuroleptics unless there is no other choice; atypical neuroleptics and then low potency agents provide less of a risk. Prompt early diagnosis with withdrawal of neuroleptics is only chance of recovery. Maneuvers to facilitate early diagnosis: observe patient walking and with protruding tongue. Ask patient to "let your arms

TABLE 9.12. (*continued*)

Side Effect	Characteristics	Management
	dive akathisia, tardive Gilles de la Tourette's disorder	hang loose at your sides" Risk factors Other neurologic disease Age > 60 years Mood disorder Prior use of anticholinergic antiparkinson agents Due to months or years of neuroleptic use; affects 30%–50% of persons with prolonged neuroleptic exposure
Neuroleptic malignant syndrome (NMS)	Cardinal features: rigidity, hyperpyrexia. Also common: sweating, hypertension, tachycardia, delirium, incontinence, mutism, stupor, catatonia, coma. Can be fatal. Laboratory tests: elevated white blood cell count (WBC) and creatinine phosphokinase (CPK) (> 300 U per cc) Elevated CPK often associated with myoglobinuria, increasing risk of death. Risk factors Large neuroleptic doses Dehydration Other co-morbid brain disease Co-prescription of lithium or anticholinergic agent Previous episode of catatonia Usually occurs within a month of inpatient admission	Discontinue neuroleptic Reduce hypothermia. Prescribe dantrolene (muscle relaxant that reduces rigidity) and a dopamine agonist (e.g., bromocriptine, amantadine, levodopa, apomorphine), or, *better still*, lorazepam or ECT
Endocrine	Gynecomastia (males and females), breast tenderness, lactorrhea, amenorrhea, false-positive pregnancy test, weight gain, reduced sex drive, male erectile or female arousal disorder	Amantadine Weight gain less likely if diet is reasonable and patient exercises
Anticholinergic	Dry mouth	Avoid sugar-containing fluids or candy (cause thrush and weight gain); commercial saliva substitute such as Moi-Stir spray twice PO PRN ad libitum, or

TABLE 9.12. Neuroleptic Side Effects and Their Management (*continued*)

Side Effect	Characteristics	Management
		pilocarpine mouth rinse 4%, 4 drops in 10 drops of water
	Constipation	Prevention: High fiber diet
		Treatment: Bulk laxatives or stool softeners
	Urinary retention most common in elderly men with benign prostatic hypertrophy (BPH)	Severe BPH contraindicates neuroleptics; mild urinary retention: bethanechol 25–50 mg PO TID
	Blurred vision due to combination of antimuscarinic-caused pupillary dilation and alpha-adrenergic–blocking pupillary constriction	Pilocarpine 1% optic solution 1 drop in each eye BID
	Fever due to reduced sweating (alpha-adrenergic blockade contributes to this)	Prevention: Adequate fluid intake; air-conditioned rooms in hot weather
	Anticholinergic delirium from overdose or polypharmacy with other drugs with anticholinergic properties (e.g., antiparkinsonians, antidepressants)	Physostigmine (see text)
Postural hypotension	Due to alpha-adrenergic blockade; onset usually within hours or days; sometimes associated with blurred vision and poor accommodation and problems with thermo-regulation (hyperthermia)	Rise slowly from lying down or sitting position
		Support hose and abdominal binder, caffeine (1–2 cups of coffee or its equivalent [200–300 mg caffeine] a day)
		If above fail, sodium chloride 0.5–1 g TID *or* fludrocortisone 0.1 mg QD or or BID or triiodothyronine 25 μg QD
Blood	Agranulocytosis: Fever usually first sign, often with sore throat; risk of death from fulminant infection	Order stat WBC for any patient on neuroleptic who develops fever If WBC <3,000 or polymorphic cells <1,000, stop neuroleptic and treat infection
	Risk factors	
	Clozapine	
	Euro-American ethnicity	
	Female gender	
	Middle age	
	Develops gradually over 2–18 weeks	
	Benign drop in WBC: asymptomatic drop of 10%–20% in WBC below baseline	No treatment needed

TABLE 9.12. (*continued*)

Side Effect	Characteristics	Management
Liver	Benign allergic intrahepatic chole-static jaundice: Jaundice, mild eosinophilia, mild elevation of alkaline phosphatase and con-jugated bilirubin	No treatment needed
Seizures	Lowered seizure threshold; sei-zures of any type	Prevention: Avoid prescribing neu-roleptics to epileptics
	Risk factors Epilepsy Other neurologic disease	For nonepileptic patients taking neuroleptics who develop sei-zures, stop the neuroleptic and look for other brain disease
Photosensitivity	Skin: Sunburn with minimal sun exposure	Prevention: Instruct patient to limit sun exposures, use sun-screen SPF 30–45
	Eyes: Photophobia	Patient should routinely wear sun-glasses on bright days
Pigmentation	Skin: Generalized grayish-blue skin pigmentation Risk factor: Phenothiazines	Prevention same as for photosen-sitivity
	Retinitis pigmentosa: Retinal pig-mentation with partial or com-plete blindness Risk factor: thioridazine >600 mg/day	Prevention: Do not prescribe thiori-dazine > 600 mg/day If pigmentary retinopathy occurs, discontinue drug
	Lens: Asymptomatic benign dis-coloration of cornea or lens usually observable only with slit lamp examinaton	Prevent with routine wearing of sunglasses on bright days. Regular follow-up ophthalmologic examinations
Sexual dysfunction	Reduced libido, male erectile dys-function, female arousal dis-order, retrograde ejaculation	If anticholinergic cause suspected, prescribe neostigmine 7.5–15 mg PO 30 min before coitus
Cardiac repolarization abnormalities	T-wave flattening, notching, split-ting, and inversion; P-Q and Q-T interval prolongation; S-T segment depression; often due to myocardial potassium depletion	Prevention: Do not prescribe neu-roleptics to persons with heart disease Treatment: If no heart disease, and with normal or low serum K^+, treat the EKG changes with high potassium foods such as bananas or apricots or oral po-tassium supplements
Sudden death	Causes altered thermoregulation due to anticholinergic drugs; cardiac arrhythmia; laryngeal dystonia, NMS	Prevention: Use neuroleptics as the last resort

TABLE 9.13. Drugs Used to Treat Neuroleptic Extrapyramidal Side Effects (EPS)

Drug	Usual Daily Oral Dose (mg)	Indication	Adverse Effects
Amantadine (Symmetrel)	100–400	Broad spectrum for all EPS and may potentiate benefit of other agents; needs BID dosing	Light-headedness, decreased concentration, jitteri-- ness, indigestion; excreted in urine, so renal function must be adequate
Benztropine mesylate (Cogentin)	2–6	Relieves muscle rigidity and sialorrhea (excess salivation, sometimes with drooling); 24-hour duration of action, so give once daily	Potent anticholinergic effects
Diphenhydramine (Benadryl)	150	Dystonia (best when used 50 mg IV)	Somnolence
Propranolol (Inderal)	30	Akathisia	Problematic drug interactions, diffuse cognitive impairment in elderly
Benzodiazepines			
Diazepam (Valium)	15	Akathisia; 10 mg IV for dystonia	Drowsiness and lethargy
Lorazepam (Ativan)	1–4	Akathisia	Time-limited because of addiction potential
Piperidines			
Procyclidine (Kemadrin)	5–30	Mild broad spectrum for all EPS	Significant peripheral anticholinergic effects, confusion in elderly
Trihexyphenidyl (Artane)	5–15	Broad spectrum, needs BID or TID dosing	Same as for procyclidine

treatment, 10% die or are left with neurologic deficits. An alternative is to treat NMS as if it were catatonia: give lorazepam (1–2 mg IM TID day 1; 2–4 mg IM TID day 2; if no response, 6–7 mg IM TID day 3; if still no response, ECT). Most patients will initially respond within a dose or two of a benzodiazepine and take fluids and become afebrile. ECT, regardless of the cause of NMS, also has dopamine agonistic effects and is the fastest (one to two treatments), the safest, and a life-saving treatment for NMS. It may then also be continued as definitive treatment for the patient's psychosis.

Tardive dyskinesia (TD) is the major concern in the use of neuroleptics because a substantial proportion of persons who take neuroleptics for 6–24 months will develop it. The motor features (see Table 9.12) can be horrendous, deforming, and terribly debilitating. Worse, TD (like many chronic basal ganglia disorders) can cause substantial cognitive impairment consistent with disrupted action brain function (e.g., poor sustained attention, poor fluency of ideas, poor cognitive flexibility, poor new learning). Other than the use of dopamine agonists (limited because of the potential for exacerbating positive symptoms) or switching to an atypical neuroleptic, there is no treatment for the cognitive impairment other than prevention. Prevention is also the best strategy for the motor features. However, if they develop, lowering the neuroleptic dose, stopping the neuroleptic, or switching to an atypical neuroleptic or a different treatment regiment can prevent further damage.

For newly developed symptoms, vitamin E (400 IU daily, increased weekly by 400 to 1,600 IU) may help and is well tolerated. For moderate symptoms, acetazolamide, a carbonic anhydrase inhibitor, may help (500 mg TID for elderly patients; 750, 750, and 500 mg daily for younger patients). Thiamine is given with it to reduce the risk of renal stones. Orange juice (8 oz) is also given to maintain potassium levels. Side effects include lethargy, loss of appetite, and parathyroid dysfunction. Allergic rash, fever, and malaise with reduced platelets can occur during the first few days of treatment. Acetazolamide increases cerebral blood flow and thus the brain uptake of neuroleptics so that lower doses may give the same therapeutic response. Vitamin E may also be used at this stage of TD.

If the TD is severe, and you can identify the involvement of specific muscle groups, then you can obtain substantial relief for the patient with botulinum toxin (Botox). Botulinum toxin prevents the presynaptic release of acetylcholine at the neuromuscular junction. Purified type A is used clinically to correct strabismus, endocrine orbital myopathy, lateral rectus paralysis, blepharospasm, hemifacial spasm, and dystonic torticollis. Patients are treated under electromyographic control to identify the specific muscle or group of fibers in spasm. The toxin is injected with tuberculin needles directly into the most involved muscle regions, doses varying depending on the size of the muscle (20 units for eye, 100 plus units for neck and shoulder muscle). For TD patients two to three treatments 1 month apart can produce dramatic improvement. Follow-up treatments every 6 months may be needed.

Patients most at risk for TD are those who (1) had acute dystonias, NMS, or substantial extrapyramidal features during acute neuroleptic treatment; (2) have co-morbid neurologic disease; (3) received intermittent rather than continuous exposure (perhaps explaining why mood disorder patients may have a higher risk than other patients); and (4) have a family history of basal ganglia disease or relatives with some basal ganglia motor features on examination. Right-handed men with positive psychiatric symptoms are reported to be at greater risk, but this may be due to higher dosing in those patients and, thus, more exposure plus the increased likelihood of secondary neurologic causes for psychoses in men (e.g., head trauma).

Avoid prescribing neuroleptics for pregnant or breast-feeding women for the same general reasons given above for other psychotropics. Avoid their use in persons with narrow angle glaucoma.

Drug-Drug Interactions

Alpha-adrenergic–blocking agents, including low potency neuroleptics, negate the effects of epinephrine and may affect treatment for asthmatics. Hepatic enzyme inducers like carbamazepine and phenytoin reduce serum neuroleptic levels, requiring higher neuroleptic doses to obtain a therapeutic effect. Antacids reduce absorption of neuroleptics.

Enzyme inhibitors like cimetidine increase serum neuroleptic levels, requiring lower neuroleptic doses to avoid side effects. Propranolol and serotonin reuptake–inhibiting antidepressants also increase neuroleptic levels. Neuroleptics potentiate the central nervous system depressant effects of sedative-hypnotics, benzodiazepines, and narcotic analgesics.

ADDITIONAL READINGS

American Psychiatric Association: Practice guideline for the treatment of patients with schizophrenia. *Am J Psychiatry 154*(suppl), 1997.

Andreasen S, Allenbeck P, Engstrom A, Rydberg U: Cannabis and schizophrenia. *Lancet 2*:1483–1486, 1987.

Andreasen NC, Arndt S, Swayze II, V, Cizadlo T, Flaum M, O'Leary D, Ehrhardt JC, Yu WTC: Thalamic abnormalities in schizophrenia visualized through magnetic resonance image averaging. *Science 266*:294–298, 1994.

Andreasen NC, Flaum M, Swayze VW II, Tyrrell G, Arndt S: Positive and negative symptoms in schizophrenia: A critical reappraisal. *Arch Gen Psychiatry 47*:615–621, 1990.

Andreasen NC, O'Leary DS, Flaum M, Nopoulos P, Watkins GL, Boles Ponto LL: Hypofrontality in schizophrenia: Distributed dysfunction circuits in neuroleptic naive patients. *Lancet 349*:1730–1734, 1997.

Andreasson S, Engstrom A, Allebeck P, Rydberg U: Cannabis and schizophrenia: A longitudinal study of Swedish conscripts. *Lancet 2*:1483–1486, 1987.

Bebbington P, Kuipers L: The clinical utility of expressed emotion in schizophrenia. *Acta Psychiatr Scand 89* (suppl 382):46–53, 1994.

Bebbington P, Kuipers L: The predictive utility of expressed emotion in schizophrenia: An aggregate analysis. *Psychol Med 24*:707–718, 1994.

Beng-Choon H, Nopoulos P, Flaum M, Arndt S, Andreasen NC: Two-year outcome in first-episode schizophrenia: Predictive value of symptoms for quality of life. *Am J Psychiatry 155*:1196–1201, 1998.

Berman KF, Zec RF, Weinberger DR: Physiologic dysfunction of dorsolateral prefrontal cortex in schizophrenia. II. Role of neuroleptic treatment, attention, and mental effort. *Arch Gen Psychiatry 43*:126–135, 1986.

Bousquet J: Neuroleptic malignant syndrome: A review of the literature. *J Clin Psychopharmacol 6*:257–273, 1986.

Bredkjaer SR, Mortensen PB, Parnas J: Epilepsy and non-organic non-affective psychosis: National epidemiologic study. *Brit J Psychiatry 172*:235–238, 1998.

Brown S, Birtwistle J: People with schizophrenia and their families: Fifteen-year outcome. *Brit J Psychiatry 173*:139–144, 1998.

Bymaster FP, Calligaro DO, Falcone JF, Marsh RD, Moore NA, Tye NC, Seeman P, Wong DT: Radioreceptor binding profile of the atypical antipsychotic olanzapine. *Neuropsychopharmacology 14*:87–96, 1996.

Caroff SN, Mann SC: Neuroleptic malignant syndrome. *Psychopharm Bull 24*:25–29, 1988.

Castle DJ, Scott K, Wessely S, Murry RM: Does social deprivation during gestation and early life predispose to later schizophrenia? *Social Psychiatry Psychiatr Epidemiol* 28:1–4, 1993.

Clementz BA, Grove WM, Iacono WG, Sweeney JA: Smooth-pursuit eye movement dysfunction and liability for schizophrenia: Implications for genetic modeling. *J Abnorm Psychol* 101:117–129, 1992.

Crawford TJ, Sharma T, Puri BK, Murray RM, Berridge DM, Lewis SW: Saccadic eye movements in families multiply affected with schizophrenia: The Maudsley family study. *Am J Psychiatry* 155:1703–1710, 1998.

Cummings JL: Organic delusions: Phenomenology, anatomical correlations, and review. *Br J Psychiatry* 146:184–197, 1985.

DeJesus Mari J, Steiner DL: An overview of family interventions and relapse in schizophrenia: Meta-analysis of research findings. *Psychol Med* 24:565–578, 1994.

DeVane CL: Drug interactions and antipsychotic therapy. *Pharmacotherapy* 16:15S–20S, 1996.

Eagles JM: Is schizophrenia disappearing? *Br J Psychiatry* 158:834–835, 1991.

Erlenmeyer-Kimling L, Cornblatt B: Biobehavioral risk factors in children of schizophrenic parents. *J Autism Dev Disord* 14:357–374, 1984.

Essen-Moller E: The concept of schizoidia. In Kloesi J (ed): *Psychiatrie und Neurologie,* vol 112. Karger, Basel, 1946, pp 258–271.

Faber R, Abrams R, Taylor MA, Kasprisin A, Morris C, Weisz R: Formal thought disorder and aphasia: Comparison of schizophrenic patients with formal thought disorder and neurologically impaired patients with aphasia. *Am J Psychiatry* 140:1348–1351, 1983.

Falloon IRH, Boyd JL, McGill CW, Razani J, Moss HB, Gilderman AM: Family management in the prevention of exacerbations of schizophrenia: A controlled study. *N Engl J Med* 306:1437–1440, 1982.

Fish B, Marcus J, Hans SL, Auerbach JG, Perdue S: Infants at risk for schizophrenia: Sequelae of a genetic neurointegrative defect: A review and replication analysis of pandysmaturation in the Jerusalem infant development study. *Arch Gen Psychiatry* 409:221–235, 1992.

Gervin M, Browne S, Lane A, Clarke M, Waddington JL, Larkin C, O'Callaghan EO: Spontaneous abnormal involuntary movements in first-episode schizophrenia and schizophreniform disorder: Baseline rate in a group of patients from an Irish catchment area. *Am J Psychiatry* 155:1202–1206, 1998.

Green MF, Bracha HS, Salz P, Christenson CD: Preliminary evidence for an association between minor physical anomalies and second trimester neurodevelopment in schizophrenia. *Psychiatry Res* 53:119–127, 1994.

Green MF, Satz P, Ganzell S, Vaclav JF: Wisconsin Card Sorting Test performance in schizophrenia: Remediation of a stubborn deficit. *Am J Psychiatry* 149:62–67, 1992.

Gur RE, Maany V, Mozley D, Swanson C, Bilker W, Gur RC: Subcortical MRI volumes in neuroleptic-naïve and treated patients with schizophrenia. *Am J Psychiatry* 155:1711–1717, 1998.

Hoffman RE, Dobscha SK: Cortical pruning and the development of schizophrenia: A computer model. *Schizophr Bull* 15:477–490, 1989.

Holden NL: Late paraphrenia or the paraphrenias? *Br J Psychiatry* 150:635–639, 1987.

Howard R, Almeida O, Levy R: Phenomenology, demography and diagnosis in late paraphrenia. *Psychol Med* 24:397–410, 1994.

Howard RJ, Graham C, Sham P, Jennehey J, Castle DJ, Levy R, Murray R: A controlled family study of late-onset nonaffective psychosis (late paraphrenia). *Br J Psychiatry* 170:511–514, 1997.

Hyde TM, Nawroz S, Goldberg TE, Bigelow LB, Strong D, Ostrem JL, Weinberger DR, Kleinman JE: Is there cognitive decline in schizophrenia? A cross-sectional study. *Br J Psychiatry* 164:494–500, 1994.

Ismail B, Cantor-Graae E, McNeil TF: Minor physical anomalies in schizophrenic patients and their siblings. *Am J Psychiatry* 155:1695–1702, 1998.

Jankovic J: Tardive syndromes and other drug-induced movement disorders. *Clin Neuropharmacol* 18:197–214, 1995.

Jankovic J, Schwartz K: Botulinum toxin injections for cervical dystonia. *Neurology* 40:277–280, 1990.

Jones RB, Rantakallio P, Hartikainen AL, Isohanni M, Sipila P: Schizophrenia as a long-term outcome of pregnancy, delivery, and perinatal complications: A 28-year follow-up of the 1966 North Finland general population birth cohort. *Am J Psychiatry* 155:355–364, 1998.

Keck PE, Pope HG Jr, Cohen BM, McElroy SL, Nierenberg AA: Risk factors for neuroleptic malignant syndrome: A case–control study. *Arch Gen Psychiatry* 46:914–918, 1989.

Keefe RSE, Silverman JM, Siever LJ, Cornblatt BA: Refining phenotype characterization in genetic studies of schizophrenia. *Soc Biol* 38:197–218, 1991.

Kendler KS: The nosologic validity of paranoia (simple delusional disorder): A review. *Arch Gen Psychiatry* 37:699–706, 1980.

Kendler KS: The genetics of schizophrenia and related disorders: A review. In Dunner DL, Gershon ES, Barrett JE (eds): *Relatives at Risk for Mental Disorder*. Raven Press, New York, 1988, pp 247–266.

Kinney DK, Yurgelum-Todd DA, Woods BT: Hard neurologic signs and psychopathology in relatives of schizophrenic patients. *Psychiatry Res* 39:45–53, 1991.

Laurie SM, Abukmeil SS: Brain abnormality in schizophrenia: A systematic and quantitative review of volumetric magnetic resonance imaging studies. *Br J Psychiatry* 172:110–120, 1998.

Lewis DA, Anderson SA: The functional architecture of the prefrontal cortex and schizophrenia. *Psychol Med* 25:887–894, 1995.

Love RC: Novel versus conventional antipsychotic drugs. *Pharmacotherapy* 16:6S–10S, 1996.

Merriam AE, Kay SR, Opler LA, Kushner SF, vanPraag HM: Neurological signs and the positive–negative dimension in schizophrenia. *Biol Psychiatry* 28:181–192, 1990.

Nasrallah HA, Schwartzkopf SB, Coffman JA, Olson SC: Perinatal brain injury and cerebellar vermal lobules I through X in schizophrenia. *Biol Psychiatry* 29:567–574, 1991.

Olbrich R, Mussgay L: Reduction of schizophrenic deficits by cognitive training: An evaluation study. *Eur Arch Psychiatry Neurol Sci* 239:366–369, 1990.

Olin SCS, Mednick SA, Cannon T, Jacobsen B, Parnas J, Schulsinger F, Schulsinger H: School teacher ratings predictive of psychiatric outcome 25 years later. *Bri J Psychiatry* 172(suppl 33):7–13, 1998.

Pakkenberg B: The volume of the mediodorsal thalamic nucleus in treated and untreated schizophrenics. *Schizophr Res* 7:95–100, 1992.

Pantelis C, Barnes TRE, Nelson HE: Is the concept of frontal-subcortical dementia relevant to schizophrenia? *Br J Psychiatry* 160:442–460, 1992.

Persaud R: The reporting of psychiatric symptoms in history: The memorandum book of Samuel Coates, 1785–1825. *History Psychiatry* 4:499–510, 1993.

Remington G, Kaput S, Zipursky RB: Pharmacotherapy of first-episode schizophrenia. *Br J Psychiatry* 172:66–70, 1998.

Russell AJ, Munro JC, Jones PB, Hemsley DR, Phil M, Murray RM: Schizophrenia or the myth of intellectual decline. *Am J Psychiatry* 154:635–639, 1997.

Sanger TM, Lieberman JA, Tohen M, Grundy S, Beasley C, Tollefson GD: Olanzapine versus haloperidol treatment in first-episode psychosis. *Am J Psychiatry* 156:79–87. 1999.

Sham PC, O'Callaghan E, Takei N, Murry GK, Hare EH, Murray RM: Schizophrenia following prenatal exposure to influenza epidemics between 1939–1960. *Br J Psychiatry* 160:461–466, 1992.

Sharma T, Lancaster E, Lee D, Lewis S, Sigmundsson T, Takei N, Gurling H, Barta P, Pearlson G, Murray R: Brain changes in schizophrenia. Volumetric MRI study of families multiply affected with schizophrenia—The Maudsley Family Study 5. *Brit J Psychiatry* 173:132–138, 1998.

Shoulson I: Huntington's disease: cognitive and psychiatric features. *Neuropsychiatry, Neuropsychol Behav Neurol 3*:15–22, 1990.

Staal WG, Hulshoff HE, Schnack H, van der Schot AC, Kahn RS: Partial volume decrease of the thalamus in relatives of patients with schizophrenia. *Am J Psychiatry 155*:1784–1786, 1998.

Stephens JH, Shaffer JW, Carpenter WT Jr: Reactive psychoses. *J Nerv Ment Dis 170*:657–663, 1982.

Sweeney JA, Haas GL, Keilp JG, Long M: Evaluation of the stability of neuropsychological functioning after acute episodes of schizophrenia: One year follow-up study. *Psychiatry Res 38*:63–76, 1991.

Tanna VL: Paranoid states: A selected review. *Compr Psychiatry 15*:454–469, 1974.

Taylor MA: The role of the cerebellum in the pathogenesis of schizophrenia. *Neuropsychiatry Neuropsychol Behav Neurol 4*:251–280, 1991.

Taylor MA: Are schizophrenia and affective disorder related? I. A selected literature review. *Am J Psychiatry 149*:22–32, 1992.

Thomas P, King K, Fraser WI, Kendell RE: Linguistic performance in schizophrenia: A comparison of acute and chronic patients. *Br J Psychiatry 156*:204–210, 1990.

Tollefson GD, Beasley CM Jr, Tran PV, Street JS, Krueger JA, Tamura RN, Graffeo KA, Thieme ME: Olanzapine versus haloperidol in the treatment of schizophrenia and schizoaffective and schizophreniform disorders: Results of an international collaborative trial. *Am J Psychiatry 154*:457–465, 1997.

Tollefson GD, Sanger TM: Negative symptoms: A path analytic approach to a double-blind placebo and haloperidol-controlled clinical trial with olanzapine. *Am J Psychiatry 154*:466–474, 1997.

Waddington JL, Youssef HA, Kinsella A: Mortality in schizophrenia: Antipsychotic polypharmacy and absence of adjunctive anticholinergics over the course of a 10-year prospective study. *Brit J Psychiatry 173*:325–329, 1998.

Wahlberg K-E, Wynne LC, Oja H, Keskitalo P, Pykalainen L, Lahti I, Moring J, Naarale M, Sorri A, Seitamaa M, Laksy K, Kolassa J, Tienari P: Gene-environment interaction in vulnerability to schizophrenia: Findings from the Finnish adoptive family study of schizophrenia. *Am J Psychiatry 154*:355–362, 1997.

Weinberger DR: Implications for normal brain development for the pathogenesis of schizophrenia. *Arch Gen Psychiatry 44*:660–669, 1987.

Weinberger DR, Aloia MS, Goldberg TE, Berman KF: The frontal lobes and schizophrenia. *J Neuropsychiatry Clin Neurosci 6*:419–427, 1994.

Weinberger DR, Berman KF, Illowsky BP: Physiological dysfunction of dorsolateral prefrontal cortex in schizophrenia. III. A new cohort and evidence for a monoaminergic mechanism. *Arch Gen Psychiatry 45*:609–615, 1988.

Weinberger DR, Berman KF, Zec RF: Physiologic dysfunction of dorsolateral prefrontal cortex in schizophrenia. I. Regional cerebral blood flow evidence. *Arch Gen Psychiatry 43*:114–124, 1986.

Welch J, Manschreck T, Redmond D: Clozapine-induced seizures and EEG changes. *J Neuropsychiatry Clin Neurosci 6*:250–256, 1994.

Williamson P, Pelz D, Merskey H, Morrison S, Conlon P: Correlation of negative symptoms in schizophrenia with frontal lobe parameters on magnetic resonance imaging. *Br J Psychiatry 159*:130–134, 1991.

Winokur G: Delusional disorder (paranoia). *Compr Psychiatry 18*:511–521, 1977.

Woods BT: Is schizophrenia a progressive neurodevelopmental disorder? Toward a unitary pathogenetic mechanism. *Am J Psychiatry 155*:1661–1670, 1998.

10

Epilepsy and Related Syndromes

Epilepsy results from excessive neuronal electrical discharges that synchronize and spread (by recruiting more neurons) through parts or all of the brain, producing a focal or generalized electrical "storm" or seizure. For there to be a seizure, instability must occur or be induced in neuronal membrane voltage-dependent sodium and chloride channels that then produce high frequency potentials. These potentials spread, producing the seizure. Dopamine and GABA stabilize these channels and can prevent the high frequency potential spread and thus the seizure.

One in 20 persons will have a seizure during his lifetime (most likely before age 5 years as a febrile convulsion or after age 60 years from stroke or metabolic disorder). The electrical seizure produces the behavioral change, the convulsion, or the fit that we clinically recognize. To be an epileptic, however, one must have more than one seizure, and 70% who have a seizure have more than one. About 0.5% of persons will develop epilepsy during their lifetime, and at any point in time there are between 4 and 10 epileptics for every 1,000 persons in the general population.

Three fourths of epileptics develop behavioral syndromes or intellectual deficits, and nearly 50% have interictal (the time between seizures) psychiatric symptoms affecting social and job functioning. About 10% of epileptics are hospitalized for psychiatric reasons, and another 20% are regularly treated in psychiatric outpatient settings. Because epilepsy is a fairly common condition and causes so many behavioral changes, you need to routinely consider seizure disorder in the differential diagnosis of many psychiatric patients.

CLASSIFICATION

Seizure disorders are classified as follows:

1. *Generalized* (the initial electrical discharge is generalized, originating from all or most centrencephalic structures): Absence (petit mal), atonic, tonic, clonic, tonic-clonic (grand mal), myoclonic, infantile spasms. Generalized seizures can be idiopathic or symptomatic of a recognized acquired morbid process

2. *Partial* (the initial electrical discharge is focal, local, or partial, cortical or subcortical, and may or may not become generalized): Simple (attacks without significant impairment of consciousness, accompanied by motor and sensory symptoms) or complex (attacks with significant impairment of consciousness accompanied by behavioral, cognitive, and affective phenomena)
3. *Mixed* forms

Complex partial seizures are sometimes termed *psychosensory* (the old term was *psychomotor*). Psychosensory seizures result from foci in the temporal (most common), frontal (next most common), or parietal lobes or related subcortical structures. Table 10.1 lists the characteristics of a partial complex seizure. Most epileptics with a behavioral syndrome have partial complex epilepsy. The majority of these foci are of temporal lobe origin, and most such persons (about 80%) are misdiagnosed as having a primary psychiatric disorder at least sometime during their illness.

Behavioral changes associated with epilepsy can directly relate to the seizure (the ictal state), the prodrome period (hours to weeks preceding the seizure), the post-ictal period (hours to days subsequent to the seizure), or to the inter-ictal period. Because the seizure rarely lasts more than 15 minutes and is most often less than 1 minute, the behaviors that lead to psychiatric hospitalization or treatment are typically nonictal.

TABLE 10.1. Characteristics of a Partial Complex Fit

Characteristic	*Typical Pattern*
Paroxysmal	From normal brain electrical activity and behavior to seizure onset takes only a few seconds; from onset to peak severity takes only a few seconds
Transient	Less than 60 seconds; frontal lobe fits often last longer than temporal lobe fits; status, although uncommon, can occur with all types and is defined by its continued length or increased frequency of fits over a 1–2 week period
Alteration in arousal	A sudden decrease in attention or responsivity usually associated with a sudden stopping of previous behavior and the sudden appearance of new behaviors
Automatisms	Complex, repetitive behaviors performed in an automatic fashion; a classic feature, but not necessary for the diagnosis
Psychosensory experiences	Paroxysmal and transient emotional, sensory, and autonomic experiences; a classic feature but not necessary for the diagnosis
Amnesia for the event	Can be total, only for details, or remembered as one remembers a dream

CLINICAL PRESENTATION: THE PRODROME

Prodrome behaviors typically last hours or less, rarely weeks. Irritability, features of nonmelancholic or atypical depression, or being ill at ease are most common. Rarely, the prodrome can be a psychosis. Prodrome psychosis is usually associated with grand mal epilepsy, and the psychosis, as other prodromal features, typically resolves with the fit. This observation lead to the development of convulsive therapy, (i.e., inducing a seizure to end psychosis similar to the way spontaneous seizures appeared to end them).

CLINICAL PRESENTATION: AURAS

Auras are sudden, intense, and brief experiences (a few seconds) that precede the full fit. Sometimes a patient will experience an aura, but the full fit never develops. Ninety percent of patients with temporal lobe foci, 60% of patients with frontal lobe foci, and 50% of patients with parieto-occipital lobe foci have auras.

Table 10.2 lists types of temporal lobe auras. Emotive and perceptual auras are referred to as *experiential phenomena* and occur in about one third of patients. Intense fear suggests amygdala involvement. Violence suggests mesial frontal and basal forebrain involvement. Perceptual disturbances are typically visual (visual

TABLE 10.2. Temporal Lobe Auras

Type	Characteristics
Emotive	Sudden unexplained sadness or elation, emotional incontinence, fear (can be confused with anxiety disorder), dysphoria, anxiety, brief panic attack, irritability, anger and sudden violence (can produce episodic dyscontrol syndrome and be misdiagnosed as a Cluster B personality disorder)
Perceptual	Hallucinations, dysmegalopsia, or dysmorphopsia (can be confused with schizophrenia)
Mnestic	Deja vu, jamais vu (can be misdiagnosed as dissociative disorder)
Arousal	Derealization (the world seems flat like a cartoon, the patient feels he is in a dream), depersonalization (the patient feels detached from his body, floating above himself) (DSM labels these dissociative disorders)
Autonomic	Brief panic attack, body temperature instability (sudden feeling of intense heat or cold), cardiovascular signs (sudden tachycardia or palpitations), flushing (can be confused with panic disorder)
Visceral	Epigastric rush, nausea, abdominal pressure, choking sensation (can be misdiagnosed as somatization disorder or Cluster B personality disorder)

TABLE 10.3. Frontal Lobe Auras

Type	Characteristics
Cephalic sensations	Light-headedness, pressure on top of the head, band around the head, vertigo, dizziness, feeling drunk, head feeling inflated
Diffuse warmth	Begins somewhere on the body and ascends into the head, entire body feels warm
Language*	Speech arrest, forced speech (an experience of control), unable to think or speak clearly or make sense
Atypical motor behavior*	Side-to-side head movement, pelvic thrusting

*May also occur during the ictal phase. When an aura, it is of shorter duration and may generalize into a tonic-clonic fit.

pathways pass through temporal lobes), but olfactory and gustatory hallucinations may also occur. Emotive, perceptual, and mnestic auras result from the direct disruption of temporal lobe function. Forty-five percent of patients experience visceral auras (e.g., abdominal coldness, hollowness, or pressure). Visceral, autonomic auras and changes in consciousness result from the seizure affecting other limbic structures and perhaps the thalamus.

Table 10.3 lists the types of frontal lobe auras. Cephalic sensations occur in about 25% of patients; 20% experience diffuse warmth. Compared with temporal lobe auras, frontal lobe auras are more likely to have a motor component and involve cognition. Patients with frontal lobe foci may also have temporal as well as frontal lobe auras because of frontotemporal connections in the uncinate fasciculus. The reverse, however, is not true, and temporal lobe foci do not produce frontal lobe signs.

Table 10.4 lists types of parieto-occipital lobe auras. Parietal lobe auras typically involve sensation and changes and distortions in body image. Occipital lobe auras can lead to self-mutilating behavior in which the patient damages his eyes.

TABLE 10.4. Parieto-Occipital Auras

Type	Characteristics
Sensory experiences	Sudden brief tingling, numbness, electric shocks, coldness, burning, unilateral pain
Body part perceptual distortion	Perceived changes in shape, size, weight, composition (made of metal, wood), location (hand in abdomen), or ownership (body part belongs to someone else, experience of alienation)
Elementary hallucinations	Seeing lights, colors, halos; tinnitus
Ocular sensations	Electric feeling in eyes, feeling eyes are being pulled out of their sockets

CLINICAL PRESENTATION: THE SEIZURE (THE ICTAL EVENT)

Table 10.5 lists typical ictal behaviors. Suspect epilepsy whenever a psychopathologic phenomenon lasts less than an hour or so. Frontal lobe foci produce additional characteristic behaviors (Table 10.6). Table 10.7 lists some features distinguishing frontal from temporal lobe epilepsy.

Many dissociative states are epilepsy related and are described below. Depersonalization and derealization are typical complex partial ictal phenomena. Petit mal and partial complex status also can produce a psychosis with an alteration in consciousness and responsivity. These rare psychoses can last for days and are characterized by disorientation or perplexity, hallucinations, vague delusional ideas, rambling speech, and agitation.

CLINICAL PRESENTATION: POST-ICTAL PHENOMENA

Post-ictal phenomena immediately follow the seizure and can last minutes to hours, rarely days to weeks. Most commonly, the patient is lethargic and some-

TABLE 10.5. Ictal Behaviors

Type	Characteristics
Automatisms	Repetitive automatic movements such as lip smacking, puckering of the lips, opening and closing the mouth, rubbing, scratching, swallowing
Autonomic signs	Bursts of pallor or flushing, salivation, sweating, tachycardia, gastrointestinal tract motility, hiccupping, belching, sneezing, gastrointestinal tract motility changes, respiratory rate changes, gasping or apnea, urinary incontinence, autonomic paroxysms (palpitations, sudden intense feelings of cold or heat)
Complex behaviors	Aimless walking, automatically doing a daily routine such as going to the refrigerator, putting on or taking off clothes, drinking and other sudden expressions of procedural memory
Psychopathology	Mundane posturing, depersonalization/derealization, forced thinking (e.g., experiences of control), emotional incontinence, dysmorphopsia and other visual hallucinations and distortions (right focus more likely), deja vu/jamais vu, auditory misperceptions and hallucinations (left focus more likely if voice), experiencing an entire life episode (as a flashback, right focus more likely), autoscopic phenomena (hallucinating oneself), sudden, transient, shallow expressions of sadness or tearfulness (nondominant focus for ictal crying), or euphoria or laughter (dominant hemisphere focus)

TABLE 10.6. Frontal Lobe Seizure Behaviors

Area of Focus	Characteristic Behaviors
Supplementary motor area	Speech arrest (mutism), forced vocalizations, grunting and mumbling, muttering, palilalia, head and eye movement (often side to side), head turned away from focus, upper limb movement (raised hand palm forward as if responding to roll call), catatonic posturing, grimacing, hand and arm postures, pedaling and kicking
Dorsolateral	Speech arrest, catatonia, altered consciousness
Anterior cingulate	Fear/terror/screaming, corprolalia (compulsive use of profanity), elementary hallucinations, complex motor behavior ("archaic": urinating, defecating, pelvic thrusting), alteration in consciousness
Orbitofrontal	Olfaction changes, visceral sensations, gestural movements, apnea, arrhythmias, flushing/pallor, hunger/thirst, incontinence

what disoriented and may be unable to focus his thoughts (suggests temporal lobe). Some patients have a great need to sleep after a fit. Orienting behaviors (fumbling and patting one's clothes, picking, rubbing, checking surroundings) are suggestive of a temporal lobe focus. Post-ictal Todd's paralysis (a transient unilateral weakness), sexually and socially inappropriate behavior (touching), undressing, and irritability suggest a frontal lobe focus. Language problems following the seizure (dysarthria, mumbling, rambling speech) suggest a left frontal focus. Aprosodias suggest a right-sided focus.

TABLE 10.7. Some Features That Distinguish Frontal From Temporal Lobe Epilepsy

Frontal	Temporal
History of head trauma	History of febrile convulsions
Often occurs at night and in clusters	Visceral aura
Often previously labeled "hysterical" (gasping, arms flailing, pedaling, waving arms)	Mouth movements and contralateral posturing; facial weakness during emotional expression (interictally) contralateral to focus
Sexual automatisms	Fumbling and picking at clothes or objects
Vocalizations	More likely to have post-ictal elevated prolactin levels
Frenetic behavior	
Multiple forms from single focus (drop attacks, psychosensory fits, absence; thalamus and surrounding areas often the focus)	

Some patients develop a post-seizure psychosis. This is most likely with grand mal epilepsy and typically begins 1–3 days after the fit following a period of seeming normality or only mild other post-ictal features. The psychosis is characterized by (1) great emotionality, (2) hallucinations in several sensory modalities, and (3) some change in alertness or responsivity (e.g., oneiroid or stuporous state).

Dissociative fugue states may occur post-ictally. Persons who abandon their lives and resurface in another place with a new life and identity do not do so because of epilepsy. Epileptic fugues last minutes and typically involve walking several hundred feet.

CLINICAL PRESENTATION: INTER-ICTAL PHENOMENA

Inter-ictal behavioral changes do not predict location of focus or type of seizure. There are four categories of inter-ictal phenomena: the psychomotor quartet, psychosis, mood disorders, and personality change.

The Psychomotor Quartet (Gastaut-Geschwind Syndrome)

Many chronic epileptics behave abnormally between seizures. The behaviors are not the direct expressions of the fits themselves, as are prodromal, ictal, and post-ictal behaviors, but are due to the long-term effects of the epileptic process on the limbic system. These behaviors also occur in 40% of chronic psychiatric patients, particularly those with bipolar mood disorder or drug-induced recurrent psychosis. There are four features:

1. *Circumstantial speech,* which is not rapid or intense as in mania, but rather is methodical in its relentless addition of detail and parenthetical comments. It is an obsessive need to give detail.
2. *Hyposexuality* can be profound and many patient's even lose the desire to masturbate.
3. *Hypergraphia* occurs, and the patient keeps copious notes, diaries, or other documentation of his ideas, feelings, experiences, and symptoms. The writing is typically pedantic, perseverative and plodding, overdetailed and cliche-ridden, much like the content of the circumstantial speech. The hypergraphia can take the form of letter writing, doodling, or drawing. It is an obsessive need to write.
4. *Pseudoprofundity* develops without previous interest or training, and the patient becomes obsessively interested in religion, philosophy, cosmology, and the like, but without any true understanding of the concepts behind the words. Patients quote the texts of their interest, obsessively underline every word, and point out passages to you as if by doing so the importance of what they are saying will suddenly be revealed. Some patients become fixated on philosophic or religious ideas and practices culturally different from their previous experience, par-

ticularly those credos that endorse a universal community or "one-ness" (e.g., transcendental meditation, joining a cult).

Inter-Ictal Psychosis (10% of Epileptics)

Some epileptics develop recurrent psychoses that are not directly related to a seizure (i.e., neither prodromal nor post-ictal). These psychoses typically begin after years (average, 5–10) of illness, and tend to increase in frequency as seizure frequency decreases. Inter-ictal epileptic psychosis is characterized by (1) acute onset; (2) emotionality (75% have an elevated or depressed mood); (3) hallucinations, often in several sensory modalities and in rare forms (e.g., elementary, extracampine, functional; see Chapter 3), and persecutory delusions (50% of patients); (4) psychosensory features; and (5) normal arousal (unlike postictal psychosis where it is often altered).

Epileptics most likely to develop inter-ictal psychoses are those with (1) an epilepsy onset around puberty; (2) frequent seizures during the first decade of illness; (3) complex partial epilepsy or complex partial epilepsy that generalizes into grand mal; (4) seizures associated with epigastric or fear auras, automatisms, and deja vu phenomena; (5) temporal lobe foci, and (6) an EEG abnormality of a spike–slow wave pattern.

Schizophrenic-like or delusional disorder epileptic psychoses are associated with left-sided (50%) or bilateral (30%) foci, more than exclusively right-sided foci (20%). Bilateral foci are associated with psychotic mood disorders. Anterior mesiobasal temporal foci (50%) are most often associated with psychosis. The patient's handedness or family history of epilepsy is not predictive of later psychosis.

Mood Disorder

Inter-ictal depression is common. These depressions are nonmelancholic and "atypical" and are characterized by an intermittent course with brief periods of intense anergia, insomnia, dysphoria, and anxiety or by a low grade, treatment-resistant late-onset dysthymia. Bipolar disorder secondary to epilepsy is less common, but also tends to be chronic and treatment resistant.

Epileptic Personality

Forty to 60% of epileptics develop permanent changes in personality. These chronic behaviors are often more disrupting to social and job functioning than are the psychoses. Although the psychomotor quartet and epileptic personality behaviors overlap, two personality patterns have been identified. The *adhesive* or *viscous* personality, first described in 1916, is characterized by perseveration, stubbornness, a narrowed field of interest and attention, loss of humor, circumstantiality, cliche-filled speech, and a pedantic, dry manner. Behaviors and cognitions are narrowed to one or two plodding, repetitive, overly valued, and constantly expressed themes (they are viscous). They are said to be adhesive because they are compelled to speak to people in some authority (e.g., employers, government officials, their doctors) about their concerns, and it is almost impossible to divert them from their theme and extremely difficult to end the conversation. They see you, make contact, and stick to you. They lose sight of basic concepts and themes and focus on minutiae. Nothing is trivial; every detail must be mulled over. This personality change is correlated with mesial temporal lobe foci.

A second personality pattern is characterized by moodiness and becoming quarrelsome, spiteful, suspicious, and malicious. These patients hold grudges, protest city hall, and file suits against neighbors. They become the neighborhood cranks. This pattern also occurs with adhesive behaviors, but is correlated with lateral temporal lobe foci.

In addition to the inter-ictal personality changes noted above, epileptic patients with complex partial fits are also more likely to meet DSM criteria for some personality disorders (schizotypal, borderline, dependent, explosive). These disorders represent a change in personality from what was typical for the patient prior to the epilepsy.

CLINICAL PRESENTATION: RELATED SYNDROMES

Nonepileptical Seizures

Nonepileptic seizures (formerly *pseudoseizures*) are episodes of abnormal behavior that look like seizures but that occur without a typical brain epileptic electrical discharge. At least 10%–20% of patients attending epilepsy centers have nonepileptic seizures, and most persons with nonepileptic seizures are persons who at other times have seizures, that is, they are epileptics. Nonepileptic seizures are characterized by

1. Prolonged duration with rapid recovery without drowsiness
2. Unresponsiveness without prominent motor features or prominent motor features with interactive conversation
3. Incongruous motor features (e.g., slow writhing movements, bilateral kicking or stomping without upper body involvement)
4. No psychosensory phenomena
5. When grand mal-like, no reflex changes, incontinence, or tongue biting
6. Post-ictal crying

Episodes are induced by suggestion and occur when others are present. Prolactin levels, almost always elevated 15–20 minutes after a grand mal fit, remain normal.

In addition to epilepsy, nonepileptic seizures are associated with premorbid personality disorder (the dramatic-emotional DSM Cluster B group), conversion disorder, somatoform disorder, dissociative disorder, mood disorder, and anxiety disorder. Epileptics with these experiences tend to be highly suggestive, dependent, and histrionic. From 10% to 70% of patients with nonepileptic seizures have a between-episode nonspecific abnormal EEG.

Epilepsy Spectrum Disorder

Some patients have many features of epilepsy, but these features do not occur in paroxysms and there is no alteration in consciousness or attention. These patients' EEGs are abnormal but not epileptic; they do not have nonepileptic seizures.

Patients typically complain of persistent dysphoria. They have angry, sometimes violent outbursts that fill them with remorse and sometimes lead to suicide. They are more likely to damage furniture or themselves than other persons. They are concerned about "going crazy," may hallucinate, and develop a nonaffective, positive symptom psychosis (see Chapter 9). They complain of illusions of peripheral movement, tinnitus, word-finding problems, speaking jargon, "confusional spells" (brief and usually unnoticed by others), memory gaps, unrecalled behavior, staring, depressive and anxiety spells, and angry outbursts. They may meet criteria for schizotypal or borderline personality disorder. Consider epilepsy spectrum disorder when a patient has persistent dysphoria and multiple complex partial seizure-like symptoms but no stereotyped spells or motor automatisms. Whether these patients are, in fact, epileptics with a deep brain undetected focus or have another temporolimbic disorder is unknown, but they respond to anticonvulsants.

Dissociative Disorders as Variants of Seizure Disorder

The validity of dissociative states as discrete disorders is unproven. These states are most often associated with specific neurologic disease (i.e., epilepsy, multiple sclerosis, traumatic brain injury) or another psychiatric disorder (e.g., anxiety disorder, psychosis, schizotypal personalities). Because of the strong association of these features with epilepsy, they are described here. *Dissociative fugue* is described above, and documented cases have an association with epilepsy, drug abuse, or sleep walking.

Depersonalization and *derealization* are associated with partial complex ictal events, any psychosis involving temporolimbic systems (e.g., bipolar mood disorder), drug abuse, and schizotypal personality disorder. Some early European diagnostic systems rely on the presence of depersonalization and derealization for the diagnosis of schizophrenia. Depersonalization and derealization also occur in persons with anxiety disorder who also have daily anxiety and several phobias or fears.

Dissociative amnesia is never like what is portrayed in fiction. It is typically of short duration during which the patient may be agitated and disoriented. These amnestic states are associated with epilepsy (ictal or post-ictal), drug abuse, abnormal metabolic states (e.g., hypoglycemia), and head injury (anterograde amnesia, i.e., the period following the head trauma when continuing brain dysfunction disrupts laying down of new memories).

Dissociative identity disorder (formerly *multiple personality*) is also never like what is portrayed in fiction and probably does not exist as portrayed in some movies (*Three Faces of Eve, Sybil*). Some patients fabricate experiences to maintain the sick role (*factitious disorder*) or malinger to avoid legal or other consequences or to get money. Some highly suggestible, dependent patients develop symptoms to please their caregivers, whose motivations also vary. Documented cases involve only two "personalities": the person's basic personality (typically introverted, passive, dependent) interspersed with sudden relatively brief periods of aggressiveness and extroversion for which there is some amnesia and that represent events during and after a seizure.

Dissociative conversion disorder is a pseudoneurologic condition involving the organs of special sense (e.g., eyes, ears), voluntary musculature, pain, or disturbed sexual functioning whose signs and symptoms incompletely resemble those of neurologic disorders. These include blindness, tunnel vision, anosmia, anesthesia, paresthesia, aphasia, paralysis, seizures, coordination disturbances, akinesia, and dyskinesia. The DSM concept includes some precipitating stress that relates to a psychological conflict or need and, thus, the emergence or exacerbation of the conversion feature, but the patient is not intentionally producing the feature.

Despite the belief that explainable pathology cannot be found in conversion disorder, 30%–50% of conversion disorder patients have diseases explaining their symptoms, and about 30% have another psychiatric disorder. For example, galactorrhea and amenorrhea, typifying pseudocyesis, are associated with hyperprolactinemia in 50%–70% of cases and with prolactinomas 35%–60% of the time. Conditions most often mislabeled as hysteria are those involving degenerative disease of skeletal, muscular, and connective tissues, the spinal cord, and peripheral nerves. Included among these are multiple sclerosis, myopathies, polyneuritis, dystonia musculorum deformans, transverse myelopathy, and thoracic outlet syndrome. Homosexual men, the psychiatrically ill, and patients with plausible psychogenic explanations for their condition are at greatest risk to be misdiagnosed, and movement disorders and paralysis are most often misdiagnosed as hysterical conversion.

Although any patient diagnosed as having a conversion symptom could be a malingerer (particularly one with antisocial personality disorder), malingering does not routinely explain conversion symptoms. Seizure disorder and nonepileptic seizures are also associated with conversion disorder. A Todd's paralysis can be mistaken for a conversion if you miss the related seizure, migraine, or other neurologic event.

For those patients whose underlying cause you cannot identify or possible comorbid condition you cannot explain, consider a combination of a highly suggestible person whose dissociations evolve from social learning and memory (often influenced by caregivers), and a predisposition to respond to excessive cortical arousal (as with stress, high stimuli environments) with synaptic inhibition in sensorimotor pathways via negative feedback between the cerebral cortex and the brain stem reticular formation. This protective functional disconnection is the form of the dissociation, whereas social learning and mimicry determine the content (e.g., conversion or depersonalization). The classic indifference to conversion conditions, or *la belle indifference,* is uncommon, and most patients are distressed.

EEG and magnetic resonance imaging (MRI) of the brain or spinal cord, lumbar puncture, electromyography, and auditory, visual, and somatosensory evoked potentials are helpful in diagnosis. Evoked potentials and MRI are the best means of diagnosing multiple sclerosis, and they reveal abnormalities in the majority of affected persons.

Most dissociative states are treated by identifying and treating any underlying or co-morbid conditions. For primary dissociative states, a Cluster B personality disorder is usually present. Treat these by (1) educating the patient that symptoms are real and can be controlled with relaxation, (2) using suggestion techniques while administering a 10% solution of sodium amobarbital, and (3) hypnosis. Long-term prognosis is poor.

Hysteria

Most patients who in the past were diagnosed as hysteric are today said to have somatoform disorder. Some of these cases, however, reflect seizure disorder. Always consider seizure disorder (a partial epilepsy that then generalizes, complex partial epilepsy with a frontal or temporal focus) when the "hysteria" is

1. *Astasia-abasia:* Total body, head and limb ataxia without other neurologic explanation
2. *Hysterical twilight state:* Oneiroid state or other apparent alterations in consciousness that occur when the patient is being noticed or confronted and during which the patient can partially respond or converse as if mimicking a trance state
3. *Ganser syndrome:* A twilight state during which the patient gives silly responses to easy questions (pseudologica fantastica) such as, what was the color of George Washington's' white horse? (Ans: brown). How many legs does a three-legged stool have? (Ans: four). Who is buried in Grant's tomb? (Ans: Kennedy).

Migraine Headache as a Variant of Epilepsy

Migraine and epilepsy can co-occur. Epileptics are twice as likely to develop migraine as are their nonepileptic relatives. Migraine is most common in epilepsy due to head trauma, but it can occur with any epilepsy. About 6% of migraineurs are epileptic compared with 0.5% of the general population. Among epileptics 10%–20% have migraine. Among the first-degree epileptic relatives of migraineurs about 25% also have migraine. Among the first-degree relatives without epilepsy about 15% have migraine. The co-occurrence is explained by a neuronal hyperexcitability, similar to kindling, common to both disorders.

Because clinical features of both conditions overlap, differential diagnosis can be difficult. Migraine is most likely if (1) the aura lasts more than 5 minutes, (2) there are no alterations in consciousness or automatisms; (3) the EEG is normal or shows an epileptic-like tracing that waxes and wanes but never fully forms an epileptic pattern, and (4) on magnetic imaging spectroscopy, migraineurs show low occipital lobe metabolism. Epileptics have low metabolism at the site of the seizure focus, which is rarely occipital. Migraine is described in detail in Chapter 16.

Phobic–Anxiety Depersonalization Disorder as an Epilepsy Variant

The phobic–anxiety depersonalization disorder (PAD) syndrome is a European term for an anxiety disorder that combines daily anxiety with agoraphobia, panic attacks, and periods of depersonalization. The condition is chronic. Patients with PAD have other psychosensory features besides depersonalization, fit-like episodes, temporal lobe structural changes, and abnormal but not necessarily epileptic-like EEGs. Antidepressants make some of these patients worse or offer no benefit. Consider anticonvulsants as an alternative treatment for those PAD patients who do not respond well to the standard treatments for anxiety disorder.

Reproductive Endocrine Disorders Associate with Epilepsy

About 50% of epileptics have reproductive endocrine disorders, and two thirds of these patients have abnormal levels of serum luteinizing hormone (elevated), follicle-stimulating hormone (decreased), and testosterone (elevated). Twenty percent of women epileptics have amenorrhea, 40% have menorrhagia or metrorrhagia, and 70% have fertility problems. *Polycystic ovarian syndrome* (amenorrhea or oligomenorrhea, hirsutism, galactorrhea, and polycystic ovaries) is correlated with left temporal lobe foci. *Hypogonadotropic hypogonadism* (amenorrhea or oligomenorrhea, low luteinizing hormone [LH], diminished LH response to gonadotropin-releasing hormone, normal-sized ovaries) and hyposexuality are correlated with right-sided temporal lobe foci. Seizure control often requires first stabilizing any endocrine abnormalities.

EPILEPSY IN CHILDREN AND ADOLESCENTS

Epilepsy is more common in children than in adults, with a prevalence rate of about 20 per 1,000. Three fourths of epilepsies begin before age 20 years, and 50% of childhood epilepsies begin before age 5. Table 10.8 describes a few childhood epilepsies.

The prognosis for idiopathic childhood epilepsy is variable, but the prevalence drops in the teenage years (in part from high mortality rates: 20% with neonatal and infantile onsets, 6%–10% with onset at ages 3–10 years). Some (benign rolandic) almost always stop by age 20. Absence seizures also may resolve and have the next best prognosis. Complex partial seizures and mixed seizures have the worst prognosis. Grand mal is intermediary. About 30% of childhood epilepsies resolve with good treatment. Good prognostic signs are (1) no identifiable etiology, (2) a normal neurologic examination, (3) no inter-ictal cognitive changes, (4) infrequent seizures, and (5) only a mildly abnormal EEG.

TABLE 10.8. Some Childhood Epilepsies

Type	Characteristics
Absence (petit mal)	1. Staring spells that rarely last more than 30 seconds, frequency can be 1–2 per week to hundreds per day 2. Onset age 5–10 years and may "outgrow" them or develop temporolimbic seizures 3. 3/sec spike–slow wave discharges characteristic 4. Autosomal dominant with variable penetrance accounts for some cases (well siblings have abnormal EEG) 5. Ethosuximide and valproate drugs of choice if frequency high
Lennox-Gastaut	1. Delayed mental development, multiple seizure types (tonic, tonic-clonic, myoclonic, absence, drop attacks, complex partial) 2. Multiple spike discharges against slow wave background
Landau-Kleffner	1. Progressive aphasia after initial language development 2. Spike discharges in deep sleep focal in dominant hemisphere speech areas
Benign Rolandic	1. Simple partial fits involving face and laryngeal muscles or arms, nocturnal seizures 2. Onset age 5–10 years, and almost all outgrow it between 12 and 20 years 3. High amplitude centrotemporal spikes and dipoles (central negative peak with anterior positive wave)
Frontal midline	1. Rhythmic leg movements, fencer's posture, bicycling leg movements, pelvic thrusting 2. Supplementary motor area focus
Juvenile myoclonic	1. Minor myoclonic seizures in morning for months before first convulsion recognized; patients think their jerks mean they are "clumsy" in the morning 2. Also occurring are absence fits, myoclonic, and generalized tonic-clinic types 3. EEG shows rapid spike waves (4–5–5/sec) and 3/sec spike wave and runs of multiple spikes

Thirty to 50% of epileptic children have a behavioral illness (conduct disorder, ADHD, mood disorder with higher suicide risks in teenagers), and other behavioral problems (nail biting, thumb sucking, stuttering, enuresis, and encopresis). Childhood psychosis due to epilepsy is virtually unknown. Adjustment disorder in adolescent epileptics is common.

DIFFERENTIAL DIAGNOSIS

Epilepsy is a clinical, not a laboratory, diagnosis; thus total reliance on EEG is misplaced. Only 40%–60% of epileptics are identified after two to three specialized EEG studies (sleep deprived, photic driving, hyperventilation, specific montages, nasopharyngeal and sphenoidal electrode placement). Twenty percent of epileptics repeatedly have normal EEGs. A careful, detailed clinical evaluation is the best way to determine if a patient is epileptic. Many conditions associated with fainting, brief memory lapses, or altered consciousness superficially mimic epilepsy.

Syncope syndromes mimic epilepsy and typically result from deceased blood flow to the brain from stress-induced vagal–vagal responses (e.g., getting blood drawn), blood shunting to large muscle groups in maladaptive flight/fight (seen in 10%–15% of anxiety disorder patients), dehydration, or hypotension from drugs or orthostasis (in some teenagers). Light-headedness and cold, clammy sweating usually precedes nonepileptic syncope. Some syncopal episodes can cause transient brain ischemic changes resulting in brief tonic or tonic-clonic seizures, but identifying and treating the underlying condition usually resolves this rare complication.

Cardiac arrhythmias also can lead to decreased brain blood flow, syncope, and sometimes convulsive syncope. Some familial arrhythmias induce syncope, and family history and EKG are diagnostic.

Transient ischemic attacks (TIAs) are most likely to occur in men over 65 years with cardiovascular disease or diabetes and no previous fit-like episodes. TIAs last longer than most seizures and are associated with disorientation and poor coordination rather than automatisms, complex behaviors, and rhythmic motor behavior. TIAs affecting the mesial temporal lobe can produce a transient global amnesia that can mimic a partial complex fit. In this type of TIA, however, the patient remains interactive and has no previous features of epilepsy.

Hypoglycemia can result in disorientation, delirium, and grand mal seizures. Look for a prodrome of hunger, sweating, and light-headedness and a history of fasting or diabetes. Correcting the problem rather than labeling the patient epileptic is the treatment goal.

Sleep disorders leading to daytime sleepiness can be mistaken for epilepsy. Narcolepsy with associated hypopompic hallucinations and sleep paralysis, sleep apnea with its associated snoring and middle-age onset, and REM behavior disorder with its early morning wild thrashing about and screaming are all identified with sleep studies and EEG (also see Chapter 16).

Movement disorders with tics and habit spasms can be confused with partial epilepsy. These behaviors, however, are under some voluntary control and usually involve more muscle groups than partial epilepsy. They are also more prolonged and may be associated with obsessive compulsive disorder in the patient or first-degree relatives. Neuroleptic-induced dystonias are associated with drug exposure and usually with other side effects.

Intermittent explosive disorders are a particular diagnostic problem because epilepsy is always part of their differential diagnosis. When a result of epilepsy, violence is typically (1) brief and occurring just before or after a seizure-like event, (2) nongoal directed and random, and (3) a lashing out at nearby objects rather than complex and premeditated.

Catatonia with its stereotypes, mannerisms and mutism can look like a seizure, and epilepsy is part of the differential diagnosis of catatonia. Unlike epileptics, however, many catatonics converse or respond during their manneristic or stereotypic behavior. Their movement abnormality lasts longer than those associated with seizure, and 50% will have past or present features of bipolar mood disorder.

Mood disorders can also be mistaken for epilepsy because they can be episodic, relatively brief, and associated with psychosensory experiences. Although associated with temporal limbic dysfunction, primary mood disorder patients do not have seizure episodes as outlined in Table 10.1.

Premenstrual behavioral syndromes can be confused with epilepsy because some partial complex fits are triggered by premenstrual hormonal changes. Epileptics will likely have (1) fits at other times; (2) no personal or family history of mood disorder (more likely in women with premenstrual syndrome); (3) epileptic EEG, SPECT, and MRI findings; and (4) elevated prolactin levels within 15–20 minutes of any discrete fit-like episode.

Drug and alcohol abuse is associated with seizures, but abstinence usually avoids any additional fits. Alcoholics can, but rarely do, have withdrawal seizures, and are at greater risk than the general population for unprovoked seizures. Too rapid withdrawal of sedative-hypnotics, benzodiazepines, and anticonvulsants, even in nonepileptics, can cause a seizure. Cocaine intoxication and overdoses of lithium and antidepressants can cause seizures.

Confusional migraine is characterized by loss of consciousness, disorientation, and sensorimotor abnormalities. These patients rarely have automatisms, but do have classic migraines at other times (also see Chapter 16).

Many epileptics with behavioral disturbances are not identified and treated appropriately. Missed diagnosis is due to (1) focusing on longer duration, often more dramatic psychopathology rather than on the brief seizures; (2) not being aware of the association between psychosensory features and epilepsy; and (3) not considering epilepsy in the differential diagnosis. Always think of epilepsy when a patient (1) has an *atypical psychiatric disorder* (e.g., panic disorder that begins for the first time after age 35 years or when attacks last only 1–2 rather than 15–30 minutes); (2) has *syncope* without a clear general medical or neurologic cause; and (3) has an *epilepsy-related diagnosis* (e.g., hysteria, pseudoseizures, conversion disorder, dissociative disorder, or other epilepsy-related conditions).

Frontal lobe epilepsy may be mistaken for obsessive compulsive disorder because these patients can have forced thinking and odd repetitive behavior. Epilepsies with psychosis can be confused with primary psychotic disorders. In addition to having seizures when compared with primary psychoses, epileptic psychoses

TABLE 10.9. Causes of Epilepsy

Cause	Characteristics
Genetic	1. Typical onset between 5 and 10 years of age; siblings most likely to be clinically concordant, or, although asymptomatic, to have EEG abnormalities
	2. A general susceptibility to have seizures has been indirectly associated with chromosomes 2, 3, and 9
	3. Look for associated features: Mental retardation, limb asymmetry, neurologic signs, multiple seizure forms;
	4. Nonspecific genotype affecting seizure threshold most common with primary generalized epilepsy (concordance rates for monozygotic and dizygotic twins 80% and 5%, respectively);
	5. 1% of epileptics have specific genotype (e.g., autosomal-recessive Krabbe's disease and Batten's disease, X-linked Aicardis syndrome, autosomal dominant tuberous sclerosis, neurofibromatosis)
Congenital malformations	1. Vascular and cavernous sinus malformations and cortical dysplasias from cell migrational abnormalities are most common and typically affect frontotemporal regions
	2. Seizure onset typically around puberty, and complex partial seizures most common with vascular, grand mal with cavernous, and partial seizures with dysplasias
	3. Look for other evidence of vascular malformations (e.g., Sturge-Weber syndrome) and MRI evidence of focally reduced structures or disrupted architecture
Birth trauma	1. Anoxia during delivery can cause substantial brain damage, resulting in spasticity, mental retardation, and seizures beginning in infancy
	2. Amman's horn sclerosis, increased risk for childhood febrile convulsions and later epilepsy, is the most common association in patients with temporal lobe seizures

tend to be (1) of shorter duration, (2) without loss of emotional expression, and (3) with an altered sensorium when post-ictal, irritability when prodromal, and with many more inter-ictal personality changes when inter-ictal.

Epilepsy is part of the differential diagnosis of borderline and schizotypal personality disorder, particularly among men patients. Look first for psychosensory features and then for the characteristics of a complex partial seizure.

TABLE 10.9. (*continued*)

Cause	Characteristics
Head trauma	1. 40% of penetrating and 15% of nonpenetrating injuries result in epilepsy, particularly focal seizures that may generalize
	2. See Chapter 11 for characteristics of a substantial nonpenetrating head injury likely to lead to behavioral syndromes.
	3. Epilepsy from head trauma results from scarring and may not develop until several years after the injury; accounts for about 5% of epileptics
Infection	1. Brain infections that produced delirium or seizures during the acute illness are also more likely to lead to later epilepsy: meningitis, encephalitis, epidural or subdural abscesses, brain abscesses
	2. Herpes virus has an affinity for temporal lobe and is implicated in monofocal sites (EEG may just show temporal lobe sharp waves)
Metabolic disorders	1. Seizures commonly confined to acute and rapid metabolic changes: hypoglycemia, electrolyte imbalance (hyponatremia, hypocalcemia), and water intoxication or dehydration
	2. Other causes are glycogen storage diseases, amino acid metabolic disorders (phenylketonuria), lipid storage disease, vitamin deficiencies (e.g., pyridoxine)
Substance abuse	1. Alcohol withdrawal, stimulant drug intoxication, glutamate receptor agonist intoxication (phencyclidine)
	2. Psychotropic drug overdoses or toxicity (e.g., lithium, antidepressants)
	3. Anticonvulsant drug withdrawal
Other neurologic	1. Neoplasms, depending on site (frontotemporal), size (large), and malignancy (low grade)
	2. Neoplasms account for about 5% of epileptic cases, and the most common are gangliogliomas and astrocytomas
	3. Degenerative disease (e.g., vascular dementia)

Epilepsy Work-Up

Seventy percent of epilepsy is idiopathic. Looking for the associated features of the remaining 30% is, however, necessary. Table 10.9 summarizes some of the more likely causes of epilepsy and their other characteristics. Physical examination findings, family history, and specific laboratory tests usually are sufficient to identify these conditions. The remaining laboratory evaluation is to confirm your clinical diagnosis. If the results are negative, and you still believe the patient is an epileptic, treat for epilepsy.

The EEG evaluation is not done to reveal a seizure (too infrequent and too short), but to find inter-ictal discharges: spikes and sharp waves that stand out from the background activity. A complete EEG assessment includes multiple assessments, 24-hour telemetry with video monitoring, and specialized EEG techniques (sleep deprived, hyperventilation, strobe light to look for photic driving [occipital spikes]), and topographic EEG (looking for rapidly changing focal areas or dipoles [a negative sharp peak with an subsequent positive wave]). A repeated focal EEG abnormality with spikes very likely indicates the seizure focus.

When a temporal lobe focus is suspected, an MRI and SPECT are helpful. Amygdala-hippocampal volumes are often reduced and inter-ictal hypometabolism often observed at the site of the focus. During a seizure (rarely captured in a laboratory test) hypermetabolism occurs at the focus. Cerebral blood flow in the temporal lobe with the focus may, however, be normal, indicating an uncoupling between metabolism and blood flow. In addition, reduced benzodiazepine receptor binding is commonly seen at an epileptic focus and in a more restricted distribution with functional MRI than the hypometabolism on SPECT or PET.

Obtain prolactin levels whenever you suspect a patient has just had a seizure. Post-ictal prolactin levels are elevated 15–20 minutes after most grand mal and after 60% of complex partial seizures.

If you suspect a nonepileptic seizure, give intravenous normal saline while doing EEG recording and tell the patient you are giving something that may induce some of his seizure behaviors. Thirty percent of patients with nonepileptic seizures will respond to suggestion and have an episode. When counseled with this evidence of "good news," that is, that they do not have epilepsy, about 50% will stop having these episodes, and among these, 60% remain episode-free, whereas 40% may have occasional recurrences. Patients with some recurrences are likely to have epilepsy or somatoform disorder. Behavior therapy focusing on reducing the reinforcers of the nonepileptic seizures further reduces their frequency. Persons with epileptic seizures, in contrast to those with nonepileptic seizures, are more likely to have (1) a normal premorbid personality; (2) inter-ictal personality changes; and (3) episodes that are random in occurrence or influenced primarily by sleep, eating, and other diurnal patterns, season, menstrual cycle, strong visceral stimuli (e.g., coitus, eating a large meal), or specific triggers (e.g., specific light or sound frequency).

Behaviors during and after a seizure are helpful (but not definitive) in localizing the focus to cortical or subcortical, dominant or nondominant hemisphere. Table 10.10 displays these modest correlations.

TREATMENT AND MANAGEMENT

The treatment and management of epilepsy is difficult and must be comprehensive if the patient is to be seizure-free. Principles of seizure control are

TABLE 10.10. Some Localizing Seizure-Related Behaviors

Cortical	Subcortical*
Ictal aphasia and thought disorder (D)	Rising epigastric sensations and elementary automatisms
Postictal dysphagia (D)	Autonomic signs
Prolonged auditory hallucinations (D)	Aura of fear or panic
Post-ictal disorientation (D)	Olfactory or gustatory hallucinations
Auditory and visual hallucinations in episodic or panoramic form (ND)	Oral automatisms
Illusions, dysmorphopsia, dysmegalopsia (ND)	Sexual behaviors
	Aggression and violence
	Learning and memory problems
	Deja vu and jamais vu
	Absence and dreamy states
	Indescribable sensory experiences
	Derealization and depersonalization

D, dominant hemisphere: ND, nondominant hemisphere.

*Particularly amygdala, parahippocampus, hippocampus, hypothalamus, and septum.

1. *Thoroughly evaluate the pretreatment seizure pattern,* which includes number and type of seizures; the presence of nonepileptic seizures; triggers; any diurnal or seasonal pattern; details of the aura, ictus, post-ictal, and inter-ictal periods; environmental stressors; cognitive/interpersonal/job functioning; personality dimensions; and personal and family strengths.
2. *Thoroughly evaluate associated behavioral syndromes* to determine
   a. To which period of epilepsy (e.g., ictal/post-ictal) they relate
   b. If the syndromes are caused by previous or present anticonvulsive treatments (e.g., 50% of epileptic children develop an attention deficit hyperactivity syndrome [ADHD] from phenobarbital and phenytoin; an adult epileptic's irritability and decreased frustration tolerance and cognitive changes adversely affecting social and job functioning may occur from phenytoin or higher doses of any anticonvulsant; phenytoin toxicity can cause psychosis)
   c. what is the behavioral syndrome (e.g., manias, depressions, anxiety disorders, etc.)
3. *Choose the best anticonvulsant under the circumstances,* maximize its dose, and if there is an initial response, stick with it if you can for at least 6 months before considering changing or adding medications. The more anticonvulsants a patient is taking the more seizures he is likely to

have; reducing anticonvulsants from several to one often leads to seizure control.

Although somewhat controversial, many epileptologists start antiepileptic medication after a single unprovoked seizure because 70% of patients will have more seizures and because treatment leads to substantial reduction in the risk of relapse. Table 10.11 lists the characteristics of some anticonvulsants. All but gabapentin and topiramate are metabolized by the liver. Most are protein bound. Gabapentin is not, and topiramate, felbamate, and primidone are only weakly protein bound (less that 30%).

4. *Minimize stressors (family, job problems) and triggers* (caffeine use, situations in which the patient is exposed to bright flickering lights, such as passing over a trestle bridge on a bright sunny day). Stress management, biofeedback, and patient and family counseling can reduce seizure frequency.

5. *Correct all co-occurring general medical conditions* because they can complicate anticonvulsant treatment (increasing side effect risks or resulting in adverse drug–drug interactions), or they may directly reduce the seizure threshold leading to poor seizure control. For some women patients whose seizures cluster during the luteal phase of menses (catamenial seizures), progesterone lozenges 200 mg TID on days 15–25 and then tapered can reduce by 50% the frequency of complex partial and secondary generalized fits, particularly if associated with dysphoric depression.

6. *For children, the three most important factors in shaping treatment and management are*
   a. *Determine the specific etiology* that is more likely knowable in childhood onset epilepsy
   b. *Identify and treat co-morbid conditions:* ADHD, oppositional defiant disorder, mood disorder, autism, spectrum disorders, learning disabilities, conduct disorder, adjustment disorders, mental retardation, communication disorders, nonepileptic seizures, psychosis
   c. *Family functioning:* provide counseling, education, support groups, caregiver holidays, home care assistance to minimize caregiver stress. Help family members deal with their expectations of their child's development and future functioning, the financial costs of care and time away from work, and time and energy required to give care and simultaneously be parents to nonaffected siblings.

7. *Cognitively assess all epileptic patients when they are in an inter-ictal, behaviorally asymptomatic state:* Some patients with childhood onset seizures are also mentally retarded, and many patients with mesial temporal lobe foci develop cognitive impairment (decreased verbal comprehension and fluency and verbal memory [dominant hemisphere focus], problems with perceptual organization). To minimize chronicity, provide cognitive rehabilitation for those patients with any deficits.

Table 10.12 lists some specific treatment suggestions for the more common behavioral syndromes associated with epilepsy. With comprehensive treatment many epileptics do well and lead normal or almost normal lives. Many U.S. states and other countries however, have placed some driving restrictions on epileptics, often depending on the duration of seizure-free periods. Frequency and type of seizures also guides any job restrictions (e.g., working with machinery, working on ladders or roofs). Epileptics who commit a crime during or around a seizure (e.g., assault) cannot plead guilty for "medical reasons," but can plead guilty by reason of insanity even though they were not psychotic.

Psychosurgery

Twenty percent of epileptics continue to have seizures, despite aggressive drug therapy. Many of these patients can benefit from psychosurgery, but only a small percentage of these patients are referred.

Epilepsy surgery requires a team of specialists working within a high-tech, high-resource epilepsy-surgery center. Extensive behavioral, neurologic, cognitive, and brain structural and functional assessments are needed to select appropriate patients. The most common procedure (for refractory complex partial with and without generalized seizures from mesial temporal lobe foci) involves removal of the amygdala and anterior part of the hippocampus, entorhinal cortex, and a small part of the temporal pole, leaving the lateral temporal neocortex intact. Other procedures include neocortical resection or lesionectomy (for refractory partial seizures), hemispherectomy and large multilobar resection (for refractory unilateral seizures from large or widespread lesions), and corpus callosotomy (for refractory drop attacks). Appropriate patients are those who have not responded to aggressive drug and adjunct behavioral treatments and who have a surgically remediable lesion (e.g., hippocampal sclerosis, vascular malformation, localized cortical dysplasia, glioma).

Two-thirds of surgically treated patients become seizure free, and another 10%–20% improve. Because most patients are in otherwise good health, surgical complications are infrequent (<2%) and are confined to bleeding and infection. Surgery does not increase behavioral problems and may ameliorate episodes of irritability and personality change (if done early in the course).

Newer surgical techniques implanting electrodes in the cerebellum or into the thalamus that then deliver a low electrical current to ameliorate seizure-related mood disturbances are experimental and unproven. An implantable (under chest skin), programmable pulse generator that delivers constant current electrical signals to the vagus nerve to abort seizures (with long prodromes or auras) also needs more study.

Outcome

Between 60% and 80% of epileptics gain full or substantial seizure control. Surgery can cure or substantially help 60%–80% of well-selected patients refractory to other treatments. Those most likely to do well with drug treatment are pa-

TABLE 10.11. Characteristics of Some Anticonvulsants

Drug	Dosing for Epilepsy	Clinical Considerations
Phenytoin (Dilantin)	1. Slow absorption, 20-hour half-life, once or twice daily 200–500 mg/day for adults, 4–7 mg/kg daily for children 2. Therapeutic level 10–20 ng/ml	1. Not directly helpful for the behavioral syndromes of epilepsy 2. Best limited for partial and grand mal 3. Can cause psychosis 4. Avoid use in children because of ADHD-like syndrome side effects, coarsening of facial features, and gum hyperplasia 5. May also cause nystagmus, lethargy, ataxia, rash, hepatitis, hirsutism, lymphodenopathy; 6. Stabilizes neural membranes, GABAergic, potentiates serotonin
Phenobarbital (Arco-Lase, Donnatal, Quadrinal, Bellatal)	Slow absorption, 100-hour half-life, once or twice a day dosing, 30–120 mg/day for adults, 3–7 mg/kg/day for children, 2–5 mg/kg/day for drug for neonates	1. Not helpful for the behavioral syndromes of epilepsy 2. A second-line drug for grand mal in children, but can cause ADHD-like syndrome in children and irritability in children and adults; 3. Can also cause lethargy, ataxia, rash, and, rarely, Stevens-Johnson syndrome and serum sickness 4. Enhances GABA inhibition of ion channels and release of excitatory amino acids (glutamate)
Primidone (Mysoline)	Rapid absorption, 12-hour half-life, but metabolizes to phenobarbital, TID dosing at 300–1,500 mg/day	Used only for children
Carbamazepine (Tegretol)	1. Pharmacology covered in Chapter 8 2. For epilepsy, 600–1,600 mg daily for adults, 5–20 mg/kg/day for children divided 2–3 times daily, 4–12 µg/ml therapeutic range	1. Drug of choice for partial seizures with or without generalization 2. Use for partial complex seizures if associated behavioral syndrome depression or irritability 3. Aplastic anemia, hepatitis, pancreatitis, rash, and hyponatremia can occur (most are rare) 4. Diplopia, dizziness, headache, and nausea most common complaints 5. Stabilizes sodium channels, GABAergic, affinity for peripheral-like benzodiazepine receptors
Valproate (Depakote, Depakene)	1. Pharmacology covered in Chapter 8	1. Broad spectrum, used for most types of generalized seizures and for complex partial seizures

TABLE 10.11. (*continued*)

Drug	Dosing for Epilepsy	Clinical Considerations
	2. For epilepsy, 375–3,000 mg/day for adults, 15–45 mg/kg/day for children divided BID or TID, 50–125 µg/ml therapeutic range	2. Use if associated behavioral syndrome bipolar-like 3. Tremor, weight gain, hair loss, and ankle swelling common side effects 4. GABA agonist that inhibits sodium and potassium conductance and suppresses kindling
Felbamate (Felbatol)	1. 20-hour half-life; 1,800–4,800 mg/day divided BID or TID for adults and 15–45 mg/kg/day for children 2. May work on aspartate receptors 3. Increases blood levels of phenytoin and valproate by 20%, valproate increases felbamate levels by 80%, carbamazepine reduces those levels; felbamate increases carbamazepine epoxide (causes neurotoxicity)	1. Used for partial seizures and as an adjunctive drug for Lennox-Gastaut syndrome 2. Can cause insomnia, anorexia, nausea, vomiting, and headache, rarely aplastic anemia and hepatic neurosis 3. Not a first-line drug
Gabapentin (Neurontin)	1. 8-hour half-life, 600–4,800 mg/day in adults, 10–30 mg/kg/day in children, TID dosing 2. May work on neurotransmitter precursors intracellularly	1. Used for partial seizures; 2. Not helpful for behavioral syndromes 3. Can cause lethargy, ataxia, dizziness, headache, ADHD-like - syndrome, and irritability in children 4. Inhibits release of excitatory amino acids
Lamotrigine (Lamictal)	1. 24-hour half-life, 200–800 mg/day for adults, 3–15 mg/kg/day for children, once or twice daily 2. Metabolism affected by valproate	1. Used for intractable partial epilepsy 2. Can cause lethargy, dizziness, slowed thinking, ataxia, renal stones (rare) 3. Works on sodium channels, inhibiting glutamate release
Clonazepam (Klonopin)	1. Peak onset 1–3 hours, 50%–80% protein bound, 20–80-hour half-life, liver metabolism with no autoinduction 2. Once a day dosing up to 16 mg	1. Used for absence, myoclonic, atonic, and infantile spasm 2. Also for Gilles de la Tourette's syndromes, restless leg syndrome, facial spasm 3. Side effects: Ataxia, drowsiness, paradoxical disinhibition 4. Potentiates GABA transmission, increases synaptic concentrations of serotonin (increases synthesis), and has affinity for benzodiazepine receptors

TABLE 10.12. Treatment Suggestions for the More Common Behavioral Syndromes Associated with Epilepsy

Syndrome	Suggested Management
Prodrome psychosis	Electroconvulsive therapy (ECT; was essentially invented for this)
Post-ictal psychosis	Several days sedation with phenobarbital or a benzodiazepine with antiseizure properties (e.g., diazepam, clonazepam); valproate; ECT
Inter-ictal psychosis	ECT, valproate, carbamazepine
Depression	ECT, selected serotonin reuptake inhibitors, with low seizure potential (sertraline), desipramine, monoamine oxidase inhibitors
Aggression (post-ictal, or intermittent explosive disorder)	Brief sedation if post-ictal with benzodiazepines with anticonvulsive properties: Clonazepam (1–4 mg), diazepam (10–25 mg); if irritability more prolonged or recurrent, evaluate for medication effect and correct; if not medication effect, but prolonged, carbamazepine; psychosurgery last resort (25%–50% improvement)
Apathy	Methylphenidate, dextroamphetamine, bromocriptine (in low doses to avoid seizure induction)
Personality change	Education, counseling, behavior modification, some improvement with psychosurgery if seizure associated with discrete focus in mesial (adhesive/vision) or lateral (irritable) temporal lobe

tients who (1) are compliant with treatment, (2) have an idiopathic epilepsy, (3) have seizures related to specific triggers (e.g., reduced sleep) that can be avoided, (4) do not drink or use drugs, (5) have partial fits only, (6) have a prolonged prodrome that gives them time to take treatment to abort or control the fit, and (7) do not have a substantial behavioral syndrome and cognitive impairment.

ADDITIONAL READINGS

Ahern GL, Herring AM, Tackenberg J, Seeger JF, Oomnen KJ, Labiner DM, Weinand ME: The association of multiple personality and temporal lobe epilepsy. Intracarotid amobarbital test observations. *Arch Neurol* 50:1020–1025, 1993.

Bear DM, Fedio P: Quantitative analysis of interictal behavior in temporal lobe epilepsy. *Arch Neurol* 34:454–467, 1977.

Benson DF, Blumer D: Psychiatric manifestations of epilepsy. In Benson DF, Blumer D (eds): *Psychiatric Aspects of Neurologic Disease*, vol 2. Grune & Stratton, New York, 1982, pp 25–47.

Benson DF, Miller BL, Signer SF: Dual personality associated with epilepsy. *Arch Neurol* 43:471–474, 1986.

Bredkjaer SR, Mortensen PB, Parnas J: Epilepsy and non-organic non-affective psychosis: National epidemiologic study. *Br J Psychiatry* 172:235–238, 1998.

Breslau N, Merikangas K, Bowden CL: Comorbidity of migraine and panic disorder. *Neurology 44* (suppl 7):S17–S22, 1994.

Brodie MJ: Established anticonvulsants and treatment of refractory epilepsy. *Lancet 336*:350–354, 1990.

Cendes F, Andermann F, Gloor P, Evans A, Jones-Gotman M, Watson C, Melanson D, Olivier A, Peters T, Lopes-Cendes I, Leroux G: MRI volumetric measurement of amygdala and hippocampus in temporal lobe epilepsy. *Neurology 43*:719–725, 1993.

Cohen RJ, Suter C: Hysterical seizures: Suggestion as a provocative EEG test. Arch Neurol *11*:391–395, 1982.

Devinsky O, Putnam F Grafman J, Bromfield E, Theodore WH: Dissociative states and epilepsy. *Neurology 39*:835–840, 1989.

Devinsky O, Vazquez B: Behavioral changes associated with epilepsy. In Brumback RA (ed): *Behavioral Neurology, Neurologic Clinics,* vol 11. WB Saunders, Philadelphia, 1993, pp 127–149.

Duncan JS: Imaging and epilepsy. *Brain 120*:339–377, 1997.

Editorial: Epilepsy and disorders of neuronal migration. *Lancet 336*:1035–1036, 1990.

Engel J Jr: Surgery for seizures. *N Engl J Med 334*:647–652, 1996.

Feindel W, Rasmussen T: Temporal lobectomy with amygdalectomy and minimal hippocampal resection: Review of 100 cases. *Can J Neurosci 18*:603–605, 1991.

Gilad R, Lampl Y, Galbay U, Eshel Y, Sarova-Pinhas I: Early treatment of a single generalized tonic-clonic seizure to prevent recurrence. *Arch Neurol 53*:1149–1152, 1996.

Gould R, Miller BL, Goldberg MA, Benson DF: The validity of hysterical signs and symptoms. *J Nerv Ment Dis 174*:593–597, 1986.

Hermann BP, Seidenberg M, Schoenfeld J, Davies K: Neuropsychological characteristics of the syndrome of mesial temporal lobe epilepsy. *Arch Neurol 54*:369–376, 1997.

Herzog AG, Seibel MM, Schomer DL, Vaitukaitus JL, Geschwind N: Reproductive endocrine disorders in women with partial seizures of temporal lobe origin. *Arch Neurol 43*:341–346, 1986.

Jackson GD, Kuzniecky RI, Cascino GD: Hippocampal sclerosis without detectable hippocampal atrophy. *Neurology 44*:42–46, 1994.

Jasper HH, Riggio S, Goldman-Rakic PS (eds): *Epilepsy and the Functional Anatomy of the Frontal Lobe, Advances in Neurology,* vol 66. Raven Press, New York, 1995.

Jensen R, Brinck T, Olesen J: Sodium valproate has a prophylactic effect in migraine without aura: A triple-blind, placebo-controlled crossover study. *Neurology 44*:647–651, 1994.

Kumar KL: Recent advances in the acute management of migraine and cluster headaches. *J Gen Intern Med 9*:339–348, 1994.

Laskowitz DT, Sperling MR, French JA, O'Conner MJ: The syndrome of frontal lobe epilepsy. Characteristics and surgical management. *Neurology 45*:780–787, 1995.

Leis AA, Ross MA, Summers AK: Psychogenic seizures. Ictal characteristics and diagnostic pitfalls. *Neurology 42*:95–99, 1992.

Lipton RB, Ottman R, Ehrenberg BL, Hauser WA: Comorbidity of migraine: The connection between migraine and epilepsy. *Neurology 44*(suppl 7):S28–S32, 1994.

Lowenstein DH, Alldredge BK: Status epilepticus. *N Engl J Med 338*:970–976, 1998.

Mace CJ, Trimble MR: Ten-year prognosis of conversion disorder. *Br J Psychiatry 169*:282–288, 1996.

Make ME Jr, Paakalnis A, Phillips BB: Neuropsychological and psychiatric correlates of intractable pseudoseizures. *Seizure 1*:11–13, 1992.

Markley HG: Verapamil and migraine prophylaxis: Mechanisms and efficacy. *Am J Med 90* (suppl SA):49S–53S, 1991.

Mathew NT, Saper JR, Silberstein SD, Rankin L, Markley HG, Solomon S, Rapoport AM, Silber CJ, Deaton RL: Migraine prophylaxis with divalproex. *Arch Neurol 52*:281–286, 1995.

Mendez MF, Doss RC, Taylor JL, Arguello R: Relationship of seizure variables to personality disorders in epilepsy. *J Neuropsychiatry Clin Neurosci 5*:283–286, 1993.

Merikangas KR, Fenton BT, Cheng SH, Stolar MJ, Risch N: Association between migraine and stroke in a large scale epidemiological study of the United States. *Arch Neurol* 54:362–368, 1997.

Mesulam MM: Dissociative states with abnormal temporal lobe EEG. Multiple personality and the illusion of possession. *Arch Neurol 38*:176–181, 1981.

Nielsen H, Kristensen O: Personality correlates of sphenoidal EEG foci in temporal lobe epilepsy. *Acta Neurol Scand 64*:289–300, 1981.

Persinger MA: Canonical correlation of a temporal lobe signs scale with schizoid and hypomania scales in a normal population: Men and women are similar but for different reasons. *Percept Motor Skills 73*:615–618, 1991.

Post RM, Silberstein SD: Shared mechanisms in affective illness, epilepsy, and migraine. *Neurology 44* (suppl 7):S37–S47, 1994.

Ramsay RE: Advances in the pharmacology of epilepsy. *Epilepsia 34*(suppl 5):S9–S16, 1993.

Rise, ML, Frankel WN, Coffin JM, Seyfried TN: Genes for epilepsy mapped in the mouse. *Science 253*:669–673, 1991.

Rubin E, Dhawan V, Moeller JR, Takikawa S, Labor DR, Schaul N, Barr WB, Eidelberg D: Cerebral metabolic topography in unilateral temporal lobe epilepsy. *Neurology 45*:2212–2223, 1995.

Sanders VJ, Felison SL, Waddell AE, Conrad AJ, Schmid P, Swartz BE, Kaufman M, Walsh GO, DeSalles AAF, Tourtellotte WW: Presence of herpes simplex DNA in surgical tissue from human epileptic seizure foci detected by polymerase chain reaction. Preliminary study. *Arch Neurol 54*:954–960, 1997.

Schenk L, Bear D: Multiple personality and related dissociative phenomena in patients with temporal lobe epilepsy. *Am J Psychiatry 138*:1311–1316, 1981.

Schwartz TH, Bazil CW, Walczak TS, Chan S, Pedley TA, Goodman RR: The predictive value of intraoperative electrocorticography in resections for limbic epilepsy associated with mesial temporal sclerosis. *Neurosurgery 40*:302–311, 1997.

Shen W, Bowman ES, Markand ON: Presenting the diagnosis of pseudoseizure. *Neurology 40*:756–759, 1990.

Shorvon SD, Reynolds EH: Reduction of polypharmacy for epilepsy. *BMJ 2*:1023–1025, 1979.

Silberstein SD, Lipton RB: Overview of diagnosis and treatment of migraine. *Neurology 44*(suppl 7):S6–S16, 1994.

Silberstein SD, Merriam GR: Sex hormones and headache. *J Pain Symptom Manage 8*:98–114, 1993.

Silberstein SD, Young WB: Migraine aura and prodrome. *Semin Neurol 15*:175–182, 1995.

Smith DB, Treiman DM, Trimble MR (eds): *Neurobehavioral Problems in Epilepsy, Advances in Neurology*, vol. 55. Raven Press, New York, 1991.

Stewart W, Breslau N, Keck PE Jr: Comorbidity of migraine and panic disorders. *Neurology 44*(suppl 7):S23–S27, 1994.

Terry RS, Tarver WB, Zabara J: The implantable neurocybernetic prosthesis system. *PACE 14*:86–93, 1991.

Toni C, Cassano GB, Perugi G, Murri L, Mancino M, Petracca A, Akiskal H, Roth M: Psychosensorial and related phenomena in panic disorder and in temporal lobe epilepsy. *Compr Psychiatry 37*:125–133, 1996.

Trimble MR: *The Psychoses of Epilepsy*. Raven Press, New York, 1991.

Trimble MR, Bolwig TG (eds): *The Temporal Lobes and the Limbic System*. Wrightson Medical Publishing, Ltd, Petersfield, 1992.

van Paesschen W, Sisodiya S, Connelly A, Duncan JS, Free SL, Raymond AA, Grunewald RA, Revesz T, Shorvon SD, Fish DR, Stevens JM, Johnson CL, Scaravilli F, Harkness WFJ, Jackson GD: Quantitative hippocampal MRI and intractable temporal lobe epilepsy. *Neurology 45*:2233–2240, 1995.

Welch KMA: Relationship of stroke and migraine. *Neurology 44*(suppl 7):S33–S36, 1994.

11

Traumatic Brain Injury and Stroke

TRAUMATIC BRAIN INJURY

Each year about 200/100,000 Americans (80% mild, 10% substantial, 10% severe) suffer a traumatic brain injury (TBI). Only 15% are hospitalized, but 50%–100% have ongoing neurologic impairment. Reduced head injury mortality has increased the number of persons with TBI-related neuropsychiatric disabilities. TBI incidence peaks between 15 and 25 years of age and again after 60 years. Males are two to three times as likely as females to be seriously injured, and 50% of persons with TBI have substantial blood alcohol levels at time of injury. About 20% of victims are left with significant disability.

Head injuries received in war are usually penetrating and lead to focal syndromes. In nonwar circumstances, closed head injuries are more common, and 90% of patients survive. The most common causes are motor vehicle accidents (more than 50%), falls (21%), violence (12%), and recreation (10%). Acceleration/deceleration of the brain is the usual injury mechanism. Closed head injuries can lead to mild changes (postconcussion syndrome or mild frontal lobe personality changes) or to more dramatic regional brain syndromes, dementia, or seizure disorder.

Head injuries are classified as penetrating or closed head, the former always severe. If the latter is associated with a skull fracture, it is severe. Closed head injuries without skull fracture are classified using the Glasgow Coma Scale: 13–15 (mild), 9–12 (moderate), and 3–8 (severe) (Table 11.1).

CLINICAL PRESENTATIONS

If a behavioral syndrome develops for the first time following an open head injury or a head injury resulting in a skull fracture, assume the TBI to be the cause of the behavioral syndrome. The greater the depth of penetration and the more brain tissue destroyed, the greater the validity of this assumption.

If at the time of injury the person's head was in motion (e.g., falls, traffic acci-

TABLE 11.1. Glasgow Coma Scale

Response	Type	Score*
Eye opening (E)	Spontaneous	4
	To speech	3
	To pain	2
	Nil	1
Best motor response (M)	Obeys	6
	Localizes	5
	Withdrawn	4
	Abnormal flexion	3
	Extensor response	2
	Nil	1
Verbal response (V)	Orientated	5
	Confused conversation	4
	Inappropriate words	3
	Incomprehensive sounds	2
	Nil	1

*Coma score (E + M + V) = 3 to 15.

dents) the likelihood of contracoup injury increases. If the head was static at injury (e.g., bullet wounds, blows), a local lesion at point of impact is likely. Contracoup and concussive injuries are rarer with penetrating than with closed head trauma.

Table 11.2 characterizes closed head injuries tending to cause neuropsychiatric disability. Consider that 10% of persons with traumatic brain lacerations and 50% of persons with traumatic brain hemorrhage do not have concurrent skull fracture, so the immediate and short-term sequelae of the injury are the most valid indications of severity. The longer and deeper the unconsciousness, the more prolonged and disabling the post concussion syndrome, and the more neurologic signs upon awakening, the worse the injury.

Most head injury patients will have some *retrograde amnesia* for the few mo-

TABLE 11.2. Characteristics of a Closed Head Injury Likely to Cause Neuropsychiatric Disability

Unconscious longer than 15 minutes

Profound coma (Glasgow Coma Scale score <12)*

Prolonged (>72 hours) postconcussion syndrome

Prolonged (>48 hours) anterograde amnesia

Neurologic signs (e.g., diplopia, seizure) immediately after injury

Prolonged (>1 week) impaired functioning following injury

*A Glasgow score more than 12, unconsciousness less than 20 minutes, and anterograde amnesia less than 48 hours characterizes a "mild" head injury, but these injuries can cause a postconcussion syndrome.

ments before the injury. These memories were not yet put into long-term storage and were literally knocked out of the patient's head. Retrograde amnesia of this type is clinically insignificant. However, substantial amnesia for large portions of the patient's life is associated with the severest head trauma. *Anterograde amnesia* (i.e., amnesia for events after the injury) highly correlates with the degree of head injury (the longer the anterograde amnesia, the worse the injury), because it results from continued active pathophysiology preventing the acquisition of new memory. During the period of anterograde amnesia the patient will appear unfocused, not remember recent conversations, may have an altered sleep–wake cycle, and be disoriented to time of day (unlike when delirious, they will not be agitated, fearful, or otherwise disoriented). A patient with a head injury resulting in the above is at substantial risk for a neuropsychiatric disorder later in life. Table 11.3 lists common behavioral complaints of TBI victims.

The *postconcussion syndrome* occurs in 80%–100% of patients with mild but clinically meaningful head injury. Most symptoms resolve within 3–6 months postinjury, but about 6% of patients may remain symptomatic for years. Postconcussion syndrome sufferers are not malingering. They are no more likely than other persons to have preexisting "neurotic" traits. They have brain dysfunction. In addition to problems with attention and new learning, and at least one feature listed in Table 11.3, these patients may show modest magnetic resonance imaging (MRI) changes (scattered punctate hyperintensities suggesting axon shearing) and brain glucose hypometabolism during cognitive tasks. Forty percent will have nonspecific EEG slowing. Most of these patients also demonstrate abnormal caloric testing, vestibular dysfunction on electronystagmography, and delayed waveforms in brain stem auditory evoked potentials.

Persistent cognitive dysfunction is the main feature in over 80% of patients with postconcussion syndrome (attention, reaction time [particularly when faced with choices], new learning, delayed response to verbal and written language). Those with mild cognitive impairment (often nondominant hemisphere and frontal in pattern) may respond to standard doses of stimulants (methylphenidate, amphetamines), monoamine oxidase inhibitors (MAOIs), or amantadine. Patients under 60 years who are irritable or assaultive, particularly in the initial phase of the syndrome, may respond to propranolol in doses as high as 320 mg daily.

TABLE 11.3. Typical Chief Complaints of Head Injury Victims with Neuropsychiatric Disability

---

Postconcussion syndrome complaints (30%–50%): Headache, fatigue, dizziness, blurred or double vision, noise and light sensitivity, insomnia, irritability

Emotional complaints (20%–50%): Feeling depressed, apprehensive, anxious, or moody with unexpected fluctuations in moods

Cognitive complaints: Trouble concentrating, forgetfulness, trouble "handling" information

Behavioral complaints: More easily angered, yelling or striking out, "personality" change, impulsive

---

Improvement from postconcussion syndrome is accelerated if you combine medication with psychotherapy. Specifically, education about signs and symptoms, their nature and causes and how to deal with them (including consumer manuals), reassurance that most patients recover fully, stress management techniques, discouraging the patient's negative biases about his symptoms, and providing a schedule for gradual resumption of preinjury activities and responsibilities with specific reinforcers for success all have a substantial therapeutic benefit. Patients who respond best are those with (1) mild injuries and no seizures, (2) no premorbid antisocial, histrionic, or other DSM Cluster B personality traits; (3) more education or other evidence of good "brain reserve"; and (4) the ApoE polymorphism gene 2/2 or 3/3 (4/4 is twice as likely as the others to have poor outcome and is the same gene that influences risk and severity for Alzheimer's disease).

Patients may also develop a "postconcussion-like" syndrome after a viral infection. Mononucleosis, viral hepatitis, and influenza without recognizable encephalitis are the viral illnesses most likely to produce this syndrome, which can become chronic or episodic. These patients may also respond to stimulants or MAOIs.

Mood disorder resulting from head injury is also common. About 60% of head injury patients have a nonmelancholic modest depression. If postconcussion depression persists beyond several weeks or is incapacitating, standard antidepressant treatment can be effective. If the depression is mostly dysphoric, carbamazepine helps. Widespread injury to nondominant frontoparietal cortex (on the lateral surface and toward the top) and subcortical connections is most likely to produce this dysphoric depression.

Anxiety disorders following TBI occur in about 60% of patients, particularly as a phobia-like response to the situation in which they were injured. Anxiety beyond 3–6 months post-TBI tends to be generalized, associated with fatigue, and is linked to situations in which demands are placed on the patient's cognitive, language, motor, and other areas with deficits. Although benzodiazepines are often used to treat short-lasting anxiety, they can cause memory impairment, ataxia, sedation, and, in rare instances, disinhibition. Long-term use leads to dependence. If generalized anxiety persists past 2 weeks or side effects become problematic, consider alternatives. These include buspirone (5 mg BID to start, 5-mg increases every 5 days to a maximum daily dose of 45 mg), propranolol (up to 80 mg BID), and naltrexone (50–100 mg daily).

Phobias and agoraphobia also can develop, usually in response to balance problems and vertigo. Treatment of the neurologic problem and then office and in vivo desensitization of the phobic situation are effective (see Chapter 15). *Social phobias* can develop as cognitive demands are placed on the patient that he cannot meet. This is particularly likely for the patient who has no obvious language or motor disorder and so is assumed to be well (e.g., a patient with frontal lobe or nondominant parietal lobe injury). Attention to matching placement, management strategies, and social and job goals with the patient's cognitive strengths and weaknesses minimizes this problem. Treatments for primary social phobia are also effective (see Chapter 15), but not as good as prevention.

Obsessive compulsive behaviors following TBI can develop with basal ganglia injury (right more than left). Treatment is the same as for primary obsessive compulsive disorder (see Chapter 14).

Irritability is a complaint of nearly 50% of head injury patients. Depending on the size and location of the brain injury, the irritability can result in tantrums and provoked or unprovoked assaults (dyscontrol syndrome). Treatment for these patients includes (1) avoiding substances that may induce irritability or agitation (e.g., alcohol, hypnotics, opiates, steroids, stimulants, anticholinergics); (2) education about the association between the head trauma and the behavioral syndrome; (3) rehabilitation, employment, and socialization planning based on assessment of cognitive strengths and weaknesses; and (4) pharmacotherapy such as anticonvulsants or lithium in doses typical for psychiatric patients or fluoxetine in standard antidepressant doses for dysphoric patients and buspirone in anti-anxiety, or higher doses.

Epilepsy can develop after TBI, and TBI patients with mild head injury have a 1.5-fold increased risk for seizures during the 5 years after injury. This risk is substantially elevated in the older TBI patient. About 5% of mild and about 12% of severe closed head injury patients develop a seizure disorder. Closed head injuries most likely causing seizures are those that include (1) a brain contusion, subdural hematoma, depressed skull fracture, or intracerebral bleed; (2) loss of consciousness of greater than 20 minutes or anterograde amnesia of more than 24 hours, (3) injury to the temporal lobes; and (4) occurrence in childhood. Standard EEGs are often abnormal, but not specifically epileptic. Nevertheless, these patients respond to carbamazepine or valproate.

Psychosis occasionally develops after head injury. Psychosis is more likely when the injury involves the temporal lobes or the orbitomesial aspects of the frontal lobes. Although many types of psychoses have been reported following TBI, the most common are (1) mood disorders, specifically mania with frontal (right more than left) or bilateral temporal lobe lesions, depression with nondominant large lesions; positive-symptom nonaffective psychoses with mesial frontotemporal lesions (left more than right); (2) epileptic psychosis; (3) paraphrenias where one psychopathologic feature predominates (auditory hallucinations with left hemisphere temporal lobe lesions; experiences of alienation and control with right parietal lobe lesions; misidentification delusions [Capgras, Fregoli's reduplicative paramnesia] with nondominant temporal parietal lobe lesions); and (4) schizophrenia-like pschosis (with subcortical bilateral fronto-temporal lesions).

Because giving neuroleptics to patients with head injury may slow neurocognitive recovery, alternative treatments are preferred for psychosis secondary to TBI. These include carbamazepine and valproate (for psychosis associated with a mood disturbance, seizures, or psychosensory features); lithium (if the psychosis is associated with manic-like behaviors or irritability); and electroconvulsive therapy (ECT; for most disorders when the injury occurred over 6 months before). If you must prescribe a neuroleptic, risperidone in doses up to 8 mg daily or low doses of haloperidol may be the least problematic choices. Recovery is not as good as in the primary syndromes.

Personality changes are commonly reported after moderate to severe closed head injury. Most commonly, these behavioral changes are not in classic personality traits (see Chapter 6), but represent chronic frontal lobe syndromes (see Chapters 1 and 12).

Table 11.4 lists the chronic behavior patterns seen after severe TBI. Patients with injuries of the temporal lobes and adjacent structures also may develop problems with sexual arousal and control (increased arousal and reduced control with excitatory lesions, decreased libido with ablating lesions).

Post-traumatic dementia can occur with severe closed head injury when mechanical forces at the moment of impact produce a shearing effect, causing diffuse axonal (i.e., white matter) injury. Whether it occurs independently or with more circumscribed effects of acceleration/deceleration lesions, this injury often results in a complex picture of a subcortical dementia (see Chapter 12) plus a regional cortical syndrome.

Post-traumatic thalamic syndrome results from a relatively circumscribed injury to the thalamus after a closed head injury. This syndrome is characterized by a variable initial period of generalized analgesia, followed by lateralized (contralateral to a unilateral lesion) or generalized spontaneous pain or pain as a response to a stimulus not usually considered pain inducing. Constant or paroxysmal symptoms can be associated with frontal lobe cognitive and language problems, thalamic-like aphasic responses, odd sensations such as formication (tactile hallucinations of itching or crawling insects under the skin) or other paresthesias, and gnawing, crushing or freezing sensations. Becoming verbally or physically abusive, using obscenities, and feeling fearful or angry at seeing unfamiliar faces also may occur. The syndrome can be mistaken for hysteria or an atypical psychosis. Diagnosis requires a particularly careful evaluation, including brain imaging studies. Carbamazepine (400–1,200 mg) and other tricyclics (e.g., amitriptyline 50–150 mg daily) help patients with this syndrome. Clonidine and beta-blockers may also help.

Hemisphere lateralization syndromes can occur with TBI. These are rarely as well demarcated as syndromes from stroke, but they follow the same basic patterns

TABLE 11.4. Chronic Behavioral Changes After Severe Closed Head Injury

Lateral frontal orbital pattern (40%)*: Irritable, immature, emotionally labile, unrealistic, lacking insight and self-direction, restless, impatient, impulsive, sensitive to noise and stress, episodic dyscontrol with nonpredatory violence, manic-like psychopathology, suspiciousness, and delusions (rare)

Dorsolateral prefrontal pattern (10%–30%): Lack of spontaneity; loss of interest, drive, and initiative; sluggish; socially isolative; easily fatigued; and dysphoric

Childishness pattern† (40%): Self-centered, insensitive to others, giddy, overtalkative and exuberant, euphoric, anosognosia, needs supervision or continued care to achieve goals

*Numbers in parentheses are percentages of modest to severe closed TBI patients reported to have the syndrome.

†May be an exaggeration of premorbid personality traits.

outlined in Chapters 1 and 4 (e.g., language related [dominant hemisphere]; visu-ospatial, visuomotor related [nondominant hemisphere]).

Assessment

Motor Behavior

Always assess the motor system from the left/right, front/back, top/bottom perspectives described in Chapter 3. Motor strength assessment is not enough for the person with TBI. Look for asymmetry, slowness, awkwardness, and inertia (trouble starting and stopping). The worse the motor function, the worse the prognosis.

Frontal Lobe Features

Because the frontal lobes are often damaged in TBI, check for frontal lobe release signs (grasp and gegenhalten, Hoffman's sign, palmomental, suck, snout, rooting reflexes). Check smell because damage to orbitofrontal cortex can damage nearby olfactory nerves. Anosmia correlates with a poor outcome for this reason. Also, the more frontal lobe features a person with TBI has, the worse the outcome. The presence of the dorsolateral prefrontal cortex or the lateral orbitofrontal syndromes predicts chronicity.

Speech and Language

Assess speech and language thoroughly. Besides predicting injury location, the more speech and language problems a person with TBI has, the worse the outcome. Classic aphasia symptoms seen in stroke are rare, and mixed aphasias are most common.

Seizures

With lacerations and contusions from closed head injury, seizures result from subsequent scarring that then develops into an excitatory focus. This process may take several years to develop so that there is often a 1–5 year lag between injury and first seizure. Those seizures developing closer to the injury are more likely associated with behavioral problems. The most common TBI-related seizure type is complex partial epilepsy. Always check for seizure-like episodes and behaviors in TBI patients with episodic behavioral problems. Always check visual fields, which can be "cut" when the temporal lobes are damaged because visual pathways pass through the temporal lobes on their way to the occipital cortex.

Drug and Alcohol Abuse

Drug and alcohol use is often a contributing cause to TBI. Use also damages the brain, and some agents (e.g., cocaine) can sensitize limbic structures. Past drug use and alcohol abuse predict a poor outcome. Continued use guarantees it. (See Chapter 13 for details.)

Personality

Personality also can contribute to TBI, as some persons tend to be impulsive and engage in high risk behavior. Personality assessment is also essential for rehabilitation: Will the patient work hard? Will he discourage easily? What will motivate and interest him? High novelty seeking with low reward dependence predicts impulsive noncompliance. High harm avoidance suggests the patient may not work hard when rehabilitation is associated with discomfort. Any relatively sudden or substantial personality change in a person over age 35 suggests brain dysfunction, disease, or damage until proven otherwise.

Cognition

Cognitive assessment of persons with TBI serves several purposes. In your initial diagnostic evaluation (trying to answer the question "Does this patient have TBI and can that explain his present behavioral syndromes?") focus on (1) speed of information processing (use digit symbol substitution, serial sevens); (2) reaction time (A-test responses); (3) cognitive flexibility (Trails A and B); and (4) memory (immediate and delayed recall of story paragraphs and the Rey-Osterreith figure).

Use the vocabulary subtest of the WAIS along with the patient's previous education and job history as a comparison to present performance. Determine previous talents and skills (e.g., typing, knitting, playing a musical instrument, painting, quilting, playing golf or tennis) and determine present functioning in these areas. Always get this information from relatives as well as the patient. Persons with TBI can over- or underestimate their abilities. Whenever possible have the patient demonstrate talents or skills because procedural is different from declarative memory (e.g., I can tell you how to ride a bike, but unless I do it in front of you, you can't know if I actually can ride a bike). More extensive neuropsychological testing is also needed to determine cognitive strengths and weaknesses that guide rehabilitation. Repeated neuropsychological testing is needed to monitor improvement. Neuropsychological testing is also used in evaluating any forensic issues involving the patient. Table 11.5 lists some of the functions and tests used in the neuropsychological assessment of persons with TBI.

Social Supports

A critical factor in the recovery of any person with TBI is the quality of his social support system. You must assess the ability of family and friends to help. Do they have the motivation, intelligence, and situational and financial resources to provide the caregiving, guidance, and comfort the patient needs? Even if they do, they too will need support. Many family members of persons with TBI (like family

TABLE 11.5. Commonly Tested Cognitive Functions in Patients with TBI

Function	Tests*
Attention and vigilance	Digit Span, WAIS, Digit Symbol Substitution, A-Test
Distractibility	Stroop Color and Word Test, Paced Auditory Serial Addition Test
Executive functions	Wisconsin Card Sorting, Trails A and B, Porteus Maze, Category Test
Visuospatial	Benton Facial Recognition, Hooper Visual Organization
Visuomotor	Rey-Osterreith Complex Figure, Benton Visual Retention, WAIS Block Design, WAIS Object Assembly
Language	Boston Diagnostic Aphasia Battery, Western Aphasia Battery
Memory	Wechsler Memory Scale, California Verbal Learning Test, Rey Auditory-Verbal Learning Test, Rey-Osterreith Complex Figure, Benton Visual Retention, Corsi Blocks

*See Lezak in Additional Readings for details.

members of almost all patients with neuropsychiatric disorders) report feeling occasionally frustrated, angry, demoralized, isolated, financially insecure, trapped, and guilty about feeling these things. How well you deal with caregivers often determines how well the patient does.

Laboratory Studies

Laboratory testing for TBI focuses on brain structure, metabolism, and information processing. Structural assessment includes skull films (fracture, acute subdural hematomas), MRI (twice as sensitive as computed tomography [CT] in diagnosing intracranial soft tissue abnormalities, except if calcified or during the first few days after injury when CT is more sensitive; MRI demonstrates the lesion in 80% of patients with substantial or serious TBI).

Metabolic assessment includes cerebral blood flow (diminished diffusely immediately after acute TBI and then locally diminished in areas of injury if arousal returns to normal), single photon emission computed tomography (findings similar to cerebral blood flow and more available), and positron emission tomography (greatest resolution, but usually available at only large academic medical centers). Magnetic resonance spectroscopy and functional MRI are likely to be helpful, but are too new to be in wide clinical use.

Information processing assessment includes EEG (localized low voltage slowing at injury site; helping assess for epilepsy) and evoked potentials (brain stem studies most helpful showing delayed waveforms).

TREATMENT AND MANAGEMENT

The long-term treatment of persons with TBI is a model for the treatment of all patients with serious neuropsychiatric disease. Principles of treatment are detailed in Chapter 5. Briefly:

1. A behavioral and neurologic assessment that, in addition to diagnosis, provides an understanding of the patient's strengths and weaknesses (i.e., behavioral and sensorimotor problems, cognitive strengths and deficits, personality patterns, social behaviors, family and environmental strengths and weaknesses)
2. The judicious use of psychotropic medication (start low, go slow, monitor behavioral and cognitive changes frequently). Take into account the brain system involved (e.g., frontal circuit versus temporal lobe), as well as the behavioral syndrome
3. Neuroleptics delay cognitive recovery in brain-damaged patient's and tardive dyskinesia is a permanent cognitive deficit as well as a motor deficit
4. Rehabilitation is almost always required and must broadly focus on improving cognition, motor skills, self-care, and interpersonal functioning
5. Treatment goals are based on the patient's specific strengths and weaknesses and prognosis for improvement, not on an idealized version of the condition the patient has. "One size fits all" treatment programs (e.g., adolescent inpatient units, post-traumatic stress disorder programs, alcohol and drug rehabilitation programs) do not work for most patients when all patients get the same biologic, behavioral, and social interventions.

Table 11.6 displays specific medication recommendations for patients with behavioral syndromes due to TBI. Some guidelines are (1) the more typical the behavioral syndrome is to its primary (idiopathic) counterpart, the more likely it will respond to typical treatments; (2) the more positive symptoms (in this case positive refers to neurologic features rather than hallucinations and delusions) a patient has (e.g., irritability, seizure-like), the more likely he will respond to an anticonvulsant, mood-stabilizing, or anxiety-reducing drug; and (3) the more apathy and avolition, bradykinesia, and bradyphrenia a patient has, the more likely he will respond to a dopaminergic stimulating drug.

STROKE

Stroke is the third leading cause of death in industrialized countries, causing 10%–12% of all deaths. Eighty-eight percent of deaths from stroke occur in people over age 65. In the United States, women may be at greater risk than men, and women are older when they have a stroke and are more likely to die from it. Risk

TABLE 11.6. Treating Behavioral Syndromes Due to TBI

Syndrome	Recommendations
Depression	1. The more typical the syndrome, the more you treat like primary depression 2. The more apathetic, the more likely stimulants will help 3. Avoid antidepressants with anticholinergic properties, as these agents interfere with cognitive function 4. Carbamazepine plays a greater role than for primary depressions 5. ECT works well and is safe
Mania	Valproate, lithium, ECT
Impulsivity and dyscontrol syndrome	1. If associated with manic-like features, begin with mood stabilizers as if mania were primary condition 2. For aggressive-violent behavior without mania, beta-blockers (lithium may also work) 3. For irritability, aggressive-violent behavior, and agitation, buspirone (15–20 mg and up to 60 mg daily) or amantadine* (200–400 mg daily)
Epilepsy	See Chapter 10. For epileptic psychosis associated with TBI: carbamazeine, valproate, ECT and clonazepam
Psychosis	1. If schizophrenia-like, olanzapine or risperidone if you do not prescribe high doses likely to cause extrapyramidal side effects; otherwise haloperidol 2. Avoid clozapine because of its anticholinergic and hypotensive properties 3. If delusional disorder, carbamazepine or antipsychotics, as above
Apathy/avolitional syndrome	Dopamine agonists (do not use if patient is also irritable or psychotic): amantadine (200–400 mg), bromocriptine (10–50 mg), pemoline (56.25–75 mg), levodopa/carbidopa (Sinemet, 30/300 to 100/1,000 mg)
ADHD-like syndromes	Stimulants (both dopaminergic and noradrenergic), e.g., methylphenidate (10–60 mg)
Anxiety disorders	Buspirone (as above), selected serotonin reuptake inhibitors

*Amantadine is an NMDA glutamate receptor antagonist and may also have some neuroprotective properties.

factors include hypertension, hypercholesterolemia, smoking, overweight, high plasma fribrinogen levels, diabetes, oral contraceptive use, and heavy alcohol use.

Stroke is a sudden event that lasts longer than 24 hours. About 25% of patients have a headache at the onset. Twenty percent of patients have a clear progression of neurologic deficits. Stroke is classified as major or minor. Minor stroke is a reversible ischemic neurological deficit (RIND) that typically lasts less than 7 days. Major stroke (typically lasting more than 3 weeks) is subtyped as ischemic (thrombotic or embolic; 80%) or hemorrhagic (20%).

Brain imaging is critical in diagnosing stroke. CT scans can demonstrate hemorrhagic stroke within hours, but cannot demonstrate the extent of a stroke for 7–10 days after the stroke. MRI (weighted T_2 images) can demonstrate ischemic stroke as early as 45 minutes after the stroke and is better at distinguishing ischemic from hemorrhagic stroke. Carotid Doppler ultrasonography (used to assess carotid stenosis), transcranial Doppler (used to assess patency of anterior, middle, and sometimes the posterior cerebral arteries), and digital subtraction angiography (for carotid artery stenosis) are also used to assess stroke. Single photon emission computed tomography may also reveal an area of hypoperfusion early in the stroke process. The more the reduced perfusion, the worse the long-term outcome. Table 11.7 lists some of the causes of stroke. Table 11.8 lists some of the vascular syndromes of stroke.

TABLE 11.7. Some Causes of Stroke

Cause	Characteristics
Hypertension	1. Hemorrhagic stroke in small parenchymal arteries of the basal ganglia (50%), thalamus (10%–15%), cerebellum (10%) pons (10%), hemispheric white matter (5%–10%) 2. Primarily affects the action brain
Carotid artery stenosis	Large arteries, producing classic major stroke ischemic syndromes (e.g., aphasias and paresis)
Subarachnoid hemorrhage	Ruptured aneurysm causing hemorrhagic stroke (most common in anterior circulation)
Heart disease	Embolic stroke affecting small and sometimes large vessels from atrial fibrillation, infarction with mural thrombus, valvular vegetations, mitral valve prolapse (stroke in young persons)
Vasculopathies	1. Amyloid and collagen diseases 2. Arteritis affecting small vessels, producing ischemic stroke
Blood disease	Hemolytic disease (e.g., sickle cell) affecting small vessels, producing ischemic stroke
Vascular anomalies	1. Congenital malformations 2. Tumors causing hemorrhagic stroke

TABLE 11.8. Vascular Syndromes

Location	Characteristics
Middle cerebral artery	Contralateral hemiplegia (particularly face and arm), aphasia, apraxia, contralateral hemianopsia
Internal capsule	Contralateral hemiplegia (face, arm, leg), contralateral hemianesthesia
Anterior cerebral artery	Paralysis and sensory impairment of contralateral leg
Posterior cerebral artery	Contralateral homonymous hemianopsia with sparing of macular vision
Basilar and vertebral arteries	Contralateral hemiplegia, ipsilateral cranial nerve signs

Ischemic stroke is managed conservatively by anticoagulation (heparin, coumadin) and antiplatelet agglutination agents (aspirin, dipyridamole [Persantine]), fibrinolysis, and calcium channel blockers (to protect neurons and relax arterial smooth muscles). Reperfusion of the ischemic area using thrombolytic drugs may also be successful in the first few hours after the stroke. Surgical procedures are also used (carotid and subclavian endarterectomy, bypass and anastomoses angioplasty).

Hemorrhagic stroke (40%–50% of patients with intracerebral bleeds die; 30%–50% are associated with hypertension) is managed by controlling the source (e.g., surgically clipping an aneurysm, removing a vascular malformation, evacuating a cyst and tying off vessels; reducing blood pressure and giving antifibrinolytic agents *before* the bleed to prevent hemorrhage). *Subarachnoid hemorrhage* typically results from a ruptured or leaking aneurysm. Hemorrhage and then vasospasm can result in seizure and death. Surgically accessible aneurysms are almost always clipped within 3 days of the bleed. Anticonvulsants, stool softeners, blood pressure control, and calcium channel antagonists (e.g., nimodipine) to counteract vasospasm are the conservative treatments for surgically less accessible aneurysms (in the anterior communicating artery or in the posterior fossa).

Rehabilitation for stroke is essential. Even 3–6 months after the stroke, when likelihood of recovery of motor functions is past, cognitive and behavioral functioning can continue to improve. The "use it or lose it" principle apples. Recovery of different functions is variable within patients. Persons likely to do best are those (1) with more education, (2) who are younger than 65 years, (3) whose strokes were relatively mild or discrete, and (4) whose aphasia, if present, is a motor not a receptive pattern. Among elderly persons, those doing best have (1) a more active pre-stroke lifestyle, (2) no post-stroke depression, (3) strong family support, and (4) minimal motor dysfunction.

Transient ischemic attacks (TIAs) are acute ischemic episodes of focal loss of cerebral or special sensory function lasting less than 24 hours. Patients with TIAs have an increased risk for ischemic stroke, and 20%–25% of TIA patients have a stroke in the next 12 months from their first TIA. Focal signs of a TIA include (1) isolated, sudden, reversible anterograde and, often, retrograde amnesia; (2) transient bilateral blindness; (3) transient dysarthria; and (4) transient diplopia, dysphagia, loss of balance, tinnitus, and scotomas. Although they occur during TIAs, loss of consciousness, dizziness, and mental "confusion" are not acceptable symptoms for the diagnosis of TIA because they occur in many other conditions.

TIAs begin suddenly; symptoms arise and spread rapidly and peak in seconds. They are distinguished from seizures by their length (much longer), their lack of associated complex behavior and psychosensory features, and the presence of more specific neurologic signs. For example, gait and posture disturbances and cranial nerve signs suggest a vertebrobasilar TIA. Aphasias and perceptual alterations suggest a carotid TIA. CT and MRI are unhelpful in classifying TIAs because there are no significant differences in clinical features and prognosis between TIA patients with and without infarcts on imaging.

CLINICAL PRESENTATIONS:
BEHAVIORAL SYNDROMES SECONDARY TO STROKE

Strokes are associated with a wide array of neuropsychiatric features, although most stroke patients do not experience these phenomena. *Depression* is the most common behavioral syndrome associated with a single stroke (30%–50% of patients), and anterior brain lesions are most likely to cause depression (dominant more than nondominant). Besides the temporal relationship to the stroke, post-stroke depression can sometimes be differentiated from primary depressions by the presence of avolition, anergia, and mood reactivity rather than the profound unremitting sadness or apprehension characteristic of primary melancholia.

Post-stroke depression often occurs when the dominant caudate and other dominant anterior structures are involved. Stroke patients with depression are typically more impaired in motor and language function than stroke patients without depression.

Post-stroke depression can be treated successfully. If the mood is sadness or apprehension, antidepressants or ECT can be dramatically effective. If avolition and anergia are present, methylphenidate or bromocriptine can help.

Mania following stroke is typically associated with a nondominant lesion. When mania and obsessive compulsive disorder co-occur after stroke, the nondominant caudate nucleus is often involved. Patients with post-stroke mania often have a family history of mood disorder.

Personality changes are also common in patients who have suffered several strokes or a large stroke in anterior brain regions. Predominant changes are in temperament: Post-stroke personality disorder is often characterized by irritability, apathy, or impulsivity. These changes may respond to treatments similar to those for head trauma personality change.

Atypical psychoses can occur following stroke. These are often positive symptom nonaffective psychoses characterized by agitation, suspiciousness, complex visual and fragmented memory-like auditory hallucinations, delusions, and denial of illness (anosognosia). Right hemisphere and perceptual integrating brain systems are most often involved. When involving the dominant hemisphere the psychosis can be associated with a fluent aphasia. Nonfluent aphasias result from more anterior strokes and are more often associated with depression. Some thalamic strokes (left more than right) can produce a schizophrenic-like psychosis with avolition, anergia, and the dorsolateral prefrontal cortex syndrome. Formal thought disorder (fluent speech with episodes of paraphasias and nonsequiturs), poor executive function, and hallucinations can also occur.

Isolated psychopathology can occur with small strokes. Musical hallucinations (e.g., a particular song or type of music as if listening to a radio) is more common with nondominant hemisphere lesions, as are panoramic visual hallucinations (as if watching a movie). Isolated auditory hallucinations are associated with temporal lobe lesions (right more than left) and are like memory fragments. Table 11.9 lists other neuropsychiatric stroke-related syndromes.

DIFFERENTIAL DIAGNOSIS

Assume any obvious stroke predating a behavioral syndrome the cause of that syndrome until proven otherwise. The likelihood of the stroke actually being the cause increases if the lesion is in (1) the frontal lobes or related subcortical structures (mood and personality disturbances), (2) the temporal or parietal lobes (psychosis), or (3) the nondominant hemisphere (irritability and violence). MRI and single photon emission computed tomography are the best methods for confirming the diagnosis.

When the stroke is obvious and followed quickly by the behavioral syndrome, making the connection is not difficult. "Masked" strokes are more problematic. Patients with masked stroke can be categorized as: (1) elderly patients with multiple system diseases and associated behavioral problems who suddenly worsen or develop a new behavioral problem, (2) psychiatric patients who later in life have a stroke with behavioral changes that are mistakenly assumed to be an expression of their longstanding psychiatric illness, and (3) psychiatric patients whose behavioral syndrome is due to a small stroke in what used to be called "a silent" area (i.e., cerebellar neocortex, pons, right thalamus, right frontal lobe). Guidelines for identifying these patients are

1. *In the elderly patient with multi-system disease,* think of stroke when there is any new behavioral change that you cannot directly attribute to medications, dehydration, or metabolic disturbance.
2. *In a psychiatric patient with a new episode or exacerbation of illness,* think of stroke (as the cause of the new, not the old behavior) whenever the following are present: hypertension, diabetes with vascular changes elsewhere in the body, left-sided heart disease that can cause an embolus, hypercholesterolemia, heavy smoking, recent heavy cocaine use, alcoholism, co-morbid migraine, oral contraceptive use, and (in a patient over age 70) constipation (and straining while trying to defecate).

TABLE 11.9. Some Neuropsychiatric Stroke-Related Syndromes

Syndrome	Characteristics
Reduplicative delusions	1. *Capgras* (delusions that familiar persons are impostors), *Fregoli* (delusions that unfamiliar persons are familiar and sometimes celebrities), *reduplicative paramnesia* (delusions that places and buildings are replications of the real thing that have been moved elsewhere) associated with anxiety, irritability, experiences of alienation or control; nondominant posterior temporal parietal lesions 2. Treat with mild sedation and good nursing care, risperidone if no resolution in 1 week
Emotional blunting (loss of emotional expression) without avolition or psychosis	1. Motor aprosodia; nondominant anterior cerebral hemisphere (action brain) lesion, particularly the basal ganglia 2. Treat with social retraining
Pathologic crying (or, less commonly, laughing)	1. Sudden, socially inappropriate, and embarrassing release of intense emotion-related motor sequences with no or only mild mood change triggered by nonspecific or only mildly specific circumstances 2. Pontine lesions most likely, followed by nondominant cerebral hemisphere (frontotemporal) 3. Low therapeutic doses of the older antidepressants (e.g., amitriptyline, nortriptyline) are effective
Frontal lobe syndromes	1. Dorsolateral prefrontal cortex avolitional syndrome, the lateral orbitofrontal disinhibited syndrome, motor aprosodia 2. Nondominant ventral lateral and dorsomedial thalamic nuclei lesions can cause apathetic syndrome with hemispatial neglect and visual memory and visual spatial dysfunction
Gerstmann syndrome	Lesion in the angular gyrus and surrounding tissue (the inferior parietal lobule) of the dominant parietal lobe, producing dysgraphia, dyscalculia, right/left disorientation, finger agnosia
Angular gyrus syndrome	Lesion disconnecting the dominant angular gyrus from the language system, resulting in a rapid-onset nonprogressive dementing picture with surprisingly good visuospatial functioning
"Right hemisphere" syndrome	Body image problems (limbs seem suddenly too large, too heavy), unsure of limb location, topographic disorientation and getting lost even on familiar routes, the world looks "confused" or jumbled
Bailint syndrome	Right temporoparietal–occipital junction lesion producing optic ataxia in which visual cues interfere with movement, making them imprecise; directed gaze is also impaired

TABLE 11.9. *(continued)*

Syndrome	Characteristics
Denial and neglect	1. Right parietal lobe lesions can cause anosognosia and neglect of the left side of space; left supplementary motor area lesions can cause neglect of the right side of space
	2. Patient may not wash, shave, or comb hair on neglected side and can be injured walking into or tripping over objects on that side
	3. Right-sided lesion associated with receptive aprosodia and suspiciousness and delusions as the patient misinterprets the emotional expressions and actions of others
	4. Severe denial can lead to the delusion of a double (Doppelganger) who is held responsible for the patient's inappropriate social behaviors
	5. Unilateral neglect may be helped by patching the eye contralateral to the neglected side, plus visually stimulating (transient stimuli moving in jerky manner) the patient in the neglected area; bromocriptine (15 mg daily) also can improve neglect, particularly if anterior structures are involved
Anton syndrome	Lesion disconnecting the occipital lobe leading to blindness and denial of the blindness; the patient can be injured walking into or tripping over objects
Chronic pain syndrome	1. About 8% of stroke patients develop regional pain
	2. Posterior lateral portions of the thalamus often involved
	3. Associated with hemianesthesia, hemiataxia, and astereognosis
	4. Pain sharp and paroxysmal on hemiplegic side
	5. Mid to posterior thalamic lesions may also be associated with cerebellar syndrome (ataxia, dysmetria, dysdiadochokinesia) plus pain and sensory loss
	6. Left anterior thalamic lesions can cause aphasic problems
	7. Transcutaneous electrical stimulation, antidepressants, and carbamazepine help
Kluver-Bucy syndrome	Bilateral large temporal lobe lesions causing placidity, hypersexuality, increased oral behaviors, and visual agnosia
Akinetic mutism	1. The patient is mute and immobile, but follows you around the room with his eyes; lesion in outer cingulate gyrus bilateral, septohypothalamic, or mesodiencephalic areas
	2. This is also catatonia

TABLE 11.9. Some Neuropsychiatric Stroke-Related Syndromes (*continued*)

Syndrome	Characteristics
Alien hand syndrome	1. Anterior corpus callosum lesion disconnects the hands, and they act independently of each other and in conflict (when one hand does something, the other hand may try to stop the action), associated with ideomotor dyspraxia in nonpreferred hand, and preferred hand having "will of its own"
	2. Dominant frontal lesion (supplementary motor area or anterior cingulate lesion) disconnects dominant hand, and it develops a "will of its own" and compulsively gropes, grasps, and does not release objects, and exhibits unilateral utilization behavior (see below)
Utilization behavior syndrome	1. Exaggerated dependency on environment for behavioral cues and breakdown in self-monitoring from frontal paramedian thalamic or basal ganglia lesions
	2. Leads to echopraxia or compulsive use of objects or overlearned situations (e.g., sees a pen, picks it up and writes with it, sees a bed and lies in it, sees a fire alarm and pulls it)
	3. Can lead to legal (shoplifting) and social (touching) problems and difficult hospital management

3. *in a psychiatric patient who is neither elderly nor has the indicators in guideline 2*, think of stroke as the cause of the psychiatric illness whenever the following are present: an atypical course particularly of late onset; the psychiatric diagnosis is based primarily on one symptom rather than a cluster of symptoms (e.g., the patient hallucinates an odor but has no other striking psychopathology); the episode pattern is substantially atypical (e.g., depression with apathy rather than sadness, apprehension, or dysphoria); there is an associated regional cortical symptom pattern (e.g., a dominant parietal lobe pattern of features); or there is a striking finding on cognitive testing (e.g., a dramatically abnormal copying of intersecting pentagons on the Mini-Mental State).

TREATMENT AND MANAGEMENT

Increased intracranial pressure from large bleeds and brain edema is an acute medical concern. Transcranial Doppler ultrasound can detect the extent of this. The elderly, with some cerebral atrophy, withstand increased intracranial pressure better than the young. With hematomas of less than 30 ml, no surgery is needed. Hematomas between 30 and 80 ml offer the best chance for surgical recovery. Endarterectomy reduces the risk for stroke after a TIA by 10-fold in appropriately se-

TABLE 11.10. Treating Behavioral Syndromes Due to Stroke

Syndrome	Recommendations
Depression	1. The more typical the depression, the more you treat like a primary depression; avoid antidepressants with anticholinergic properties, as they interfere with cognitive function; if depression is melancholic, ECT is the safest treatment for ischemic stroke and for hemorrhagic stroke after 6 weeks post-stroke if blood pressure is controlled
	2. For depression with apathy and no irritability or psychosis, use dopamine agonists, (amantadine [200–400 mg], bromocriptine [10–50 mg], pemoline [56.25–75 mg], levodopa/carbidopa [Sinemet 30/300–100/1000 mg]), or methylphenidate (10–60 mg)
	3. For depression with dysphoria, use carbamazepine
	4. For depression with anxiety, use antidepressant/buspirone combinations based on recommendations in Chapters 7 and 15 for depression and anxiety
Mania or the disinhibition syndrome	1. Valproate or ECT in typical antimanic doses
	2. Other anticonvulsants have modest effect
	3. Avoid lithium, as it may exacerbate stroke features
Irritability/violence	1. Buspirone (15–60 mg), carbamazepine (400–1,600 mg) beta-blockers (e.g., propanolol 160–320 mg), amantadine (20–400 mg)
	2. Avoid lithium
Delusional disorder	1. Risperidone (<8 mg daily)
	2. Avoid clozapine because of its anticholinergic side effects
Nonaffective, positive symptom psychosis	1. Anticonvulsants, ECT
	2. Risperidone, olanzapine (if no irritability or agitation) in typical antipsychotic doses
Anxiety disorder	Same as for primary anxiety disorders (see Chapter 15)
Obsessive compulsive disorders	Same as for primary obsessive compulsive disorder and its variants (see Chapter 14)
Personality disorder	1. If schizotypal: Anticonvulsants, risperidone, olanzapine
	2. If borderline: Valproate, carbamazepine
	3. Doses between one-half and full dose for mood disorder or psychosis

lected patients. Three hundred milligrams of aspirin reduces the risk by 20%. Ticlopidine is 20% more effective than aspirin in preventing stroke, but can cause neutropenia and requires biweekly blood counts.

Rehabilitation training during acute recovery may prevent loss of function to cortex adjacent to the damaged motor cortex and facilitates the reorganization of the adjacent cortex to recover some of the functional loss. Almost all stroke patients require long-term rehabilitation. Physical therapy helps for at least 6 months after the stroke. Cognitive rehabilitation can help improve and maintain functioning for a much longer time. In general, the recovery from stroke increases when there is minimal motor deficits, intact proprioception and balance, and adequate cognition (orientation, attention and concentration, and memory [particularly new learning]). Always assess these functions in a stroke patient. Once the acute post-stroke period is over, chances for prolonged institutionalization can be predicted by simple cognitive tests (drawing a house, person, clock).

The management of the behavioral syndromes due to stroke includes (1) prevention of future strokes; (2) motor, sensory, and cognitive rehabilitation of any deficits due to the stroke; 3) all the psychotherapy and family strategies suggested for TBI; and (4) specific pharmacotherapy. Table 11.10 summarizes the specific pharmacologic interventions for behavioral syndromes due to stroke.

ADDITIONAL READINGS

Anneggers JF, Hauser A, Coan SP, Rocca WA: A population-based study of seizures after traumatic brain injuries. *N Engl J Med* 338:20–24, 1998.
Beckson M, Cummings JL: Neuropsychiatry aspects of stroke. *Int J Psychiatry Med* 21:1–15, 1991.
Benson DF: Psychiatric aspects of aphasia. *Br J Psychiatry* 123:555–566, 1973.
Blumbergs PC, Scott G, Manavis J, Wainwright H, Simpson DA, McLean AJ: Staining of amyloid precursor protein to study axonal damage in mild head injury. *Lancet* 344:1055–1056, 1994.
Bogousslevsky J, Regli F, Assal G: The syndrome of unilateral tuberothalamic artery territory infarction. *Stroke* 17:434–441, 1986.
Brown SJ, Fann JR, Grant I: Post-concussion disorder: Time to acknowledge a common source of neurobehavioral morbidity. *J Neuropsychiatry Clin Neurosci* 6:15–22, 1994.
Caplan LR: New therapies for stroke. *Arch Neurol* 54:1222–1224, 1997.
Davison K, Bagley CR: Schizophrenia-like psychoses associated with organic disorders of the central nervous system: a review of the literature. *Br J Psychiatry* Spec Pub No. 4:113–184, 1969.
Gilman S: Imaging the brain. First of two parts. *N Engl J Med* 338:813–820, 1998.
Goldstein LB: Potential effects of common drugs on stroke recovery. *Arch Neurol* 55:454–456, 1998.
Greverson GC, Gray CS, French JM, James OFW: Long-term outcome for patients and careers following hospital admission for stroke. *Age Aging* 20:337–344, 1991.
Hier DB, Mondlock J, Caplan LR: Behavioral abnormalities after right hemisphere stroke. *Neurology* 33:337–344, 1983.
Karbe H, Kessler J, Herholz K, Fink GR, Heiss WD: Long-term prognosis of post-stroke aphasia studied with positron emission tomography. *Arch Neurol* 52:186–190, 1995.
Kogure T, Kogure K: Molecular and biochemical events within the brain subjected to cerebral ischemia (targets for therapeutic intervention). *Clin Neurosci* 4:179–183, 1997.

Kraus MF, Maki PM: Effect of amantadine hydrochloride on symptoms of frontal lobe dysfunction in brain injury: Case studies and review. *J Neuropsychiatry Clin Neurosci 9:*222–230, 1997.

Krieglstein J: Mechanisms of neuroprotective drug actions. *Clin Neurosci 4:*184–193, 1997.

Kuroda S, Siesjo BK: Reperfusion damage following focal ischemia: Pathophysiology and therapeutic windows. *Clin Neurosci 4:*199–212, 1997.

Lezak MD: *Neuropsychological Assessment*, 3rd ed. Oxford University Press, New York, 1995.

Lishman WA: Brain damage in relation to psychiatric disability after head injury. *Br J Psychiatry 114:*373–410, 1968.

McAllister TW: Neuropsychiatric sequelae of head injuries. *Psychiatric Clin North Am 15:* 395–413, 1992.

Merskey H, Woodforde JM: Psychiatric sequelae of minor head injury. *Brain 95:*521–528, 1972.

Mittenberg W, Zielinski RE, Fischera S: Recovery from mild head injury: A treatment manual for patients. *Psychother Private Pract 12:*37–52, 1993.

Nudo RJ, Wise BM, SiFuentes F, Milliken GW: Neural substrates for the effects of rehabilitative training on motor recovery after ischemic infarct. *Science 272:*1791–1794, 1996.

Parikh RM, Robinson RG, Lipsey JR, Starkstein SE, Fedoroff P, Price TR: The impact of post-stroke depression on recovery in activities of daily living over a 2-year follow-up. *Arch Neurol 47:*785–789, 1990.

Pimental PA, Kingsbury NA: *Neuropsychological Aspects of Right Brain Injury*. PRO-ED, Inc., Austin, TX, 1989.

Plum F: Extension of fundamental stroke research into clinical care. *Clin Neurosci 4:*175–178, 1997.

Price BH, Mesulam M: Psychiatric manifestations of right hemisphere infarctions. *J Nerv Ment Dis 173:*610–614, 1985.

Prigatano GP: Personality disturbances associated with traumatic brain injury. *J Consult Clin Psychol 60:*360–368, 1992.

Rowe MJ, Carlson C: Brainstem auditory evoked potentials in postconcussional dizziness. *Arch Neurol 37:*679–683, 1980.

Rustin MJ: Stroke rehabilitation: A geropsychological perspective. *Arch Phys Med Rehab 71:*914–922, 1990.

Robinson RG, Parikh RM, Lipsey JR, Starkstein SE, Price TR: Pathological laughing and crying following stroke: Validation of a measurement scale and a double-blind treatment study. *Am J Psychiatry 150:*286–293, 1993.

Sandercock P, Williams H: Medical treatment of acute ischemic stroke. *Lancet 339:*537–539, 1992.

Schott GD: From thalamic syndrome to central post-stroke pain (editorial). *J Neurol Neurosurg Psychiatry 61:*560–564, 1995.

Schousboe A, Belhage B, Frandsen A: Role of CA^{++} and other second messengers in excitatory amino acid receptor mediated neurodegeneration: Clinical perspectives. *Clin Neurosci 4:*194–198, 1997.

Shewan CM, Kertesz A: Effects of speech and language treatment on recovery from aphasia. *Brain Lang 23:*272–299, 1984.

Signer S, Cummings JL, Benson DF: Delusions and mood disorders in patients with chronic aphasia. *J Neuropsychiatry 1:*40–45, 1989.

Silver JM, Yudofsky SC, Hales RE: Depression in traumatic brain injury. *Neuropsychiatry, Neuropsychol Behav Neurol 4:*12–23, 1991.

Silver JM, Yudofsky SC, Hales RE: *Neuropsychiatry of Traumatic Brain Injury*. American Psychiatric Press, Washington, DC, 1994.

Solomon DA, Barohn RJ, Bazon C, Grissom J: The thalamic ataxia syndrome. *Neurology 44:*810–814, 1994.

Teasdale GM, Nicoll JAR, Murray G, Fiddes M: Association of apolipoprotein E polymorphism with outcome after head injury. *Lancet 350:*1069–1071, 1997.

12

Dementia

Five percent of persons over age 65 years, and 20% or more of those over age 80 years, are demented. Dementia, however, is not an inevitable outcome of aging, although cognitive decline is. Dementia is characterized by widespread cognitive impairment, usually of slow onset, and, in the early stages, a clear sensorium. Some dementing processes can resolve if identified and treated (e.g., due to depression, medications, hypothyroidism). Most end in a chronic defect state.

THE ELDERLY PATIENT AND NORMAL AGING

The U.S. population is aging. Today, 12% are over age 65 years. By 2030, 22% will be over 65 years. About 12% of the elderly have a psychiatric illness, most often depression, dementia, anxiety disorder, and alcoholism. Common general medical conditions that affect brain function in the elderly include hypertension, ischemic heart disease, diabetes, and arteriosclerosis. Twenty percent of the elderly with a general medical illness also have a psychiatric disorder. Sometimes this psychiatric disorder co-occurs by chance. Often, however, the behavioral syndrome is caused by the same pathophysiology that caused the general medical condition. For example, hypertension can cause stroke, and the stroke can cause a secondary depression. Despite high risk for disease, the prognosis is excellent for recovery from many behavioral and general medical conditions of the elderly. Failure to distinguish illness from normal aging, however, can lead to a failure to recognize clinical features of treatable conditions. The principles of diagnosis and treatment for the elderly are identical to those for the young.

The exact nature of aging is unknown. Some cell lines seem genetically programmed to die after a fixed and predetermined number of cell replications. Among brain cells, death is programmed to occur by default unless suppressed by signals from other cells, because dependence on specific signals for survival is a simple way for the brain to eliminate misplaced cells and for regulating cell numbers (i.e., neuronal pruning). Aging involves a combination of several processes: DNA damage, mutation, formation of free radicals, formation of cross-linkages between molecules, wear and tear, accumulation of toxic metabolites, and impaired supply of nutrients.

Aging causes decline in physiologic function (actual numbers of active metabolic cells and cellular functions decrease over the life span), but the rate of decline varies considerably. For almost every test of general health or brain function, variability is greater among the elderly than among the young. Thus, many persons can function outstandingly to advanced ages. The decline of organ systems also varies, so that an elderly person can be doing poorly in one area (e.g., chronic arthritis), but well in another (e.g., brain and heart functioning).

Table 12.1 lists some aging changes. In addition, aging may result in shortened stature, stooped posture resulting in part from inadequate dietary calcium and decalcification of bones, depigmentation and loss of hair, wrinkling of skin, decreased muscle mass and strength, slowing of movements and halting of gait, redistribution of fat, loss of teeth, altered facial architecture, loss of high-frequency hearing, decreased visual acuity, increased systolic blood pressure, reduced heart and lung function, reduced blood flow to the brain (20%) and brain weight (10%), reduced fibers in nerves (30%–40%), and reduced metabolic rate (15%). The kidneys, lungs, and skin age more rapidly than do the heart and liver.

Although aging effects can be detected after age 40, in many persons marked decline is not apparent until their late 70s or early 80s. This decline can be substantially ameliorated by general good health practices plus aerobic exercise training, which has substantial positive cardiovascular, pulmonary, and cognitive effects in older persons. The regular playing of video games also improves visuoperceptual performance. Brain development continues with experience, and the more an elderly person is cognitively "busy," the more likely brain development (dendritic arborization, less pruning) continues. "Use it or lose it" is the process.

There are also substantial genetic influences on aging. For example, among elderly twins, genes explain 60% of general cognitive function, 50% of verbal and 30% of spatial function, and 60% of speed of information processing. The apolipoprotein E (ApoE) genotype is also associated with cognitive decline in community dwelling, nondemented elderly persons. 4/4 (homozygous) predicts the worse cognitive decline. Intelligence and education also predict cognitive decline, with higher pre-age 40 IQ scores and more education associated with better functioning after age 65.

Dizziness and falling are particular problems for the elderly. The former is the most common presenting complaint in primary care practice for patients over 75 years. The latter is the sixth leading cause of death among people over 65, and 30% of persons over 65 living in their community fall each year, resulting in substantial disability, fearfulness, or institutionalization. Some treatable causes of dizziness are (1) medication related orthostasis, (2) fear and anxiety initiated vasovagal attacks, (3) hyperventilation (even mild), and (4) decreased cardiac output.

Feeling off-balance and unsteady when walking (dysequilibrium) is due to (1) vestibular system disease, (2) proprioceptive and somatosensory loss from peripheral neuropathy or thalamic or parietal lesions, and (3) motor system lesions.

TABLE 12.1. Some Physiologic Changes of Aging

Change	Neuropsychiatric Implications
Osteoporosis	Increased risk of hip fracture from falling secondary to orthostatic hypotension from many drugs, particularly psychotropics
Increased body fat	1. Increased concentration of plasma lithium and water-soluble drug metabolites
	2. Decreased plasma concentration of lipid-soluble drug metabolites, but increased total body distribution and prolonged elimination half-life
Liver changes	
Decrease in albumen	Increased bioavailability at same total plasma levels of many drugs
Decreased enzyme activity	Decreased demethylization of tertiary amine, partially specific reuptake-inhibiting antidepressants, and benzodiazepines with active demethyl metabolites
Decreased hepatic blood flow (50%)	Some reduction in first-pass metabolism and prolonged half-lives and bioavailability of first-pass drugs
Kidney Changes	
Decreased renal blood flow	1. Decreased clearance of lithium and antidepressant metabolites
Decreased glomerular filtration rate	
Decreased renal tubular secretion	2. Capacity to conserve sodium declines (osmoreceptor sensitivity produces more vasopressin and water retention and an antidiuretic hormone secretion syndrome)

Viral infections and Meniere syndrome also contribute to complaints of vertigo or dysequilibrium. Whatever the behavioral syndrome, assess all elderly patients for their risk of falling. Specific interventions (e.g., gait training, balance and strength exercise, cautious use of medications that cross the blood–brain barrier, removing household hazards) can substantially reduce the risk of falls. The list of medications that can adversely affect the elderly producing delirium, depression or dementia is staggering. Table 12.2 lists some of them.

CLINICAL PRESENTATION

In the early stages of dementia, signs and symptoms often are ambiguous and behavioral changes may be most prominent. Patients are often misdiagnosed as suffering from major depression, dysthymia, or schizophrenia.

During the early stages of dementias with insidious onset (e.g., Alzheimer's)

TABLE 12.1. *(continued)*

Change	Neuropsychiatric Implications
	3. Reduced ability to compensate for acid–base and electrolyte abnormalities, increasing risk for metabolic induced deliria
Decreased intestinal motility	1. May delay peak blood levels
	2. Increased risk for paralytic ileus with drugs with anticholinergic properties
Prostatic hypertrophy	Increased risk for urinary retention with drugs with anticholinergic properties
Diminished thyroid reserves	Increased risk for hypothyroidism with lithium treatment
Brain changes	1. Decreased total sleep time and stage four (deep) sleep, EEG slowing in all frequencies, ventricular enlargement (decreased numbers and size of dendrites, decreased extracellular space), and white matter hyperintensities on MRI (20%), decreased frontal lobe cerebral blood flow; normal aging changes make EEG and MRI less helpful in the differential diagnosis of primary from secondary behavioral syndromes in persons over age 75
	2. Biogenic amine neurotransmitters decrease, dopamine decreases (but monoamine oxidase increases), and norepinephrine increases at rest and in response to stress; has little practical effect on pharmacotherapy
	3. Women tend to have more hippocampal and parietal lobe changes, while men tend to have more frontal and whole-brain changes

frequent complaints include fatigue, mild sadness, headache, poor concentration, and loss of efficiency. Patients will frequently show a decline in their general activities and lose interest in sports and hobbies. They may report a vague difficulty using words (particularly the expression of polysyllabic words) and in word finding. They may become lost in familiar places and lose efficiency in previously learned skills (e.g., cooking, typing, driving in heavy traffic). Denial of illness is frequently observed, and patients may offer outlandish excuses for their poor performance of simple cognitive tasks. A general lack of spontaneity and mild recent memory problems are also common. Because women are at greater risk than men for most nonalcohol-related and noncardiovascular dementias, and because many dementing processes begin in the sixth decade or later, the early stages of dementia are most often confused with major depression. Such patients may even have a mild or transient improvement with antidepressant medication or electroconvulsive therapy (ECT).

In the latter stages of dementia, the profound memory deficit, disorientation,

TABLE 12.2. Some Drugs That Can Adversely Affect the Elderly

Delirium/Dementia/Depression	Agitation	Psychosis/Mania
Anticholinergics (antidepressants, antiparkinsonians, neuroleptics)	Sympathomimetics (including cold preparations)	Stimulants
Antihistamines (cold and sleep preparations)	Thyroid hormones	Anticholinergics
Antiarrhythmics (quinidine)	Antidepressants	Anticonvulsants
Sedative-hypnotics	Levodopa/bromocriptine	Antidepressants
Lithium carbonate	Cardiac drugs	Digitalis/quinidine
Narcotic analgesics	Anticonvulsants	Caffeine
H$_2$ receptor blockers (cimetidine)	Benzodiazepines	Corticosteroids
Digitalis	Antihistamines	Beta-blockers
Anticonvulsants	Anticholinergics	H$_2$ blockers
Beta-blockers	Theophylline	Theophylline
Antihypertensives	Narcotics	Thyroid hormones
Corticosteroids	Antitubercular drugs	
Antibiotics		
Metaclopramide		
Benzodiazepines		

and readily observed nonbehavioral neurologic features help in diagnosis. Patients are disoriented to time and place, amnestic, and occasionally psychotic (vascular dementia the likely cause). Demented persons can be tactless, cruel, ill-mannered, and ill-groomed, particularly when they have a frontal lobe dementia. Their speech is perseverative, cliche ridden, and stereotyped. They are often restless (rubbing, tapping, and folding hand movements are common) and occasionally severely agitated. Emotional lability, Witzelsucht (a shallow, silly, fatuous mood), emotional blunting, or emotional incontinence (sudden and unexpected brief outbursts of laughter or crying often unassociated with the corresponding mood) can occur. They have multiple soft neurologic signs, anosmia, changes in muscle tone (often weakness and rigidity without cogwheeling), a puppet-like gait, nystagmus, the Kluver-Bucy syndrome, urinary incontinence, and pupillary changes. Frontal, temporal, and parietal lobe cognitive syndromes can occur. Seizures of all types may occur. Table 12.3 lists common diagnostic features of dementia.

DIFFERENTIAL DIAGNOSIS

Dementia is a clinical, not a laboratory, diagnosis. Once you have identified the syndrome, your next step is to identify the specific type of dementia. Although

TABLE 12.3. Common Diagnostic Features of Dementia

Feature	Operational Definition
Clear sensorium	<5 errors on letter cancellation, the A-test
Cognitive impairment	Mini-Mental State score of 22 or less in early stages, or <20 in later stages
Impairment in memory	Problems with new learning *and* recall with Alzheimer's disease; problems with recall with frontal disease;* scattered problems with vascular or generalized problems in all memory functions; use paragraph recall and Rey-Osterreith figure immediate and delayed recall
Impairment in thinking	Difficulty with verbal and visual absurdities, similarities, and problem solving

*After rehearsing a list of 10 words, Alzheimer's patients cannot recall them or pick them out from a list of 20 words, 10 of which they rehearsed. Patients with frontal lobe dementia can identify many of the 10 words from the list of 20, but cannot spontaneously recall them. They need help. Alzheimer's patients do not benefit from this cuing.

Alzheimer's disease is the most common (50%), the etiologic probabilities differ by age group. Table 12.4 lists the most likely types by age.

Reversible Dementias

The first step in the differential diagnosis of dementia is to consider potentially reversible dementias. *Drug-induced dementia* (see Table 12.2) is the largest group of potentially reversible dementias, and any elderly person receiving a medication that crosses the blood-brain barrier and can produce dementia should be considered suffering from a drug-induced dementia until proven otherwise. Drug-induced dementia most often results from the physician not considering side effects in prescribing, polypharmacy, or drug–drug metabolic interactions.

The single most common condition producing a reversible dementia in patients 65–75 years old is depression (5%–20% of demented inpatients), and distinguishing *pseudodementia* or major depression in the elderly from the other dementias is the next step, and Chapter 7 details this. Depression in the elderly responds as well to treatment as depression in younger patients.

The third concern is to look for suggestive historical and physical examination findings of other partially reversible dementias. The elderly are especially sensitive to *metabolic imbalance,* and chronic electrolyte changes, dehydration, and renal and hepatic failure can produce dementia. Acute change causes delirium. When identified early and depending on their severity, these dementias are partially reversible. Periodic monitoring of cognition can detect these dementias early.

Hypoxemia from obstructive sleep apnea (see Chapter 16), chronic obstructive pulmonary disease, and congestive heart failure can also cause dementia. The degree of reversibility depends on the severity and duration of the hypoxia and in correcting the primary condition.

TABLE 12.4. Likely Dementias by Age Group

Under 50 Years	50-70 Years	Over 70 Years
Infection	Depression (pseudo-dementia)	Alzheimer's disease
Alcoholism		Prescription or over-the-counter drug toxicity
Head trauma	Prescription or over-the-counter drug toxicity	
Normal pressure hydrocephalus	Vascular	Vascular
		Metabolic imbalance
Nutritional	Basal ganglia diseases (Parkinson's)	Hypoxemia
Endocrinopathies	Hypoxemia	
Pick's disease	Space-occupying lesions	
Collagen-vascular disease	Cancer and cancer therapy	
Multiple sclerosis and other white matter dementias	Nutritional	
Basal ganglia diseases (Huntington's, and Wilson's diseases)	Non-Alzheimer neuro-degenerative disease (olivo-pontocerebellar, progressive supra-nuclear palsy, amyo-trophic lateral sclerosis, non-diffuse Lewy body disease)	
Prion disease* (Creutzfeldt-Jakob, Kuric, Scrapie, familial fatal insomnia)		

*Prion is an infectious protein structure without nucleic acid that produces spongiform encephalopathy, gliosis, and senile plaques; acts as if it were autosomal dominant, producing rapidly progressing dementia, ataxia, tremor, and rigidity.

Endocrinopathy (e.g., thyroid, parathyroid, adrenal, pituitary adenoma, steroid therapy) causing dementia is very rare (<1% of dementias). Unless the patient has suggestive symptoms or early onset atypical dementia features, automatic laboratory testing is a waste of time and money. When present, however, the dementia is fully reversible if the primary condition is treated.

Nutritional dementias (e.g., pernicious anemia [B_{12}], megaloblastic anemia [folate], beriberi or Korsakoff's dementia [thiamine], and pellagra [niacin]) are rare in industrial countries unless the patient is alcoholic, or has a malabsorption syndrome or anorexia nervosa. For other patients automatic testing is of no benefit unless the patient has suggestive symptoms. The degree of reversibility with vitamin replacement therapy depends on the severity and duration of the process. For pernicious anemia, look for peripheral neuropathy, optic atrophy, and an atypical mood disorder because anemia and macrocytosis may not occur until late in the course. The dementia pattern will also be subcortical (see below) because white matter is primarily affected.

Alcoholism causes two types of dementia: frontal lobe dementia (see below for features) and Korsakoff's dementia. The frontal lobe dementia results from the direct neurotoxic effects of alcohol (50%–70% of sober, once chronic alcoholics have cognitive problems). It is partially reversible after a year or two if abstinence can be maintained. Korsakoff's dementia results from the alcoholic being vulnerable to low thiamine levels because of an autosomal gene unrelated to alcoholism but that leads to low levels of fibroblast transketolase, an enzyme needed to bind thiamine. Korsakoff's patients have gross new learning problems, poor episodic and other anterograde memory difficulties (e.g., forgetting new information after 1–2 minutes with preserved immediate recall), and patchy retrograde amnesia. Depending on other factors (e.g., personality), they may confabulate events (a minority of patients) to fill their memory gaps. Also commonly present are VIth cranial nerve palsy, cerebellar ataxia, and peripheral neuropathy. Thiamine in high doses only modestly improves the condition.

Infection can produce an acute onset dementia. These dementias are rarely fully reversible even with specific treatment (e.g., antibiotics, antiviral agents), but vigorous treatment can minimize damage. AIDS patients can develop an apathetic syndrome with bradyphrenia and a white matter dementia. They are more at risk for neurosyphilis (5% of AIDs patients, thus, look for pupils that react to accommodation but not to light [Argyll-Robertson pupil]) and neurotuberculosis. Cryptococcosis is the most likely fungal and toxoplasmosis the most likely parasitic infection to produce dementia, and both are also more likely in AIDS patients. Lyme neuroborreliosis can also produce a partially reversible dementia, as can *collagen-vascular damaging disorders* such as systemic lupus erythematosus, rheumatoid vasculitis, and sarcoidosis. These disorders are rare, their systemic signs are usually also present, and the dementia's response to steroid treatment is variable.

Normal pressure hydrocephalus can produce a dementia. Urinary incontinence or ataxia are early signs. Ataxia and altered arousal predict a good response to ventricular-venous shunting. Ten percent of patients are alcoholics; many have head injuries or infection as the cause.

Finally, *space-occupying lesions, cancer,* and *cancer therapy* can produce dementia. Frontal and temporal pole slow-growing tumors or bilateral chronic subdural hematomas cause 3%–5% of all dementias. Personality change and problems with recall are early signs of anterior masses. Magnetic resonance imaging (MRI) will reveal these, and surgically removable masses offer the best chance for recovery. Surgical evacuation of the subdural hematoma (seen best with computer tomography scanning) can also resolve the dementia.

Some carcinomas produce neurotoxic substances, causing demyelination and a subcortical dementia pattern. Cancer chemotherapy and radiation can cause necrosis and diffuse leukoencephalopathy with periventricular edema and cortical atrophy. If detected early, these dementias partially respond to corticosteroids.

Nonreversible Dementias

Many nonreversible dementias initially affect specific brain systems, and thus the early pattern of the dementia can help in diagnosis. After considering potentially reversible dementias, consider if the dementia has initially affected the action or perceptual-integrating brain. If symptoms suggest action brain, consider if the pattern is consistent with cortical or subcortical involvement. If subcortical, consider if the pattern suggests basal ganglia or white matter disease. Table 12.5 displays dementias initially affecting different brain systems. Alzheimer's disease is the most common dementia (50% of patients). Action brain dementias form the next largest group, and vascular dementia is the second most common single cause of dementia. Variants of Lewy body disease affect the action and the perceptual-integrating brain and cortical and subcortical structures.

Perceptual-Integrating Brain Dementia: Alzheimer's Disease

The earlier the onset of Alzheimer's disease, the faster the decline. Death usually results from secondary infection. Prevalence increases with age, from 5% of the population at age 65 years to 25%–35% by age 90 years. Women are slightly more at risk than men.

Risk factors for Alzheimer's disease are

1. Family history of dementia, Down syndrome, myeloproliferative disease, or Parkinson's disease
2. Prior head injury with unconsciousness doubles the risk for Alzheimer's disease (perhaps due to release of beta-amyloid peptide by injured neurons)
3. Late onset depression doubles the risk
4. Previous hypothyroidism also increases the risk

TABLE 12.5. Some Dementias Initially Affecting Specific Brain Systems

Action Brain	*Perceptual-Integrating Brain*
Cortical	Alzheimer's disease
Primary frontal degeneration	Lewy body dementia
Alcohol dementia	Creutzfeldt-Jakob disease
Lewy body dementia	Korsakoff's encephalopathy
Pick's disease	
Creutzfeldt-Jakob disease	
Subcortical	
White matter dementia	
Vascular	
AIDS	
Nutritional	
Multiple sclerosis	
Basal ganglia dementia	
Parkinson's disease	
Lewy body dementia	
Huntington's disease	
Wilson's disease	

Possible protective factors are

1. Education beyond high school (mildly protective), perhaps because people with more education tend to have more dendrites, axons, and synapses (i.e., brain reserve, requiring more damage before dysfunction is obvious)
2. The frequent use of nonsteroidal anti-inflammatory agents (mildly protective) at usual dosages may ameliorate decline, perhaps by slowing the brain's inflammatory response to amyloid accretion
3. The use of postmenopausal estrogen replacement therapy, perhaps because estrogen is needed in neuronal repair

The findings that Alzheimer's disease is less common among cigarette smokers and therefore nicotine (the known psychoactive ingredient) is protective are likely artifactual, resulting from cigarette smokers developing chronic lung and heart disease or stroke and either dying from those conditions before developing Alzheimer's or having a vascular or metabolic dementia or other neurologic syndrome that rules out the Alzheimer diagnosis.

Alzheimer's progresses through three overlapping stages. In *stage 1*, speech becomes progressively empty and ideas restricted. Patients may have problems following conversations with more than one person, leading to complaints of hearing loss beyond any actual deficit. Also commonly observed are anomia and word finding problems, mild dysgraphia, poor verbal fluency, mild memory impairment (forgetting to remember, e.g., chores, turning off lights and gas stoves; inability to learn simple instructions), and visuospatial problems (getting into auto accidents, unable to copy geometric shapes and designs, misidentifying people, getting lost). Depression with avolition and loss of interest, rather than profound sadness, occurs in about 25% of patients. MRI and single positron emission computed tomography (SPECT) show modest temporoparietal changes. EEG may be normal or show nonspecific, low voltage slowing.

In *stage 2*, action and perceptual-integrating systems are involved, and cognitive and behavioral deterioration increases. Fluent aphasia may occur. Memory impairment is marked. Periods of agitation, loss of some grooming and hygiene skills, and a coarsening of personality also occur. Most patients will have an abnormal EEG and MRI, and SPECT findings are grossly abnormal. Those patients with aphasia (particularly receptive) are most likely to develop psychotic features and have a more rapid rate of decline. Psychotic patients also are more likely to have the early onset form. The presence of extrapyramidal signs (e.g., muscle rigidity) is also an indicator of rapid decline. In *stage 3*, severe deterioration develops, incontinence is common, and constant care is necessary.

Five Alzheimer's variants have been identified:

1. Duke variant, representing 60%–80% of all cases, with late onset and typical pathology
2. Seattle variant, representing 2%–5% of all cases, with early onset and chromosome 14 linkage

3. Boston variant, representing 1% of all cases, with early onset, amyloid overproduction, and chromosome 21 and ApoE involvement
4. Down's variant, representing 1% of all cases, with early onset, amyloid overproduction, associated with trisomy 21, and seen in 5%–100% of Down syndrome patients
5. Idiopathic form, representing 10%–20% of all cases, that is, sporadic

Although there is the "sporadic" (nonfamilial) form of Alzheimer's disease, and many twin pairs are discordant for it, clinically assume all patients have the familial form until proven otherwise so that family member evaluation and subsequent monitoring can be done and potentially preventative or onset delaying treatment started.

About half of first-degree relatives will be affected by their mid-80s. Also, a familial relationship to Down syndrome and to some myeloproliferative disorders (e.g., leukemia) suggests a common accelerated aging problem in specific cell lines. Deviant genotypes identified are on chromosomes 1, 14, 19, and 21. Mitochondrial DNA may also be involved in sporadic Alzheimer's disease, but confirmation of this is needed. Also implicated are a polymorphism on chromosome 12 (late onset familial type with sporadic susceptibility) and 17 (a frontotemporal type dementia that clinically resembles Alzheimer's disease). Chromosomes 1 and 14 polymorphisms are associated with an uncommon, early onset (about age 50), rapidly deteriorating form, with several first-degree relatives usually also developing the illness. The chromosome 21 polymorphism leads to increased accretion of amyloid in blood vessels and neurons. The ApoE gene on chromosome 19 may contribute to 25%–40% of all cases. The ApoE 4/4 homozygote (2%–3% of the population) leads to the highest risk (50%); 2/3, 3/3, and 3/4 (about 10%, 60%, and 20% of the population, respectively), an intermediary risk; and 2/2 (1% of the population), a risk no greater than that of the general population.

Once a person gets Alzheimer's disease, the presence of ApoE 4 does not predict rate of decline. ApoE is expressed in the lipoprotein structure of neuronal membranes and neurofibrils, and the 4/4 homozygote may produce lipoprotein that is particularly vulnerable to the neural inflammatory response to accumulating amyloid, or lipoprotein less effective in repair of neuronal damage. In addition to neocortical lesions, many patients have degeneration of the hippocampus, parahippocampus, and substantia nigra; dorsal raphe nucleus, nucleus basilis of the basal forebrain, and its cholinergic projections to the cortex; and the locus ceruleus and its noradrenergic projections. The pathophysiologic process seems to initially involve the accretion of intra- and extracellular amyloid. This causes a neuroinflammatory response and the release of excitatory toxic amino acids (e.g., glutamate). In an individual whose neuronal lipoprotein is particularly vulnerable to the neuroinflammatory response and cannot properly help in neural repair, structural breakdown occurs, leading to cell death and neurofibrilatory tangles.

Early detection and correct diagnosis are the only hope of delaying or modifying the rate of decline. Some treatment strategies benefit persons at risk, so the diagnostic effort is worth the initial cost. MRI is helpful in distinguishing Alzheimer's disease from pseudodementia in persons under age 65, with the former more likely to have decreased temporal lobe volumes. MRI hyperintensities are seen in the elderly and in depressed patients and do not discriminate them from Alzheimer's disease patients. SPECT is more helpful for demonstrating mesial temporal lobe hypoperfusion in stage 1. Temporoparietal hypoperfusion is more often seen in the later stages. Cognitive testing may identify dementia, *even several years before clinical features are obvious.* The Mini-Mental State is useful, with scores dropping to 27 or 26 suggestive. Digit Symbol Substitution and Similarities on the WAIS, Delayed Visual and Verbal Recall, Object Memory, and Selective Reminding are some of the cognitive tests that are helpful in this early detection.

These or other cognitive tests detect about 85% of persons who will become demented in 4 years. About 5% of persons whose early testing is suggestive do not become demented. These are false positives, whose cognitive decline may be functionally important but not due to Alzheimer's disease. Positron emission tomography (PET) with radiolabeled acetylcholinesterase can also identify the substantially reduced parietotemporal acetylcholine activity that is found in Alzheimer's disease patients.

The very early predictive ability of cognitive tests cannot be overemphasized. For example, in a group of nuns, autobiographies written in their early 20s predicted Alzheimer's disease almost 60 years later. Low idea density was the best predictor. In fact, cognitive testing plus family perceptions of the patient's condition are the best predictors of the diagnosis.

Although the A-Test (a letter cancellation test) is the most sensitive bedside test for delirium, more difficult forms of cancellation are sensitive to "preclinical" dementia when used about every 6 months to avoid improvement by practice. Figure 12.1 displays a digit cancellation test you can use to evaluate persons you suspect are at high risk for Alzheimer's disease.

Once the dementia is obvious, the diagnostic likelihood of Alzheimer's disease substantially increased when SPECT shows posterior hypometabolism, EEG shows nonspecific slowing and low voltage activity, and MRI findings are normal, nonspecific, or indicate reduced temporal lobe volumes. The atropinic agents in eye drops, producing greater dilation in Alzheimer's patients, is still an experimental test, but pupillary dilation in response to tropicamide may identify carriers of ApoE 4 who are at greater risk for the disease. This test should be reserved for relatives who want to know more specifically their individual risks. Testing for an elevated intraneuronal protein (41-KD protein AD7C-NTP) is also experimental. Specific genetic testing for ApoE can improve diagnostic accuracy. Its use in otherwise healthy and cognitively normal older persons has no proven screening benefit.

Because early detection provides an opportunity to begin treatment with nonsteroidal anti-inflammatory agents and these agents can delay or ameliorate the decline, assess and follow up every first-degree relative of an Alzheimer's disease patient. Periodic SPECT and MRI in those with cognitive change or other risk factors can also help monitor the patient's response to anti-inflammatories. Consider this: A delay of only 5 years in the typical Alzheimer's onset or stage 2 of the illness would mean that 60% or more of persons likely to get Alzheimer's disease would die of something else *before* the illness develops or is at its worse.

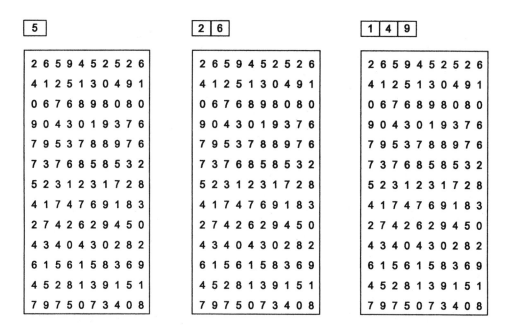

Figure 12.1. Digit Cancellation Test with target digits at the top of each set. Rectangle reproduction should be 21 cm long and 13 cm wide. Three sets of random numbers (0–9) are used. In the first set there is one target number, and the patient has to cross out all of these. In the second set there are two numbers to cross out, and in the last set there are three numbers to cross out. Tell the patient to scan each line from left to right starting at the top, as if reading. Do not allow the patient to use a finger or pencil to scan. The total of correctly crossed out numbers minus the number of any incorrect cross outs within 45 seconds is the score for each set. The first two lines of each set are for practice, the remaining 11 are the test with top scores of 10, 20, and 30, respectively. Cut-off scores are 6, 9, and 8, respectively. Normal persons typically achieve scores of 9, 13, and 16 or more. About 30% of Alzheimer's patients will perform below 6, and 50% will perform below 9 and 8, respectively. (After Della Sala, et al; *Psychol Med* 22:885–901, 1992.)

Action Brain Dementias: Frontal Lobe Dementias

Many conditions (Table 12.6) can produce frontal lobe dementia, and as a group they are the second most common dementia syndrome after Alzheimer's disease. Frontal lobe dementia involves the action brain, and its clinical features reflect a disruption in action (e.g., too little as in avolition, too much as in disinhibition). Alzheimer's disease initially involves the perceptual-integrating brain, and its clinical features reflect this (e.g., poor spatial functioning and facial recognition). Table 12.7 summarizes the differences between frontal lobe dementia and Alzheimer's disease.

Once you have established that the patient has a frontal lobe dementia, your next step is to determine cause. First, try to establish if the dysfunction has a subcortical pattern. If so, then white matter or basal ganglia disease becomes more likely. If the dysfunction appears mostly cortical, then primary cortical degeneration or traumatic brain injury becomes more likely. Table 12.8 lists some of the fea-

TABLE 12.6. Causes of Frontal Lobe Type or Action Brain Dementia Syndrome

Most white matter dementias (progressive multifocal leukoencephalopathy, multiple sclerosis, metachromatic leukodystrophy, AIDS, vitamin B$_{12}$ deficiency, Binswanger's disease)

Basal ganglia dementias (Huntington's, Parkinson's, Wilson's diseases)

Non-Korsakoff's alcohol dementia

Stroke (to anterior or action brain systems, hypertension more likely than diabetes; other causes are severe hyperlipidemia, sickle cell disease, thrombocytosis, polycythemia, ruptured aneurysm)

Amyloid angiopathy (thickened arterial walls lead to white matter and cortical infarcts and dementia)

Antiphospholipid antibody syndrome (women more than men; an autoimmune-like proneness to thrombosis syndrome with lupus anticoagulant and anticardiolipin abnormalities causing strokes, pulmonary embolism, phlebothrombosis, arthralgias, spontaneous abortions, lupus-like cardiac valvular abnormalities, migraine-like headache, thrombocytopenia, and dementia)

Cancer (a white matter dementia from myelotoxic producing carcinomas)

CADASIL (Cerebral Autosomal Dominant Arteriopathy with Subcortical Infarcts and Leukoencephalopathy); locus on chromosome 19, causing eosinophilic and granular material build up in blood vessel walls resulting in early onset (ages 30–50 years) TIAs, strokes, migraine-like headaches, pseudobulbar palsy, and dementia)

Chromosome 17 autosomal dominant dementia (an unclear process that leads to rapidly progressive frontotemporal cortical degeneration and gliosis with onset around age 50 and death within 3 years; akinesia, leg apraxias, muscle rigidity, loss of spontaneous speech and nonfluent aphasia, dementia)

Progressive supranuclear palsy (a diencephalic neurodegenerative process that affects the superior colliculi, substantia nigra, striatum, and limbic system; hypersomnia, somatic complaints, loss of interest, crying spells can be mistaken for depression; dementia with eye movement problems in a nonalcoholic)

Pseudoxanthoma elasticum (blood vessel wall deterioration leading to white matter dementia with multiple small strokes and progressive motor abnormalities; like Binswanger's disease without hypertension and more motor signs)

Space-occupying lesions (syphilis [frontal gumma], tumors [typically meningioma impinging on frontal lobe poles], frontal subarachnoid and intracerebral traumatic bleeds, vascular malformations [usually with secondary hemorrhaging], can cause long-standing subtle behavioral changes that eventually progress with increasing cognitive decline to dementia)

Idiopathic frontal lobe degeneration (a non-Pick's disease process with degeneration of the frontal cortex and caudate nuclei and frontal myelin; clinically similar to Pick's disease and often misdiagnosed as Pick's disease, Alzheimer's disease, or schizophrenia)

TABLE 12.7. Differences Between Frontal Lobe Type (an Action Brain Dementia) and Alzheimer's Disease (a Perceptual-Integrating Brain Syndrome)

Frontal Lobe Dementia	Alzheimer's Disease
Early personality change: apathy and emotional blunting, disinhibition, coarsening	Early temporoparietal pattern of problems: Visuospatial difficulties (auto accidents), poor facial recognition, getting lost; memory problems early and worse than frontal: Forgetting events, loss of details in giving history, cuing does not help with new learning tasks
May become hypochondriacal, obsessional, and gluttonous; persecutory delusions and irritability, loss of social graces, and social withdrawal	
Less intellectually impaired on testing, which is better than predicted by their behavior: do better on short delay recall of new information, cuing helps, more perseverative errors, loss of sequences of events but not details in giving history; spatial abilities preserved, but attentional shifts, poor abstraction, poor category formation	Auditory comprehension and naming problems
	More "neurologic" signs: Rigidity, akinesia, myoclonus
	Abnormal EEG
Decreased verbal fluency, more verbal stereotypes, decreased speech spontaneity, eventually profound paucity of speech	SPECT shows temporoparietal hypoperfusion
EEG often normal	MRI shows reduced temporal lobe volumes
SPECT shows hypofrontality	30–50% of patients will have positive family history: Alzheimer's disease, Down syndrome, leukemia
MRI may be normal or shows anterior brain lesions	

tures helpful in this differentiation. Because cerebellar-pontine systems are part of the action brain, disease in this area can also produce a mild frontal lobe dementia, with cerebellar rather than basal ganglia or frontal motor signs.

Frontal Lobe Dementia: Initial Cortical Pattern

Among the conditions to consider is *idiopathic frontal lobe degeneration.* The majority of patients are not diagnosed until autopsy and are clinically misdiagnosed as having Pick's or Alzheimer's disease or schizophrenia. However, it is clinically distinct from Alzheimer's disease, and Alzheimer's plaques and neurotangles are absent. It is initially clinically similar to Pick's disease, but the clinical progression remains frontal, whereas in Pick's disease the initial frontal lobe pattern is compounded with additional temporoparietal features as the disease progresses. Neuroanatomically, Pick's is characterized by swollen neurons with displaced nuclei and round argentophilic intraneuronal inclusions (Pick's bodies), whereas idiopathic frontal lobe degeneration is characterized by frontal cortical gray matter,

TABLE 12.8. Features Helpful in Circumscribing Frontal Lobe Type Action Brain Dementia Causing Lesions

Prefrontal Cortex	Basal Ganglia	Thalamus	White Matter	Cerebellum-Pons
Pure avolitional or disinhibition syndrome	Depression (L)	Apathy or irritability	Loss of spontaneity and apathy	Mild avolition or mild disinhibition
Delusions	Obsessive compulsive disorder (R)	Formal thought disorder (L), psychosis	Emotional lability	Learned movements are no longer automatic, patient must think about doing them (sequencing done slowly)
Coarsening of personality	Mania (R)	Pathologic crying	Perseverations	
Loss of spontaneous speech and fluency speech (L)	Trouble starting movement sequences and, once started, trouble stopping	Hypersomnia	Bradykinesia *without* rigidity or tremor	
Apraxias	Muscle stiffness	Pseudobulbar palsy as strokes in thalamus can affect surrounding areas (poor vertical gaze, up worse than down, slow saccades)	Dysarthria	Other cerebellar signs (nystagmus, past-pointing, intention tremor, dysdiadochokinesia)
Confabulation	Other motor signs (resting tremor, propulsive gait)		Muscle weakness (legs worse than arms)	
Poor motor sequencing			Small-stepped gait	Urinary incontinence (pontine lesion)
Practice improves motor performance			Grasp reflex	
			Urinary incontinence	Glossopharyngeal nerve problems (trouble swallowing)
			Altered consciousness	
			Initial hemiparesis or hemiplegia that resolves quickly	Practice does not improve motor performance
				Trouble generating and using verbs

L, left; R, right.

caudate nuclei, and frontal myelin degeneration, with secondary astrocytic gliosis.

Pick's disease (frontotemporal dementia) accounts for 5% of dementias. Most Pick's disease patients are not identified until autopsy, after being clinically diagnosed as having Alzheimer's disease. Men are somewhat more at risk than women. Onset age is usually 40–60 years. Although Pick's and Alzheimer's diseases have overlapping features, in Pick's disease dysfunction begins frontotemporally (more left than right) and progresses posteriorly. Personality change occurs early with marked executive function problems, but relative sparing of new learning. Patients can become avolitional or disinhibited. Speech becomes cliche filled and perseverative. The dorsolateral prefrontal cortex syndrome combined with the higher risk for men, occasionally results in the misdiagnosis of Pick's disease as late onset schizophrenia. Food craving and compulsions may also develop, explaining some accounts of schizophrenia with obsessive compulsive disorder. EEG and imaging findings circumscribed to frontotemporal areas (including frontal hypoperfusion on SPECT) help to distinguish Pick's disease from Alzheimer's disease and schizophrenia. Alzheimer's disease has an early temporoparietal pattern, whereas schizophrenia has more diffuse structural changes, although a SPECT pattern similar to that for Pick's disease. Patients with Pick's disease may have increased spinal fluid globulins. In both Pick's disease and Alzheimer's disease, bilateral hippocampal degeneration can cause the Kluver-Bucy syndrome.

Patients with behavioral syndromes due to Pick's disease are treated as if they had the primary syndrome (e.g., mood stabilizers for the disinhibited syndrome, selected serotonin reuptake inhibitors for obsessive compulsive disorder). Some patients develop a cortical-basal ganglia variant with neuronal degeneration. Apraxia, cortical-sensory loss, alien limb, parkinsonian features, dystonia, and myoclonus can develop, with neuronal loss and basophilic inclusions in achromatic neurons in the substantia nigra compacta.

Frontal Lobe Dementia with Basal Ganglia Disease

Parkinson's, Huntington's, and Wilson's diseases form the majority of extrapyramidal disorders causing dementia. Tardive dyskinesia (discussed elsewhere in the text) also can cause a modest frontal lobe syndrome. The dementia associated with these disorders differs somewhat in pattern (termed *subcortical*) from those dementias directly affecting the cerebral cortex, although frontal lobe features are prominent because frontal lobe–basal ganglia–thalamic circuits are disrupted. There is substantial symptom overlap between cortical and subcortical dementia; nevertheless, the subcortical pattern, when clear, helps in diagnosis. The subcortical pattern is (1) bradykinesia; (2) memory impairment; (3) bradyphrenia (i.e., the slowing of cognitive processes leading to poor performance on many tests); (4) mood disturbances, most commonly an avolitional nonmelancholic depression; (5) motor abnormalities; and (6) absence of apraxia, aphasias, and agnosias.

Parkinson's disease (PD) is the most common basal ganglia disorder associated with dementia. PD affects 2% of the population and as many as 20% of persons over age 65. Thirty percent of PD patients become demented. Although street drugs (methylphenyl-tetrahydropyridine [MPTP]), viral infection, toxins, and trauma can cause a parkinsonian syndrome, in most patients the etiology is unknown. In these patients widespread brain areas are involved (ventral tegmental area, brain stem raphe nuclei, substantia innomenata, hypothalamus, locus ceruleus, and dorsal motor nucleus of the vagus), with the effect on the nigrostriatal system being most pronounced. Neuronal loss and Lewy body neuronal inclusions are the typical pathologies and are sometimes indistinguishable from Alzheimer's disease. Also, about 30% of Alzheimer's patients develop muscle rigidity.

Some distinguishing clinical features are (1) PD patients can recall when prompted, but Alzheimer's disease patients cannot; (2) PD patients do not have aphasia, whereas Alzheimer's disease patients can develop transcortical sensory aphasia; (3) poor psychomotor speed and bradyphrenia are common in PD, but normal in early stages of Alzheimer's disease; (4) a dorsolateral prefrontal cortex syndrome is seen in PD, but not in Alzheimer's disease; (5) depression is common in PD, less so in Alzheimer's disease; and (6) PD patients have a frontal cognitive impairment pattern with frontal hypometabolism and delayed waves on evoked potential, whereas Alzheimer's disease patients have a temporoparietal pattern with temporoparietal hypometabolism, temporal lobe atrophy, and reduced wave amplitude on evoked potential.

Classic features of PD include (1) motor disturbances (bradykinesia, rigidity, resting tremor that can begin in one limb, often the preferred arm or leg); (2) mood disturbances (nonmelancholic major depression in 50% of patients, mania in 5%); and (3) memory and cognitive deficits, including bradyphrenia (slow cognition) and impaired recall with spared recognition.

The depression in PD is a "neurologic" dysfunction, not simply demoralization, and the severity of the depression does not correlate with the severity of motor impairment. Having a family history of PD (about 15% of patients), a prior head injury with unconsciousness, and chronic exposure to insecticides and herbicides increases the risk for PD. PD patients are less likely to be smokers, perhaps because they are less sensitive to the dopamine-stimulating properties of nicotine. Also, there appears to be an association between PD and amyotrophic lateral sclerosis, with both co-occurring in the same families. A susceptibility gene on the long arm of chromosome 4 that codes for a presynaptic protein and is thought to be involved in neuronal plasticity has been implicated in PD.

Levodopa (up to 600 mg) or levodopa plus a decarboxylase inhibitor (e.g., carbidopa) is the treatment of choice for the motor features of PD. Further treatment includes adding a dopamine agonist (bromcriptine) to levodopa rather than increasing the levodopa dosage. This strategy minimizes the likelihood of levodopa side effects, including nausea and hypotension (usually early), dyskinesias, cognitive impairment, psychosis (often manic-like), and fluctuating mobility problems. Bromocriptine may also modestly improve the bradyphrenia associated with PD, so cognition benefits somewhat. The use of levodopa within 3 years of diagnosis substantially reduces the mortality rate of PD patients. Apomorphine challenge and SPECT help predict levodopa responsivity. The apomorphine test requires administering 20 mg of the peripheral dopamine-receptor antagonist domperidone TID for 24 hours (to prevent side effects), followed by 2–5 mg of apomorphine subcutaneously. A positive test is the transient but unequivocal improvement in motor symptoms. SPECT, using I^{123} or similar agents, can reveal proportionally greater infusion frontally than in basal ganglia.

ECT is also helpful, even in PD patients without depression. Selegiline (deprenyl), a monoamine oxidase B inhibitor, also ameliorates the progression of disability and may be added to levodopa therapy. For those patients who no longer respond to medication or ECT, stereotactic ventral pallidotomy can substantially help with minimal mobility or mortality. Fetal adrenal tissue transplant surgery remains experimental.

Huntington's disease (HD) is the most commonly recognized form of familial chorea. It typically begins between 30 and 50 years of age, is progressive, and usually leads to death within 15–20 years of the first symptoms. There is a juvenile form with prominent muscle rigidity and a late onset form with less progressive deterioration with cognitive impairment but no dementia. HD reflects the autosomal dominant transmission of a trinucleotide repeat (CAG)* on the short arm of chromosome 4, which when more than 36 repeated sequences occurs, results in varying degrees of bilateral neuronal loss in the caudate, putamen, and other brain structures. Typically, the more repeats, the worse the neuronal loss and the more progressively dementing the condition. Repeats can go as high as 150.

HD has substantial clinical variation. Those with the highest number of repeats have an early onset (juvenile form), whereas those with the fewest repeats (but still more than 36), have the later onsets and the best prognosis, sometimes avoiding dementia. About one-third of patients develop a nonmelancholic, avolitional depression early in the illness course when none or only subtle motor signs are present (mild finger overflow, mild dysarthria when excited or speaking fast). A small proportion become manic or psychotic, and these too may occur early before the motor features are obvious. Early signs of cognitive impairment include a sense of reduced efficiency and indecisiveness (perhaps reflecting problems with executive functions and reduced cognitive speed) and vague memory concerns with modest reduced performance in verbal learning. Cerebral atrophy is modest at first, but in later stages bilateral caudate atrophy produces a "butterfly" pattern of ventricular enlargement on CT scan.

Like most diseases affecting the basal ganglia, the HD pattern is abnormal movements, memory problems, and mood disturbances. Suspect HD in any person under age 50 with this triad. Conditions that must be ruled out are (1) neuroa-

---

*Some of the base consequences in genes are repeats, usually three bases repeating themselves (e.g., CAG, CAG, CAG). When repeats get too long (the threshold length varies with the amino acids involved) that section of the genetic sequence becomes chemically different. For example, in the CGG repeat of the fragile X syndrome, when the repeats number over 230, that string of repeats is methylated and becomes genetically silent. Because the repeat section of the genetic code is now different it results in different (abnormal) protein formation or protein not being produced, and cells, receptors, neurotransmitters, and so forth, become abnormal in some way leading to disease. There are several diseases that result from trinucleotide repeats, e.g., HD (CAG 30–150 repeats), fragile X syndrome (230–2,000 CCG repeats), myoclonic dystrophy (99–2,000 CTG repeats), and Friedrich's ataxia (200–1,000 CAA repeats).

canthrocytosis (an autosomal recessive disorder that produces an HD pattern plus anemia with distorted red cells or acanthrocytes); (2) Wilson's disease (look for Kayser-Fleischer rings and test blood for ceruloplasmin); (3) pernicious anemia (measure B_{12} and folic acid levels); (4) multiple sclerosis (has two incidence peaks, in the 20s and 40s, and the latter may initially look like mild HD; look for cerebellar more than basal ganglia problems, plus MRI white matter lesions, evoked potential increased wave latencies, and increased spinal fluid globulin); (5) familial striatal degeneration (measure antinuclear antibody levels); (6) Fahr's disease (bilateral basal ganglia calcifications from trauma, infection, hemorrhagic stroke, carbon monoxide poisoning); and (7) exposure to agents that damage the basal ganglia (e.g., neuroleptics, MPTP).

Treatment for HD is similar to the nonspecific treatments for Alzheimer's disease (see below). Haloperidol can control some of the dyskinetic movements of HD.

Wilson's disease can be partially reversed if identified early. Onset is at ages 15–25 years, characterized by frontal lobe features, facial bradykinesia (expressionless), tremors, limb rigidity, dysarthria, choreoathetosis, and arm movements like the beating of wings. Seizures can occur later in the course. Kayser-Fleischer rings (golden brown copper pigmentation along the edge of the cornea) are not always present. Liver degeneration also occurs, so the pattern is (1) early onset cognitive decline with frontal lobe features, (2) motor abnormalities, and (3) liver dysfunction with cirrhosis. Liver function tests, MRI findings in the basal ganglia, and elevated serum ceruloplasmin level are diagnostic. Early treatment with D-penicillamine helps.

Frontal Lobe Dementia Associated With White Matter Disease

The pattern of white matter dementia is (1) a dementia usually developing before age 70 years, (2) mild progression of cognitive impairment, (3) sparing of personality, and (4) a subcortical dementia pattern. Frontal lobe features predominate, so white matter dementias are one cause of the frontal lobe dementia syndrome. Several morbid processes affecting white matter can cause dementia.

Vascular dementia accounts for 10%–15% of dementia patients. African-Americans are at greater risk for vascular dementia than are Euroamericans. Even though frontal lobe dementias form the second largest group of dementias, next to Alzheimer's disease, vascular brain changes are the second single most common *cause* of dementia. Many vascular dementias have a frontal lobe pattern.

Onset of vascular dementia usually occurs during the 50s or 60s; men are more at risk. Vascular dementia usually results from sustained hypertension that causes necrosis and occlusion of cerebral arterioles, with erratic but progressive disruption of cognitive function. Atherosclerosis of large blood vessels, vascular inflammatory conditions, and hematologic disorders (e.g., sickle cell anemia, polycythemia) are other causes. Hemispheric white matter is most often affected (Binswanger's disease). The thalamus, basal ganglia, and internal capsule may also be involved. Compared with Alzheimer's disease patients, patients with vascular dementia are more apt to have bradykinesia (psychomotor retardation), psychosis, depression (when dominant frontal circuits are involved), or anxiety. SPECT shows focal hypoperfusion, and MRI shows multiple white matter hyperintensities. Treatments of the underlying condition may slow progression of the disorder. Anticoagulants or aspirin may prevent thrombus formation.

Other white matter dementias are *progressive multifocal leukoencephalopathy* (almost always associated with chronic lymphoma, myeloproliferative disease, or papovavirus infection), multiple sclerosis (later onset peak in the 40s with optic atrophy or cerebellar signs), *metachromatic leukodystrophy* (with peripheral neuropathy from an autosomal recessive gene), *adrenoleukodystrophy* (onset in childhood), *AIDS* (HIV positive and overt AIDS features), *vitamin B12 deficiency* (early atypical apathetic depression, spinal cord posterior column signs, and megaloblastic anemia), *traumatic brain injury* (diffuse axonal injury), and *neurotoxicity* (e.g., from toluene, alcohol). Most patients with these conditions avoid dementia unless the white matter involvement is extensive. For example, although 50%–75% of HIV/AIDS patients have some cognitive impairment, the prevalence and severity of the impairment increases with illness severity, so dementia develops only in later stages of AIDS. In addition to specific laboratory testing, MRI and evoked potentials are the most helpful laboratory assessments.

Dementias Initially Affecting Both Action and Perceptual Integrating Brains

Creutzfeldt-Jakob disease is a degenerating process of the action and the perceptual-integrating brain systems. Other than for outbreaks associated with conditions such as "mad cow" disease, this rapidly progressive dementia is rare. The more severe form usually occurs after age 65, is characterized by initial ataxia, myoclonus, dementia, and death in 1–2 years. An early onset variant (<age 30) is characterized by early sensory complaints (e.g., post-pain leg dysathesias, cold feet), early behavioral problems (avolitional depression), and later motor problems (unsteadiness, involuntary movements, cerebellar signs), and cognitive decline (visuoperceptual function and memory) followed by rapid overall decline and death. EEG shows periodic slow triphasic complexes due to spongiform encephalopathy from prion inclusions (codon 129), usually acquired from eating meats contaminated with prion-containing brains and spinal cords of sheep.

Lewy body dementia is a neuropatholic designation for dementing conditions associated with the presence of small rounded cytoplasmic esosinophilic inclusions near the neuronal nucleus or in dendrites. Four subtypes represent differences in the distribution of the Lewy bodies:

1. Subcortical type, the most common, with brain stem and basal ganglia involvement and clinically identical to Parkinson's disease
2. Cortical type, with only a cerebral cortex distribution that mimics frontotemporal dementias (e.g., Pick's disease, idiopathic frontal lobe degeneration)
3. Mixed type, found in 10%–15% of Alzheimer's disease patients (often without a family history for Alzheimer's disease, the "sporadic" type)

4. Diffuse type, with cortical and subcortical inclusions, which has a fluctuating course and an early positive symptom nonaffective psychosis that can be mistakenly labeled late onset schizophrenia.

Diffuse type patients have substantial problems with memory retrieval; thus, unlike Alzheimer's patients, their recall is helped by cuing. Early after onset they also have motor problems (resting tremor, rigidity, and myoclonus) and can be mistaken for having Parkinson's disease. Unlike Parkinson's disease patients, their EEGs may show early frontotemporal bursts of slow waves and MRI frontal atrophy. Recognizing this condition is important because 50%–80% of these patients are hypersensitive to neuroleptics and, if given neuroleptics, will develop severe motor side effects. If you cannot avoid using a neuroleptic, use risperidone in low doses.

MANAGEMENT

Specific Treatments

The treatment of dementia rarely targets the cause. Etiologically specific treatments include D-penicillamine for Wilson's disease, vitamin and hormone replacement for nutritional and endocrine disorders, ventricular shunting for normal pressure hydrocephalus, penicillin for neurosyphilis, and surgery for vascular malformations and subdural hematoma.

Patients with Alzheimer's disease have cholinergic deficits, and thus some treatments focus on *enhancing cholinergic function.* Although none of these treatments has proved consistently helpful, physicians and family members will try almost any therapy, particularly early in the disease. Tacrine and donepezil, cholinesterase inhibitors, are the most commonly used drugs, but they are only modestly helpful during stage 1 of the illness, when a critical number of cholinergic neurons are still functional. Tacrine (Cognex) is given in doses below 100 mg daily to minimize liver damage. It is highly lipophilic and thus concentrates in the brain. It inhibits muscarinic receptors, increases acetylcholine release, and has some MAO and monoamine reuptake-inhibiting properties. Side effects include nausea, belching, diarrhea, sweating, and bradycardia.

Donepezil (Aricept) given 5–10 mg once daily has less side effects (syncope, nausea, diarrhea, vomiting). A test dose of physostigmine (1–2 mg subcutaneously), a short-acting (2-hour half-life) cholinesterase inhibitor, can help determine if the longer acting drugs are likely to work. A substantial but transient improvement in memory test performance is a good sign.

Lecithin and choline, acetylcholine precursors, are sometimes added as dietary supplements. Naltrexone stimulates acetylcholine release by inhibiting endorphins and is sometimes added as an enhancer during stage 1. The postsynaptic acetylcholine receptor stimulators arcoline, succinimide, and velnacrine are used in stages 2 and 3 as they do not require an intact presynaptic system.

Among other drug strategies, selegiline (10 mg daily), an irreversible MAOI

TABLE 12.9. Treatment Strategy for Alzheimer's

PHASE 1:

The High Risk Patient in the "Preclinical" Stage (the guiding principle is prevention or delay of onset)

1. Base-line SPECT, EEG, and MRI
2. Monitor preventative efforts with cognitive testing
3. Begin nonsteroidal anti-inflammatory agents, vitamin E, and, for women, estrogen replacement
4. Aerobic and cognitive exercises
5. Patient and family education and counseling; link family with a support group or organization

PHASE 2:

Clinical Alzheimer's Stage 1 (the guiding principle is to moderate the decline)

1. Monitor treatment efforts with cognitive testing
2. Maintain nonsteroidal anti-inflammatory agents, vitamin E, and estrogen
3. Treat with a cholinergic enhancing drug
4. Continue aerobic and cognitive exercises
5. Continue patient and family counseling
6. Begin to structure patient's living situation

PHASE 3:

Clinical Alzheimer's Stages 2 and 3 (the guiding principle is to maximize the patient's quality of life)

1. Monitor treatment efforts with cognitive testing
2. Value of continuing nonsteroidal agents, vitamin E, and estrogen unclear
3. As decline has continued, cholinergic enhancement less likely to be of benefit; switch to selegiline and postsynaptic receptor stimulators
4. Treat behavioral problems
5. Continue aerobic and cognitive exercises
6. Provide interesting sensory excursions and activities to punctuate needed structure and routine
7. Continue family counseling and support group

specific for the MAO-B isoenzyme, may benefit some patients by improving cognition; reducing depression, psychotic features, agitation, and anxiety; and alleviating caregiver stress. Its use and side effects are similar to those of other MAOIs. MAOI dietary and drug restrictions are followed, but the risks of tyramine-induced hypertension at low doses is minimal. Its use becomes the responsibility of the caregivers, as selegiline is used in the later stages of the illness, when patients will not be able to adhere to detailed dietary instructions. As mentioned above, nonsteroidal anti-inflammatory agents may delay the onset and slow the

TABLE 12.10. Treatments for Frontal Lobe Type Action Brain Dementia Behavioral Problems

Problem	Suggested Treatment(s)
Anxiety and agitation	Buspirone 10–15 mg daily
Aggressiveness and violence	Beta-blockers, lithium, carbamazepine in doses similar to those used to control these behaviors due to traumatic brain injury
Disinhibited syndrome	The more manic-like, the more you treat like a primary mood disorder (e.g., valproate, carbamazepine, lithium)
Pathologic crying	1. Sudden, short, but often frequent crying outbursts that the patient does not experience as a depression
	2. If associated with basal ganglia motor features, particularly stiffness, use carbidopa/levodopa; if no stiffness or other basal ganglia signs, use an antidepressant; low doses usually work (e.g., nortriptyline 50–75 mg, desipramine 50–100 mg)
Depression	1. The more like a typical depression, the more you manage with typical antidepressant treatments
	2. The more avolition and anergia rather than a typical mood of depression, the more likely stimulants alone or combined with an antidepressant will work best
	3. Do not use stimulants if the patient is psychotic or agitated
Avolition and anergia	1. Stimulants often improve these features as well as overall cognitive performance as bradyphrenia resolves
	2. Methylphenidate (15–30 mg daily), bromocriptine (30 mg TID), amantadine* (400 mg daily)
	3. If associated with an apathetic depression, bupropion in standard doses
	4. Do not use stimulants if patient is psychotic or agitated
Psychosis	1. When manic-like, use mood stabilizers, ECT, neuroleptics (haloperidol [5–10 mg daily], resperidone [<8 mg daily)
	2. When schizophrenic-like, use resperadone

*Amantadine facilitates dopamine release, delays its reuptake, and increases or alters postsynaptic dopamine receptors; it also decreases cholinergic transmission (do not use in Alzheimer's disease) that relatively increases dopamine as it is a glutamate receptor antagonist and may protect against secondary neuronal damage from too much glutamide release; best when dementia due to traumatic brain injury.

TABLE 12.11. Guidelines for Psychosocial and Behavioral Care of the Demented Patient

Area of Concern	What to Do
Caretaker's behavior	1. Pace interactions to match patient's response time
	2. Act calmly during patient's overly emotional reactions to inability to perform tasks ("catastrophic response")
	3. Use distraction, not confrontation, to control irritable or socially inappropriate behavior
	4. Expect denial of symptoms and be firm but nonconfrontational in maintaining injury prevention procedures
	5. Pitch voice to lower, easier-to-hear register that also sounds less stressed
	6. Use short, simple sentences
	7. Explain all interactions and activities and, as much as possible, include patient in decision making
	9. Avoid distractions, such as more than one person speaking at a time
Living area	1. Keep area uncluttered, tidy, well lit, unchanging, and familiar
	2. Use night lights and reflecting tape to facilitate nighttime perception
	3. Use a system of clearly displayed, simply written instructions, reminders, and directions
Self-care	1. Simplify and routinize all self-care tasks (bathing, dressing, cleaning living area)
	2. Rely on less complex utensils and clothes (velcro straps instead of laces or buttons, clip-on ties)
	3. Stress procedural strengths
	4. Use home care, visiting nurses, and daycare to delay going into nursing home for as long as possible
Activities	1. Establish a daily routine for meals, medication, exercise, recreation, and hobbies
	2. Match activities to patient's cognitive abilities
	3. Schedule special activities with pleasurable sensory theme (food, pets, music, visits to park or botanical garden) to highlight a low stimulus environment
Sleep disturbance	1. Morning bright light therapy (the same system that is used for seasonal affective disorder), time-release melatonin at bedtime, daily exercise, good sleep hygiene, flexible environment that expects and tolerates sleep problems

TABLE 12.11. (*continued*)

Area of Concern	What to Do
	2. Avoid sedative-hypnotics, as they increase the risk for delirium and falls
	3. As last resorts, try aspirin if not contraindicated (has mild sedating effect in some elderly persons), a nicotine patch, or short-acting benzodiazepines in low doses
Memory problems	1. Educate caregivers to the patient's specific memory deficits
	2. Use constant repetition of concrete information about date, time of day, activities
	3. Use signs and word pictures, clocks and calendars, list of daily and special activities, labeled photographs of persons important to the patient
	4. Sequence medications based on staging: Vitamin E and nonsteroidal anti-inflammatory agents and aerobic exercise throughout, cholinergic enhancers early (lecithin, choline, tacrine, donepezil), naltrexone to stimulate acetylcholine early, selegiline in stage 2, cholinomimetic agents late (arecoline, succinimide, velnacrine)
Restlessness and agitation	1. Educate caregiver to expect this and how to remain as relaxed, friendly, and calm as possible; educate caregiver about catastrophic reactions
	2. Exercise can replace some agitation, and a calm and uncluttered environment can minimize it
	3. Background music may reduce agitated periods
	4. Educate about wandering (particularly at night); use exercise/ID bracelet/secured living environment to minimize wandering
	5. Buspirone rather than benzodiazepines or sedative-hypnotics
Violence	1. Structured, friendly, respectful caregiving is best preventative
	2. Use buspirone rather than sedative-hypnotics
Psychosis	1. Determine if psychosis is co-occurring delirium and if so treat the delirium
	2. If no delirium, use risperidone for nonaffective psychoses, haloperidol second choice
	3. If mood disorder, ECT is safest treatment, lithium and valproate second choices

decline. Vitamin E, estrogen replacement in women, and aerobic and cognitive exercises all have some benefit and should be routinely used with Alzheimer's patients. Estrogen may inhibit amyloid accretion; vitamin E may help with neuronal repair. Table 12.9 displays the overall strategy for treating patients with Alzheimer's disease.

What *does not* work for Alzheimer's disease patients are vasopressin (thought to play a role in normal memory), piracetam (thought to enhance memory), nerve growth factor (does not cross the blood–brain barrier), ergoloid mesylates (e.g., Hydergine, widely used to improve cognition but, if effective, only at highest doses), psychostimulants (to reduce apathy, but cause anxiety), chelators (hoped to bind excessive aluminum in the brains of Alzheimer's patients, but side effects are substantial without demonstrated benefit), and neurotransmitter precursors (tyrosine, 5-hydroxytryptophan, and carbidopa, all producing side effects with little improvement).

Because prevention or at least a substantial delay in symptoms is now possible, patients 65 years or older with a family history of Alzheimer's disease or associated diseases (especially if they have additional risk factors noted above) should (1) receive genetic counseling and, if assessed as being able to deal well with "the news," may be tested for the ApoE and perhaps the amyloid genotype; (2) be periodically screened with cognitive testing (Mini-Mental State, Digit Span, and Digit Symbol Substitution; story paragraph recall and recall of a complex geometric figure; digit cancellation); (3) have baseline metabolic (look for temporoparietal hypoperfusion on SPECT) and structural (look for some decrease in MRI temporal lobe volume) assessments; and (4) if their risk seems moderate to high, begin a regular dose of an anti-inflammatory agent and, for women, estrogen replacement if their risk seems moderate to high.

Nonspecific Treatments

Nonspecific treatments for frontal lobe dementias are similar to those for Alzheimer's disease (see below). More specific treatments focus on controlling or eliminating the cause (e.g., controlling hypertension, giving aspirin to reduce risk for ischemic stroke, removing a tumor) and ameliorating the behavioral syndrome likely to be present with a frontal lobe dementia. Table 12.10 lists some treatment guidelines.

Nonspecific treatment also remains important in the care of patients with other dementias. Nonspecific pharmacologic treatment includes low-dose neuroleptics for psychosis (risperidone less than 8 mg daily is a good choice to minimize extrapyramidal side effects). However, whenever possible, avoid neuroleptics because their use may hasten cognitive decline in dementia. Avoid the newer neuroleptics with substantial anticholinergic properties (clozapine, olanzapine) that are poorly tolerated in the elderly. Also, because the early strategy for Alzheimer's disease is to *enhance* cholinergic function, anticholinergic drugs are counterproductive. For seizures, use anticonvulsants. The type of seizures determines anticonvulsant choice. ECT for psychoses due to dementia also can be effective, particularly when depressive or manic features predominate.

Hospital or nursing home care must be structured. Often, demented patients neglect their self-care and food intake. Much effort is required to maintain their hygiene and to provide an adequate diet. Continued physical activity in structured exercise and sports and socialization programs can delay deterioration and enrich a patient's life. Participation in frequent "special events" (picnics; visits to museums, botanic gardens, zoos) may delay cognitive decline. Encourage family members and friends to visit often and participate in these activities. Physicians and ward staff often underestimate the capabilities of demented patients. Encourage patients to participate in activities consistent with their cognitive, behavioral, and physical abilities Activity programs should be interesting. Do not treat elderly and demented patients as children. Table 12.11 provides some psychosocial and behavioral guidelines for caring for demented patients.

ADDITIONAL READINGS

Alessi CA: Managing the behavioral problems of dementia in the home. *Geriatric Home Care* 7:787–801, 1991.

American Psychiatric Association: Practice guideline for the treatment of patients with Alzheimer's disease and other dementias of late life. *Am J Psychiatry* 5(suppl), 1997.

Baloh RW: Dizziness in older people. *J Am Geriatr Soc* 40:713–721, 1992.

Beck KD, Hefti F: Neurotrophic factor therapy of Alzheimer's disease. *Clin Neurosci* 1:219–224, 1993.

Bennett DA, Beckett LA, Murray AM, Shannon KM, Goetz CG, Pilgrim DM, Evans DA: Prevalence of Parkinsonian signs and associated mortality in a community population of older people. *N Engl J Med* 334:71–76, 1996.

Black SE: Focal cortical atrophy syndromes. *Brain Cogn* 31:188–229, 1996.

Blacker D, Tanzi RE: The genetics of Alzheimer disease: Current status and future prospects. *Arch Neurol* 55:294–296, 1998.

Blumenthal JA, Emery GF, Madden DJ, George LK, Coleman RE, Riddle MW, McKee DC, Reasoner J, Williams RS: Cardiovascular and behavioral effects of aerobic exercise training in healthy older men and women. *J Gerontol* 44:147–157, 1989.

Bonte FJ, Hom J, Tintner R, Weiner MF: Single photon tomography in Alzheimer's disease and the dementias. *Semin Nucl Med* 20:342–352, 1990.

Brandt J, Welsh KA, Breitner JCS, Folstein MF, Helms M, Christian JC: Hereditary influences on cognitive functioning in older men. A study of 4000 twin pairs. *Hered Cogn Funct* 50:599–603, 1993.

Bredesen DE: Potential role of gene therapy in the treatment of Parkinson's disease. *Clin Neurosci* 1:45–52, 1993.

Bryson HM, Benfield P: Donepezil. *Drugs Aging* 10:234–241, 1997.

Calne DB: Treatment of Parkinson's disease. *N Engl J Med* 329:1021–1027, 1993.

Campbell JJ III, Duffy JD, Salloway SP: Treatment strategies for patients with dysexecutive syndromes. *J Neuropsychiatry Clin Neurosci* 6:411–418, 1994.

Caplan LR: Binswanger's disease—revisited. *Neurology* 45:626–633, 1995.

Carlen PL, Wortzman G, Holgate RC, Wilkinson DA, Rankin JG: Reversible cerebral atrophy in recently abstinent chronic alcoholics measured by computed tomography scans. *Science* 200:1076–1078, 1978.

Clark RF, Goate AM: Molecular genetics of Alzheimer's disease. *Arch Neurol* 50:1164–1172, 1993.

Claus JJ, Ongerboer de Visser BW, Walstra GJM, Hijdra A, Verbeeten B Jr, van Gool, WA: Quantitative spectral electroencephalography in predicting survival in patients with early Alzheimer disease. *Arch Neruol* 55:1105–1111, 1998.

Corder EH, Lannfelt L, Voiitamen M, Corder LS, Manton KG, Winblad B, Basun H: Apolipoprotein E genotype determines survival in the oldest (85 years or older) who have good cognition. *Arch Neurol* 53:418–422, 1996.

Corder EH, Saunders AM, Strittmatter WJ, Schmechel DE, Gaskell PC, Small GW, Roses AD, Haines JL, Pericak-Vance MA: Gene dose of apolipoprotein E type 4 allele and the risk of Alzheimer's disease in late onset families. *Science* 261:921–923, 1993.

Couch JR Jr: Physical conditioning in the elderly. In Good DC, Couch JR Jr (eds): Handbook of Neurorehabilitation. Marcel Dekker, New York, 1994, pp 63–72.

Cummings JL, Benson DF: *Dementia: A Clinical Approach,* 2nd ed. Butterworth-Heinemann, Boston, 1992.

Darvish S, Freedman M: Subcortical dementia: A neurobehavioral approach. *Brain Cogn* 31:230–249, 1996.

DeLong MR, Wichmann T: Basal ganglia–thalamocortical circuits in parkinsonian signs. *Clin Neurosci* 1:18–26, 1993.

Della Sala S, Laiacone M, Spinnler H, Ubezio C: A cancellation test: Its reliability in assessing attentional deficits in Alzheimer's disease. *Psychol Med* 22:885–901, 1992.

Dogali M, Fazzini E, Kolodny E, Eidelberg D, Sterio D, Devinsky O, Berie A: Stereotactic ventral pallidotomy for Parkinson's disease. *Neurology* 45:753–761, 1995.

Dustman RE, Emmerson RY, Steinhaus LA, Shearer DE, Dustman TJ: The effects of video game playing on neuropsychological performance of elderly individuals. *J Gerontol Psychol Sci* 47:P168–P171, 1992.

Ebly EM, Hogan DB, Parhad IM: Cognitive impairment in the nondemented elderly. Results from the Canadian study of health and aging. *Arch Neurol* 52:612–619, 1995.

Edwards RH: Pathogenesis of Parkinson's disease. *Clin Neurosci* 1:36–44, 1993.

Ellis RJ, Jan K, Kawas C, Koller WC, Lyons KE, Jeste DV, Hansen LA, Thal LJ: Diagnostic validity of the dementia questionnaire for Alzheimer disease. *Arch Neurol* 55:360–365, 1998.

Fabrigoule C, Rouch I, Taberly A, Letenneur, L, Commenges D, Mazaux JM, Orgogozo JM, Dartigues JF: Cognitive process in preclinical phase of dementia. *Brain* 121:135–141, 1998.

Fink JS: Neurobiology of basal ganglia receptors: Targets for future therapy in Parkinson's disease. *Clin Neurosci* 1:27–35, 1993.

Graybiel AM: Functions of the nigrostriatal system. *Clin Neurosci* 1:12–17, 1993.

Geldmacher DS, Whitehouse PJ: Evaluation of dementia. *N Engl J Med* 335:330–336, 1996.

Geokas ML, Conteas CN, Majumdar APN: The aging gastrointestinal tract, liver, and pancreas. *Clin Geriatr Med* 1:177–206, 1985.

Golbe LI: The genetics of Parkinson's disease: A reconsideration. *Neurology* 40(suppl 3):7–16, 1990.

Gottlieb GL, Kumar A: Conventional pharmacologic treatment for patients with Alzheimer's disease. *Neurology* 43 (suppl 4):S56–S63, 1993.

Greenough WT, Black JE, Wallace CS: Experience and brain development. *Child Dev* 58:539–559, 1987.

Grilli M, Pizzi M, Memo M, Spano P: Neuroprotection by aspirin and sodium salicylate thought blockade of NF-KB activation. *Science* 274:1383–1385, 1996.

Hakim AA, Petrovitch H, Burchfiel CM, Ross GW, Rodriguez BL, White LR, Yano K, Curb D, Abbott RD: Effects of walking on mortality among nonsmoking retired men. *N Engl J Med* 338:94–99, 1998.

Henderson VW, Paganini-Hall, A, Emanuel CK, Dunn ME, Buckwalter G: Estrogen replacement therapy in older women. Comparison between Alzheimer's disease cases and nondemented control subjects. *Arch Neurol* 51:896–900, 1994.

Higuchi S, Matsushita S, Hasegawa Y, Muramatsu T, Arai H, Hayashida M: Apolipoprotein E4 allele and pupillary response to tropicamide. *Am J Psychiatry* 154:694–696, 1997.

Ishii N, Nishihara Y, Imamura T: Why do frontal lobe symptoms predominate in vascular dementia with lacunes? *Neurology* 36:340–345, 1986.

Jacobs DM, Sano M, Dooneief G, Marder K, Bell KL, Stern Y: Neuropsychological detection and characterization of preclinical Alzheimer's disease. *Neurology 45:*957–962, 1995.

Jagust WJ: Functional imaging in dementia: A review. *J Clin Psychiatry 55*(suppl 11):5–11, 1994.

Jason GW, Suchowersky O, Pajurkova EM, Graham Z, Klimek ML, Garber AT, Poirier-Heine D: Cognitive manifestations of Huntington disease in relation to genetic structure and clinical onset. *Arch Neurol 54:*1081–1088, 1997.

Jonker C, Schmand B, Lindeboom J, Havekes LM, Launer LJ: Association between apolipoprotein E4 and the rate of cognitive decline in community-dwelling elderly individuals with and without dementia. *Arch Neurol 55:*1065–1069, 1998.

Kalaria RN: Cerebral microvasculature and immunological factors in Alzheimer's disease. *Clin Neurosci 1:*204–211, 1993.

Katzman R: Clinical and epidemiological aspects of Alzheimer's disease. *Clin Neurosci 1:*165–170, 1993.

Kempermann G, Kuhn HG, Gage FH: More hippocampal neurons in adult mice living in an enriched environment. *Nature 386:*493–495, 1997.

Kertesz A, Munoz D: Pick's disease, frontotemporal dementia, and Pick complex. *Arch Neurol 55:*302–304, 1998.

Kim E, Rovner BW: Depression in dementia. *Psychiatr Ann 24:*173–177, 1994.

Knopman DS, Christensen KJ, Schut LJ, Harbaugh RE, Reeder T, Ngo T, Frey WH II: The spectrum of imaging and neuropsychological findings in Pick's disease. *Neurology 39:*362–368, 1989.

Lang AE, Lozano AM: Parkinson's disease: First of two parts. *N Engl J Med 339:*1044–1053, 1998.

Lang AE, Lozano AM: Parkinson's disease: Second of two parts. *N Engl J Med 339:*1130–1143, 1998.

Lapalio LR, Sakla SS: Distinguishing Lewy body dementia. *Hosp Pract 33:*93–108, 1998.

Linn RT, Wolfe PA, Bachman DL, Knoefel JE, Cobb JL, Belanger AJ, Kaplan EF, D'Agostino RB: The preclinical phase of probable Alzheimer's disease. A 13-year prospective study of the Framingham cohort. *Arch Neurol 52:*485–490, 1995.

Litvan I, MacIntyre A, Goetz CG, Wenning GK, Jellinger K, Verny M, Bartko JJ, Jankovic J, McKee A, Brandel JP, Ray Chaudhuri K, Lai EC, D'Olhaberriague L, Pearce RKB, Agid Y: Accuracy of the clinical diagnoses of Lewy body disease, Parkinson disease, and dementia with Lewy bodies: A clinicopathologic study. *Arch Neurol 55:*969–978, 1998.

Locascio JL, Growdon JH, Corkin S: Cognitive test performance in detecting, staging and tracking Alzheimer's disease. *Arch Neurol 52:*1087–1099, 1995.

Lopez OL, Becker JT, Brenner RP, Rosen J, Bojulaiye OI, Reynolds CF: Alzheimer's disease with delusions and hallucinations. *Neurology 41:*906–912, 1991.

Lyketsos CG, Chen L-S, Anthony JC: Cognitive decline in adulthood: An 11.5-year follow-up of the Baltimore epidemiologic catchment area study. *Am J Psychiatry 156:*58–65, 1999.

Mace NL, Rabins PV: *The 36-Hour Day: A Family Guide to Caring for Persons With Alzheimer's Disease, Related Dementing Illness, and Memory Loss in Later Life.* Johns Hopkins Press, Baltimore, 1982.

Markesbery WR, Ehmann WD: Aluminum and Alzheimer's disease. *Clin Neurosci 1:*212–218, 1993.

Markham CH (ed): *Parkinson's Disease: Clinical Neuroscience, vol 1.* Wiley-Liss, New York, 1993.

Markham CH, Diamond SG: Clinical overview of Parkinson's disease. *Clin Neurosci 1:*5–11, 1993.

Martinez M, Campion D, Brice A, Hannequin D, Dubois B, Didierjean O, Michon A, Thomas-Anterion C, Puel M, Frebourg T, Agid Y, Clerget-Darpoux F: Apolipoprotein E 4 allele and familial aggregation of Alzheimer disease. *Arch Neurol 55:*810–816, 1998.

Masliah E, Terry RD: Role of synaptic pathology in the mechanisms of dementia in Alzheimer's disease. *Clin Neurosci 1:*192–198, 1993.

Masur DM, Sluvinski M, Lipton RB, Blau AD, Crystal HA: Neuropsychological prediction of dementia and the absence of dementia in healthy elderly persons. *Neurology 44:*1427–1432, 1994.

Mayberg HS: Clinical correlates of PET and SPECT identified defects in dementia. *J Clin Psychiatry 55*(suppl 11):12–21, 1994.

Mayeaux R, Stern Y, Rosen J, Benson DF: Is "subcortical dementia" a recognizable clinical entity? *Ann Neurol 14:*278–283, 1983.

Mazziotta J: Neuroimaging in Parkinson's disease. *Clin Neurosci 1:*53–63, 1993.

McClearn GE, Johansson B, Berg S, Pedersen NL, Ahern F, Petrill SA, Plomin R: Substantial genetic influence on cognitive abilities in twins 80 or more years old. *Science 276:*1560–1563, 1997.

McShane R, Keene J, Gedling K, Fauburn C, Jacoby R, Hopi T: Do neuroleptic drugs hasten cognitive decline in dementia? Prospective study with necropsy follow-up. *BMJ 314:*266–270, 1997.

Mendez ME, Selwood A, Mastri A, Frey WH II: Pick's disease versus Alzheimer's disease: A comparison of clinical characteristics. *Neurology 43:*289–292, 1993.

Miller BL, Cummings JL, Villanueva-Meyer J, Boone K, Mehringer CM, Lesser IM, Mena I: Frontal lobe degeneration; clinical, neuropsychological, and SPECT characteristics. *Neurology 41:*1374–1382, 1991.

Mishima K, Okawa M, Hishikawa Y, Hozumi S, Hori H, Takahashi K: Morning bright light therapy for sleep and behavior disorders in elderly patients with dementia. *Acta Psychiatr Scand 89:*1–7, 1994.

Moellentine C, Rummans T, Ahlskog JE, Harmsen WS, Suman VJ, O'Connor MK, Black JL, Pileggi T: Effectiveness of ECT in patients with parkinsonism. *J Neuropsychiatry Clin Neurosci 10:*187–193, 1998.

Mori E, Hirono N, Yamashita H, Imamura T, Ikejiri Y, Ikeda M, Kitagaki H, Shimomura T, Yoneda Y: Premorbid brain size as a determinant of reserve capacity against intellectual decline in Alzheimer's disease. *Am J Psychiatry 154:*18–24, 1997.

Murphy DGM, DeCarli C, McIntosh AR, Daly E, Mentis MJ, Pietrini P, Szczepanik J, Schapiro MB, Grady CL, Horwitz B, Rapoport SI: Sex differences in human brain morphometry and metabolism: An in vivo quantitative magnetic resonance imaging and positron emission tomography study on the effect of aging. *Arch Gen Psychiatry 53:*585–594, 1996.

Murphy GM Jr, Taylor J, Kraemer HC, Yesavage J, Tinklenberg JR: No association between apolipoprotein E4 allele and rate of decline in Alzheimer's disease. *Am J Psychiatry 154:*603–608, 1997.

Nasrallah HA, Schwartzkopf SB, Coffman JA, Olson SC: Perinatal brain injury and cerebellar vermal lobules I through X in schizophrenia. *Biol Psychiatry 29:*567–574, 1991.

Neary D, Snowden J: Fronto-temporal dementia: Nosology, neuropsychology and neuropathology. *Brain Cogn 31:*176-187, 1996.

Neary D, Snowden JS, Northen B, Goulding P: Dementia of frontal lobe type. *J Neurol Neurosurg Psychiatry 51:*353–361, 1988.

Nutt JG: Pharmacotherapy of Parkinson's disease. *Clin Neurosci 1:*64–68, 1993.

Orrell MW, Sahakian BJ (editorial): Dementia of frontal lobe type. *Psychol Med 21:*553–556, 1991.

Ott A, Slooter AJC, Hofman A, van Harskamp F, Witteman JCM, van Broeckhoven C, van Duijn CM, Breteler MMB: Smoking and risk of dementia and Alzheimer's disease in a population-based cohort study: The Rotterdam study. *Lancet 351:*1840–1843, 1998.

Papka M, Rubio A, Schiffer RB: A review of Lewy body disease, an emerging concept of cortical dementia. *J Neuropsychiatry Clin Neurosci 10:*267–279, 1998.

Parkin AJ, Walter BM: Recollective experience, normal aging, and frontal dysfunction. *Psychol Aging* 7:290–298, 1992.

Perry G, Smith MA: Senile plaques and neurofibrillary tangles: What role do they play in Alzheimer's disease? *Clin Neurosci* 1:199–203, 1993.

Plassman BL, Welsh KA, Helms M, Brandt J, Page WF, Breitner JCS: Intelligence and education as predictors of cognitive state in late life. A 50-year follow-up. *Neurology* 45:1446–1450, 1995.

Polymeropoulos MH, Lavendan C, Leroy E, Ide SE, Dehejia A, Dutra A, Pike B, Root H, Rubenstein J, Boyer R, Stenroos ES, Chandrasekharappa S, Athenassiadou A, Papapetropoulos T, Johnson WG, Lazzarini AM, Duvoisin RC, Di Iorio G, Golbe LI, Nussbaum RL: Mutation in the alpha synuclein gene identified in families with Parkinson's disease. *Science* 276:2045–2047, 1997.

Prince M, Cullen M, Mann A: Risk factors for Alzheimer's disease and dementia: A case–control study based on the MRC elderly hypertension trial. *Neurology* 44:97–104, 1994.

Prohovnik I, Mayeaux R, Sackeim HA, Smith G, Stern Y, Alderson PO: Cerebral perfusion as a diagnostic marker of early Alzheimer's disease. *Neurology* 38:931–937, 1988.

Prusiner SB: Genetic and infectious prion diseases. *Arch Neurol* 50:1129–1153, 1993.

Raff ML: Social controls on cell survival and cell death. *Nature* 356:397–400, 1992.

Rapp PR, Amaral DG: Individual differences in the cognitive and neurobiological consequences of normal aging. *TINS* 15:340–345, 1992.

Ritchie K: Establishing the limits of normal cerebral ageing and senile dementias. Current conceptualisations of 'normal' cerebral ageing. *Brit J Psychiatry* 173:97–101, 1998

Roses AD: Genetic testing for Alzheimer disease: Practical and ethical issues. *Arch Neurol* 54:1226–1229, 1997.

Rubenstein DC (editorial): Apolipoprotein E: A review of its roles in lipoprotein metabolism, neuronal growth and repair and a risk factor for Alzheimer's disease. *Psychol Med* 25:223–229, 1995.

Rubin EH, Storandt M, Miller JP, Kinscherf DA, Grant EA, Morris JC, Berg L: A prospective study of cognitive function and onset of dementia in cognitively health elders. *Arch Neurol* 55:395–401, 1998.

Rumble B, Retallack R, Hilbich C, Simms G, Multhaup G, Martins R, Hockey A, Montgomery P, Beyreuther K, Masters CL: Amyloid A4 protein and its precursor in Down's syndrome and Alzheimer's disease. *N Engl J Med* 320:1446–1452, 1989.

Saint-Cyr JA, Taylor AE, Lang AE: Neuropsychological and psychiatric side effects in the treatment of Parkinson's disease. *Neurology* 43(suppl 6):S47–S52, 1993.

St. George-Hyslop PH: Recent advances in the molecular genetics of Alzheimer's disease. *Clin Neurosci* 1:171–175, 1993.

Sano M, Ernesto C, Thomas RG, Klauber MR, Schafer K, Grundman M, Woodbury P, Growdon J, Cotman CW, Pfeiffer E, Schneider LS, Thal LJ, for members of the Alzheimer's Disease Cooperative Study: A controlled trial of selegiline, alpha-tocopherol (vitamin E) or both as a treatment for Alzheimer's disease. *N Engl J Med* 336:1216–1222, 1997.

Schneider LS: Clinical pharmacology of aminoacridines in Alzheimer's disease. *Neurology* (suppl 4) 43:S64–S79, 1993.

Schupf N, Kapell D, Lee JH, Ottman R, Mayeaux R: Increased risk for Alzheimer's disease in mothers of adults with Down's syndrome. *Lancet* 344:353–356, 1994.

Schwartz J, Tatsch K, Arnold G, Trenkwalder C, Kirsch CM, Oertel WH: ^{123}I-Iodobenzamide-SPECT in 83 patients with de novo parkinsonism. *Neurology* 43(suppl 6):S16–S20, 1993.

Scinto LFM, Daffner KR, Dressler D, Ransil BI, Renz D, Weintraub S, Mesulam M, Potter H: Potential noninvasive neurobiological test for Alzheimer's disease. *Science* 266:1051–1054, 1994.

Selkoe DJ: Alzheimer's disease: Genotypes, phenotype, and treatments. *Science* 275:630–631, 1997.

Semchuk KM, Love EJ, Lee RG: Parkinson's disease: A test of the multifactorial etiologic hypothesis. *Neurology* 43:1173–1180, 1993.

Shay KA, Roth DL: Association between aerobic fitness and visuospatial performance in healthy older adults. *Psychol Aging* 1:15–24, 1992.

Sisodia SS, Price DL: Amyloidogenesis in Alzheimer's disease. *Clin Neurosci* 1:176–183, 1993.

Snowdon DA, Kemper SJ, Mortimer JA, Greiner LH, Wekstein DR, Makesbery WR: Linguistic ability in early life and cognitive function and Alzheimer's disease in late life; findings from a nun study. *JAMA* 275:528–532, 1996.

Solomon PR, Hirschoff A, Kelly B, Relin M, Brush M, DeVeaux RD, Pendlebury WW: A 7 minute neurocognitive screening battery highly sensitive to Alzheimer's disease. *Arch Neurol* 55:349–355, 1998.

Sultzer DL, Levin HS, Mahler ME, High WM, Cummings JL: A comparison of psychiatric symptoms in vascular dementia and Alzheimer's disease. *Am J Psychiatry* 150:1806–1812, 1993.

Swartz JR, Miller BL, Lesser IM, Darby AL: Frontotemporal dementia: Treatment response to serotonin selective reuptake inhibitors. *J Clin Psychiatry* 58:212–216, 1997.

Tang M-X, Jacobs D, Stern Y, Marder K, Schofield P, Gurland B, Andrews H, Mayeaux R: Effect of estrogen during menopause and risk and age at onset of Alzheimer's disease. *Lancet* 348:429–432, 1996.

Taylor S, McCracken CFM, Wilson KCM, Copeland JRM: Extent and appropriateness of benzodiazepine use. Results from an elderly urban community. *Brit J Psychiatry* 173:433–438, 1998.

Thapa PB, Gideon P, Cost TW, Milam AB, Ray WA: Antidepressants and the risk of falls among nursing home residents. *NEJM* 339:875–882, 1998.

Thrach WT: On the specific role of the cerebellum in motor learning and cognition: Clues from PET activation and lesion studies in man. *Behav Brain Sci* 19:411–431, 1996.

Tierney ML, Szalai JP, Snow WG, Fisher RH: The prediction of Alzheimer disease: The role of patient and informant perceptions of cognitive deficits. *Arch Neurol* 53:423–427, 1996.

Tinetti ME, Baker DI, McAvay G, Claus EB, Garrett P, Gottschalk M, Koch ML, Trainor K, Horwitz RI: A multifactorial intervention to reduce the risk of falling among elderly people living in the community. *N Engl J Med* 331:821–827, 1994.

Trojanowski JQ, Schmidt ML, Shin RW, Bramblett GT, Goedert M, Lee VMY: PHF$_t$ (A68): From pathological marker to potential mediator of neuronal dysfunction and degeneration in Alzheimer's disease. *Clin Neurosci* 1:184–191, 1993.

Weiner WJ, Lang AE (eds): *Behavioral Neurology of Movement Disorders, Advances in Neurology*, vol 65. Raven Press, New York, 1995.

White K, Grether ME, Abrams JM, Young L, Farrell K, Steller H: Genetic control of programmed cell death in *Drosophila*. *Science* 264:677–683, 1994.

Yaffe K, Cauley J, Sands L, Browner W: Apolipoprotein E phenotype and cognitive decline in a prospective study of elderly community women. *Arch Neurol* 54:1110–1114, 1997.

Yan SD, Soto JF, Chen X, Zhu H, Al-Mohanna F, Collison K, Zhu A, Stern E, Saido T, Tohyama M, Ogawa S, Roher A, Stern D: An intracellular protein that binds amyloid-B peptide and mediates neurotoxicity in Alzheimer's disease. *Nature* 389:689–695, 1997.

13

Substance-Induced Neuropsychiatric Disorders

About 10% of U.S. women and 20% of U.S. men have abused alcohol (lifetime risks), and about 4% of U.S. women and 10% of U.S. men are dependent on alcohol. Alcohol abuse is highest in 20–35 year olds, Hispanic men and Native Americans, urbanites, persons living in states outside the "deep south," and tobacco users. European-Americans and African-Americans have similar lifetime rates. Waiters, bartenders, longshoremen, musicians, authors, reporters, and police have relatively high rates of consumption and abuse. Among general medical patients, about 40% have alcohol-related problems.

About 10% of the adult U.S. population (men more than women) seriously abuse drugs. The lifetime prevalence rate for nonalcohol drug abuse is about 6%. Marijuana is the most commonly used illicit drug (33% of the population over age 12), followed by cocaine (11%). About 12% of persons misuse prescription psychotropics. Nonalcoholic drug abuse is highest among males, persons 18–25 years old, urbanites, persons living in the western half of the United States, and the poor and unemployed.

Although caffeine and nicotine are not officially considered drugs of abuse, many persons are addicted to them. These addictions also have substantial health risks and are as difficult to treat as are addictions to alcohol and illicit drugs. Most definitions of substance abuse require continued use of a psychoactive substance despite awareness that it has caused interpersonal, social, job, or health problems. Dependence also requires (1) physiologic tolerance (increased amounts needed to obtain desired effect or markedly reduced effect from same amount of substance); (2) withdrawal syndrome when use of substance is abruptly stopped; (3) interpersonal, social, job, or health problems from use; time and energy devoted to obtaining and using the substance interferes with functioning; and (4) No. 1, 2, or 3 occurs within a 12-month period. Although the DSM tries to separate abuse from addiction, this dichotomy reflects the pharmacology of the specific substance being used and the severity of abuse rather than different illnesses.

Alcohol in moderation has no clear adverse health effects (except during pregnancy) and may even be protective for some cardiovascular disease because it raises high-density cholesterol. Some illicit drugs, however, used once can kill (cocaine seizure or fatal arrhythmia), cause acute psychosis (lysergic acid diethylamide [LSD], phencyclidine [PCP], peyote, mescaline, "designer" drugs), or cause a recurrent psychosis even without further drug use (PCP, LSD, most other hallucinogens). Consequences depend on doses taken, impurities in the street drug, and the user's constitutional vulnerability (e.g., family history of mood disorder, past psychiatric or neurologic disorder).

Tables 13.1 lists some of the clinical indicators of alcohol abuse. Other factors increasing the likelihood of use are (1) high novelty seeking personality characterized by being impulsive, disorderly, easily bored, quick-tempered, excitable, fickle, risk-taking, and unconventional; (2) a family history of alcoholism; and (3) being a tobacco or street drug user. Table 13.2 lists some clinical indicators of nonalcohol substance abusers. Other factors increasing the likelihood of use are (1) high novelty seeking personality; (2) unexplained erratic behavior; (3) personality change after age 30 years characterized by increased irritability and suspiciousness; (4) a family history of nonalcohol drug abuse; and (5) being a gang member. Substance-related neuropsychiatric syndromes include intoxications with and without delirium or acute psychosis, withdrawal states, dementia, and recurrent or chronic psychosis.

CLINICAL PRESENTATIONS: ALCOHOL-RELATED SYNDROMES

Acute alcohol intoxication is characterized by facial flushing, slurred speech, ataxia, nystagmus, mild diffuse cognitive impairment, talkativeness, circumstantial and rambling speech, euphoria (initially), irritability, sadness, and emotional lability. Intoxication is directly related to the blood alcohol level, which depends on the amount and rate of alcohol consumed, body weight and degree of pharmacologic tolerance. Medical care is usually sought because of combative or suicidal behavior.

Management focuses on controlling self-destructive or assaultive behavior. A calm, firm, reassuring manner works for most patients. Restraints and benzodiazepine sedation occasionally may be needed. Little potentiation occurs, and you can give doses of chlordiazepoxide as high as 50–100 mg. Monitor vital signs, obtain blood alcohol levels, and observe the patient to prevent aspiration from vomiting. If blood levels exceed 300 mg% (usually producing stupor or coma), high doses of intravenous fructose can lower them significantly. Alcohol is metabolized at a rate of about 1 ounce per hour, and the acutely intoxicated but otherwise healthy person recovers spontaneously in a short time.

Death from acute alcohol intoxication usually is associated with simultaneous ingestion of sedatives or central nervous system (CNS) depressants. Always obtain a urine drug screen in stuporous or comatose patients with acute alcohol intoxication. Diabetic acidosis or hypoglycemia (best treated with intravenous glucose) or alcohol-disulfiram reactions (flushing, tachycardia, hypotension, headache and dizziness, nausea and vomiting—best treated with presser agents,

TABLE 13.1. Clinical Indicators of Alcohol Abuse

	Information		
Area of Focus	Suggestive	Likely	Definite
1. Pattern of use	Heavy drinking: more than 3 drinks almost daily with occasional intoxications at parties	4 or more drinks daily with more than 1 intoxication per month; any binge	Heavy drinking interfering with social, job, or recreational activities
2. Behaviors of use	Drinking and obtaining alcohol an important part of social interactions	Persistent desire or unsuccessful efforts to cut down; occasional driving while intoxicated	Much time spent in activities obtaining alcohol or recovering from its effects; job or social problems due to drinking
3. Social, legal, and occupational consequences of use	Driving under the influence once	Driving under the influence more than once	Injuries from drinking while doing hazardous things (e.g, driving, using machinery)
4. Physical examination and related findings	Male erectile dysfunction, female arousal disorder, full head of white hair before age 55 years	Acne rosacea, palmar erythema; peripheral neuropathy, abducens nerve palsy	Enlarged painless liver* or cirrhotic liver (5%–10% of older chronic alcoholics) with reduced lower limb strength and sensations (barrel chest and pot belly in person with thin limb musculature); cigarette burns between index and middle fingers, scars and bruises from repeated falls, injuries, and fights; bouts of pancreatitis

* Carbohydrate-deficient transferrin (CDT) serum levels is a highly sensitive measure of recent alcohol use and is probably better than the older measure, gammaglutamyltransferase (GGT).

TABLE 13.2. Clinical Indicators of Nonalcohol Drug Abuse

Area of Focus	Information		
	Suggestive	Likely	Definite
1. Pattern of use	Any substance used more than twice	Any substance used weekly, or any substance injected	Any substance used several times weekly
2. Behaviors of use	Using drug as an important part of social interactions	Unsuccessful efforts to cut down; occasional driving while under the acute effects of the drug	Much time spent in activities obtaining the drug or recovering from its effects; job or social problems due to drug use
3. Behavioral consequences of use	Experimentation with any drug other than marijuana	Any arrest for possession or use	More than 2 arrests for possession or use; loss of work due to use; family disruption due to use
4. Physical examination and related findings	Otherwise medically unexplained impaired lung function in a person under 40 years (marijuana)	Stroke in a young person with no history of migraine, or placental abruption (cocaine); early onset dementia-like syndrome with tremor, ataxia, peripheral neuropathy, or loss of visual acuity (inhalants); excoriated skin (cocaine)	Nasal septal ulcers (cocaine), sclerotic skin blemishes (opiates), sclerotic veins (opiates)

ascorbic acid, and antihistamines) are life-threatening conditions that can masquerade as simple alcohol intoxication.

The *alcohol withdrawal syndrome* is associated with a sudden, precipitous drop in alcohol consumption. Most commonly the patient continues to drink, but switches from high- (liquor) to low-alcohol containing (beer) beverages. The syndrome is serious in 5% of patients (delirium tremens [DTs]) and, when severe, is characterized by coarse tremors of the hands, tongue, and eyelids; nausea and vomiting; weakness and malaise; tachycardia; sweating; hypertension and orthostatic hypotension; dysphoria and irritability; some alteration in consciousness; diffuse cognitive impairment, insomnia, agitation, and, at times, psychosis. Visual hallucinations are most common, but auditory hallucinations also occur. Severity of withdrawal depends on the degree and duration of alcohol consumption and the patient's general health (the worse the health, the more severe the withdrawal). Always look for other illness in a patient with DTs. These include pancreatitis, infection, hepatic insufficiency, subdural hematoma, fractures, and vitamin deficiencies. DTs usually begin 6–8 hours after the marked reduction in alcohol intake, peak in 24–36 hours, and may take 10–14 days to subside. The worse the patient's hepatic function, however, the slower the metabolism of alcohol, so that in these patients and elderly alcoholics withdrawal onset can be delayed for several days.

Initial emergency treatment may require temporary restraints. Prolonged restraints are contraindicated, because patients with DTs may struggle against them to exhaustion. Rapidly sedate with benzodiazepines. Titrate doses against the patient's initial response, with mild sedation the goal. An initial dose of 15–20 mg of diazepam IV temporarily controls the typical withdrawal delirium and provides an indication (based on the patient's sedative response) for a definitive withdrawal drug schedule. Doses as high as 120 mg of diazepam may be needed. Spontaneous withdrawal seizures ("rum fits") are less likely to occur with diazepam, because it has more anticonvulsant properties than other sedating benzodiazepines.

Once you determine the mildly sedating daily dose, you can then use the benzodiazepine to "detoxify" the patient through a slow tapered withdrawal period of 7–10 days. Intravenous or intramuscular, and then oral, carbamazepine during the detoxification period offers minimal additional seizure protection, but it does help ameliorate withdrawal symptoms and craving. Giving anticonvulsants beyond the detoxification period is not justified. Hospitalization is always required. Additional treatment with thiamine 100 mg IM BID (alcoholics often have a mild malabsorption syndrome) and multivitamins, particularly B complex and C, may prevent Wernicke-Korsakoff syndrome. Beta-blockers (propranolol, atenolol) or alpha$_2$-agonists (clonidine, lofexidine) may ameliorate peripheral sympathomimetic features. Clonidine, an alpha-adrenergic agonist, 0.1–0.3 mg BID or TID, may be sufficient for mild to moderate withdrawal states. A magnesium sulfate solution to prevent seizures from hypomagnesemia is of questionable benefit. Fluid and electrolyte administration is rarely needed unless the hematocrit is elevated and there are other signs of dehydration. Most alcoholics are overhydrated, and unnecessary intravenous fluids may cause seizures. Avoid intravenous glucose.

Neuroleptics are contraindicated during the withdrawal delirium. They have no cross-tolerance with alcohol, suppress the immune system (already compromised in many alcoholics), lower the seizure threshold, tax hepatic metabolism, and increase morbidity and mortality rates. Barbiturates, used in some medical centers, are not recommended because they are myocardial irritants, and withdrawing alcoholics often have arrhythmias.

When hallucinations persist after the delirium has ended, the patient is said to have *alcoholic hallucinosis,* the etiology of which is unclear. There is no relationship, however, to schizophrenia in outcome (90% recover by 6 months) or family history (low for schizophrenia, high for alcoholism). Because these patients' psychoses have not responded to benzodiazepines during the delirium phase of their disorder, neuroleptics may now be needed. Haloperidol is preferred if the patient is agitated or has intense psychotic features. If the hallucinosis is relatively mild, risperidone is the alternative. Electroconvulsive therapy (ECT) will also work.

Wernicke's syndrome is characterized by sudden onset of ophthalmoplegia (most often abducens nerve/external rectus palsy), nystagmus (almost always present), ataxia, memory loss, altered consciousness, and diffuse cognitive impairment. Peripheral neuropathy and myocarditis also may be present, and a history of Korsakoff's syndrome is typical. Wernicke's syndrome most commonly occurs in alcoholics, but any profound thiamine deficiency (e.g., gastric carcinoma, pernicious anemia, hyperemesis gravidarum, malnutrition, anorexia nervosa) can produce the syndrome in a genetically vulnerable person (an autosomal gene unrelated to alcoholism).

The acute phase usually remits rapidly with IV (400–1,500 mg) and then IM (100 mg BID) thiamine and multivitamins. Five percent of patients die. Residual Korsakoff's syndrome is the most common sequela. Emergency treatment consists of restraints when necessary; thiamine; sedation with a benzodiazepine (e.g., diazepam 10–15 mg PO or IV, lorazepam 2–4 mg PO or IM) and hospitalization. As in the treatment of alcohol withdrawal, do not automatically give intravenous fluids and electrolyte replacement (see Chapter 12 for details and Korsakoff's dementia)

Alcohol-related delusional disorder usually occurs in men who are chronic heavy drinkers with few alcohol-related difficulties until age 50–60 years, when they become increasingly suspicious, sullen, irritable, and finally delusional. Delusions usually involve themes of a spouse's infidelity, a relative's dishonesty, a neighbor's "dirty tricks," or a municipality's illegal action. They may also experience auditory hallucinations. These patients become neighborhood cranks who are finally hospitalized when local authorities run out of patience from constant complaints or litigation or family members become exasperated or fear that the patient may hurt someone. These patients do not appear depressed or manic.

Many patients with alcohol-related delusional disorder exhibit mild to moderate cortical atrophy and cognitive impairment. A frontal lobe dementia due to the direct neurotoxic effects of alcohol may develop. Neuroleptics may be required if the delusions do not resolve fully with abstinence and multivitamins.

Alcohol Co-Morbidities

Alcoholism co-occurs with several conditions, and one third of alcoholics have another nonsubstance-related lifetime psychiatric diagnosis. Most common are antisocial personality disorder (14%), recurrent, usually nonmelancholic depressions (20%), bipolar mood disorder (10%–15%), and anxiety disorder (20%). All these conditions are familial with substantial heritability, but transmission of each of these co-morbidities is independent of alcoholism.

In most patients the antisocial personality, bipolar disorder, or anxiety disorder predates the alcoholism. Among men alcoholics, alcoholism predates depressions, whereas among women alcoholics, depression typically predates the alcoholism. Thus, women who become alcoholics are more likely to have depressive illness and may be drinking to self-medicate (the alcoholism is a consequence of the mood disorder), whereas in many men alcoholics the depression is more likely a consequence of the alcoholism. Among persons with alcoholism and anxiety disorder, the alcoholism is likely to be a consequence of repeated attempts at self-medication.

Treatment of Alcoholism

Most alcoholics and other drug abusers do not voluntarily seek treatment for substance abuse. When they do, they are usually concerned about the health (e.g., hepatitis in an intravenous drug user, arrhythmias in a caffeine user) or social (e.g., legal) consequences of their abuse. Sometimes they are forced by their family to seek treatment. In most situations, motivation is poor for stopping use, and about 90% relapse. Success rates improve when abstinence is linked to continued or new employment. In most psychiatric settings, alcoholics are hospitalized because of their co-morbid condition.

The long-term successful management of the alcoholism typically requires a combination of treatments. For some patients, counseling, AA, or a similar program may work, particularly if linked to employment (as in many police department programs). If you decide to treat alcoholic patients, you will likely need to combine rehabilitative psychotherapy (see Chapter 5) with medications. Regular assessment of carbohydrate-deficient transferrin (CDT) serum levels can be used to monitor abstinence.

There are some general steps for psychotherapy with alcoholics:

1. Do not accept *any* minimizing or denying of the condition. If any treatment is to be successful, the patient must fully recognize that he is an alcoholic.
2. Educate and counsel family members not to facilitate the patient's drinking by covering up for the patient with employers or in meeting other responsibilities, including treatments and appointments.
3. Encourage family members to participate in alcohol support groups such as Al-Anon.

4. Educate the patient and the family *together* about all your findings and their consequences and about what you or they need to do about each finding. Do this periodically so that no "second-hand" information gets transmitted.

5. Encourage family expressions of concern and deal with attempts to place blame; educate the family to the concept that the patient has an illness.

Several medications have been used to treat alcoholism. *Disulfiram* is still used as a pharmacologic deterrent to drinking. The rationale is that because disulfiram blocks acetaldehyde dehydrogenase, ingested alcohol is metabolized only to acetaldehyde, causing nausea and flushing. If the impulsive alcoholic regularly takes disulfiram he will fear drinking despite a sudden craving for alcohol. Once the craving subsides the alcoholic will continue the disulfiram because it helped and because subsiding of the craving frees him to continue treatment. However, most alcoholics are not offered or do not accept disulfiram, and of those who do, many discontinue it and resume drinking.

Recently, pharmacologic treatments of alcoholism have focused on craving, using this rationale:

1. Many alcoholics have co-occurring depression or anxiety disorder, and because these conditions respond to medications, perhaps the alcoholism might also.

2. A neurotransmitter (dopamine) affected by alcohol is also implicated in depression.

3. As there seems to be a genetic predisposition for alcoholism, biochemical and physiologic expressions of that disposition may respond to biologic treatment.

4. Alcohol affects reward systems in the brain and has antianxiety properties; thus substituting other agents for alcohol might achieve the same results without the adverse consequences, paralleling the rationale for methadone maintenance for heroin addiction.

5. Because alcoholism can be viewed as a compulsion to drink, it might respond to treatments for other compulsions.

Several agents have been or could be used to treat alcoholism. *Naltrexone,* an opiate antagonist, 50 mg daily, reduces relapse rates and amounts of alcohol consumed during relapses; and, for primary alcoholics with intact personalities and good general health, it is the agent of choice to minimize craving. *Nalmefene,* another opiate antagonist, also has a substantial effect. *Dopamine agonists* (e.g., bromocriptine) have a mild to moderate effect and may work best with patients who are impulsive with high novelty seeking. *Thymoleptics* (e.g., lithium, valproate) have a mild effect and become particularly important if the patient has comorbid mood disorder. Specific serotonin reuptake inhibitors (SSRIs) have a mild effect and may work best in patients with high harm avoidance. Agents that work on NMDA receptor-mediated glutamate neurotransmission (e.g., acamprosate) also reduce alcohol craving, but are not available in the United States.

Which heavy drinkers or alcoholics will respond to these compounds is unclear. However, the patient's temperament patterns may be helpful, as not all alcoholics are alike. Those with normal personality traits (i.e., no personality disorder) or with high dependency are likely to respond to naltrexone, AA, and other supportive rehabilitation programs. Those who are typically anxious, shy, and worriers may do best when detoxification and rehabilitation are combined with an SSRI. Those who are impulsive, excitable, and risk takers may do best with a dopamine agonist such as bupropion or bromocriptine (see Chapter 6 for a rationale for these choices). If there is a co-occurring mood or anxiety disorder, these must be successfully treated first if there is to be any hope of resolving the alcoholism.

Long-term results of treatments for alcoholism are not good, but this fact needs to be tempered by recognizing that many treatment programs are not comprehensive or provide one set of treatments to all patients, as if "one size fits all." Combinations of treatments using anticraving strategies seem to be achieving better results. What past studies do show, however, is (1) the likelihood of drinking again is highest in alcoholics with a family history of alcoholism and persons who had a substantial behavioral response to alcohol (e.g., a "high") *before* becoming a heavy drinker; (2) alcoholics who are abstinent for 5 years have very low rates of future relapse; and (3) over a 40-year follow-up (age 20–60) of college alcohol abusers, abstinent rates are between 10% and 30%, death rates are between 20% and 30%, and controlled drinking about occurs in 10%. City dwellers are more likely to die, but also to become abstinent.

CLINICAL PRESENTATION: DRUG ABUSE

Early diagnosis of nonalcohol substance abuse requires an evaluation similar to that for alcohol. Table 13.3 lists common drugs of abuse. Drug screening for initial diagnosis and to monitor long-term treatment is essential. Know the method of testing in the laboratory you use and the list of drugs tested. Ask the laboratory to report even traces of a drug. Thin-layer chromatography is the least expensive and least sensitive assay method. Immunoassay (radio, enzyme, fluorescent polarization) is the preferred method. Urine is the typical sample choice. Detection after last day of use is shortest for cocaine (5–12 hours) and longest for cannabis (2–6 weeks). Other detection limits in days are amphetamines (1–2), barbiturates (3–5, short-acting; 10–14, long-acting), benzodiazepines (2–9), opiates (1–2), and phencyclidine (2–8). Most other laboratory tests are nonspecific.

Sedative-Hypnotics and Benzodiazepines: Intoxication and Withdrawal

Sedative-hypnotics, all synthetic, are general CNS depressants that produce sedation in small doses and sleep in larger doses. Meprobamate and methaqualone have particularly high abuse potential, and their overdoses are particularly lethal. Do not prescribe them. Persons who habitually use sedative-hypnotics tend to be

TABLE 13.3. Common Drugs of Abuse

SEDATIVES-HYPNOTICS AND ANXIOLYTICS

Chloral hydrate

Barbiturates
   a. Longer acting (phenobarbital [Luminal])
   b. Shorter acting (secobarbital [Seconal], pentobarbital [Nembutal], amobarbital [Amytal])

Methyprylon (Noludar)

Ethchlorvynol (Placidyl)

Ethinimate (Valmid)

Meprobamate (Miltown, Equanil)

Methaqualone (Quaalude)

Benzodiazepines
   a. Longer acting (chlordiazepoxide, diazepam)
   b. Shorter acting (lorazepam, oxazepam)

OPIATES AND OPIOIDS

Opium (10% morphine)

Heroin (diacetylmorphine)

Morphine

Meperidine (Demerol)

Oxymorphone (Percodan)

Codeine (methylmorphine)

OPIATE-LIKE

Pentazocine (Talwin)

D-Propoxyphene (Darvon)

SYMPATHOMIMETICS

Cocaine

Amphetamines
   a. Amphetamines (Benzedrine)
   b. Dextroamphetamine (Dexedrine)

TABLE 13.3. (*continued*)

  c. Methamphetamine (Methedrine)

  d. Methylenedioxy methamphetamine ("Ecstasy")

Amphetamine congeners

  a. Methylphenidate (Ritalin)

  b. Phenmetrazine (Preludin)

Hallucinogens

D-Lysergic acid diethylamide-25 (LSD)

Peyote

Mescaline (trimethoxyphenylethylamine)

Psilocybin (related to serotonin)

Corymbos (morning glory seeds [related to LSD])

Myristica (nutmeg)

Arylcyclohexylamines

Phencyclidine (PCP)

Marijuana

Cannabis (marijuana [tetrahydrocannabinol])

Inhalants

Glue

Spray paints, lacquers (e.g., toluene)

Paint thinner (e.g., turpentine)

Cleaning fluids

Refrigerants (e.g., Freon)

Lighter fluids

Gasoline

Adhesives

Solvents (e.g., acetone)

Aerosols

Nitrous oxide

Nitrites

young, antisocial males, or middle-aged, often middle-class persons who are initially prescribed a sedative-hypnotic for anxiety or insomnia and then continue
to use the drug as dependence, physiologic tolerance, and, eventually, addiction
develops.

Sedative-hypnotic intoxication resembles simple alcohol intoxication. The patients, however, tend to be healthier than alcoholics. Behavioral management is
similar to that for alcohol intoxication. High blood levels of a sedative-hypnotic,
unlike those of alcohol, are likely to induce respiratory arrest, and very lethargic
patients are treated in critical care units. Like alcohol, barbiturate pharmacodynamic effects are widespread. At anesthetic doses the molecule dissolves into cell
membranes, altering lipid configurations. Barbiturates affect multiple types of ion
channels and so have multiple neurotransmitter effects. Their strongest effect is
on GABA receptors.

In mild intoxication, behavioral treatment includes a safe, quiet environment
where the patient's behavior, vital signs, and level of consciousness are regularly
observed. Restraints may initially be necessary for agitated patients. The semico-
matose or comatose patient is intubated and ventilated after gastric lavage. Activated charcoal may be introduced into the stomach to absorb any remaining drug.
The urine may be alkalinized with sodium bicarbonate infusion if phenobarbital
intoxication is suspected. If meprobamate is the offender, 20% IV solution of man-
nitol at 50 ml/hour is administered, and fluid and electrolyte balances are maintained. Aqueous or lipid hemodialysis can remove most of the sedative-hypnotic
from the blood. If the specific coma-causing drug is not known, and the patient is
not an alcoholic, IV naloxone (0.4 mg) and 50 ml of 50% glucose are given.

Sedative-hypnotic withdrawal is similar to alcohol withdrawal, but coarse tremor
is not always present and grand mal seizures (also observed in alcohol withdrawal) may occur early in 5%–20% of withdrawals. Obsessive compulsive disorder–like behaviors can also occur during benzodiazepine withdrawal. Symptoms
begin 12–48 hours after the last dose but may be delayed as long as 7–10 days for
long-acting compounds. Severity of symptoms is directly related to daily dose
and duration of use. With most sedative-hypnotics, suspect physiologic dependence if daily use at therapeutic doses or higher has occurred for more than 30
days. After 90 days of use at or above the therapeutic dosage range, addiction is
virtually guaranteed (for benzodiazepines, dependence reaches virtual certainty
at 4 months). Treatment requires hospitalizing and mildly sedating the patient
with a long-acting sedative-hypnotic and then withdrawing that compound by
8%–10% per day over 10–12 days.

Detoxification from barbiturates is best accomplished in a hospital with pentobarbital. Initially give a 200-mg test dose by mouth and then again every 2 hours
until the patient exhibits mild ataxia, dysarthria, nystagmus, and lethargy. If a
daily total of 400 mg or less produces intoxication, no further treatment is needed.
If a daily total of 600 mg or more is needed for intoxication, prescribe that daily
amount in divided doses given every 6 hours. After 24 hours, start dose reduction
with the morning and mid-day doses, with the time of dose reduction rotating so
that the evening dose is retained as long as possible.

Benzodiazepine withdrawal usually does not require hospitalization. However, the withdrawal takes a long time. It is done using the benzodiazepine being taken by the patient. Any co-morbid axis I condition must be resolved first if withdrawal is to be effective. Use of low dose antidepressants, selection based on personality traits, may help. Begin with the patient's usual daily dose. The first 50%–75% of that dose can be reduced over 2–4 weeks. Taper the remaining dose over several months just as you would an antidepressant.

Chronic use of CNS depressants may cause cognitive impairment and EEG changes that persist long beyond cessation of drug use. Benzodiazepines, like barbiturates, have widespread CNS effects. They work on a benzodiazepine–GABA receptor complex that opens chloride channels, leading to hyperpolarization and neuronal inhibition.

Opiate Intoxication and Withdrawal

Opiate addiction in western countries primarily involves heroin and dolophine (methadone). The latter is often obtained at methadone clinics. Heroin may be sniffed ("snorting") or injected subcutaneously ("skin popping") or intravenously ("mainlining"). Methadone is usually taken orally. The number of addicted persons is not known, although estimates suggest at least 500,000 in the United States. Urban African-Americans and Hispanic-Americans comprise the majority of opiate addicts. Physicians and nurses form the next largest group. Opiates have widespread pharmacodynamic effects. One concentration of receptors is in the median forebrain bundle and the dopaminergic mesolimbic reinforcement system, including the nucleus accumbens and ventral tegmental area.

Opiate intoxication is characterized by euphoria or dysphoria followed by apathy, psychomotor retardation, slurred speech, impaired attention, concentration and memory, and then somnolence. Initially, intravenous administration produces flushing and a lower abdominal sensation, described as similar to orgasm ("the rush"). The second stage is a period of drowsiness ("the nod"), during which vivid mental images in a semi-awake state occur ("opium dreams"). Pupillary constriction is always present initially, but in comatose anoxic patients pupillary dilation can occur. Other signs of severe intoxication are respiratory distress, apnea with cyanosis, cold limbs, areflexia, hypotension, and tachycardia. Pulmonary edema and grand mal seizures can occur. Needle tracks, or scarring of veins, a classic finding, result from repeated intravenous injection. Look for these on the forearms, behind the knee, on the feet and between the toes, and under the tongue.

Treatment for opiate intoxication includes maintaining adequate oxygenation, preventing aspiration of vomitus, and maintaining cardiac output and blood pressure. Naloxone (0.4 mg IV, diluted in 10 ml of sterile normal saline) is an extremely safe narcotic antagonist that is given immediately to any patient suspected of medically dangerous opiate intoxication. This dose is repeated three to four times within the first 10 minutes if no response is seen. Jugular or femoral vein administration is required when the usual intravenous sites are scarred and unusable. Pupillary dilation is often the first sign of a response. Apply restraints before injecting naloxone because, if it is effective, the patient awakes in severe withdrawal and is agitated, disoriented, and irritable. Control severe delirium with intravenous benzodiazepines. As most opiates have a longer half-life than naloxone, repeat doses may be needed. To prevent respiratory arrest, constant observation is essential during the next 24 hours.

Opiate withdrawal is rarely life threatening (an exception is the fetus of an addicted mother) and virtually never as dramatic as depicted in movies. Because most opiates are short acting, withdrawal signs, even if mild, begin within 8–12 hours after the last dose. Peak severity occurs 48–72 hours before withdrawal symptoms start to abate. Residual features, such as restlessness, fatigue, and insomnia, last for several weeks.

The withdrawal syndrome begins with restlessness, dysphoria, lethargy, and fitful sleep, followed by tearing, nasal discharge, sweating, yawning, and deep sighing. These features can all be self-induced (plucking a nasal hair produces tearing and nasal discharge) or feigned, so do not begin treatment until you see piloerection by stroking the patient's forearm. If severe addiction remains untreated, chills, muscle and joint pain, abdominal cramps, vomiting and diarrhea, tachycardia, hypertension, fever, anorexia, insomnia, anxiety, and agitation can occur.

Opiate abusers are treated in specialized hospital units where staff is trained to deal with the frequent manipulative, disruptive, dishonest, and intimidating behaviors of these patients. Often drug-related conditions (e.g., hepatitis, HIV, thrombophlebitis, subcutaneous abscesses, endocarditis, pulmonary infection or emboli, osteomyelitis) are the major treatment concern, rather than the typically mild withdrawal.

Detoxify with oral methadone. If an initial test dose of 20 mg causes intoxication, no further treatment is needed. Rarely does a patient need more than 40 mg daily, divided into morning and evening doses, with a withdrawal schedule reducing the dose by 5 mg each day. Administer flurazepam 30 mg PO for sleep throughout the withdrawal period. Clonidine (Catapres) (0.1–0.3 mg TID for up to 2 weeks), an alpha$_2$-adrenergic agonist that reduces noradrenergic activity in the locus ceruleus, has a modest adjunct effect in alleviating opiate withdrawal.

The course of opiate addiction depends on factors other than the pharmacologic effects of opiates. Relapse is more likely if the detoxified person returns to the environment in which he used drugs, and conditioned craving develops (i.e., the conditioned abstinent syndrome in which familiar drug-related environmental cues trigger craving). Methadone maintenance (1–2 years) substantially reduces the criminal activity of prior heroin addicts. For optimal results 60–80 mg daily is needed. Monitor blood levels and maintain the patient on 150–600 mg/ml, with 400 being the model level. Do not use with drugs that increase methadone metabolism and lower blood levels (e.g., carbamazepine, barbiturates). Cimetidine slows metabolism and increases levels. Valproate has little effect. One-third of patients who remain on methadone maintenance eventually become abstinent after stopping treatment. Some patients on methadone maintenance, however, abuse cocaine or alcohol, and some save part of their doses for street sales.

Buprenorphine (an agonist) and naltrexone (an antagonist) have also been successfully used to reduce craving. Naltrexone can be given 50 mg daily or 100 mg Monday and Wednesday and 150 mg Friday. It has long-acting mu opioid antagonism and can block craving if the patient can be compliant for at least 60 days of treatment. Buprenorphine can also be substituted for methadone to "detoxify" a patient from methadone maintenance. Two to 4 mg of buprenorphine equals 20–30 mg of methadone. Buprenorphine has less abuse potential than heroin and methadone, so use it as the last stage of maintenance before the patient is fully drug-free.

Stimulants

The two major stimulants of abuse are cocaine and amphetamine. Cocaine has no cross-tolerance with amphetamine. Regular cocaine use can be physiologically addicting, but most users do not become addicted. However, crack and free-based cocaine, for which the HCl molecule is split off, are highly addicting. Cocaine use in the United States is of epidemic proportions and now affects all ethnic and social groups, urban and nonurban. It can be absorbed by being rubbed on mucous membranes, inhaled as a powder ("snorted"), dissolved in water, injected intravenously, or smoked as an ether extract ("free-basing"). Most street cocaine is adulterated ("cut") with talcum powder or dry milk. Crack is highly potent and can cause placental abruption and stroke, cardiac arrhythmia, myocardial infarction, and cardiac arrest even in young persons with normal hearts. Because of cocaine's short, intense euphoric effect, some persons readminister the drug frequently (every 10 minutes) over a period of 8–12 hours. Such binges cause rapid mood changes. The annual U.S. death rate from cocaine is 5/1,000 deaths.

Cocaine, a monoamine reuptake inhibitor, works in minutes, and its acute euphoric effect lasts 45 minutes. Its plasma half-life is 90 minutes. *Cocaine intoxication* is characterized by peripheral vasoconstriction, increased body temperature and metabolic rate, excessive sweating, mydriasis, increased heart rate and blood pressure, and a sense of expansiveness, unlimited energy, and euphoria. Acute use may also cause hypersexuality, hyperactivity, and repetitive compulsive-like behaviors. Intoxication sometimes produces irritability, suspiciousness, fearfulness, jerky agitation (like actors in silent movies), stereotypies, tactile hallucinations of insects crawling on or under the skin (cocaine bugs or formication), visual hallucinations (classically of geometric shapes and patterns), and violence. Respiratory depression, hyperpyrexia, hypertension, and seizures can occur, and each can cause sudden death.

Cocaine withdrawal is called the "crash." It usually follows binge use and is characterized by anergia, anhedonia, anxiety, agitation, somnolence and dysphoria, and a craving for carbohydrates and sweets. During withdrawal or when the chronic user is acutely intoxicated, dystonias, chorea, akathisia, and choreoathetoid movements can develop. When dramatic, this is referred to as "crack dancing," presumably due to receptor hypersensitivity. Withdrawal begins shortly after the last dose, peaking during the next 12–96 hours. Treat the patient in a controlled, calm setting, and let the patient sleep. Bromocriptine, methylphenidate, and carbidopa/levodopa can each ameliorate cocaine withdrawal. For example, start bromocriptine at 1.25 mg BID, increase to TID in 2–3 days, then 2.5 mg BID and then TID for 2 and 4 days, respectively, and then 5 mg BID thereafter until the acute phase is over (about 4 weeks). Bromocriptine is then tapered and stopped. Maintenance treatment with standard doses of desipramine, bupropion, or carbamazepine are of modest benefit.

Amphetamine and *dextroamphetamine* are synthetic substitutes for ephedrine. Oral and intravenous doses of amphetamine and its congeners methlyphenidate and phendimetrazine have acute effects similar to cocaine, although longer lasting and milder. Physical tolerance also develops to amphetamine. Amphetamine (to a lesser extent methlyphenidate) is a strong dopamine reuptake inhibitor. Amphetamine also has presynaptic autoregulatory effects, increasing dopamine production and monoamine oxidase inhibition. Amphetamine is also a moderate reuptake inhibitor of serotonin and reduces noradrenergic activity in the locus ceruleus.

Massive doses of cocaine and amphetamine can produce a neurotoxic metabolite (6-hydroxydopamine) that may account for the continued cognitive impairment seen in some chronic users even after years of abstinence. Chronic amphetamine or cocaine use can also cause a delusional, hallucinatory disorder that can mimic schizophrenia or chronic mania. Stereotypic movements and emotional unresponsiveness are characteristic. These patients also move in a jerky, bird-like manner, and continuously look around as if scanning for danger. They can be violent. Chronic users, when not intoxicated or in withdrawal, may at other times appear parkinsonian, as if they have tardive dyskinesia, or Gilles de la Tourette's syndrome.

Withdrawal is characterized by prolonged sleep with increased REM time, fatigue, apathy, headache, sweating, muscle cramps, and increased appetite. Desipramine is helpful for this syndrome. Chronic users do poorly on cognitive tests, even though not intoxicated at the time of testing. They have problems with abstract thinking, problem solving, verbal memory (poor paragraph recall), and mental math. Cerebral metabolism is bilaterally reduced frontally. After detoxification, metabolism remains low (left more so than right). They may have a frontal lobe avolitional or disinhibited syndrome. In additon to its neurotoxic metabolites, chronic use can cause long-term vasospasm and subsequent cell loss, further explaining these chronic brain changes.

In addition to the standard behavioral strategies for treating acute drug intoxications, sympathomimetic drug intoxication may require (1) neuroleptics for psychosis (haloperidol), (2) standard cooling treatments for hyperpyrexia to prevent cardiovascular collapse and seizures, (3) acidification of the urine with ammonium chloride 500–1,000 mg every 4 hours to enhance drug excretion, and (4) phentolamine 1–5 mg IV for severe hypertension. The psychosis secondary to chronic abuse may continue for weeks. ECT can resolve this condition. Outpatient rehabilitation programs using behavioral and psychosocial techniques also benefit some patients.

There are three stages of treatment for a patient with cocaine abuse but without other major behavioral syndromes:

1. *Detoxification* (1–4 weeks) using dopaminergic agents to control withdrawal symptoms and minimize craving. These agents include bromocriptine, methylphenidate, carbidopa/levodopa, pergolide, and amantadine. Do not use these agents if the patient is also bipolar or psychotic because they can exacerbate these conditions. Buprenorphine can also be used (one 4–8 mg sublingual dose may reduce the crash effect, so abstinence is more tolerable).
2. *Maintenance of recovery* (3–6 months) using agents that are dopaminergic or serotonergic to reduce craving. These include desipramine, imipramine, bupropion, fluoxetine, sertraline, and phenelzine, all in standard antidepressant doses. Naltrexone (100 mg Monday and Wednesday, 150 mg Friday) and carbamazepine (200–800 mg) have also been used.
3. *Long-term treatment* with an anticraving drug and urine testing.

Always couple stages 2 and 3 with trying to change environmental drug using factors.

Caffeine and *nicotine* are also stimulant, highly addicting drugs. Caffeine in high doses clinically mimics amphetamine use and anxiety disorder. In high doses it can exacerbate mania, lower the seizure threshold, and exacerbate the behavioral symptoms of epilepsy. Caffeine and nicotine induce liver enzymes and can lead to lower doses of liver metabolized psychotropics. Caffeine may also increase cholesterol levels, but also may have a neuroprotective effect (as an adenosine competitive antagonist) during ischemic stroke. Nicotine combined with alcohol increases the risk for subarachnoid hemorrhage.

Hallucinogens

Lysergic acid diethylamide (LSD), a synthetic ergot alkaloid derivative; *peyote* and *mescaline*, extracted from a Mexican cactus; *psilocybin*, extracted from a Mexican mushroom; and *corymbus* and *myristica*, from morning glory seeds and nutmeg, respectively, are hallucinogens primarily used by middle- and upper-class young adults.

LSD is structurally related to serotonin (5-HT) and it inhibits 5-HT_{1A} (autoreceptor) firing in the dorsal raphe nucleus. DMT (*N,N,*-dimethyltryptamine) and psilocybin also do this. Although this effect may relate to some anxiety-producing properties of these drugs, it does not correlate with hallucinogenic potency. This effect appears related to LSD and similar agents' effects on 5-HT_2 postsynaptic receptors in the neocortex, nucleus accumbens, and other forebrain structures. Mescaline and other phenthylamine-like agents do not have substantial serotonergic properties.

Acute effects of LSD include altered perception of shape, color, and stimulus intensity, synesthesias (a perception in one sensory modality caused by a stimulus in another), parasthesias, altered consciousness, dizziness, weakness, tremors, and nausea. Intense moods (particularly anxiety), mood lability, distorted time sense, dream-like states, states of religious and philosophic ecstasy, hallucinations (particularly visual), delusional moods and ideas, incoordination, and general cognitive impairment also may occur.

Uncomplicated and mild adverse intoxications rarely require hospitalization. A calm, structured, pleasant environment with moderate light and sound and a calm supportive staff are usually enough to resolve all symptoms. Benzodiazepines and, for some psychotic but nonexcited patients, a single low dose of a neuroleptic may be needed. Because several hallucinogens have serotonergic properties, atypical neuroleptics would be logical choices, especially risperidone. Risperidone use, however, is limited, because it does not yet come in an intramuscular form. Although it is not FDA approved for this purpose, cyproheptadine is a potent 5-HT_2 antagonist and can block LSD hallucinations.

Patients who are extremely agitated and excited or whose symptoms persist past 4–6 hours need hospitalization. ECT is the safest, most rapid and effective treatment for these drug-induced psychoses. Depending on the intensity of mood (the more the better), mood stabilizers (valproate, carbamazepine, lithium) would be the next choice. Neuroleptics are the last resort. Because many illicit drugs have anticholinergic properties, as do some neuroleptics, choose a neuroleptic with low muscarinic effects.

In some persons, particularly those who have "bad trips" (usually frightening psychotic states), vulnerability to the neurotropic effects of hallucinogens is presumed, and a single dose of any hallucinogen can cause permanent brain dysfunction. Certainly, repeated use of hallucinogens can cause cognitive impairment, recurrent psychoses, chronic hallucinosis, and a chronic avolitional state, each of which may persist long after discontinuation of the drug. There are many patients in their 30s or 40s with chronic emotional blunting, speech and language impairments, and sporadic auditory hallucinations who, in their late teens or early 20s, used hallucinogenic drugs for 1–2 years. Despite no further drug use (confirmed by family, friends, and medical observation), these schizophrenia-like symptoms persist. A family history of mood disorder may be a particular vulnerability, as persons with chronic drug-induced psychoses have rates of mood disorder in their families that are three to four times that of the general population. The presence of avolition and formal thought disorder are particularly poor prognostic signs in these patients.

Arylcyclohexylamines

Phencyclidine (PCP) is a white crystalline powder that may be mistaken for cocaine, and "cheap" cocaine highs are commonly reported by patients intoxicated with PCP. Two to three million Americans (most under age 25 years) have used PCP ("angel dust," "hog," "crystal," and "weed"), which can cause an usually intense euphoria with feelings of unlimited power and energy, but also intense depression, psychosis, and violence. PCP users commonly use other illicit drugs and alcohol and have drug-related arrests. PCP may be snorted, smoked, or injected. Once distributed in body fat, as much as 94% of a given dose remains in body tissue indefinitely. "Flashbacks" have been attributed to temporary mobilization of the molecule from fat to brain. PCP is a dissociative anesthetic that induces catalepsy and analgesia but leaves the person's eyes open as if awake. Because of this property, it was used as an animal tranquilizer, as shown in nature programs on TV. PCP appears to work on sigma type opiate receptors and a more specific PCP receptor.

Because PCP has an affinity for the vestibulocerebellar system, intoxication is usually characterized by dizziness, nystagmus, and incoordination. Tachycardia and hypertension are also common. Pupils are normal in size or narrow. A delirium with intense anxiety, suspiciousness, irritability, and violence is characteristic. Psychosis most often appears as a typical drug-induced psychotic state or mania. Chronic psychoses and cognitive deficits can occur. Definitive care is similar to that for cocaine.

Cannabis

Marijuana, a form of cannabis derived from the hemp plant, is the most widely used illicit drug. It can be smoked, brewed in a tea, or made into cakes or candy. Nearly 60% of U.S. high school graduates have used it. Its main active ingredient is delta-9-tetrahydrocannabinol (THC). There is some cross-tolerance with alcohol. Cannabis is very lipid soluble. It binds with adrenoceptors, dopaminergic and opioid receptors. Hashish, another form of cannabis, has a high concentration of THC. Onset of action is within minutes, and its effect can last 2–3 hours. Physiologic tolerance has not been established, but psychologic dependence can occur, as can a withdrawal syndrome of anorexia, anxiety, agitation, irritability, dysphoria, tremor, and insomnia. This response mimics an atypical depression, and some patients seek admission for this hoping to be prescribed other drugs. Observation is the best treatment with symptoms, usually resolving in several days.

Acute effects of cannabis include a high or euphoria, increased heart rate and blood pressure, conjunctival infection, reduced concentration and new learning, diminished reaction time and time sense (events appear slower than they actually are), and impaired coordination, balance, and judgment. Some persons, particularly first-time users, experience acute panic, disorientation, dysphoria, irritability, suspiciousness, delusions, hallucinations, and body image distortions. Chronic effects from heavy use include an uncommon "amotivational" syndrome of apathy, loss of drive and ambition, and mild general cognitive impairment. Persons with a family history of psychosis or mood disorder are most prone to the avolitional syndrome and may also develop a chronic schizophrenia-like psychosis.

Long-term use probably impairs lung function and suppresses the immune system. Heavy cannabis smokers are at greater risk for lung cancer and fungal infections than are smokers of equivalent amounts of tobacco. Reproductive and chromosomal aberrations also have been reported with chronic use.

Treatment for the acute syndrome rarely requires sedation. A quiet, structured environment with a friendly, calm staff usually resolves the patient's symptoms. Benzodiazepines help in severe anxiety, but neuroleptics are virtually never required unless the acute psychosis lasts more than a few hours, in which case a single dose neuroleptic usually works. If hospitalization is required for a prolonged psychosis, management is similar to that for hallucinogens.

Inhalants

Seven million Americans have used inhalants (volatile substances, organic solvents), most of which are hydrocarbons found in substances like gasoline, lighter fluids, fuel gases, spray paints, typewriter correction fluid, cleaning fluids, and adhesives. Inhalant use is more common among young poor persons, and more common among European-Americans and Hispanic-Americans than among African-Americans.

The majority of inhalant abusers abuse other substances, and large numbers eventually use intravenous drugs and have antisocial personality disorder. Most inhalants are easy to purchase legally. Inhalation rapidly produces behavioral effects, and users can titrate doses more readily than persons taking drugs orally. Inhalants can be sniffed from a container or from a soaked rag.

General physical findings may include a papular rash around the nose and mouth ("glue sniffer's rash"), an odor of paint or solvent on clothes, skin, or breath, and thermal burns. Inhalant intoxication resembles alcohol intoxication but is of shorter duration. Any inhalant can cause aggressive, assaultive behavior requiring restraints and sedation. Diazepam 10–30 mg PO or 10–15 mg IV may be needed. As many as 40% of persons who regularly use organic solvent inhalants develop severe cognitive impairment from the chemical's toxic effect on the brain. Chronic use also may affect peripheral nerves and kidney and liver function. There is also a greater risk for brain tumors. Acute intoxication is characterized by delirium, tinnitus, ataxia, tremors and fasciculations, distortions of body image, and visual hallucinations, often of colorful images and geometric shapes. These patients may be violent. Nitrites chemically unrelated to other inhalants specifically produce a transient alteration in consciousness and are used primarily in association with sexual behavior.

THE NEUROBIOLOGY OF SUBSTANCE ABUSE

Alcoholism is familial and apparently is specifically transmitted from parent to child whether or not the child is exposed to the alcoholic parent. The rates for alcoholism may be higher in parents of female alcoholics than in the relatives of male alcoholics. There is also a threefold increase of alcoholism among the adopted daughters of alcoholic biologic mothers compared with control daughters. There is also an excess of alcohol abuse among the daughters of biologic alcoholic fathers. Fathers who are alcoholic and criminal (both characteristics reflecting an underlying antisocial personality disorder) probably have no excess of alcoholic daughters. In addition to having a family history of alcoholism, women alcoholics are also more likely to be depressed, to be impulsive, and to have a partner who abuses alcohol.

About 25% of fathers and brothers of alcoholics are alcoholic. Monozygotic twins have higher concordance rates for alcoholism than do dizygotic twins. Biologic relatives of alcoholic adoptees are more likely to become alcoholic than are relatives of control adoptees. However, children without alcoholic biologic relatives and who are reared by alcoholic adoptive parents are no more likely to become alcoholics than are other children.

Two forms of familial alcoholism, with distinct genetic and environmental causes and with different associations with criminality and severity, have been proposed. The least common type appears to be highly heritable over the entire range of social backgrounds and is associated with severe alcohol abuse and criminality, particularly in fathers and their sons. The more common type, although heritable, is influenced more by environmental factors (pre- and postnatal in particular) and is associated with mild alcohol abuse in fathers and mothers, but not with criminality. Eighty percent of alcoholics show some signs of it before age 30 years, although for some patients the full expression of the condition may not occur until their 30s or 40s.

Acutely administered alcohol stimulates brain reward systems through the release of dopamine. DNA samples from the brains of the highly heritable severe-type alcoholics and nonalcoholics find a D_2 dopamine receptor gene on chromosome 11 to be significantly more frequent in the alcoholics (70%–80%) than the nonalcoholics (about 20%). This finding needs further confirmation.

Thus, alcohol abuse appears to be heterogeneous, representing (1) a behavior pattern associated with some illnesses (e.g., alcoholism with mood or anxiety disorder); (2) a sporadic late onset disorder with some genetic predisposition and substantial environmental causative factors; and (3) an early onset highly heritable syndrome.

What biologic processes the genes of alcohol abuse might influence leading to increased alcohol consumption are unknown. Theories generally revolve around the pharmacologic fact that alcohol in low doses is initially a CNS stimulant, whereas in high doses it is a CNS depressant that can lead to physiologic tolerance. Theories also try to incorporate the apparent common use of alcohol by alcoholics and nonalcoholics in stressful social settings, particularly approach–avoidance conflict situations.

The highly heritable form of alcoholism may be associated with the personality traits of high novelty seeking and low harm avoidance and reward dependence (see Chapter 6). This is similar to the pattern observed in antisocial personality, which would explain the association between this form of alcoholism and criminality. Low basal dopaminergic activity, proposed as an underlying neurotransmitter pattern in high novelty seeking, may lead to increased sensitivity to dopamine agonists (cocaine, alcohol, opiates). The sporadic form of alcoholism may be associated with low novelty seeking, and high harm avoidance and reward dependence (dependent personality). High basal serotonergic turnover, leading to behavioral inhibition and anxiety that is relieved by some drugs, particularly alcohol, has been proposed as an underlying neurotransmitter pattern for high harm avoidance.

The sporadic-type alcoholic when abstinent is hypervigilant and apprehensive and displays a typical high resting anxiety level EEG pattern (minimal alpha, excessive fast activity, and poor synchrony). In response to alcohol, the EEGs of these individuals show a marked increase in alpha, which is associated with a sense of calm attention and well-being. Hypervigilance and avoidance behaviors are consistent with high harm avoidance and reward dependence traits. On the other hand, abstinent early onset high heritability alcoholics are hypovigilant with high novelty seeking traits. When studied with evoked potentials, and when asked to respond to stimuli, they demonstrate reduced amplitude in late component waves (P300) as compared with controls, even though they do not make more errors than controls. This response is also observed in nonalcoholic sons of alcoholic fathers and suggests a heritable deficit in ability to allocate significance to the target stimuli. Furthermore, such alcoholics also show increasing amplitudes to stimuli of increasing intensity rather than the more common reducing pattern.

TABLE 13.4. Factors in Addiction

Determinants of Use	Determinants of Abuse	Determinants of Abstinence (Recovery)
1. Availability of drugs	1. Effects of drug on brain reward system (see Fig. 13.1)	1. Specific pharmacologic intervention to properly detoxify and reduce craving
2. Peer or partner pressure	2. Continued availability, acceptance, pressure	2. Control of co-occurring conditions
3. Acceptance and frequency of use in subculture	3. Severity of co-occurring conditions (e.g., depression, anxiety disorder)	3. Treatment of brain and general medical problems from the drug abuse
4. Personality traits that influence experimentation (high novelty seeking most important)	4. Effect of drug on other brain functions (e.g., frontal damage from alcohol leads to poor executive function and less self-control)	4. Personality traits that particularly influence compliance (harm avoidance, persistence, cooperativeness)
5. Gene/endophenotypic modifiers (e.g., patterns of function of brain systems involved in reward, information processing [IQ], other personality traits [harm avoidance, self-directedness, self-transcendence, cooperativeness])	5. General medical effects of drug	5. Removal from environments of high availability and peer, partner, subcultural pressures
6. Co-occurring conditions increasing probability of self-medication (e.g., mood disorder, anxiety disorder)		6. Repair of social and job damage caused by abuse

Because alcohol has an excitatory effect on neurons of the ventral tegmental areas (the brain's putative reward system; see below), its use may produce a pharmacologic reward. Individuals with high novelty seeking traits and thus high dopaminergic responsivity will be particularly prone to this ethanol reward. The increased use of stimulant drugs in persons with high novelty seeking is consistent with this relationship. This alcohol and drug seeking behavior is thus a special kind of exploratory appetitive behavior. With frequent and continued use, however, tolerance develops, and abuse becomes addiction.

Alcohol is also anxiolytic. Those individuals with high harm avoidance traits, under circumstances not understood, may begin to use alcohol to relieve anxiety. As anything that quickly reduces anxiety is a strong reinforcer, those individuals who also have high reward dependence traits will tend to continue to use the reinforcing anxiety-lowering agent. Again, frequent and continued use would lead to tolerance, and abuse becomes addiction.

Substance abuse and dependence is also familial, and the use of alcohol, tobacco, stimulants, benzodiazepines, analgesics, cannabis, caffeine, nicotine, and

TABLE 13.5. Brain Reward System Implicated in Drug Addictions

Neurotransmitter	Anatomy	Actions
Dopamine	Mesocorticolimbic reticular activating system, particularly the VTA in the midbrain and the nucleus accumbens in the forebrain	1. All addicting substances have direct or indirect effect on this system 2. The primary system for operant conditioning (biochemical substrate for addiction) 3. Response to biochemical conditioning underlies tolerance and withdrawal phenomena
Opioids	Widespread, particularly spinal cord and medial thalamus (pain), periacqueductal gray; modifies dopaminergic system and stressors (a positive reinforcer)	Endogenous opioid peptides (beta-endorphin, enkephalins, dynorphin) act to modulate: 1. Nociceptive response to pain stimuli 2. Dopaminergic reward system in VTA and nucleus accumbens 3. Hippocampal and hypothalamic response to DA reward system activity 4. Homeostatic adaptive functions, (e.g., food and water need, temperature regulation)
GABA	Widespread	Anxiety regulation; interacts with other systems enhancing anti-anxiety effects

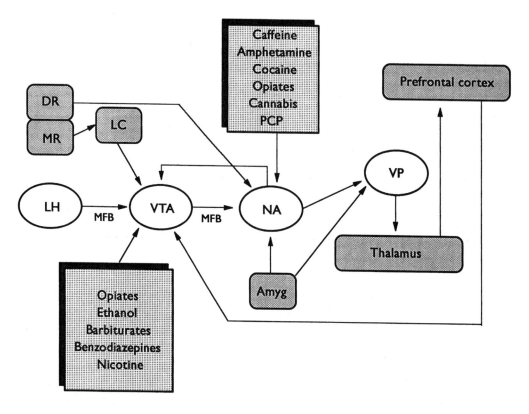

Figure 13.1. Brain reward system. LH, lateral hypothalamus; MFB, medium forebrain bundle; VTA, ventral tegmental area; NA, nucleus accumbens; VP = ventral pallidum; Amyg, amygdala; DR = dorsal raphe nucleus; MR, medial raphe nucleus; LC, locus ceruleus.

other illicit drugs by parents predicts their use in children. Studies with twins (including those reared apart) also suggest a significant genetic contribution to drug taking. One adoption study also suggests that the familialness of substance abuse results, in part, from genetic factors. Antisocial personality and behaviors consistent with high novelty seeking, low harm avoidance, and reward dependence are also observed in drug abusers, suggesting a similar set of relationships to that of familial alcoholism.

An additional problem is the effects of maternal drug use on the developing fetus. The effects of alcohol are well known, but cocaine also has profound adverse effects, among others lowering uterine blood supply (via vasoconstriction), decreasing placental transport of essential amino acids, inducing early gene transcription factors (Fos and Jun), and retarding the development of some neurotransmitter systems (e.g., serotonin). Newborns exposed to intrauterine cocaine have multiple neuromotor, cognitive, and behavioral problems and are more prone to violence (see Chapter 16). The exposure to cocaine during critical phases of neural development may also contribute to increased drug use in later life, thus increasing the penetrance and expression of any genetic predisposition to drug use.

Table 13.4 summarizes the many factors that contribute to drug use and abuse. These factors broadly reflect three processes:

1. The availability and pressures to use
2. Personality traits characterized by tendencies to be behaviorally active in novel, stressful, or frustrating nonrewarding situations
3. The brain's reward system's biochemical response to drugs of abuse

The more intense these three factors, the more likely the person will use and abuse drugs.

In addition to the specific treatments mentioned above, the neurobehavioral construct of drug abuse suggests that to successfully treat these patients you must (1) be as pharmacologically specific as possible, and for persons with multiple drug usage err on the side of modifying the dopaminergic system; (2) consider the interactive effects of the patient's personality on the likelihood of use and abuse, maintenance of use, and response to and compliance with treatments; and (3) address the environmental factors that reinforce drug use and pressure the patient to continue drug use.

Table 13.5 summarizes the brain's mesotelencephalic reward system. The heart of this system appears to be dopamine, and its source is the mesolimbic/anterior reticular activating system, which merges into the ventral tegmental area (VTA) and innovates the lateral hypothalamus. The VTA projects to the forebrain: nucleus accumbens, septal area, frontal cortex, olfactory tubercle. The nucleus accumbens projects to the ventral striatum. The ventral striatum gets limbic input and converts emotional limbic information into action and motivation by its integration within the frontal lobe–basal ganglia–thalamic circuits. The frontal cortex then sends both excitatory and inhibitory feedback to the VTA. Figure 13.1 shows that reticular activating system dopaminergic (DA) input to the lateral hypothalamus continues via the median forebrain bundle to the VTA (step 1 in reward). DA innervation continues from the VTA via the median forebrain bundle to the nucleus accumbens (step 2 in reward). The nucleus accumbens then stimulates the ventral pallidum via GABAergic and endogenous opiate (enkephalin) pathways (step 3 in reward). The ventral pallidum then activates frontal circuitry. This reward system is modified by limbic input (e.g., emotional input from the amygdala), noradrenergic input from the locus ceruleus, and serotonergic input from the raphe nuclei (the median raphe serotonergic fibers modify locus ceruleus activity and parallel noradrenergic projections to the limbic system; the dorsal raphe serotonergic fibers modify the nucleus accumbens, and its serotonergic fibers parallel DA projections).

An operant reward is any reinforcer likely to increase the probability of a response. The likelihood of response increases when the reward is associated with positive affective coloring (i.e., pleasure). Thus, drugs that activate the mesotelencephalic reward system and induce a sense of pleasure while reducing anxiety are

TABLE 13.6. Neurobiology of Drugs of Abuse

Drug	Anatomy	Pharmacodynamics	Behavior
Cocaine	1. Activates nucleus accumbens, medial prefrontal cortex, medial caudate 2 Depresses firing in dorsal raphe nucleus and locus ceruleus	1. Potent DA, 5-HT, norepinephrine reuptake inhibitor; DA inhibition via direct presynaptic membrane competition (with secondary effect on postsynaptic D_1 receptors), and presynaptic D_2 agonistic effect; 2. Acts on presynaptic 5-H2_{1A}, 5-HT_2, and alpha$_2$-adrenoceptors; 3. Chronic administration leads to decreased DA synthesis via autoreceptor effects	1. *Acute effects:* increased motor activity, euphoria, heightened operant conditioning 2. *Chronic effects:* stereotypies; and limbic sensitization (*fos* gene changes); diminished short-term memory, working memory, attention; chronic use reduces frontal 5-HT, DA, and neuropeptides
Opiates	1. Receptors widespread; with concentrations of receptors in median forebrain bundle and mesolimbic DA system 2. Excites DA neurons in ventral tegmental area and this leads to DA release in nucleus accumbens	1. Three receptors (mu, delta, kappa) coupled with G proteins leads to reduced cyclic AMP activity and opens potassium channels, causing hyperpolarization, inhibition of firing, and widespread inhibition of neurotransmitter release 2. Also act as alpha$_2$-agonists (autoreceptors), leading to presynaptic inhibition in the locus ceruleus and thus decreased anxiety	1. Euphoria independent of analgesic effect 2. Reduced motor behavior followed by increased motor behavior
Alcohol	Widespread	1. Enhances action of 5-HT and 5-HT_3 receptors,	Initial euphoria at low doses (with increased

strong operant rewards and are likely to be used and abused. Table 13.6 lists the effects of some drugs of abuse on this system. These drugs appear to affect different aspects of the reward system as shown in Figure 13.1.

On a molecular level, drugs of abuse initially inhibit cAMP systems. With chronic use a compensatory upregulation occurs that may underlie tolerance. Withdrawal from opiates is thought to work this way, specifically leading to increased noradrenergic activity in the locus ceruleus and the peripheral and central features of anxiety characteristically seen in withdrawal. Upregulation of cAMP

TABLE 13.6. *(continued)*

Drug	Anatomy	Pharmacodynamics	Behavior
		acetylcholine, and nicotinic cholinergic receptors that activate ion channels	DA and norepinephrine activity); large doses lead to CNS depression
		2. Inhibits glutamate at receptor (NMDA) level, inhibits voltage-sensitive calcium channels and enhances GABA action	
		3. Chronic use increases GABA receptors	
		4. Acute use enhances cyclic AMP activity, chronic use reduces it	
		5. Chronic use directly affects cell membranes, changing their lipid composition	
Cannabis	1. Activates nucleus accumbens, medial forebrain bundle, prefrontal cortex 2. May also affect basal ganglia, hippocampus, cerebellum	1. Presynaptic release of mesolimbic DA via action on mu opioid receptor 2. Second-messenger action inhibiting cyclic AMP and G-protein effects	1. Initial sense of well-being, sedation, perceptual distortions acute panic and susdoses 2. Conjunctival injection, tachycardia (no sub stantial change in appetite or blood pressure), hypothermia and hypoactivity, analgesia, catalepsy, ataxia, and poor new learning at high doses

systems leads to increased G-protein activity, which has been implicated in D_1 receptor hypersensitivity that is seen with chronic cocaine use. In addition, chronic drug use can induce Fos and Jun gene transcription factors, resulting in gene changes and permanent cellular functional change.

ADDITIONAL READINGS

Abood ME, Martin BR: Neurobiology of marijuana abuse. *TiPS* 13:201–206, 1992.
Aghajanian GK: Serotonin and the action of LSD in the brain. *Psychiatric Ann* 24:137–141, 1994.

American Psychiatric Association: *Practice Guidelines for the Treatment of Patients with Nicotine Dependence*. American Psychiatric Association, Washington, DC, 1996.

Balfour DJK: The effects of nicotine on brain neurotransmitter systems. *Pharmacol Ther* 16:269–282, 1982.

Blum K, Cull JG, Braverman ER, Comings DE: Reward deficiency syndrome. *Am Sci* 84:132–145, 1996.

Bohman M, Sigvardsson S, Cloninger CR: Maternal inheritance of alcohol abuse. Crossfostering analysis of adopted women. *Arch Gen Psychiatry* 38:965–969, 1981.

Bolla KI, Cadet J-L, London ED: The neuropsychiatry of chronic cocaine abuse. *J Neuropsychiatry Clin Neurosci* 10:280–289, 1998.

Cadoret RJ, O'Gormon TW, Troughton E, Heywood E: Alcoholism and antisocial personality. *Arch Gen Psychiatry* 42:161–167, 1985.

Cadoret RJ, Troughton E, O'Gorman TW, Heywood E: An adoption study of genetic and environmental factors in drug abuse. *Arch Gen Psychiatry* 43:1131–1136, 1986.

Cadoret RJ, Yates WR, Troughton E, Woodworth G, Stewart MA: Adoption study demonstrating two genetic pathways to drug abuse. *Arch Gen Psychiatry* 52:42–52, 1995.

Cardoso F, Jankovic J: Movement disorders. *Neurol Clin Neurol Compl Drug Alcohol Abuse* 11:625–638, 1993.

Childres AR, McLellan AT, O'Brien CP: Abstinent opiate abusers exhibit conditioned craving, conditioned withdrawal and reductions in both through extinction. *Br J Addict* 81:655–660, 1986.

Chiriboga C: Fetal effects. *Neurol Clin Neurol Compl Drug Alcohol Abuse* 11:707–728, 1993.

Cloninger CR: Neurogenetic adaptive mechanisms in alcoholism. *Science* 236:410–416, 1987.

Cook WL, Goethe JW: The effect of being reared with an alcoholic half-sibling: A classic study reanalyzed. *Fam Proc* 29:87–93, 1990.

Cornelius JR, Salloum IM, Ehler JG, Jarrett PJ, Cornelius MD, Perel JM, Thase ME, Black A: Fluoxetine in depressed alcoholics. *Arch Gen Psychiatry* 54:700–705, 1997.

Day NL, Cottreau CM, Richardson GA: The epidemiology of alcohol, marijuana, and cocaine use among women of childbearing age and pregnant women. *Clin Obstet Gynecol* 36:232–245, 1993

DiChiara G, North RA: Neurobiology of opiate abuse. *TiPS* 13:185–193, 1992.

Dinwiddie SH, Cloninger CR: Family and adoption studies in alcoholism and drug addiction. *Psychiatr Ann* 21:206–214, 1991.

Fibiger HC, Phillips AG, Brown EE: The neurobiology of cocaine-induced reinforcement. *1992 Cocaine: Scientific and Social Dimensions* (Ciba Foundation Symposium 166). Wiley, Chichester, 1992, pp 96–124.

Fletcher JM, Page JB, Frances DJ, Copeland K, Naus MJ, Davis CM, Morris R, Krauskopf D, Salz P: Cognitive correlates of long-term cannabis use in Costa Rican men. *Arch Gen Psychiatry* 53:1051–1057, 1996.

Fowler JS, Volkow ND, Wang G-J, Pappas N, Logan J, MacGregor R, Alexoff D, Shea C, Schlyer D, Wolf AP, Warner D, Zezulkova I, Cilento R: Inhibition of monoamine oxidase B in the brains of smokers. *Nature* 379:733–736, 1996.

Galanter M, Kleber HD (eds): *American Psychiatric Press Textbook of Substance Abuse Treatment*. The American Psychiatric Press, Inc., Washington, DC, 1994.

Gawin FH, Ellinwood EH JR: Cocaine and other stimulants, actions, abuse, and treatment. *N Engl J Med* 318:1173–1181, 1988.

George FR: Genetic models in the study of alcoholism and substance abuse mechanisms. *Prog Neuro-Psychopharmacol Biol Psychiatry* 17:345–361, 1993.

Gerstein DR: The effectiveness of drug treatment. In O'Brien CP, Jaffe JH (eds): *Addictive States*. Raven Press, New York, 1992, pp 253–282.

Glantz JC, Woods JR Jr: Cocaine, heroin, and phencyclidine: Obstetric perspectives. *Clin Obstet Gynecol* 36:279–301, 1993.

Gold MS: The epidemiology, attitudes, and pharmacology of LSD use in the 1990s. *Psychiatr Ann 24*:124–126, 1994.

Gomberg FSL: Women and alcohol: Use and abuse. *J Nerv Ment Dis 181*:211–219, 1993.

Gorelick DA: Serotonin uptake blockers and the treatment of alcoholism. *Recent Dev Alc 7*:262–281, 1989.

Grove WM, Eckert ED, Heston L, Bouchard TJ Jr, Segal N, Lykken OT: Heritability of substance abuse and antisocial behavior: A study of monozygotic twins reared apart. *Biol Psychiatry 27*:1293–1304, 1990.

Heath AC, Jardine R, Martin NG: Interactive effects of genotype and social environment on alcohol consumption in female twins. *J Stud Alcohol 50*:38–48, 1989.

Hrubec Z, Omenn GS: Evidence of genetic predisposition to alcoholic cirrhosis and psychosis: Twin concordances for alcholism and its biological end points by zygosity among male veterans. *Alcoholism Clin Exp Res 5*:207–215, 1981.

Hurt RD, Sachs DPL, Glover ED, Offord KP, Johnston JA, Dale LC, Khayrallah MA, Schroeder DR, Glover PN, Sullivan R, Croghan IT, Sullivan PM: A comparison of sustained-release bupropion and placebo for smoking cessation. *N Engl J Med 337*:1195–1202, 1997.

Huseby NE, Bjordal E, Nilssen O, Barth T: Utility of biological markers during outpatient treatment of alcohol-dependent subjects: Carbohydrate-deficient transferrin responds to moderate changes in alcohol consumption. *Alcohol Clin Exp Res 321*:1343–1346, 1997.

Jonas JM, Gold MS: The pharmacologic treatment of alcohol and cocaine abuse. *Pediatr Clin North Am 15*:179–190, 1992.

Kalivas PW, Samson HH (eds): *The Neurobiology of Drug and Alcohol Addiction,* New York Academy of Sciences, New York, 1992.

Kanzler HR, Burleson JA, Del Boca FK, Babor TF, Korner P, Brown J, Bohn MJ: Buspirone treatment of anxious alcoholics. A placebo-controlled trial. *Arch Gen Psychiatry 51*:720–731, 1994.

Kendler KS, Heath AC, Neale ML, Kessler RL, Eaves LJ: A population-based twin study of alcoholism in women. *JAMA 268*:1877–1882, 1992.

Kleber HD: Treatment of cocaine abuse: Pharmacotherapy. *1992 Cocaine: Scientific and Social Dimensions* (Ciba Foundation Symposium 166). Wiley, Chichester, 1992, pp 195–206.

Knop J, Goodwin DW, Jensen P, Penick E, Pollack V, Gabrielli W, Teasdale TW, Mednick SA: A 30-year follow-up study of the sons of alcoholic men. *Acta Psychiatr Scand (Suppl)* 370:48–53, 1993.

Koob GF: Drugs of abuse: Anatomy, pharmacology and function of reward pathways. *TiPS 13*:177–184, 1992.

Koob GF: Neurobiological mechanisms in cocaine and opiate dependence. In O'Brien CP, Jaffe JH (eds): *Addictive States.* Raven Press, New York, 1992, pp 79–92.

Koponen H, Hurri L, Stenback U, Mattila E, Soininen H, Riekkinen PJ: Computed tomography findings in delirium. *J Nerv Ment Dis 177*:226–231, 1989.

Kornetsky C, Porrino LJ: Brain mechanisms of drug-induced reinforcement. In O'Brien CP, Jaffe JH (eds): *Addictive States.* Raven Press, New York, 1992, pp 59–77.

Kosten TA, Ball SA, Rounsaville BJ: A sibling study of sensation seeking and opiate addiction. *J Nerv Ment Dis 182*:284–289, 1994.

Kosten TR, Kleber HD (eds): *Clinician's Guide to Cocaine Addiction: Theory, Research, and Treatment.* Guilford Press, New York, 1992.

Kosten TR, Rosen MI, Schottenfeld R, Ziedonis D: Buprenorphine for cocaine and opiate dependence. *Psychopharmacol Bull 28*:15–19, 1992.

Kuhar MJ: Molecular pharmacology fo cocaine: A dopamine hypothesis and its implications. *1992 Cocaine: Scientific and Social Dimensions* (Ciba Foundation Symposium 166). Wiley, Chichester, 1992, pp 81–95.

Levkoff SE, Besdine R, Wetle T: Acute and confusional states (delirium) in the hospitalized elderly. In Eisdorfer C (ed): *Annual Review of Gerontology and Geriatrics,* vol 6. Springer Publishing, New York, 1986, pp 1–26.

Longstreth WT Jr, Nelson LM, Koepsell TD, van Belle G: Cigarette smoking, alcohol abuse, and subarachnoid hemorrhage. *Stroke 23:*1242–1249, 1992.

Lowinson JH, Ruiz P, Millman RB, Langrod JG (eds): *Substance Abuse: A Comprehensive Textbook,* 3rd ed. Williams & Wilkins, Baltimore, 1997.

Malcolm R, Hutto BR, Phillips JD, Ballenger JC: Pergolide mesylate treatment of cocaine withdrawal. *J Clin Psychiatry 52:*39–40, 1991.

Mendelson JH, Mello NK: Management of cocaine abuse and dependence. *N Engl J Med 334:*965–972, 1996.

Merikangas KR, Risch NJ, Weissman MM: Comorbidity and co-transmission of alcoholism, anxiety and depression *Psychol Med 24:*69–80, 1994.

Meyer RE, Kranzler HR (guest eds): Neurobiology of alcoholism. *Clin Neurosci 3:*141–188, 1995.

Miller NS: *Comprehensive Handbook of Drug and Alcohol Addiction.* Marcell Dekker, New York., 1991.

Nestler EJ: Cellular responses to chronic treatment with drugs of abuse. *Crit Rev Neurobiol 7:*23–39, 1993.

Nestler EJ, Arghajanian GK: Molecular and cellular basis of addiction. *Science 278:*58–63, 1997.

O'Connor PG, Schottenfeld RS: Patients with alcohol problems. *N Eng J Med 9:*592–602, 1998.

O'Malley SS: Integration of opioid antagonists and psychosocial therapy in the treatment of narcotic and alcohol dependence. *J Clin Psychiatry 56(suppl 7):*30–38, 1995.

O'Malley SS, Adamse M, Heaton RK, Gawin FH: Neuropsychological impairment in chronic cocaine abusers. *Am J Drug Alcohol Abuse 18:*131–144, 1992.

O'Malley SS, Jaffe AJ, Change, G, Rode S, Schottenfeld RS, Meyer RE, Rounsaville B: Six-month follow-up of naltrexone and psychotherapy for alcohol dependence. *Arch Gen Psychiatry 53:*217–224, 1996.

Pick EM, Pagliusi SR, Tessari M, Talabot-Ayer D, von Huysduynen RH, Chiamulera C: Common neural substrates for the addictive properties of nicotine and cocaine. *Science 275:*83–86, 1997.

Pickens RW, Svikis DS, McGue M, Lykken DT, Heston LL, Clayton PJ: Heterogeneity in the inheritance of alcoholism. *Arch Gen Psychiatry 48:*19–28, 1991.

Pontieri FE, Tanda G, Orzi F, Di Chiara G: Effects of nicotine on the n. accumbens and similarity to those of addictive drugs. *Nature 382:*255–257, 1996.

Porrino LJ, Dworkin SI, Smith JE: Basal forebrain involvement in self-administration of drugs of abuse. In Napier TC, et al (eds): *The Basal Forebrain.* Plenum Press, New York, 1991, pp 339–351.

Prescott CA, Kendler KS: Genetic and environmental contributions to alcohol abuse and dependence in a population-based sample of male twins. *Am J Psychiatry 156:*34–40, 1999.

Richardson GA, Day NL, McGauhey PJ: The impact of prenatal marijuana and cocaine use on the infant and child. *Clin Obstet Gynecol 36:*302–318, 1993.

Rodnitzky RL, Keyser DL: Neurologic complications of drugs. *Psychiatr Clin North Am 15:*491–510, 1992.

Samson HH, Harris RA: Neurobiology of alcohol abuse. *TiPS 13:*206–211, 1992.

Schuckit MA, Smith TL: An 8 year follow-up of 450 sons of alcoholic and control subjects. *Arch Gen Psychiatry 53:*202–210, 1996.

Sigvardsson S, Bohman M, Cloninger CR: Replication of the Stockholm adoption study of alcoholism: Confirmatory cross-fostering analysis. *Arch Gen Psychiatry 53:*681–687, 1996.

Singer LT, Garber R, Kliegman RM: Neurobehavioral sequelae of fetal cocaine exposure. *J Pediatr 119:*667–672, 1991.

Substance Abuse and Mental Health Services Administration/Center for Substance Abuse Treatment: *Assessment of Patients with Coexisting Mental Illness and Alcohol and Other Drug Abuse.* DHHS Publication No. (SMA) 95-3061. U.S. Department of Health and Human Services, Public Health Services, Rockville, MD, 1994, reprinted 1995.

Tanda G, Pontieri FE, Di Chiara G: Cannabinoid and heroin activation of mesolimbic dopamine transmission by a common mu opioid receptor mechanism. *Science 276:* 2048–2050, 1997.

Thomas H: Psychiatric symptoms in cannabis users. *Br J Psychiatry 163:*141–149, 1993.

Tutton CS, Crayton JW: Current pharmacotherapies for cocaine abuse: A review. *J Addict Dis 12:*109–127, 1993.

Vaillant G: A long-term follow-up of male alcohol abuse. *Arch Gen Psychiatry 3:*243–249,1996.

Volkow ND, Hitzemann R, Wang G-J, Fowler JS, Wolf AP, Dewey SL, Handlesman L: Long-term frontal brain metabolic change in cocaine abusers. *Synapse 11:*184–190, 1992.

Volkow ND, Wang G-J, Fischman MW, Foltin RW, Fowler JS, Abumrad NN, Vitkuns S, Logan J, Galley SJ, Pappas N, Hitzemann R, Shea CE: Relationship between subjective effects of cocaine and dopamine transporter occupancy. *Nature 386:*827–830, 1997.

Volkow ND, Wang G-J, Fowler JS, Logan J, Gatley SJ, Hitzemann R, Chen AD, Dewey JL, Pappas N: Decreased striatal dopaminergic responsiveness in detoxified cocaine-dependent subjects. *Nature 386:*830–833, 1997.

Volpicelli JR, Clay KL, Watson NT, O'Brien CP: Naltrexone in the treatment of alcoholism: Predicting response to naltrexone. *J Clin Psychiatry 56(suppl 7):*39–44, 1995.

Volpicelli JR, Rhines KC, Rhines JS, Volpicelli LA, Alterman AI, O'Brien LP: Naltrexone and alcohol dependence. *Arch Gen Psychiatry 54:*737–742, 1997.

Weis RD, Mirin SM: Tricyclic antidepressants in the treatment of alcoholism and drug abuse. *J Clin Psychiatry (Suppl) 50:*4–11, 1989.

Withers NW, Pulvirenti L, Koob GF, Gillin JC: Cocaine abuse and dependence. *J Clin Psychopharmacol 15:*63–78, 1995.

Woolverton WL, Johnson KM: Neurobiology of cocaine abuse. *TiPS 13:*193–200, 1992.

Yudofsky, SC, Silver JM, Hales JE: Cocaine and aggressive behavior: Neurobiological and clinical perspectives. *Bull Meninger Clin 57:*218–226, 1993.

14

Obsessional Syndromes

Several seemingly distinct syndromes, upon close scrutiny, share the common feature of recurrent, intrusive thoughts or actions. These syndromes include obsessive compulsive disorder (OCD), Gilles de la Tourette's disorder (GTS), trichotillomania, kleptomania, pathologic gambling, some extreme forms of hypochondriasis (particularly when limited to one or a few recurrent health concerns), hoarding, some sexual disorders (e.g., exhibitionism), self-mutilation behavior, and some patients with substance abuse, anorexia nervosa (and perhaps bulimia), and posttraumatic stress disorder (PTSD). Table 14.1 lists OCD syndromes.

CLINICAL PRESENTATION: CLASSIC OCD

Obsessions are recurrent, unwanted thoughts or impulses recognized (at least initially) by the sufferer as senseless and unpleasant, but irresistible. Compulsions are repetitive, ritualistic acts, often but not always driven by obsessive thoughts. The sufferer is virtually never sated, nor is anxiety substantially reduced following completion of the compulsive behavior.

OCD subtypes have been proposed, but sufferers often have mixed obsessions and compulsions. Obsessionals can be cleaners and washers, checkers and doubters, orderers, repeaters and counters, hoarders, ritualizers, and pure obsessionals who experience thoughts and impulses but do not engage in ritualistic behavior. Anxiety in OCD is usually related to a fear of contamination, of failing to do something important that might lead to harm, or of doing something that might harm others. Two to 3% of the general population is affected, men and women equally (childhood onset affects boys more than girls). Onset is usually in the late teens or early twenties and can be acute or insidious. The course can be unremitting (about 50% of cases), episodic (about one third of cases), or mixed.

The relationship between OCD and obsessive compulsive personality disorder is unclear. Although most patients with OCD have abnormal premorbid personalities, these are as often avoidant or dependent as they are obsessive. The distribution in Cluster C personality types among OCD patients does not differ sub-

TABLE 14.1. Obsessive Compulsive Conditions

Obsessive compulsive disorder (classic syndrome)

Eating disorders (anorexia nervosa, bulimia nervosa)

Gilles de la Tourette's syndrome/chronic and transient tic disorders

Impulse control disorders (kleptomania, pyromania, pathologic gambling, trichotillomania)

Obsessive hoarding

Body dysmorphic disorder (in DSM, somatiform category)

Hypochondriasis (in DSM, somatiform category)

Self-mutilation behavior (some patients)

Paraphilias (exhibitionism, voyeurism, compulsive masturbation, bestiality)

Binge drinking

Substance abuse (some patients)

Post-traumatic stress disorder (chronic form; some patients)

Secondary OCD (basal ganglia disease, epilepsy, chronic stimulant drug abuse, benzodiazepine withdrawal, mania, catatonia, schizophrenia, right frontal lobe infarcts)

stantially from that of patients with anxiety disorders. OCD patients do, however, tend to have premorbid traits of low novelty seeking, high harm avoidance, high persistence, resistance to change, need for perfection, and rigid and high levels of morality. Thus, like anxiety disorder patients and persons with Cluster C avoidant/dependent characteristics, they have high harm avoidance, but, rather than inhibiting behavior to avoid anxiety, their anxiety is associated with uncontrollable, persistent behaviors to control or counter anxiety-provoking thoughts or situations.

Nonmelancholic depression is the most common OCD co-morbidity (60%), usually occurring later in the illness course. Lack of vegetative signs and a nonmelancholic mood distinguish this depression superimposed on obsessions and compulsions from primary melancholia with depressive ruminations and perseverative motor behaviors. When in doubt, always diagnose melancholia, because its high suicide risk will be immediately highlighted (hopefully preventing suicide) and because melancholia is more responsive to treatment than is OCD. Other OCD co-morbidities include generalized anxiety disorder and social phobia, attention deficit disorder, tic disorder, alcoholism, hypochondriasis, body dysmorphic disorder, and eating disorders. Persons who develop OCD are more likely to have had childhood fears and learning disabilities.

OCD onset before puberty is often associated with bipolar mood disorder, GTS, or infection. Beta-hemolytic streptococcal A is most likely and produces a syndrome termed *PANDAS: pediatric autoimmune neuropsychiatric disorder associated with strep* infection. Boys are affected more often than girls, onset age is about 6–7 years, symptoms include ADHD-like behaviors (squirms and is anxious and worried rather than jumpy and distractible), nonmelancholic depressive features, nighttime fears and separation anxiety, tics, and OCD. Anorexia nervosa may also develop. *Sydenham's chorea,* also from Strep A, is associated with lability of mood, irritability, perseverativeness, and OCD. In PANDAS and Sydenham's chorea, antineuronal antibodies lead to striatal inflammation (large volume on MRI during acute phase) that must be vigorously treated to avoid chronic dysfunction. Treatment includes early recognition (vital), plasmapheresis (plasma exchange), intravenous immunoglobulin (second choice), and corticosteroids. In adult OCD patients with early onsets (<10 years old) look for childhood Strep, abrupt OCD onset, and a family history of autoimmune disease (e.g., Grave's disease, rheumatoid arthritis).

OCD onset after age 35 years is usually secondary. Think of basal ganglia disease (stroke, Strep, toxins, and Parkinson's, Wilson's, and Huntington's diseases), epilepsy (frontal or temporal lobe foci most likely), chronic stimulant abuse, and benzodiazepine withdrawal (OCD onset will be acute).

OCD appears to be familial. However, although the risk for OCD is high in the families of OCD patients, so too are the risks for other disorders, especially generalized anxiety disorder and GTS. First-degree relatives of OCD patients are also at greater risk for other chornic tic disorders, phobic disorders, mood disorders, suicide, and possibly alcohol abuse. About 10% of first-degree relatives of OCD patients also have OCD, and an additonal 10% have obsessional traits. Twin concordnace rates for OCD are 30%–60% for monozygotic and 10%–30% for dizygotic twins. Patients with OCD may also have a significantly higher prevalence of type A and a significantly lower prevalence of type B blood groups, all suggesting that the familialness of OCD is of genetic origin.

THE NEUROLOGY OF OCD

OCD has been associated with dysfunction in the frontal lobes, basal ganglia, and limbic systems. Secondary OCD follows temporal lobe epilepsy, Sydenham's chorea, Parkinson's disease, Huntington's disease, and basal ganglia lesions secondary to carbon monoxide poisoning. Primary OCD patients also have more neurologic soft signs than do normal persons. On positron emission tomography (PET), primary OCD patients have increased levels of glucose metabolism in anterior cortical areas, cingulate gyrus, and caudate nuclei. Some, but not all, primary OCD patients have ventricular enlargement and small caudate nuclei volumes on CT scans. Some have less white matter and greater cortical volume than comparison groups. Others have enlarged caudate volumes. Also observed are prolonged magnetic resonance imaging (MRI) T_1 values in right frontal white matter, and T_1 asymmetries (right greater than left) in orbital frontal cortex correlating positively with symptom severity. Bifrontal stereotactic tractotomy of the orbital cortex significantly reduces symptoms in about 50% of OCD patients refractory to other treatments.

Electrophysiologic abnormalities have also been recorded in OCD patients. EEG shows decreased alpha and increased beta activities, and evoked potentials show shorter latencies during discrimination tasks. These findings suggest that OCD patients may be in a hyperaroused, overfocused state.

OCD patients also have deficits in visuospatial recall, recognition, and sequencing (particularly in OCD patients with a family history of OCD). These findings are not due to co-occurring anxiety or depression, are consistent with non-dominant hemisphere and basal ganglia dysfunction, and correspond with the anatomic brain imaging and metabolic findings in OCD patients.

Some abnormality in serotonergic systems has been suggested as a biochemical basis for OCD. Serotonin has been implicated as a mediator for repetitive behaviors, impulsivity, and aggression. Serotonin reuptake inhibitors (e.g., clomipramine, fluoxetine, fluvoxamine, zimelidine) are effective in ameliorating OCD symptoms. Symptom reduction has also been correlated with a reduction in platelet serotonin and serotonin metabolites in cerebrospinal fluid.

OCD may be due to a disruption in behavioral inhibition mediated by frontal-subcortical circuits. The behavioral inhibition system (also underlying harm avoidance) receives substantial projections from 5-HT neurons from the dorsal raphe nuclei. Serotonin mediates responses to conditioned punishment and frustrative nonreward stimuli. The more activated this system, the more behavior is inhibited. Deficits in this system can lead to OCD features. One model specifically implicates the dorsal (DRN) and medial (MRN) raphe nuclei (a major source of serotonin neurons) (Fig. 14.1). The DRN primarily projects to the forebrain (basal ganglia prefrontal cortical circuits) and modulates dopaminergic mesocortical systems. The MRN primarily projects to the limbic system and hypothalamus

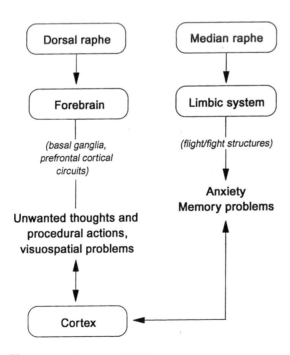

Figure 14.1. Proposed OCD pathophysiology.

(and thus also influences the sympathetic nervous system) and modulates the noradrenergic flight/fight system.

Deficits in DRN and MRN serotonin function disinhibits dopaminergic and noradrenergic systems, respectively, presumably resulting in (1) unwanted repetitive thoughts and procedural actions no longer fully controllable (from DRN-reduced modulation of prefrontal, posterior parietal, and basal ganglia disinhibition); (2) simultaneous high levels of anxiety (from MRN-reduced modulation of the limbic system and from secondary cortical cognitive discordance of being "compelled" to think and do unwanted things); and (3) fears of danger and visuospatial and memory problems in flight/fight hippocampal and parahippocampal and perhaps parietal lobe functions (from disrupted inputs from frontal circuitry).

Thus, obsessions, compulsions, and accompanying anxiety can result from disrupted serotonergic modulation of forebrain and limbic systems or from dysfunction intrinsic to these systems. In both cases, increasing serotonin modulation by reuptake inhibition should ameliorate symptoms. However, because treatment response to specific serotonin reuptake inhibitors (SSRIs) is good but not great and because clomipramine with noradrenergic and some dopaminergic affinity, as well as serotonergic affinity, is still the best drug for OCD, a serotonin problem cannot be the only explanation for OCD. Some intrinsic forebrain problem seems likely. Lateralization of this forebrain dysfunction in OCD, however, is unclear, and the metabolic, structural, and cognitive patterns detailed above suggest as overactive dominant (left) circuitry interfering with nondominant functions or primary nondominant dysfunction inducing an overcompensation by dominant systems. An imbalance between the two may be the most parsimonious explanation.

Animal models for OCD are consistent with findings in patients and with an intrinsic forebrain problem in OCD. Species-specific repetitive automatic and dysfunctional complex feeding, grooming, social, sexual, and predatory behaviors have been documented and associated with a genetic component, onset around puberty, exacerbation under stress, and response to SSRIs. For example, compulsive self-grooming and licking by dogs leading to hair loss and skin lesions (canine acral lick syndrome) can be successfully treated with SSRIs. Other canine OCD-like behaviors, performed daily for hours and that can be treated with SSRIs or opioid antagonists (clonidine), include running in circles to grasp tail, nail and foot biting, snapping at imaginary flies, repetitive chewing and sucking on objects or self, polydipsia and polyphagia with pica, repetitive digging or floor scratching, pacing, and rhythmic barking.

Some captive birds feather-pick sometimes to the point of self-mutilation (i.e., avian trichotillomania). Some horses compulsively chew corral fences and crib (grasp fence rail or stable ledge and lean back tensing neck muscles and then air swallowing). Pigs, cows, primates, bears, and elephants have also been observed in hours of repetitive, dysfunctional behavior (biting, chewing, licking, tongue rolling, masturbating, hair pulling, pacing in a specific pattern). Childhood onset OCD (30% of all OCD cases) is phenomenologically similar (more ritualistic) to nonhuman repetitive behavior disorders, suggesting that adult OCD behaviors have been modified in content by maturation and acculturation, and human OCD behaviors are elaborations of phylogenetically old behavior patterns.

CLINICAL PRESENTATION: GTS

Tics are sudden, involuntary movements or sounds that can be suppressed only temporarily and with difficulty. Tic disorders can involve simple tics, complex tics, or multiple tics. GTS is the most complex form of multiple tics on this spectrum. The accepted prevalence of 0.5/1,000 for GTS is probably an underestimation. GTS is found in all cultures and racial groups, but is rare among African-Americans. It is found in all social classes and is more common in males than in females (9:1).

Onset is usually before age 15 years, and typically begins around age 7 years. A prepubertal exacerbation is common, followed by teenage attenuation and then an adult stabilization of symptoms. The illness is lifelong, with phases of exacerbation during periods of stress. Stress is not of etiologic importance. Symptoms are also exacerbated by psychostimulant drugs. Contrary to previous thought, tics do not disappear during sleep. There is mixed evidence that birth complications or first trimester maternal stress (e.g., hyperemesis) may play an etiologic role in some patients (about 33%).

Tics are the core feature of GTS, and tics involving the eyes and head are the most frequent initial feature (about half of cases). Vocalizations, most frequently repeated throat-clearing, is the initial symptom in one third of cases. Eventually, almost all GTS patients have head, eye, and vocal tics. Coprolalia (uncontrollable paroxysms of profanity) is a late feature, but is eventually observed in about 60% of severely affected patients and in 30% of all GTS patients. Vocalizations also include grunting, coughing, barking, snorting, screaming, hissing, clicking, and inarticulate bursts of sounds.

GTS patients demonstrate a variety of complex semipurposeful repetitive movements other than tics. These include sniffing, squinting, touching, hitting or striking, jumping or stamping of feet, head banging, lip biting, eye gauging, smelling of hands or objects, retracing steps, twirling, deep knee bends, or squatting. About one third of GTS patients substantially injure themselves. Echolalia and echopraxia are seen in about one third of patients.

About 50% of GTS patients have hyperactivity, attention deficit syndromes, learning disabilities, and related school and social problems: fighting, disruption of class, temper tantrums, mood swings, hyperactivity. Ten to 30% have antisocial behaviors, including inappropriate sexual activity and aggressivity, hurting others, and killing animals. Sleep disturbances are common and include insomnia, talking during sleep, nightmares and night terrors, somnambulism, and bruxism. As many as one third of patients may have been enuretic, and 20% have phobias. Most (75%–90%) have uncomfortable sensory experiences (termed sensory tics) that are temporarily relieved by performing a tic. From 50% to 75% have typical OCD features.

GTS appears to be familial when the concept of the syndrome is broadened to incorporate pure and chronic tic disorders. About one third of GTS patients have a positive family history for GTS, and an additional one third have a positive family history of other less severe forms of tic disorder. Male relatives are more at risk than are female relatives. First-degree relatives of patients with GTS are also at greater risk for attention deficit hyperactivity disorder. Concordance rates for GTS are about 60% for monozygotic and about 10% for dizygotic twins. When GTS and chronic tics are combined, concordance rates increase to about 75% and 25%, respectively. Familial illness patterns are consistent with an autosomal dominant genotype with sex-specific penetrance.

THE NEUROLOGY OF GTS

Thirty to 60% of GTS patients have nonspecific EEG abnormalities. Evoked potential studies suggest deficits in attention, with a response pattern consistent with increased brain stem interneuron excitability.

Only 10% of computed tomography (CT) scans of GTS patients are abnormal, with mild ventricular dilation and some cortical atrophy. MRI may show reduced basal ganglia volume. PET findings in GTS patients indicate that some patients have hypometabolism in frontal cingulate and insular cortices and in the corpus striatum. Some single positron emission computed tomography studies show reduced left caudate and anterior cingulate hypoperfusion; others show increased right hemisphere cerebral blood flow.

Patients with GTS also have mild deficits in motor and sensory perceptual performance. The last is similar to problems noted in OCD. The neurochemical problem in GTS is assumed to be increased mesolimbic/mesocortical dopaminergic drive, leading to more available dopamine and secondary postsynaptic D_2 receptor hypersensitivity. This idea is primarily based on the observations that D_2 blockade (with pimozide or haloperidol) decreases symptoms, whereas stimulants increase symptoms.

THE RELATIONSHIP BETWEEN OCD AND GTS

OCD and GTS share a common liability. For example, many of the symptoms of GTS appear to be forms of compulsions, and 30%–75% of GTS patients have typical OCD symptoms. About 20% of OCD patients have tics (particularly patients with early onset or hoarding, violent, or sexual OCD). Both are associated with coprolalia and self-mutilation, and about 70% of OCD patients have either a personal or family history of tics.

The courses of the two syndromes are also similar: early age of onset, lifelong course with waxing and waning of symptoms, involuntary intrusive unwanted behaviors, worsening with depression and anxiety, and co-occurrence of nonmelancholic depression and anxiety disorders. Unlike OCD, drugs acting on the serotonergic system do not relieve tics. However, both can show a positive response to treatment with clonidine and behavior therapy.

The prevalence of OCD is elevated in the first- and second-degree relatives of GTS patients, and GTS patients with a family history of OCD have more tics. The family evidence is consistent with a single major gene accounting for tics in some patients and OCD in others, with penetrance weighted toward tics in males and OCD in females.

Evidence points to both disorders being related to dysfunction in the basal ganglia or limbic system: glucose metabolism abnormalities in frontal lobes and basal ganglia and similar neuropsychological deficits on measures of visuospatial functioning. For both OCD and GTS, basal ganglia dysfunction disrupting specific frontal-subcortical circuits has been proposed as common pathophysiologies. The dorsolateral prefrontal cortex circuit (involved with new learning), the lateral orbitofrontal circuit (involved with focused attention and cognitive flexibility), and the anterior cingulate circuit with its limbic connections (involved in emotion and flight/fight behavior) are metabolically abnormal in OCD/GTS patients. OCD may involve a right more than left imbalance, whereas GTS may involve a left more than right imbalance.

CLINICAL PRESENTATION: EATING DISORDERS*

Anorexia nervosa is an uncommon but serious condition in which the patient, typically a teenage girl, develops a gross misperception or overvalued idea that she is significantly overweight and that she must diet or use other means (e.g., self-induced vomiting, exercise programs, use of diuretics or laxatives) to lose large amounts of weight. She consequently experiences massive weight loss and associated physiologic changes (most but not all of which are due to starvation).

Anorexia nervosa may be increasing in incidence, which is about 2–4/100,000 population/year. About 95% of anorexia nervosa patients are women. Male anorexics are often homosexual or bisexual, and this is particularly true if the anorexia is associated with bulimia. Some male anorexics will have a history of PANDAS. Anorexia nervosa is more common among middle and upper socioeconomic groups and is less common among African-Americans. Eighty-five percent of patients develop the illness between the ages of 13 and 20 years, and onset is rare below the age of 10 or over 30.

Despite the weight loss causing cachexia, the anorexic does not perceive herself as gaunt, continues to fear gaining weight, and (until there are profound effects of starvation) remains physically active, even overactive. Despite the term *anorexia*, the patient usually maintains a good appetite and may be preoccupied with food, a collector of recipes, a reader of cookbooks, and an enthusiastic cook for others. She may at times gorge herself with food and avoid weight gain by immediately inducing vomiting.

The diagnosis of anorexia nervosa requires: (1) a refusal to maintain body weight to 15% or less of an age and height norm; (2) intense fear of gaining weight

---

* The DSM presents them as a separate category of their own.

or of becoming fat, although being underweight; and (3) a disturbed body image in which the person "feels" fat.

In females, the absence of at least three consecutive expected menstrual cycles is also required. Amenorrhea is extremely common among anorexics, and for some patients the amenorrhea precedes significant weight loss. Usually, but not always, menses return when weight is restored. Pregnancy is a rare explanation of the amenorrhea, as conception has been reported during periods of prolonged amenorrhea. Libido is considerably decreased. Additional behavioral problems include insomnia, diminished concentration, sad mood, suicidal ideation and attempts, and denial of serious illness and the danger of dying. With advanced weight loss, delirium may occur. Co-occurring depression is common and typically nonmelancholic.

Constipation is frequent, as is diarrhea in patients who abuse laxatives. In addition to gauntness, findings can include narrowing of the shoulders and hips, reduced basal body temperature, dry skin, and loss of scalp hair with retention of pubic and axillary hair. Lanugo hairs (blond, short, "downy" hairs) are seen on cheeks, neck, forearms, and thighs. Repeated vomiting can lead to dental problems because of gastric acidity dissolving the enamel. Also observed are parotid gland enlargement (from repeated bouts of emesis and hypochloremic alkalosis); edema; acrocyanosis (a circulatory problem in which the hands or feet are persistently cold, blue, and sweaty); Raynaud's phenomenon (a circulatory problem in which the fingers or toes become pale and painful when exposed to cold temperatures); orange pigmentation of palms and soles (probably due to dietary faddism with overingestion of carotene-containing foods); moderate anemia with associated pallor or petechiae (because of reduced numbers of platelets); and, in rare cases, beriberi, pellagra, vitamin K deficiency, or Korsakoff's encephalopathy.

The course of anorexia nervosa is not benign. Laxative abuse may lead to electrolyte abnormalities and consequent weakness, cardiac arrhythmias, tetany, or convulsions and death. Vomiting can lead to gastric bleeding or rupture. An unusual complication is duodenal compression by the superior mesenteric artery that can occur in patients with weight loss from any cause and that causes postprandial abdominal pain or intractable vomiting. The probable mechanism is the dissolution of the fat pad lying between the duodenum and the superior mesenteric artery, which crosses it, as well as the bogginess and lack of coordinated contraction of the duodenum during starvation.

Other complications of starvation include bronchopneumonia or other infections, renal failure, cardiac failure, electrolyte abnormalities resulting from vomiting and the use of purgatives, and complications of invasive medical treatments, gastric dilation from too rapid feeding, aspiration of tube feedings, and electrolyte imbalance from intravenous fluids.

Over 40% of patients fully remit, and 30% are considerably improved at follow-up. At least 20% are unimproved or seriously impaired, and 9% die over 10 years of illness. The prognosis is worse if age of onset is after 20 years or if the patient has (1) failed to respond to previous treatment, (2) has bulimia, or (3) had a significant behavior problems prior to the onset of anorexia nervosa.

The laboratory abnormalities observed in patients with anorexia nervosa are mostly due to starvation and disappear when weight normalizes. No abnormality is pathognomonic. They include hypokalemia (a serious complication of vomiting or diuretic abuse), hyponatremia, hypochloremic alkalosis, hypercholesterolemia, hypercarotenemia, anemia, thrombocytopenia, leukopenia, hypofibrinogenemia, increased blood urea nitrogen, diminished glomerular filtration rate, decreased basal metabolic rate, decreased erythrocyte sedimentation rate, EEG and electrocardiographic abnormalities, reversible ventricular enlargement on computerized tomographic brain scan, and delayed gastric emptying. Some anorexics, however, may have persistent gray matter volume deficits even when weight gain is maintained.

The first-degree relatives of anorexics have an increased prevalence of "neuroses," and about 10% of female relatives are also anorexic. In addition, parents of anorexia patients (16% of mothers, 23% of fathers) have "weight phobias" or significantly reduced adolescent weight. They also are at greater risk for alcoholism, substance abuse, and nonmelancholic depression. Bipolar mood disorder is the particularly prevalent illness in their families. Monozygotic and dizygotic twin anorexia nervosa concordance rates are about 50% and 10%, respectively.

Bulimia means binge eating. Bulimia is a feature of anorexia nervosa and some neuroendocrine disorders (e.g., Kline-Levin syndrome). *Bulimia nervosa* is characterized by (1) episodes of uncontrollable binge eating; (2) episodes of self-induced vomiting, dieting and fasting, and extreme exercise to prevent weight gain; and (3) overvalued ideas regarding body shape and weight. The DSM also requires at least two binge eating episodes a week for at least 3 months, but in practice this number should be a guideline rather than a requirement for diagnosis and treatment.

Bulimics typically alternate between binge eating and weight-loss activities that are compulsive. Obsessive thought content is focused on their eating habits and body weight and shape. Unlike the obsessive early on, the bulimic does not consider her preoccupation with food and weight to be undesirable.

Bulimics are often overweight and may have co-occurring depression, kleptomania, drug and alcohol abuse (25%–30%), anxiety disorders (30%–50%), and personality disorder (30% with anxious and fearful premorbid personalities). General medical complications include hypokalemic acidosis (from vomiting and increased renal excretion of potassium), dental problems, parotid gland enlargement and esophageal tears (also from vomiting), and metabolic acidosis (particularly from laxative abuse). During weight-loss phases, bulimics may be dehydrated, weak, lethargic, and develop cardiac arrhythmias.

Bulimia nervosa begins in the decade following puberty and rarely is observed to start after age 30. Its demography and epidemiology are similar to those of anorexia nervosa. Bulimia nervosa is a chronic disorder with high rates of relapse (40%–60%), and many patients experience continuous mild symptomatology. In addition to an association with OCD, bulimia nervosa is associated with some mood disorders, and about 50% of bulimics will have one or more depressive episodes.

The etiology of bulimia nervosa is unknown. However, it may be familial. There is a small increase in risk for bulimia in relatives of bulimic patients compared with relatives of controls (about 4% vs 2%). Monozygotic and dizygotic twin concordance rates are about 25% and 10%, respectively. Because attitudes about eating, dieting, and thinness have high heritability (about 50%), persons with a heritable tendency to be dissatisfied with their body shape and weight and to perceive themselves as overweight may be most prone to eating disorders.

Laboratory studies in bulimics are difficult to interpret because of the effects of chronic binging and purging on many neurotransmitter systems and organ structures. Nevertheless, serotonin neuronal systems modulate appetitive behaviors. Furthermore, serotonin agonists or agonist-like treatments tend to produce satiety, whereas serotonin antagonist or antagonist-like compounds increase food consumption and weight gain. Thus, it has been hypothesized that bulimia nervosa patients suffer from unstable serotonergic balance. However, other neurotransmitters (norepinephrine), some neuropeptides (PYY), and some endogenous opioids also play roles in eating behavior. Nevertheless, the serotonin hypothesis of bulimia nervosa is particularly interesting, as a similar hypothesis has been proposed for OCD and GTS. In this OCD/GTS hypothesis, a major gene (or genes) is theorized to result in low central nervous system serotonin levels that leads to limbic system and frontal lobe disinhibition and a spectrum of impulsive, compulsive, addictive, sleep, attentional, mood, memory, and anxiety disorders.

Bulimic Epilepsy

A small number of bulimics binge eat as a feature of limbic epilepsy. These patients often report odd abdominal sensations, flashes of light, unusual smells, or increasing anxiety immediately prior to binge eating. They describe their binges as unpredictable and out of their control. Some episodes occur during a depersonalized state. Following the binge eating, these patients will have post-ictal symptoms, such as prolonged sleep, altered consciousness, disorientation, and headaches. Irritability and violent outbursts can occur, as can episodes of dizziness, paresthesias, deja vu, and dysmegalopsia. These patients have abnormal EEGs, and their bulimia will improve with anticonvulsant treatments.

Relationship to OCD

Eating disorders have been traditionally viewed as a form of obsessive or compulsive behavior, and patients with anorexia nervosa often develop a pervasive, obsessive interest in exercise and engage in ritualistic eating behaviors. Patients with anorexia nervosa have many obsessive and compulsive behaviors, and some obsessional patients have a history of anorexia nervosa. Among OCD patients, as many as 10% of the women may have anorexia nervosa. These patients have an earlier age of onset of OCD than do those without co-occurring anorexia. Male OCD patients rarely have a history of anorexia, but may have other obsessions and eating compulsions. Male OCD patients are more likely to have tics. In rodents, lesions in the striatum result in prolonged anorexia and weight loss in females but not in males. This is consistent with studies implicating basal ganglia dysfunction in OCD. Patients with anorexia nervosa often have preexisting obsessional personality traits.

CLINICAL PRESENTATION: OTHER OBSESSIVE SYNDROMES

Post-traumatic stress disorder (PTSD) is characterized by recurrent, intrusive thoughts similar to obsessional thinking, and some of these patients meet diagnostic criteria for OCD (see Chapter 15 for details of PTSD). *Trichotillomania*, compulsive hair pulling, although classified as an impulse control disorder, may also be related to OCD, as is *kleptomania* (a compulsion to steal unneeded and often worthless objects), *pathological gambling* (a compulsion to gamble), *pyromania* (an obsessiveness about fire and a compulsion to set fires), *body dysmorphic disorder* (obsessive preoccupation with one's body often leading to multiple cosmetic surgeries), *hypochondriasis* (obsessiveness about one's health), and *hoarding, paraphilias,* and *self-mutilation* (compulsions to collect objects, do specific sexually related behavior [e.g., exposing oneself], and to injure oneself).

The DSM puts these conditions in other diagnostic categories,* but in their symptom pattern, course, and treatment responsiveness they seem to be variants of OCD. These conditions are often co-occurring with OCD, wax and wane like OCD, and are associated with anxiety and nonmelancholic depression. Some variants are more obsessional (e.g., the hypochondriac worries about being ill, the "more typical" OCD patient worries about getting ill, the body dysmorphic patient worries about some physical defect), whereas others are more compulsive (e.g., the patient is compelled to pull at his hair, steal, set fires, self-injure, engage in abnormal sexual behavior, gamble, use a drug, hoard objects). Persons with these conditions often also meet criteria for OCD (about one third) and often respond to SSRIs and other treatments for OCD. Although probably multidetermined syndromes, unless there is a specific reason not to do so, consider these patients as having OCD and their labels *the content* of their disorder rather than its form. Thus, treat them for OCD. Such an approach offers them the best chance for a substantial recovery.

Some *paraphilias* can also be conceptualized as sexual obsessions and compulsions. These paraphilics experience their symptoms as intrusive or senseless rather than pleasurable, have normal sexual behaviors at other times, and think of the paraphilia as interfering with their normal sexuality. They may also have other more classic OCD complaints. Paraphilias that may be OCD variants include bestiality, voyeurism, exhibitionism, and compulsive masturbation. SSRI treatment may benefit 70% of these patients.

---

* PTSD (acute and chronic) is among the *anxiety disorders;* trichotillomania, kleptomania, pathological gambling, and pyromania, are placed in the category *impulse control disorders, not otherwise specified;* the paraphilias that may relate to OCD are in the paraphilia subcategory of *sexual and gender identity disorders;* hypochondriasis and body dysmorphic disorder are placed among the *somatoform disorders;* self-mutilation has no category, and the DSM considers it a symptom rather than a specific disorder (and of course it is both an OCD variant and a feature of other conditions).

Some *self-mutilation* behavior can be considered a variant of OCD. This is particularly true if the patient perceives the associated obsessions and damaging behavior as unwanted, embarrassing, and as a sign of illness. These patients respond to typical treatments for OCD as do persons with trichotillomania and kleptomania. Some self-mutilation behavior, although compulsive, is not associated with specific thoughts. These include nail and finger biting, cheek and lip chewing, and scratching. Mutilating injury can occur, although these are seen most commonly in children with developmental disorders. These behaviors in adults as well as children may respond to naltrexone (50–150 mg daily). Starting clonidine several weeks before the naltrexone decreases the sympathetic arousal that can occur with naltrexone. Liver damage is the main adverse effect, but is uncommon. Some self-mutilating behavior is experienced as pleasurable. This paradoxical response (pain asymboly) suggests secondary OCD, and look for a parietal lobe or thalamic lesion.

OCD AND PSYCHOSIS

OCD has been associated with psychosis. Although very few typical OCD patients become psychotic, 10% of schizophrenics are reported to have OCD symptoms. Because schizophrenics can have catatonic stereotypes and mannerisms, whether these behaviors have been misinterpreted as OCD symptoms or are in fact OCD related is unclear. Schizophrenics with OCD symptoms are reported to be less emotionally blunted than those without these features. If the course of the combination illness is episodic and emotional expression is intact, ECT is the recommended treatment. Atypical antipsychotics with their serotonergic blockade may worsen the OCD features.

Schizotypal behaviors have also been described in patients diagnosed as having OCD, and their presence predicts poor response to SSRIs and behavior therapy. The combination, however, is uncommon, and patients rarely meet criteria for schizotypal personality disorder. Look for co-morbid drug or alcohol abuse or mood disorder. Also look for epilepsy and epilepsy spectrum disorder as the primary condition.

OCD can also co-occur with bipolar mood disorder. These patients have either a childhood onset of both conditions that may become chronic and is difficult to treat or a late onset condition usually due to a stroke in nondominant brain systems, particularly the basal ganglia. Treatments for mood disorder, including ECT, or combined mood disorder–OCD treatments are needed for these patients.

OCD has also been described among epileptics. Typically the patient will not meet all OCD criteria and will seem atypical. Among schizophrenics with OCD, always assess for epilepsy that can explain both conditions.

Tic disorder has also been associated with a schizophrenic-like psychosis. The onset is in childhood and usually is associated with gestational or parapartum problems, chromosomal aberrations (e.g., fragile X), or other developmental disorders. Treatment for this chronic condition is symptomatic.

MANAGEMENT

Treatments for OCD and related disorders are psychopharmacologic and behavioral. Combined therapy is usually needed, and full remission is rare. Unfortunately, most OCD sufferers experience a substantial delay (15–20 years) between symptom onset and diagnosis and treatment. The earlier the diagnosis is made and treatment begun, the better the outcome.

Pharmacotherapy: OCD and Its Variants

Drugs that effectively reduce OCD symptoms inhibit serotonin reuptake. Clomipramine (200–300 mg daily for at least 12 weeks), a chlorinated tricyclic antidepressant, may still be the best drug for OCD (about 70% of patients have a substantial response, although full remission is uncommon). Fluvoxamine (Luvox) (also about 300 mg daily), fluoxetine (at 60–80 mg daily), and venlafaxine (225 mg) are also effective. Paroxetine works at 40–60 mg daily (use for eating disorders), but 20 mg daily does not. Buspirone, a piperazine-like sedative compound, also has serotonergic action and has been used *with* (alone it has little effect) fluoxetine or fluvoxamine in the treatment of OCD. Daily doses range from 15–60 mg. Buspirone (60 mg daily) may also help PTSD patients whose comorbidities strongly suggest anxiety disorder with some OCD features. The more specific SSRIs, however, may not work as well as the less specific (e.g., clomipramine, sertraline [200 mg daily], venlafaxine, nefazodone). This distinction suggests that neurotransmitter systems other than serotonin may be involved in OCD.

Because of the tendency of OCD patients to focus on side effects, begin with low doses, and go slowly. In choosing the drug, consider the type of side effects most likely to be troublesome for the specific patient (e.g., the anticholinergic side effects of clomipramine or the sexual dysfunction and weight loss side effects of fluoxetine and fluvoxamine).

Successful treatment requires maintaining the therapeutic dose for at least 1 year to prevent relapse. After 1 year, if the patient is *in remission*, taper medication (over a 3-month period) and then discontinue. If relapse occurs, reinstitute medication and maintain for an additional year. If the patient is once again in remission, attempt a second withdrawal. Some patients who do not fully remit or who relapse when taken off medications will need to be on pharmacotherapy indefinitely. Combining drugs with cognitive–behavior therapy (usually done by a cognitive therapy specialist) may reduce the number of patients who relapse.

Because OCD is often initially resistant to treatment, consider the following.

1. The initial drug of choice (often with neurotransmitter properties in addition to serotonin reuptake inhibition) needs to be given at therapeutic doses for 12 weeks before declared a failure.
2. Three different drug trials (choose different types, e.g., clomipramine, fluoxetine, venlafaxine) with combined behavioral intervention need to fail before categorizing the patient as treatment resistant.

3. Nonresponse to one agent does not predict nonresponse to others, so be optimistic. Unlike for depression, the efficacy is unclear for using drug combinations or enhancers to treat OCD patients when your first choice drug achieves only a partial response. Nevertheless, if the patient's response is less than 40%, switch. If the patient's partial response is greater than 40%, consider pindolol (2.5 mg TID) or mirtazapine (15–50 mg divided BID or once daily). Pindolol works on presynaptic 5-HT autoreceptors, preventing feedback reduction in 5-HT metabolism. Mirtazapine works on presynaptic 5-HT and noradrenergic autoreceptors.

4. For treatment-resistant patients, IV clomipramine over a two to three week period (doses given over one hour starting at 25 to 50 mg and increasing to 200 to 250 mg) can substantially relieve symptoms for weeks or months in some patients or can make a previously unresponsive patient much more responsive to oral clomipramine. However, do not do this if you are concerned about a seizure disorder, or if the patient has heart disease. Repeated intravenous dosing over a 1–2 year period may be needed before trying to discontinue the drug.

5. MAOI (phenelzine 90 mg daily) should be tried for those patients not responding to reuptake inhibitors (do not combine with SSRIs), and a small proportion of treatment-resistant OCD patients will respond.

6. Dopamine agonists (e.g., amphetamine 10–20 mg or bromocriptine 12.5–30 mg daily) may also work for a small proportion of patients with mostly pure obsessions due to coarse basal ganglia disease. Do not use if the patient or family has tic disorder, as it will worsen that condition.

7. Clonidine (0.25–1 mg daily), a presynaptic alpha$_2$-agonist that decreases norepinephrine release, may help in tic disorder and can be combined with clomipramine for OCD. Some OCD patients may get worse with clonidine, but some substantially improve (20%). Sedation and orthostasis are the major side effects of clonidine. Clonidine is also used for GTS, and 40%–60% of patients respond over an 8–12 week course of treatment. Associated attention deficit and OCD symptoms will also improve.

8. Benzodiazepines are helpful for short-term relief of anxiety until other drugs work or as a sleep aid. Clonazepam 4–10 mg daily also has some serotonergic properties and may more specifically benefit some patients (20%). Lithium carbonate may help if the OCD is associated with a mood disorder. Carbamazepine and valproate may help if you suspect epilepsy or epilepsy spectrum disorder.

9. Agents that have been used unsuccessfully in the treatment of OCD include tryptophan (a serotonin precursor amino acid), trazodone, mianserin, bupropion, and dyphenhydramine.

Neuroleptics have also been used to treat OCD patients who also have tics. Because of the risk for tardive dyskinesia, these should be drugs of last resort, and pimozide the neuroleptic of choice followed by haloperidol. Doses are the same as when used for GTS. Pimozide (2–12 mg) and haloperidol (6–16 mg) help 70% of GTS patients. For most patients, pimozide is preferred because of less extrapyramidal side effects. Because pimozide can cause prolonged Q–T cardiac conduction problems, it is not used in patients with heart block arrhythmias. Fluoxetine (20–40 mg daily) may also benefit patients with GTS.

Behavioral Therapy: OCD and Its Variants

Behavioral therapy appears to work best for OCD patients with well-defined compulsive rituals. Treatment centers on in vivo systematic stepwise exposure (habituation) to the obsessional fear coupled with prevention from carrying out the associated compulsive behavior (response prevention). Relaxation techniques are used to facilitate exposure and restraint, as are thought-stopping techniques (the therapist interrupting the obsessions by shouting "stop") and paradoxical intention and mass practice (the patient is instructed to continuously think of the obsession to the point of fatigue). Fifty percent of patients may benefit from these procedures, and long-term benefit correlates best with longer (6 weeks) treatment schedules. For GTS patients, habit reversal techniques are also used; that is, when sensing a tic, the patient immediately tries to suppress the tic by tensing the opposite muscle group (the patient is taught to do this for each specific tic and rehearses the technique). Patients who respond well to combined medication and behavior therapy are less likely to need long-term medication than those who receive medication alone.

Psychosurgery

Stereotactic capsulotomy, anterior cingulotomy, or subcaudate tractotomy have been used for over 25 years to treat OCD patients who have failed to respond to all other treatments (including modern pharmacotherapy). As patients who undergo this procedure for OCD are typically in good general health and have no other neurologic disease, side effects from neurosurgery (bleeding, infection, seizures) are infrequent and, when they occur, remediable. An additional side effect is a 2–3 month postoperative period of fatigue, decreased initiative, and mild bradyphrenia that correlate with the degree of the transient edema from surgery. Long-term cognitive problems have not been demonstrated, but if present are far outweighed by the therapeutic response. Patients whose personalities and family support structure remain intact are the best candidates, and about 40%–50% will experience substantial improvement.

Management of Eating Disorders

Anorexics and bulimics may require hospitalization on units with a specialized eating disorder program. Admitting an anorexic patient to a general treatment unit without specific eating disorder treatment protocols and trained staff usually ends in chaos. Limit setting without power struggles and a staff with a unified approach and that "speaks with one voice" are essential. A daily activity structure is needed, which includes (1) mandatory bed rest after meals (to prevent vomiting); (2) exercise (to keep the patient fit but not overexercising to lose more weight); (3) a required daily food intake that begins low (1,500 calories) and increases only when the patient finishes each meal; (4) teaching good eating habits; (5) a reward system for weight gain; and (6) a 10–12 week after-care program that follows through on all of the above.

If the anorexic is also depressed (usually nonmelancholic), and antidepressants must be used, or if antidepressants are used to treat the obsessions of the eating disorder, clomipramine is the first choice, although it can cause nausea and constipation in these patients. Dietary fiber and stool softeners and increasing the dose slowly can help prevent gastrointestinal problems. If clomipramine is not tolerated, paroxitine is the specific SSRI of choice as it has the least weight loss effect of this class of drugs. Bulimics respond to SSRIs, phenelzine, and perhaps carbamazepine.

ADDITIONAL READINGS

Azrin N, Peterson A: Habit reversal for the treatment of Tourette syndrome. *Behav Res Ther* 26:347–351, 1988.

Asbahr FR, Negrao AB, Gentil V, Zanetta DMT, da Paz JA, Marques-Dias MJ, Kiss MH: Obsessive-compulsive and related symptoms in children and adolescents with rheumatic fever with and without chorea: A prospective 6-month study. *Am J Psychiatry* 155:1122–1124, 1998.

Baer L: Factor analysis of symptom subtypes of obsessive compulsive disorder and their relation to personality and tic disorders. *J Clin Psychiatry* 55(suppl 3):18–23, 1994.

Baer L, Minichiello W: Behavior therapy for obsessive compulsive disorder. In Jenike M, Baer L, Minichiello W (eds): *Obsessive-Compulsive Disorders: Theory and Management*. PSG Publishing, Littleton, MA, 1986, pp 45–76.

Baker RW, Bermanzohn PC, Wirshing DA, Chengappa KNR: Obsessions, compulsions, clozapine, and risperidone. *CNS Spectrums* 2:26–45, 1997.

Baumgarten HG, Grozdanovic Z: Role of serotonin in obsessive-compulsive disorder. *Brit J Psychiatry* 173 (suppl 35):13–20, 1998.

Baxter LRJ, Phelps ME, Mazziotta JC, Guze BH, Schwartz JM, Selin CE: Local cerebral glucose metabolic rates in obsessive-compulsive disorder. *Arch Gen Psychiatry* 44:211–218, 1987.

Bebbington PE: Epidemiology of obsessive-compulsive disorder. *Brit J Psychiatry* 173 (suppl 35):2–6, 1998.

Beumont PJV, Russell JD, Touyz SW: Treatment of anorexia nervosa. *Lancet* 341:1635–1640, 1993.

Boone KB, Ananth J, Philpott L, Kaur A, Djenderedjian A: Neuropsychological characteristics of nondepressed adults with obsessive-compulsive disorder. *Neuropsychiatry Neuropsychol Behav Neurol* 4:96–109, 1991.

Bornstein RA, Baker GB, Bazylewich T, Douglass AB: Tourette syndrome and neuropsychological performance. *Acta Psychiatr Scand* 84:212–216, 1991.

Carlat DJ, Camargo CA Jr, Herzog DB: Eating disorders in males: A report on 135 patients. *Am J Psychiatry* 154:1127–1132, 1997.

Clarke DJ: Psychopharmacology of severe self-injury associated with learning disabilities. *Br J Psychiatry* 172:389–394, 1998.

Cohen DJ, Bruun R, Leckman JF (eds): *Tourette's Syndrome and Tic Disorders.* John Wiley, New York, 1988.

Coleman E: The obsessive compulsive model for describing compulsive behavior. *Am J Prev Psychiatry Neurol 2:*9–14, 1990.

Comings DE, Comings BG: A controlled family history study of Tourette's syndrome III: Affective and other disorders. *J Clin Psychiatry 51:*288–291, 1990.

Crisp AH, Hsu LKG, Harding B Hartshorn J: Clinical features of anorexia nervosa: A study of 102 cases. *J Psychosom Res 24:*179–191, 1980.

Cummings JL, Frankel M: Gilles de la Tourette syndrome and the neurological basis of obsessions and compulsions. *Biol Psychiatry 20:*1117–1126, 1985.

Devor EJ: Untying the Gordian knot: The genetics of Tourette's syndrome. *J Nerv Ment Dis 178:*669–679, 1990.

Delgado PL, Moreno FA: Different roles for serotonin in anti-obsessional drug action and the pathophysiology of obsessive-compulsive disorder. *Brit J Psychiatry 173 (suppl. 35):*21–25, 1998.

Diaferia G, Bianchi I, Bianchi ML, Cavedini P, Evzegovesi S, Bellodi L: Relationship between obsessive-compulsive personality disorder and obsessive-compulsive disorder. *Compr Psychiatry 38:*38–42, 1997.

Eccleston D, Doogan DP (eds): Serotonin in behavioral disorders. *Br J Psychiatry 155(suppl 8),* 1989.

Fallon BA, Liebowitz MR, Campeas R, Schneier FR, Marshall R, Davis S, Goetz D, Klein DF: Intravenous clomipramine for obsessive-compulsive disorder refractory to oral clomipramine: A placebo-controlled study. *Arch Gen Psychiatry 55:*918–924, 1998.

Fuse-Nagase Y, Boku M: Psychotic symptoms and a diagnosis of schizophrenia follow an initial diagnosis of tic disorder. *J Psychiatry Neurosci 21:*346–348, 1996.

George MS, Trimble MR, Costa DC, Robertson MM, Ring HA, Ell PJ: Elevated frontal cerebral blood flow in Gilles de la Tourette syndrome: A [99]Tc[M]-HMPAO SPECT study. *Psychiatry Res Neuroimaging 45:*143–151, 1992.

Gilenberg AJ (ed): Obsessive-compulsive spectrum disorders. *J Clin Psychiatry 56(suppl 4),* 1995.

Greist JH, Jefferson JW: Pharmacotherapy for obsessive-comuplsive disorder. *Brit J Psychiatry 173 (suppl. 35):*64–70, 1998.

Greist JH, Jefferson JW, Kobak KA, Katzelnick DJ, Serlin RC: Efficacy and tolerability of serotonin transport inhibitors in obsessive-compulsive disorder: A meta-analysis. *Arch Gen Psychiatry 52:*53–60, 1995.

Hand I: Out-patient, multi-modal behaviour therapy for obsessive-compulsive disorder. *Brit J Psychiatry 173 (suppl 35):*45–52, 1998.

Herzog DB (ed): Recent advances in bulimia nervosa. *J Clin Psychiatry 53(suppl),* 1991.

Hollander E: Treatment of obsessive-compulsive spectrum disorders with SSRIs. *Br J Psychiatry 173(suppl 35):*7–12, 1998.

Hollander E, Stein DJ (eds): *Obsessive Compulsive Disorders.* Marcel Dekker, New York, 1997.

Hymas N, Lees A, Bolton D, Epps K, Head D: The neurology of obsessional slowness. *Brain 114:*2203–2233, 1991.

Insel TR, Akiskal HS: Obsessive-compulsive disorder with psychotic features: A phenomenologic analysis. *Am J Psychiatry 143:*1527–1533, 1986.

Jampala VC: Anorexia nervosa: A variant form of affective disorder? *Psychiatr Ann 15:*698–704, 1985.

Jenike MA: Neurosurgical treatment of obsessive-compulsive disorder. *Brit J Psychiatry 173 (suppl 35):*79–90, 1998.

Jimerson DC, Wolfe BE, Metzger ED, Finkelstein DM, Cooper TB, Levine JM: Decreased serotonin function in bulimia nervosa. *Arch Gen Psychiatry 54:*529–534, 1997.

Kerbeshian J, Burd L: Are schizophreniform symptoms present in attenuated form in children with Tourette disorder and other developmental disorders? *Can J Psychiatry 32:*123–135, 1987.

Keuthen NJ, O'Sullivan RL, Goodchild P, Rodriguez D, Jenike MA, Baer L: Retrospective review of treatment outcome for 63 patients with trichotillomania. *Am J Psychiatry* 155:560–561, 1998.

Knell ER, Comings DE: Tourette's syndrome and attention-deficit hyperactivity disorder: Evidence for a genetic relationship. *J Clin Psychiatry* 54:331–337, 1993.

Kolada JL, Bland RC, Newman SC: Obsessive-compulsive disorder. *Acta Psychiatr Scand (Suppl)* 376:24–35, 1994.

Koran LM, Sallee FR, Pallanti S: Rapid benefit of intravenous pulse loading of clomipramine in obsessive-compulsive disorder. *Am J Psychiatry* 154:396–401, 1997.

Lambe EK, Katzman DK, Mikulis DJ, Kennedy SH, Zipursky RB: Cerebral gray matter volume deficits after weight recovery from anorexia nervosa. *Arch Gen Psychiatry* 54:537–542, 1997.

Leckman JF, Dolansky ES, Hardin MT, Clubb M, Walkup JT, Stevenson J, Pauls DL: Perinatal factors in the expression of Tourette's syndrome: An exploratory study. *J Am Acad Child Adolesc Psychiatry* 29:220–226, 1990.

Leckman JF, Grice DE, Boardman J, Zhang H, Vitale A, Bondi C, Alsobrook J, Peterson BS, Cohen DJ, Rasmussen SA, Goodman WK, McDougle CJ, Pauls DL: Symptoms of obsessive-compulsive disorder. *Am J Psychiatry* 154:911–917, 1997.

McDougle CJ, Goodman WK, Leckman JF, Lee NC, Heninger GR, Price LH: Haloperidol addition in fluvoxamine-refractory obsessive-compulsive disorder. *Arch Gen Psychiatry* 51:302–308, 1994.

Mindus P, Rasmussen SA, Lindquist C: Neurosurgical treatment for refractory obsessive-compulsive disorder: Implications for understanding frontal lobe function. *J Neuropsychiatry Clin Neurosci* 6:467–477, 1994.

Nee LE, Caine ED, Polinsky RJ, Eldridge R, Ebert MH: Gilles de la Tourette syndrome: Clinical and family study of 50 cases. *Ann Neurol* 7:41–49, 1980.

Nestadt G, Samuels JF, Romanoski AJ, Folstein MF, McHugh PR: Obsessions and compulsions in the community. *Acta Psychiatr Scand* 89:219–224, 1994.

Nordahl TE, Benkelfet C, Semple WE, Gross M, King AC, Cohen RM: Cerebral glucose metabolic rates in obsessive-compulsive disorder. *Neuropsychopharmacology* 2:23–28, 1989.

Pauls DL, Towbin KE, Leckman JF, Zahner GEP, Cohen DJ: Gilles de la Tourette's syndrome and obsessive compulsive disorders: Evidence supporting a genetic relationship. *Arch Gen Psychiatry* 43:1180–1182, 1986.

Peterson BS: Considerations of natural history and pathophysiology in the psychopharmacology of Tourette's syndrome. *J Clin Psychiatry* 57(Suppl 9):24–34, 1996.

Pigott TA: OCD: Where the serotonin selectivity story begins. *J Clin Psychiatry* 57(suppl 6):11–20, 1996.

Pigott TA, Altemus M, Rubenstein CS, Hill JL, Bihar, K, L'Heureux F, Bernstein S, Murphy DL: Symptoms of eating disorders in patients with obsessive compulsive disorder. *Am J Psychiatry* 148:1552–1557, 1991.

Primeau F, Fontaine R: Obsessive disorder with self-mutilation: A subgroup responsive to pharmacotherapy. *Can J Psychiatry* 32:699–701, 1987.

Purcell R, Maruff P, Kyrios M, Pantelis C: Neuropsychological deficits in obsessive-compulsive disorder. *Arch Gen Psychiatry* 55:415–423, 1998.

Rapoport JL: The neurobiology of obsessive compulsive disorder. *JAMA* 360:2888–2890, 1988.

Rapoport JL, Ryland DH, Kriete M: Drug treatment of canine acral lick: An animal model of obsessive-compulsive disorder. *Arch Gen Psychiatry* 49:517–521, 1996.

Rauch SL, Savage CR, Alpert NM, Dougherty D, Kendrick A, Curran T, Brown HD, Manzo P, Fischman AJ, Jenike MA: Probing striatal function in obsessive-compulsive disorder: A PET study of implicit sequence learning. *J Neuropsychiatry Clin Neurosci* 9:568–573, 1997.

Riddle M: Obsessive-compulsive disorder in children and adolescents. *Brit J Psychiatry* 173 (suppl 35):91–96, 1998.

Robertson J: Sex addiction as a disease: A neurobehavioral model. *Am J Prev Psychiatry Neurol 2*:15–18, 1990.

Robertson MM: The Gilles de la Tourette syndrome: The current status. *Br J Psychiatry 154*:147–169, 1989.

Robertson MM, Gourdie A: Familial Tourette's syndrome in a large British pedigree: Associated psychopathology, severity and potential for linkage analysis. *Br J Psychiatry 156*:515–521, 1990.

Rutherford J, McGuffin P, Katz RJ, Murray RM: Genetic influences on eating attitudes in a normal female twin population. *Psychol Med 23*:425–463, 1993.

Salkovskis PM, Forrester E, Richards C: Cognitive-behavioural approach to understanding obsessional thinking. *Brit J Psychiatry 173 (suppl. 35)*:53–63, 1998.

Sallee FR, Nesbitt L, Jackson C, Sine L, Sethuraman G: Relative efficacy of haloperidol and pimozide in children and adolescents with Tourette's disorder. *Am J Psychiatry 154:* 1057–1062, 1997.

Sandor P: Gilles de la Tourette syndrome: A neuropsychiatric disorder. *J Psychosom Res 37:* 211–226, 1993.

Saxena S, Brody AL, Schwartz JM, Baxter LR: Neuroimaging and frontal-subcortical circuitry in obsessive-compulsive disorder. *Br J Psychiatry 173(suppl 35)*:26–37, 1998.

Schneider LH, Cooper SJ, Halmi KA (eds): *The Psychobiology of Human Eating Disorders: Preclinical and Clinical Perspectives.* New York Academy of Science, New York, 1989.

Schwartz JM: Neuroanatomical aspects of cognitive-behavioural therapy response in obsessive-compulsive disorder. An evolving perspective on brain and behaviour. *Brit J Psychiatry 173 (suppl 35)*:38–44, 1998.

Shapiro AK, Shapiro ES, Young JG, Feinberg TE: *Gilles de la Tourette Syndrome,* 2nd ed. Raven Press, New York, 1988.

Stein MB, Forde DR, Anderson G, Walker JR: Obsessive-compulsive disorder in the community: An epidemiologic survey with clinical reappraisal. *Am J Psychiatry 154*:1120–1126, 1997.

Stein DJ, Shoulberg N, Helton K, Hollander E: The neuroethological approach to obsessive-compulsive disorder. *Compr Psychiatry 33*:274–281, 1992.

Steinhausen H-CH, Rauss-Mason C, Seidel R: Follow-up studies of anorexia nervosa: A review of four decades outcome research. *Psychol Med 21*:447–454, 1991.

Swedo SE, Leonard HL: Childhood movement disorders and obsessive compulsive disorder. *J Clin Psychiatry 55(suppl 3)*:32–37, 1994.

Swedo SE, Pietrini P, Leonard HL, Schapiro MB, Rettew DC, Goldberger EL, Rapoport SI, Rapoport JL, Grady CL: Cerebral glucose metabolism in childhood-onset obsessive compulsive disorder: Revisualization during pharmacotherapy. *Arch Gen Psychiatry 49*:690–694, 1992.

The Tourette Syndrome Classification Study Group: Definitions and classification of tic disorders. *Arch Neurol 50*:1013–1016, 1993.

Wolf SS, Jones DW, Knable MB, Gorey JG, Lee KS, Hyde TM, Coppola R, Weinberger DR: Tourette syndrome: Prediction of phenotypic variation in monozygotic twins by caudate nucleus D2 receptor binding. *Science 273*:1225–1227, 1996.

Zald DH, Kim SW: Anatomy and function of the orbital frontal cortex I: Anatomy, neurochemistry, and obsessive compulsive disorder. *J Neuropsychiatry Clin Neurosci 8*:125–138, 1996.

Zielinski CM, Taylor MA, Juzwin KR: Neuropsychological deficits in obsessive-compulsive disorder. *Neuropsychiatry Neuropsychol Behav Neurol 4*:110–126, 1991.

15

Anxiety Disorders

Anxiety disorders are common (5%–10% of persons have severe forms, and an additional 10%–15% have specific phobias). Anxiety is also a feature of many traditional neurologic and general medical illnesses, so that *secondary anxiety disorder* is also common, and about half the patients in general medical practice have anxiety symptoms as part of their chief complaint. Table 15.1 displays the DSM-IV anxiety disorders. Although official, this classification offers little guidance for patient care and has conceptual problems. For example:

1. Agoraphobia without panic disorder does not substantially differ from agoraphobia with panic disorder, suggesting that they are variations of the same pathophysiology.
2. Persons with specific phobias clinically and physiologically differ from persons with other anxiety disorders, suggesting that specific phobias differ fundamentally from the others.
3. Post-traumatic stress disorder (PTSD) is a heterogeneous category, and patients with it often have co-occurring conditions that may, in fact, be their primary disorder.
4. Gilles de la Tourette's disorder (GTS) is not listed among the anxiety disorders, but is related to obsessive compulsive disorder (OCD), which is listed as an anxiety disorder, but which seems fundamentally different from them.

Some characteristics of anxiety disorders are (1) women are affected more than men, almost 2 to 1 (exceptions: OCD and social phobia, in which both genders are equally affected); (2) peak onset age is 15–25 years, with few primary conditions occurring for the first time after age 35 or before school age (exception: specific phobias occur before puberty); (3) the disorders are familial, but several forms can occur in the same families; (4) over 50% of patients have a preexisting personality disorder characterized by anxiousness and fearfulness and being overly cautious, pessimistic, apprehensive, a worrier, inhibited, quiet, and reserved; (5) most will have an occasional nonmelancholic depression, and some will abuse alcohol or

TABLE 15.1. DSM-IV Anxiety Disorders

Agoraphobia without panic disorder

Panic disorder without agoraphobia

Panic disorder with agoraphobia

Specific phobia

Social phobia

Obsessive compulsive disorder

Post-traumatic stress disorder

Acute stress disorder

Generalized anxiety disorder (includes overanxious disorder of childhood)

Anxiety disorder due to a general medical condition

Substance-induced anxiety disorder (coded by substance abuse category)

Anxiety disorder not otherwise specified

---

benzodiazepines to self-medicate; and (6) most patients treated early and well will improve substantially or remit.

THE NEUROLOGY OF ANXIETY

Acute anxiety is an adaptive physiologic state that is part of flight/fight behavior to avoid or defend against danger (see Fig. 15.1). In humans, at least, it occurs with a subjective experience of fear. The flight/fight system is activated by strong, typically sudden and often unexpected stimuli, or stimuli that evoke memories associated with previous anxiety or danger. Makers of horror movies are expert at using sudden loud noise or movement or familiar stimuli that evoke audience anxiety (e.g., the eerie music as the heroine goes into the dark basement, the close-up of running water in the bathtub that signals the mad killer is in the house and the hero is undressed and vulnerable).

Flight/fight mechanisms are integrated with the brain's arousal system. Sleep to full wakefulness occurs with the activation of the reticular activating system (RAS) and locus ceruleus interacting with the thalamus. The thalamus projects this arousal tone to the cortex and helps focus cortical attention to stimuli for further processing and action. Too much or too little arousal can lead to attentional problems. Intoxications and delirium are examples of disrupted arousal causing problems with attention.

Cortical processing in flight/fight involves attribution, e.g., this pattern of stimuli is good, that pattern is bad or sad or potentially dangerous. For example, you are supposed to fly to another city for a professional meeting, but it is snowing. You know plane crashes, although rare, tend to occur in bad weather. This knowledge (learned information in your memory) attaches a degree of danger to

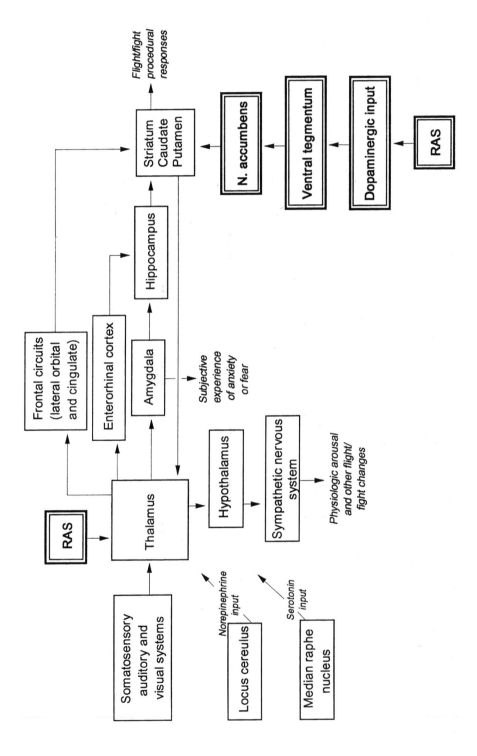

Figure 15.1. Neural circuitry of anxiety. RAS, reticular activating system.

the snow. Depending on your personality and other factors (e.g., IQ, specific experiences in your life), you might decide to cancel your trip. On the other hand, it is snowing and you want to go cross-country skiing tomorrow. You know you need snow on the ground for that, and so the same snow is attributed as a good thing. The worse the cortical attribution, however, the stronger the cortical feedback to the thalamus, the more likely that cortical feedback will invoke anxiety (flight/fight mechanisms). This is termed *cognitive anxiety.*

If the stimuli are sudden, unexpected, intense, or novel, however, the thalamus initially bypasses the cortex and sends this information directly to the amygdala, hippocampus, and parahippocampus, like express mail, for very rapid processing. Getting to the cortex and having it process this information before initial action takes too long, and our ancestors would have been lunch had they depended on the cortex to make the initial decision about flight/fight. The hippocampus/parahippocampus try to match the stimulus pattern with past patterns (memories) for danger. Even an approximate match (e.g., a dark shadow on a lonely lane at night) will trigger the hippocampus to alert the basal ganglia leading to flight/fight behavior. Simultaneously, the thalamus sends the new potentially dangerous information to the nucleus accumbens, septal nuclei, and cerebral cortex. Through a feedback loop, the hippocampus/parahippocampus get further information from the amygdala about the emotion that is being attached to the stimulus pattern. This information is also sent to the nucleus accumbens, septal nuclei, and striatum.

The thalamus also simultaneously sends the stimulus information to the hypothalamus. This input plus feedback from the amygdala/hippocampus/parahippocampus (feedback loop not shown in Fig. 15.1) stimulates the hypothalamus to arouse the sympathetic nervous system to produce the physiologic state necessary for rapid, intense activity. The system is fueled by dopamine in the RAS arousal system and mediated by norepinephrine from the locus ceruleus. Serotonin projections from the median raphe nucleus modify the system.

The intensity of the stimulus pattern, the degree of danger and fear that the hippocampus/parahippocampus/amygdala attach to the stimulus pattern, the greater the flight/fight reaction. This process relates to what is termed *somatic anxiety.* A mild reaction might be limited to a turning of the head toward the stimulus pattern source with slightly dilated pupils, small increase in heart rate, blood pressure, and muscle tension. A substantial reaction is the startle response, which includes large changes in heart rate and blood pressure, shunting of blood to large muscle groups and away from the body's surface, and muscle tension with flexion (i.e., the sudden crouch as if ducking out of the way of danger). The cortical loops are by now fully activated as is the cerebellum. Motor neurons have been recruited for flight/fight actions, and if the stimulus pattern is strong enough these motor programs are released. For example, a loud unexpected noise will startle almost any social mammal and it will immediately flex, become physiologically aroused, and run at least a few feet away from the noise before knowing the source or if the noise represents danger. At this point cortical attribution may predominate and may stop the flight/fight response (the sudden noise is 20 people in your darkened apartment yelling "surprise" on your birthday) or may lead to complex defensive behavior (the sudden noise in your darkened apartment is followed by "I've go a gun, don't move").

Flight/fight behavior, therefore, involves several parallel steps:

1. Arousal
2. Thalamic channeling of the stimulus pattern
3. Hippocampus/parahippocampus/amygdala processing
4. Basal ganglia and septal nuclei motor programming and attention
5. Cortical processing and attribution
6. Action brain integrated responses

The parallel steps in the flight/fight process also is a framework for reorganizing the DSM anxiety disorders into more clinically meaningful groupings and for developing more specific treatment strategies for primary and secondary anxiety-related conditions.

Several neurotransmitter systems are involved in flight/fight, which is one reason why different drugs can alleviate anxiety (e.g., antidepressants, benzodiazepines, alcohol, buspirone). Table 15.2 displays some of the better known relationships among norepinephrine (NE), serotonin (5-HT), and gamma-aminobutyric acid (GABA) and anxiety. Anxiety disorder probably arises from the flight/fight system's hypersensitivity to stimuli. The more ambiguous, novel, or potentially dangerous the stimulus pattern, the more intense the response. Thus, the flight/fight system in anxious patients responds to stimuli that do not produce a flight/fight response in nonanxious persons (the threshold is lower). It also over-responds to stimuli that produce a modest response in nonanxious persons (once over the threshold, the response is more intense and of greater duration).

NE appears to be the initiating factor in flight/fight, and its activity underlies many of the central and peripheral features of anxiety. 5-HT activity underlies many homeostatic processes and appears to modulate NE activity with dorsal and medial raphe nuclei projections to the locus ceruleus and again to the thalamus/parahippocampus/hippocampus/septal system. Too much NE activity can produce central and peripheral anxiety. Too much serotonergic activity reduces the inhibition of the NE system and leads to central features of anxiety. GABA distribution in the brain is more widespread than that of NE or 5-HT. Its involvement in anxiety disorder is probably indirect and as a modulating factor (i.e., high or low activity will influence the affects of NE/5-HT on flight/fight systems). It is also a chronicity factor: The longer lasting or more severe the anxiety disorder, the more likely GABAergic function is disrupted, the more likely excitatory amino acids are released and limbic sensitization with its behavior (psychosensory features) and cognitive (memory problems) consequences is likely to occur.

CLINICAL PRESENTATION

Panic Attack

Almost all patients with anxiety disorder have one or more panic attacks. Table 15.3 lists the behaviors observed in a panic attack. Many features are adaptive, and these will also appropriately occur in flight/fight situations. For example, some pupillary dilation and exophthalmus lets more light into the eyeball and increases the range of eyeball movement, aiding vision. Vascular shunting reduces blood flow to the periphery and thus reduces potential blood loss should injury occur. Blood flow also increases to large muscle groups. The changes observed in a panic attack are essentially no different from those observed in flight/fight situations except that there is no real threat and the symptoms evolve beyond adaptation.

Specific Phobia

A phobia is an irrational or exaggerated fear of a specific object, place, situation, or activity. Specific phobia (e.g., flying, heights, blood, or injury) differs from other anxiety disorders. The phobia is the only abnormal behavior experienced by most sufferers, and patients with a specific phobia usually fear only the one thing. When the patient does not anticipate contact with the phobic object or situation, he is usually comfortable and his behavior is normal. For this reason, many persons with specific phobias need no treatment. For example, a resident of Chicago is not likely to seek treatment of a snake phobia.

Although persons with specific phobia are presumed to be more vulnerable to becoming phobic than are nonphobics, no specific physiologic or other predisposing abnormalities have been demonstrated in these patients. Because of this, and the fact that specific phobia is so common (about 12% of the population, 25% if mild forms are included) and typically begins in childhood (may then resolve and recur in young adulthood), its underlying mechanism is presumed to be classic conditioning: Some intense stimulus produces a severe startle response and anxiety, which is linked to the situation, object, or activity associated with the intense stimulus. Subsequent exposure reinforces the link, and the person is now phobic. Thus, specific phobics may have nothing wrong with their flight/fight system, but rather a greater likelihood of being conditioned under certain circumstances. This is also why deconditioning (see below) is the treatment of choice for these patients.

The course of specific phobia also differs from other anxiety disorders; it begins in childhood (school phobia being the most common). The younger the age at onset of specific phobia, the better the prognosis. Half of childhood onset patients are symptom free within 5 years of expression, and virtually all improve somewhat. Adolescent and adult onset specific phobics are respectively less likely to be symptom free after 5 years, with only 5% of adult onset phobics being asymptomatic at follow-up. Women are at greater risk than are men (3 : 2).

Social Phobia, Agoraphobia, and Generalized Anxiety Disorder

Social phobia, agoraphobia, and generalized anxiety disorder (GAD) are probably variations of the same pathophysiologic process. Social phobics and GAD patients are less housebound and may function better than agoraphobics, but patients in each group fear losing self-control. Treatment is basically the same for all.

The three conditions begin in the early or mid-20s. Onset (if primary) is almost

TABLE 15.2. Neurochemistry of Anxiety

System	Anatomy	Behavioral Results	Pharmacologic Considerations
Noradrenergic (NE)	1. 70% of the brain's NE comes from the locus ceruleus with projections to hippocampus, thalamus, hypothalamus, amygdala, brain stem, spinal cord, and sympathetic and parasympathetic systems 2. Lateral tegmental area is next largest source of NE	1. Subjective feeling of apprehension and, when severe, impending doom 2. All the peripheral signs of panic from increased beta-adrenergic activity 3. Trait proneness to reinforcement, and once behaviors established they are maintained and spontaneous resolution of maladaptive behavior less likely 4. Mediates fear conditioning and associative memories	1. Yohimbine (an alpha$_2$- adrenoceptor antagonist) prevents inhibition of NE release and produces a panic attack in anxiety disorder patients. 2. Beta-blockers relieve peripheral signs of anxiety but not the underlying driving force 3. Chronic administration of NE reuptake inhibitors (e.g., some antidepressants) downregulate or decrease numbers of beta-adrenergic receptors; this only happens if 5-HT system is intact
Serotonergic (5-HT)	1. Dorsal (DRN) and median (MRN) raphe nuclei are the brain's most prominent sources of 5-HT projections	1. Homeostasis (sleep, feeding, sex, learning and memory, sensory processing); mediates adaptive responses to aversive events	1. Benzodiazepines reduce 5-HT turnover 2. Buspirone works first as a presynaptic 5-HT$_{1A}$ agonist; then, when 5-HT less

	2. DRN parallels DA projections to cerebral cortex, hypothalamus, thalamus, amygdala, basal ganglia 3. MRN parallels NE projections to septo-hippocampal system, amygdala, locus ceruleus (5-HT increases NE turnover here)	2. Too much activity (turnover) associated with anxiety; too little activity associated with depression, suicide, irritability, aggression 3. Trait proneness to inhibit behavior when faced with potential or real danger or nonreward, tendency to be anxious and fearful in many situations	available, works as partial postsynaptic 5-HT$_{1A}$ agonist with subsequent downregulation producing antianxiety effect, so not good for acute panic; works on DRN/MRN and hippocampus; buspirone metabolite 1 (2 pyrimidinyl)-piperazine is an alpha$_2$-antagonist
GABAergic	Throughout the brain and spinal cord; coupled with benzodiazepine receptors in chloride channel complex	1. Widespread inhibition modifies effects of NE and 5-HT 2. Antikindling and sensitization 3. Antiseizure	1. Benzodiazepines act on benzodiazepine receptor, coupled with GABA receptor, and together they regulate chloride channel opening and closing. Their increased activity leads to presynaptic inhibition of excitatory amino acids (e.g., glutamate) 2. Alcohol and barbiturates act on GABA receptors and directly on the chloride channel 3. Valproate acts on GABA receptors

Table 15.3. Panic Attack

Domain Affected	Manifestation
Mood	Apprehension, fear
Flight/fight phenomena	Dilated pupils, exophthalmus, piloerection, increased muscle tone, tachycardia, sweating, vascular shunting
Nonadaptive features	Tremors, dry mouth, blurred vision, chest pain/ discomfort, palpitations, air hunger, feeling of choking, dyspnea, hyperventilation, parasthesias, flushes or chills, weakness, fatigue, easy fatigability, inner shakiness, lump in throat, vascular throbbing, in creased bowel motility, nausea or abdominal distress, dizziness or syncope
Cognition	Notion of impending doom; fear of dying, losing control, going crazy; inability to concentrate; depersonalization, derealization

never before puberty or after age 35 (about 80% of patients have onsets before 30). Once developed, symptoms wax and wane, but many patients tend to become progressively isolated with social and employment deterioration. GAD patients and social phobics can also become housebound, but are not as limited as are patients with agoraphobia. All may have panic attacks, and some GAD patients develop additional phobias. About 3% of women and 1%–2% of men develop agoraphobia, and 6% of persons (men somewhat more than women) develop GAD.

Agoraphobics, social phobics, and patients with GAD have signs of physiologic hyperarousal even at rest. This includes increased systolic blood pressure and heart rate. They have poor arousal habituation to repeated stimuli (i.e., they respond to the tenth stimulus as strongly as to the first). Subsequent spontaneous panic attacks can occur, even if the patient is not in a feared situation. There is little clinical, laboratory, or familial difference between agoraphobia with and without panic attacks.

Social phobia involves fear of losing self-control in a social situation where there may be some scrutiny. When not in a social situation the patient is usually comfortable, although the number of anxiety-provoking situations can become substantial, causing daily anxiety and affecting work and interpersonal relations. Twenty percent of social phobics are alcoholics. Social phobias include such things as speaking on the telephone, eating in public, using a public toilet, test taking, working while being observed, public speaking, stage fright, speaking in a meeting, making a date, going to a party, meeting strangers, and returning purchases.

Agoraphobia differs from social phobias in that sufferers have daily, or almost daily, anxiety to any venture outside their home. Agoraphobics fear situations in which they might have a panic attack and lose self-control by crying, screaming, fainting, becoming incontinent, or dying. They fear being alone in crowds, elevators, malls, restaurants, theaters, crowded rooms, tunnels, bridges, or airplanes. Onset can be (1) sudden with a panic attack while away from home, (2) insidious as a response to frequent panic attacks and the fear of being away from home when they happen, (3) from the accumulation of social phobias that progressively restrict activities, or (4) as primary slowly progressive pattern of behavior.

GAD patients have a more gradual onset and are less housebound than agoraphobics. However, they worry more and are more likely to have nonmelancholic depressions than agoraphobics. They also are more likely to complain of fatigue, easy fatigueability, headache, insomnia, nausea, and palpitations.

Panic Disorder

Patients with pure panic disorder have recurrent, apparently unprovoked acute anxiety attacks, with little generalized anxiety or agoraphobia. Diagnosis requires recurrent, frequent (1–2 per week) attacks, associated with persistent concerns about having more attacks or worries about having a heart attack or "going crazy." During an attack, tachycardia, light-headedness, facial pallor, and hyperventilation often occur. Hyperventilation is associated with respiratory alkalosis (low Pco_2 and serum bicarbonate) and hypocalcemia, the latter leading to fasciculations, weakness, and muscle spasms. About 2% of women and 1% of men have panic disorder. Onset is in the early or mid-20s and usually begins during a period of stress. Later attacks are more often spontaneous (i.e., no stress needed).

Acute Stress Disorder

Patients with acute stress disorder have anxiety symptoms immediately or shortly (always less than 1 month) after being in a situation that is horrifying or that threatens life or could have caused serious injury. Initially the patient may feel depersonalized (numb, detached, lacking emotional responses, "in a daze," or "in a dream"). Then generalized anxiety symptoms develop, often with panic attacks. The traumatic event is often obsessively discussed and thought about, although the patient usually tries to avoid the setting in which the event occurred (e.g., not using the highway where the car was totaled). Patients may have recurrent images of the event (i.e., flashbacks). Nightmares and insomnia are common. Most persons develop some features of this disorder after a severe traumatic event (e.g., rape, serious automobile accident) and then recover within a year.

Chronic PTSD

Chronic PTSD differs from acute stress disorder in that it lasts longer. There is no evidence for onset delayed beyond 1 month, and if a patient describes a prolonged delayed onset (e.g., several years) most likely the symptoms are due to a co-occurring condition such as antisocial personality disorder, alcohol or other substance abuse, anxiety disorder, OCD, or mood disorder (usually depression). Over 85% of patients with chronic PTSD have co-occurring conditions.

The diagnosis of PTSD requires (1) exposure to an unequivocal traumatizing event (e.g., rape); (2) the traumatic event is persistently reexperienced in ruminations, imagery, or dreams; (3) stimuli associated with the trauma are avoided; (4) increased arousal not present before the trauma is now present (the DSM gives the following examples, which obviously incorporate more than arousal features: insomnia, irritability, poor concentration, hypervigilance, exaggerated startle response); and (5) disturbed social, job, and interpersonal functions.

Differential Diagnosis

Many anxiety disorder patients initially see a generalist physician because of the physiologic features of anxiety. Chief complaints include fainting and dizziness, difficulty breathing, headaches, and fears of heart disease because of palpitations, tachycardia, or chest pain. Panic attacks often result in emergency room treatment because of fears of having a heart attack. Parasthesias may be mistaken for spinal cord or peripheral nerve disease. Nausea and abdominal cramps can lead to fears of having ulcers or cancer.

The diagnosis of anxiety disorder is usually straightforward. The two important diagnostic questions are whether the disorder is secondary and what to make of co-occurring conditions.

Table 15.4 lists common causes of secondary anxiety disorder. In addition, suspect a secondary anxiety disorder if (1) onset is after age 35; (2) the patient is male who is *not* an alcoholic or heavy drinker; (3) the patient has motor disturbances; and (4) panic attacks are short (less than 5 minutes) and occur several times daily or are associated with irritability or an altered sensorum.

Laboratory Findings

There are no clinical diagnostic tests helpful in identifying idiopathic anxiety disorders. Twenty to 40% of panic patients, however, have abnormal MRIs versus 10% of controls, with some atrophy particularly observed in the right temporal lobe horn. Mild to moderate atrophy is observed on computed tomographic (CT) scan in some patients, but these abnormalities may be related to the amount of benzodiazepine these patients have used. Reduced cerebral cortex blood flow (particularly in the temporal lobes) with exposure to phobic stimuli needs confirmation.

EEG findings in anxiety patients are also inconclusive. Nonepileptic EEG abnormalities are found in a small proportion of patients and some have epileptic-like abnormalities. Atypical panic and panic associated with irritability increase the likelihood of this type of EEG; treat these patients for seizure or epilepsy spectrum disorder. Atypical panic attacks are those that are of short duration (less than 5 minutes) and associated with psychosensory features or neurologic signs such as focal paresis, problems with speech and language, and altered consciousness. However, the majority of panic patients have normal EEGs.

Laboratory-Induced Panic

Intravenous infusion of a 500 mmol solution of sodium lactate will induce a panic attack in 90% of anxiety disorder patients. Other substances that do this include

CO_2, bicarbonate, yohimbine, and isoproterenol. Laboratory-induced panic is dramatic and controllable. It provides an excellent paradigm for studying the physiologic processes of anxiety, persons with different degrees of risk for anxiety disorder, and novel treatments of anxiety disorder. It is not an accepted clinical diagnostic test.

Co-Occurring Conditions

Irritable bowel syndrome may affect over 10% of the general population, and up to 70% of these patients may have psychiatric symptoms, most commonly anxiety and depression. When irritable bowel co-occurs with anxiety disorder, treatment with monoamine reuptake-inhibiting antidepressants can resolve both conditions. It is unclear, however, whether this co-occurrence represents a common etiology and pathophysiology or, if not, which syndrome is primary.

Mitral valve prolapse has a symptom pattern similar to that of GAD: anxiety, palpitations, chest discomfort, fatigue. As many as 25% of anxiety patients have some prolapse, whereas only 10% of the general population has this cardiac deviation. The clinical significance of this relationship is unclear, but true co-morbidity seems unlikely.

Adjustment disorder is a group of conditions that develop rapidly in response to a relatively modest stress (e.g., moving to a different city; starting a new job) and resolve within the DSM prescribed 6 months or sooner if the stress resolves. The patient's symptoms cannot be explained by another condition (e.g., they cannot be bipolar or have antisocial personality disorder). Eight subtypes are defined by the predominant feature (e.g., depressed, anxious, conduct disturbance). These conditions tend to occur in adolescents and young adults in response to events few would consider overwhelming. Those patients who do not recover within 6 months tend to develop more serious disorders (e.g., mood disorder, anxiety disorder, drug abuse). Perhaps 5% of the population is at risk. Persons with anxious-fearful behavioral traits (e.g., high harm avoidance and low novelty seeking [see Chapter 6 for details], introverted rather than extroverted, low sociability, and impulsivity) are more likely to develop the anxious type of adjustment disorder and then subsequently develop a longer lasting anxiety disorder.

Nonmelancholic depression is the most common condition co-occurring with anxiety disorder. About 50% of patients with panic disorder will have a major depression during their lifetime; most patients with anxiety disorder (of any type) will have occasional, often atypical depressions; and 3%–4% of the general population will have both anxiety disorder and mood disorder during their lifetime.

Although relatives of patients with pure anxiety states do not have an increased risk for depression, relatives of patients with co-occurring anxiety and depression do. Some clinical heterogeneity seems likely. Nonmelancholic depressives whose illnesses begin with panic disorder have depressions that appear to be either states of demoralization or depressive-like states that are variants of the primary panic disorder. They have no increased risk for mood disorder in their first-degree relatives. Personality factors may underlie the co-occurrence of anxi-

TABLE 15.4. Conditions Causing Secondary Anxiety Disorder

Condition	Manifestations
TRADITIONAL NEUROLOGIC	
Temporal lobe epilepsy	1. Multiple daily panic attacks, short panic attacks (less than 5 minutes), psychosensory features, brief transient episodes of altered awareness or memory gaps 2. Mimics panic disorder
Parkinson's disease	1. Late onset (after age 60) anxiety disorder, resting tremor, and increased muscle tone with bradykinesia 2. Mimics GAD
Postconcussion syndrome	1. Recent head trauma, dizziness without syncope, concentration problems 2. Mimics GAD
Multiple sclerosis	1. Vague and fluctuating presentation incorporating cerebellar signs, optic neuritis, and weakness 2. Incidence peaks in young adults and again in persons over age 40 3. Mimics GAD
GENERAL MEDICAL	
Endocrine disorders	1. Late onset, any classic symptom or sign (particularly of hyperthyroidism, Cushing's disease, diabetes with hypoglycemia) 2. Mimics panic disorder, GAD
Cardiovascular disease	1. Late onset, any classic symptom or sign of angina pectoris, arrhythmias, congestive heart failure, hypertension, hypovolemia, myocardial infarction, syncope (multiple causes), valvular disease, vascular collapse (shock), hypertension 2. Mimics GAD
Mitral valve prolapse	Mimics panic disorder, GAD
Pulmonary embolus	1. Any classic symptom or sign 2. Mimics panic disorder

ety disorder and nonmelancholic depression, and 40%–60% of anxiety disorder patients have anxious premorbid traits.

Other co-occurrences with the anxiety disorders seem related, in part, to misdiagnosis. For example, some patients with dysthymia and significant anxiety, and melancholics with apprehension receive double diagnoses even though the features of anxiety are expressions of the depressive process. Some patients with

TABLE 15.4. *(continued)*

Condition	Manifestations
Asthma	1. Classic pulmonary and chest signs, history of allergies
	2. Mimics panic disorder
Chronic obstructive pulmonary disease	1. Dyspnea, large anterior-posterior chest diameter, irritability and personality change
	2. Mimics panic disorder and GAD
Hypoglycemia	1. History of diabetes
	2. Mimics panic disorder, GAD
Irritable bowel syndrome	1. Bowel syndrome will be obvious, and anxiety disorders often co-occur
	2. Mimics panic disorder, GAD
Secreting tumors (pheochromocytoma, carcinoid, insulinoma)	1. Always mentioned, rarely found
	2. Inconsistent symptoms and course
	3. Intermittent hypertension (which beta-blockers prescribed for anxiety will mask)
	4. Mimics panic disorder
Withdrawal states	1. Anxiety can be the first sign of benzodiazepine or other sedative-hypnotic withdrawal; narcotic and alcohol withdrawal also cause substantial anxiety
	2. Mimic panic disorder, GAD
Caffeinism	1. Heavy coffee use and an inconsistent waxing and waning of symptoms
	2. Mimics panic disorder, GAD
Drug use (stimulants, dopaminergics, sympathomimetics, and anticholinergics)*	1. Antisocial personality or history of other risk-taking and impulsive behavior
	2. Mimics panic disorder
Anemia	1. Weakness or chronic fatigue, hemorrhagia, and eating disorders
	2. Mimics GAD

*Stimulants: amphetamine, aminophylline, caffeine, cocaine, methylphenidate, theophylline; sympathomimetics: ephedrine, epinephrine, phenylpropanolamine, pseudoephedrine; anticholinergics: benztropine mesylate (Cogentin), diphenhydramine (Benadryl), meperidine (Demerol), oxybutynin (Ditropan), propantheline (Pro-Banthine), many psychotropics and antiparkinsonian agents; dopaminergics: amantadine, bromocriptine, levodopa (L-dopa), levodopa/carbidopa (Sinemet).

complex partial seizures may also have depressive and anxiety symptoms that are separately labeled, the seizure disorder going unrecognized. Self-medication with stimulant drugs by some depressives may also lead to the drug-related symptoms being misdiagnosed as anxiety. The clinical rule is, always consider the more serious or life-threatening condition as the primary condition unless there is clear evidence otherwise (e.g., the other condition occurred years earlier, and there is also a family history of it). Thus, dysthymia takes precedence over anxiety disorder, as does melancholia and seizure disorder. You would treat such patients for these conditions even if they also meet criteria for an anxiety disorder.

MANAGEMENT

Most anxiety disorder patients receive outpatient treatment. Pharmacologic and behavioral interventions are usually combined. Psychosurgery may benefit some chronic patients who have not responded to all other treatments. Education of anxiety disorder patients includes (1) *correcting misconceptions* (e.g., that the condition results from masturbation); (2) *resolving secondary fears* (e.g., of going crazy, of having a dangerous medical problem such as heart disease); (3) *providing a reasonable explanation for their condition* (e.g., symptoms are real and reflect physiologic hypersensitivity in the brain resulting in an abnormal flight/fight response); and (4) *offering a detailed discussion of the treatments* (e.g., what modalities, what each is supposed to do, side effects)

Table 15.5 lists guidelines for treating patients with anxiety disorder. During the acute phase of treatment, drug side effects are the biggest therapeutic challenge. During maintenance treatment, the patient's personality is often the biggest therapeutic challenge.

Pharmacotherapy

The pharmacologic treatment of anxiety disorder is remarkably similar to that for depression. The main differences are that dosing is done more slowly for anxiety disorder patients, and side effects are more problematic; and response takes longer and is not as good for anxiety disorder.

Reuptake-inhibiting antidepressants work with social phobia, agoraphobia, generalized anxiety, and panic disorder. The nonspecific and partially specific reuptake inhibitors are the best studied, but the selective monoamine reuptake inhibitors (e.g., fluoxetine, sertraline) are also effective. Which drug you choose

TABLE 15.5. Guidelines for Treating Patients With Anxiety Disorders

High sensitivity to drug side effects requires low starting doses and small dose increases. Educating the patient and family is essential if compliance is to be maintained. The same check-in strategies to treat mood disorder patients apply equally to patients with anxiety disorders

Full response may take weeks or several months; do not give up prematurely

Once maximum improvement has been obtained, maintenance treatment may be needed indefinitely

Compliance and perhaps quality of improvement is maximized by counseling, encouragement, and support

Combined medication plus behavioral techniques is best for severely ill patients depends on many factors, such as the patient's personality and co-morbid conditions.

Although there is no evidence that one reuptake inhibitor is better than another, most clinicians have their favorites. Table 15.6 lists rationales for choosing. If the reuptake inhibitor does not lead to remission and the otherwise healthy patient is receiving a nonspecific or partially specific reuptake inhibitor, then adding an MAOI can be effective.

Whatever your choice, the initial dose should be on the low side and increased gradually. Thus, starting doses will be half or less of what is usually given for depression, and increases will be one to two steady-state durations apart. For a small number of patients, even the smallest tablet dose available will be poorly tolerated (too excitatory or too severe side effects), and you may have to break the tablet (literally hit it with a hammer and give the largest piece). Final therapeutic doses will be in the low to mid therapeutic range for depression. Somewhere between 50% and 75% of patients will have a marked response. Once remission is achieved, maintain the patient on the same dose for 1 year to prevent relapse. After 1 year of remission, gradually taper the dose and, if possible, discontinue it over 3 months. About 60% of patients will not require immediate dose build up. Some, however, will require indefinite treatment.

Most reuptake-inhibiting antidepressants can be given once daily, and none has dietary restrictions similar to MAOIs. However, in addition to the anticholinergic side effects of the nonspecific and partially specific agents and the sexual problems caused by the specific agents, the use of these drugs with anxiety disorder patients can cause an initial hyperstimulatory response (agitation, anxiety, irritability, severe inner restlessness, tachycardia, and palpitation). Low and slow dosing can minimize this occurrence, and beta-blockers can control it. The reaction usually resolves over several weeks, so try to prepare the patient, and if it occurs get the patient through it rather than stopping the drug. The nonspecific and partially specific agents often lead to large weight gain, so prepare patients to exercise and watch their caloric intake.

Beta-Adrenergic Blocking Agents (e.g., Propranolol)

Beta-adrenergic blocking agents may be added to or substituted for the antidepressants. Dosage range for propranolol is 30–130 mg daily in divided doses. Reduction in consuming food and drink with caffeine is also helpful, but often hard to achieve because caffeine is addicting. Caffeine is a competitive antagonist of adenosine and chronic use upregulates adenosine receptors. Withdraw caffeine gradually using a withdrawal schedule, and substituted decaffeinated coffee. This withdrawal may take as long as 6 months.

Monoamine oxidase inhibitors (MAOIs) can be effective, even if reuptake-inhibiting antidepressants do not produce a substantial improvement. Phenelzine, for example, is as good as other antidepressants in treating patients with GAD or agoraphobia. A typical initial dose is 15 mg daily, increased by 15 mg in 2–3 days and then by 15 mg each week. If the patient can tolerate it, give a single daily morning dose. Therapeutic doses range from 45 to 120 mg daily. In addition to a

TABLE 15.6. Rationale for Choosing Antidepressants in Treating Anxiety Disorder Patients

Drug	Considerations
Nonselective and Partially Selective Reuptake Inhibitors Imipramine, amitriptyline	1. Most of the efficacy studies have been done with these drugs; they work for all types of anxiety disorders 2. Anticholinergic side effects and sedation remain the main problem, so they are best for younger or otherwise healthy patients 3. Use is exactly the same as for depression, only slower dosing
Desipramine/nortriptyline	1. A good compromise between the anticholinergic problems of the nonselective reuptake inhibitors and the sexual side effects and serotonin excitatory response of the SSRIs* 2. If insomnia is a problem, once a day nighttime dosing can help, taking advantage of any sedation side effect without needing a second medication for sleep
Clomipramine	Effective for panic disorder
Selective Reuptake Inhibitors Sertraline	1. Broad therapeutic spectrum; less sexual side effects than other SSRIs 2. Well tolerated by older anxiety disorder patients 3. Good choice if depression also present
Venlafaxine	1. Broad therapeutic spectrum 2. Good choice if depression also present
Paroxetine	1. Good choice for panic disorder 2. SSRI of choice if weight loss needs to be avoided (less likely than other SSRIs)
Fluoxetine	1. Effective for GAD and agoraphobia 2. Most likely SSRI to cause an excitatory serotonin response
Nefazodone	Good choice if insomnia side effect of other drugs becomes a problem, but not well studied in the treatment of anxiety disorders
Monoamine Oxidase Inhibitor Phenelzine	1. Second-line choice for pure anxiety disorder because of diet restrictions (other MAOIs may avoid this, but have not been widely studied for efficacy) 2. Good choice for otherwise healthy patient with anxiety disorder associated with nonmelancholic or atypical depression

*SSRIs, specific serotonin reuptake inhibitors.

tyramine/stimulant-restricted diet, the concomitant administration of amitriptyline (25 mg orally at bedtime, begun *before* starting the MAOI) may decrease MAOI-induced insomnia and reduce the risk of a hypertensive tyramine reaction in patients who do not fully adhere to their diet or who unknowingly eat a high-tyramine food. Stimulants, including those in over-the-counter cold preparations, must be avoided, as must opiods (synthetic opiates, like meperidine). Although MAOIs may be added to reuptake-blocking antidepressants, do not do the reverse, as it may precipitate an adrenergic crisis with delirium or seizures. If one MAOI is substituted for another, there should be a 14-day MAOI-free interval between drugs to avoid a hypertensive episode. The patient should always carry several 10 mg tablets of nifedipine for sublingual use should a hypertensive reaction begin (sudden throbbing headache, sweating and flushing, nausea and vomiting, photophobia). See Chapter 7 for foods to avoid with MAOIs.

As with other antidepressants, maintenance lasts about 1 year followed by the tapering of the daily dose (one tablet per 1–2 weeks) until the patient is drug free. If relapse occurs, reintroduce the MAOI. A lower dose may work in the second course of treatment. Maintain for another year, and again try to withdraw the drug. Some patients require indefinite MAOI treatment and after many years can relapse quickly if the drug is stopped.

A hyperstimulatory response and weight gain can also occur with MAOIs. Use the same precautions and management as with reuptake inhibitors. As both MAOIs and reuptake inhibitors have delayed responses, benzodiazepines can be used to control anxiety during that period.

Benzodiazepines (see below for details) are the drugs of choice for acute panic attacks.* One or two oral or intravenous doses usually work. Often, they are also needed for several weeks until the antidepressant begins to work. Long-term use (beyond 3 months) will cause dependence, and withdrawal is extremely difficult. Buspirone† (30–60 mg daily), a $5-HT_{1A}$ presynaptic autoreceptor agonist with additional postsynaptic effects, takes longer to work than benzodiazepines, but is nonaddicting and can be given over a longer period of time if anxiety symptoms are particularly severe.

Alprazolam, a high-potency agent, is the most commonly used benzodiazepine for initial management of panic disorder (3–10 mg daily). It also relieves anxiety in agoraphobia and works as well as some antidepressants. Tolerance, however, may not develop to alprazolam in panic disorder patients, similar to the use of barbiturates in epilepsy. Clonazepam (1.5–5 mg daily) and lorazepam (6–10 mg daily) are also used. Alprazolam requires three to four daily doses. Lorazepam and clonazepam are longer acting and can be given twice a day.

---

* Low intravenous doses can immediately stop an attack and the patient usually sleeps for 30–60 minutes. If the patient is hyperventilating, rebreathing into a paper bag ameliorates the somatic effects of low blood Co_2 levels. When the attack is abated, send the patient home with 1–3 days doses of a intermediate- or long-acting benzodiazepine as the patient may experience several days of post-attack high levels of anxiety. Education of the patient about the attack and referral for definitive treatment is also important.

† Buspirone (Buspar) is rapidly absorbed, peaks in 1 hour, is metabolized in the liver, and has a 2–4 hour half-life requiring several doses daily. Dizziness, restlessness, nausea, and headache are some common side effects. Sedation and dysarthria may occur at high doses.

Mood stabilizing anticonvulsants, valproate and carbamazepine, have been used to treat patients with anxiety disorder. Valproate at doses between 1,000 and 2,000 mg daily may help some panic disorder patients (response in 2–3 weeks), and in those patients it may be needed indefinitely. Valproate's GABAergic properties are the rationale for use. Panic patients likely to respond have abnormal, nonepileptic EEGs and might better be described as having an epileptic spectrum disorder with panic attacks. Carbamazepine's effectiveness for panic is unclear. Both, however, are helpful in the relief of anxiety (and other features) of alcohol withdrawal.

Behavior Therapy

Behavior therapy of anxiety disorder includes relaxation training, rebreathing training, and systematic desensitization. *Relaxation training* involves learning how to reduce muscle tension in large muscle groups. The idea behind this is that an anxious person will have increased muscle tension (common, but not universal) and that by reducing tension they will relax and be less anxious (it often works, and some actors use this technique—tensing and then relaxing—to help relax before performances). *Rebreathing training* involves learning how to diaphragmatically breath on cue. Almost anyone can learn this when instructed not use the chest muscles (lie prone and splint the chest by crossing arms over the chest) and to move their abdomen in and out. This ability is very helpful in preventing hyperventilation that can occur during panic attacks. The combination of muscle relaxation and diaphragmatic breathing can abort some panic attacks that develop slowly. Teach all anxiety disorder patients how to do these procedures.

Systematic desensitization involves exposing the phobic person to increasing "doses" of the phobia while they are relaxed. The idea is that you cannot simultaneously be relaxed and anxious. The increasing "doses" can be through imagery in the therapist's office or by in vivo exposure (in the real world). Desensitization is typically done in collaboration with a behavior therapist and is the treatment of choice for specific phobia, with 70% of patients having a moderate to marked response within 2–4 months.

Fairly rapid in vivo exposure is valuable for patients with agoraphobia who have few panic attacks and for patients with social or specific phobias. Anxiety levels can be minimized by relaxation training and low dose benzodiazepines. Family members, friends, office staff, and the therapist can all participate in literally taking the patient into the anxiety-provoking situation for increasingly longer and more intense exposures. For more severely ill patients, pharmacotherapy is done first, followed by behavioral therapy if needed. About 75% of patients have over a 50% reduction in symptoms with exposure techniques. Table 15.7 summarizes the behavioral treatments for anxiety disorder. Tables 15.8 and 15.9 list combined strategies for treating anxiety disorder patients. Behavioral and pharmacologic treatments may act on similar brain receptors. Some antidepressants downregulate beta-adrenergic postsynaptic receptors, and repeated in vivo exposure to stress in rodents also downregulates these receptors.

PTSD is different from the other DSM anxiety disorders. It is heterogeneous, and treatment is best based on the co-morbid condition that is likely to be pri-

TABLE 15.7. Behavioral Techniques Used in the Treatment of Anxiety Disorders

Technique	Purpose
Relaxation training	1. May reduce general levels of anxiety and moderate or abort a panic attack
	2. Helps during office and in vivo exposure to permit visualization or phobic exposure while relaxed, thus breaking the conditioned connection between the phobia and the anxiety
Rebreathing training	1. May reduce general levels of anxiety
	2. Helps during in vivo exposure
	3. May prevent or abort panic attacks precipitated by hyperventilation
Systematic desensitization (office, in vivo)	1. Treatment of choice for specific phobia
	2. Essential adjunct treatment for social phobia and agoraphobia
Response prevention	1. Helpful for OCD
	2. May be combined with other prevention techniques, such as stop thought and satiation
Education, counseling	Required for all patients to reinforce all other treatments and deal with additional social problems that arise
Cognitive psychotherapy	May help with patients with social phobia and patients with co-morbid Cluster C personality disorder (e.g., the social phobic's fear that he will be found wanting is not justified because, in fact, he is very competent, etc.)

mary. Thus, if you think the PTSD represents OCD, treat for that. If you think it represents drug and alcohol abuse in a person with antisocial personality disorder, deal with that. This approach reflects the clinical aphorism that if you will do no harm diagnose the condition for which you have effective treatments. Specific PTSD treatment programs are analogous to drug abuse rehabilitation programs, often "one size fits all." Basing PTSD treatment on the co-morbid condition offers more specific treatments with proven efficacies.

Psychosurgery

Psychosurgery (e.g., limbic leukotomy, subcaudate tractotomy) can benefit some patients with chronic anxiety disorder. About 50%–60% of patients who have *failed* all other treatments alone and combined may improve or recover. The best results are obtained in patients who have supportive families, who do not abuse drugs or alcohol, and who have not exhibited any personality deterioration. As patients undergoing this procedure are usually in good general health, surgical side effects are minimal and typical of any neurosurgical procedure.

TABLE 15.8. Treating Anxiety Disorder

Disorder	Suggestions
Panic Disorder	
Mild	1. Relaxation and rebreathing training
	2. Refer for cognitive psychotherapy or focus your psychotherapy on patients' coping skills and cognitive strengths, as they fear loss of control in public and subsequent embarrassment
	3. If medication necessary, follow plan below for moderate panic
Moderate	1. Relaxation and rebreathing training
	2. Give an antidepressant listed in Table 15.6
	3. If response unsatisfactory, consider an MAOI or a non- or partially specific reuptake inhibitor–MAOI combination (nonspecific reuptake inhibitor/ MAOI combination introduced in that order, never the reverse, as that causes hypertensive crisis)
	4. Alprazolam or clonazepam can be used for the first 4–6 weeks until other treatments take effect; benzodiazepines more likely needed if SSRI used, less likely needed if non- or partially specific reuptake inhibitor used
Severe	1. Relaxation and rebreathing training
	2. Initially use alprazolam or clonazepam to control symptoms
	3. Introduce an antidepressant listed in Table 15.6; if good response, gradually taper and then stop benzodiazepine (e.g., alprazolam about 0.5 mg less each week)
	4. If response unsatisfactory, consider a reuptake inhibitor–MAOI combination
	5. If step 4 does not work, consider valproic acid

BENZODIAZEPINES

Pharmacodynamics

Benzodiazepines share some of the properties of barbiturates: addiction/habituation, seizure suppression (and withdrawal seizures after prolonged high dosage), and inhibition of spinal interneuronal transmission (muscle relaxation). Compared with barbiturates, however, benzodiazepines are less likely to suppress respiration and rapid eye movement sleep or induce hepatic enzymes. They have a wide margin of safety in the event of overdose.

Benzodiazepines have an affinity for benzodiazepine receptors (at least five different types). By binding to these receptors, benzodiazepines increase the ac-

TABLE 15.8. (*continued*)

Disorder	Suggestions
With depression	1. Begin with an antidepressant listed in Table 15.6
	2. If response unsatisfactory, consider an MAOI, or an nonspecific or partially specific reuptake inhibitor–MAOI combination
	3. When depression resolved, relaxation and rebreathing training
With patient with high abuse potential	1. Avoid benzodiazepines and substitute buspirone when appropriate
	2. Steps 1, 2, and 3 for moderate panic
Social Phobia/Agoraphobia/GAD	1. Relaxation and rebreathing training
	2. In vivo exposure to phobic problems accompanied by a "safe person"
	3. Systematic office and in vivo desensitization if phobias are very specific
	4. If mild, use beta-blockers or buspirone; if moderate, use antidepressants listed in Table 15.6; if severe, begin with alprazolam or clonazepam, and then introduce antidepressant
	5. If response unsatisfactory, consider a reuptake inhibitor–MAOI combination, and finally valproic acid
	6. If response still unsatisfactory, consider psychosurgery
Specific Phobia	1. Relaxation and rebreathing training
	2. In office and in vivo systematic desensitization
	3. Beta-blockers, buspirone, or alprazolam can be used during the treatment period if exposure to phobia likely, but drug is then tapered and discontinued when desensitization is complete

tions of GABA at $GABA_A$ receptors. Thus, benzodiazepines affect chloride channels (i.e., $GABA_A$/benzodiazepine receptor activity opens the channel and increases chloride conductance into the neuron, inhibiting firing).

Pharmacokinetics

Benzodiazepines have differential absorption rates from the gut. Diazepam and clorazepate are quickly absorbed, oxazepam and alprazolam are slowly absorbed, and the rest have intermediary rates of absorption. As a group, they are absorbed well, and other than in emergencies, when intravenous administration is needed,

TABLE 15.9. Long-Term Treatment of Anxiety Disorders

PHASE 1 (4–6 WEEKS)

Behavioral techniques learned; begin coverage with benzodiazepines

Antidepressant begun

Counseling and education

PHASE 2 (6 WEEKS TO 12 MONTHS)

Behavioral techniques monitored to ensure they are being done correctly and are helpful

Taper and then stop benzodiazepine by 3 months to avoid addiction*

Antidepressant (adjust dose)

Counseling; cognitive psychotherapy

PHASE 3 (OPEN-ENDED; AFTER FIRST YEAR)

If patient is asymptomatic for about 12 months, taper and then stop antidepressant†

If patient remains asymptomatic, discharge from treatment, reminding the patient he can always use behavioral techniques or return to treatment

If symptoms recur, begin medications and other treatments again

*Nevertheless, a patient who is addicted to a benzodiazepine but who is virtually asymptomatic and is functioning again is better off than a nonaddicted, nonfunctioning patient.

†Try to stop medication only with asymptomatic patients; the rest require continued treatment indefinitely.

use oral rather than intramuscular administration where absorption is poor. Lorazepam is an exception to this and is absorbed well intramuscularly. Serum levels do not correlate with clinical effect, and degrees of lipid solubility (extensive redistribution to fatty tissues) determines their duration of action. This redistribution roughly divides this class into three subgroups. Table 15.10 outlines these subgroups, some compounds in each, and the general properties of each. Regardless of duration of action, most benzodiazepines are biotransformed to desmethyldiazepam, an active metabolite with a very long (several days) half-life. Flurazepam has a long half-life by virtue of its conversion to the slowly excreted active metabolite desalkylflurazepam. In contrast, lorazepam and oxazepam are excreted unconjugated, or as the glucuronide, and have a half-life of 12–18 hours.

During dose adjustment, likely benzodiazepine side effects include sedation, headache, dizziness, and some problems with new learning. Once steady state of the therapeutic dose is reached, these effects usually resolve. At high doses a typical sedative-hypnotic intoxication (i.e., drunkenness) develops. Physiologic dependence also occurs, and detoxification is very difficult. You can taper the first 50%–75% of the patient's dose fairly easily over 4 weeks. The last 25%–50% usually takes months.

TABLE 15.10. Benzodiazepines

Subtype	Characteristics
Short-acting Triazolam (Halcion) Midazolam (Versed)	1. Used for sleep 2. Little antianxiety and no anticonvulsant properties 3. At higher doses, triazolam can cause prolonged altered consciousness without sedation
Intermediate-acting Alprazolam (Xanax) Lorazepam (Ativan) Oxazepam (Serax) Temazepam (Restoril) Clonazepam (Klonopin) Clorazepate (Tranxene)	1. Alprazolam and oxazepam are generally equivalent, with weak but broad-spectrum properties; alprazolam is used in the treatment of anxiety disorder, oxazepam is particularly safe for persons with liver disease 2. Lorazepam has significant antianxiety and anticonvulsant properties and is used to treat acute panic and catatonia and as a sedative to control agitation and violence 3. Temazepam is used primarily for sleep 4. Clonazepam is used as an anticonvulsant and for treating severe somnambulism or night terrors 5. Clorazepate has some antianxiety properties but little hypnotic or anticonvulsant properties
Long-acting Chlordiazepoxide (Librium) Diazepam (Valium) Flurazepam (Dalmane)	1. Chlordiazepoxide has only antianxiety properties and is used for alcohol withdrawal 2. Diazepam has significant antianxiety and hypnotic properties and some anticonvulsant properties and is used in ECT to stop post-ECT delirium, as a muscle relaxant, and in alcohol withdrawal 3. Flurazepam is used primarily for sleep

Benzodiazepines are widely used as hypnotics. Triazolam (0.125–0.250 mg), temazepam (10 mg), and flurazepam (15–30 mg) are short- and intermediate-acting drugs useful to treat insomnia, but for only short periods (less than 2 weeks) or intermittently. Dependence is the most serious concern in using these compounds for longer than 3–4 months. Acute anterograde amnesia can occur with benzodiazepines at prescribed doses, particularly with triazolam.

Benzodiazepines are also used to treat alcohol withdrawal. Diazepam and chlordiazepoxide are commony used because of their long half-lives. Diazepam also has anticonvulsant properties. Doses as high as 400–600 mg daily of chlordiazepoxide are used, with tapered withdrawal over 2 weeks. Side effects of benzodiazepines include drowsiness, ataxia, and slurred apeech. Addiction can occur with long-term use (>4 months), and obsessive compulsive behaviors, anxiety and agitation, seizures, and delirium can occur after abrupt withdrawal from long-term use.

Benzodiazepines are the treatment of choice for acute anxiety. Intravenous or oral administration is best. Substantial intravenous dosages may be needed (e.g., 15–20 mg of diazepam, 25–50 mg of chlordiazepoxide), but doses rarely have to be repeated in a single day because of the long half-life of most benzodiazepines. Treatment for more than 2 days is rarely needed, and the drug can be stopped abruptly. Long-term pharmacologic treatment for anxiety disorders is discussed above. Lorazepam is also a useful temporizing treatment for catatonia and a useful treatment for agitation in a newly admitted undiagnosed patient.

ADDITIONAL READINGS

American Psychiatric Association: Practice guideline for the treatment of patients with panic disorder. *Am J Psychiatry (Suppl)* 155:1–34, 1998.

Andrews G, Crino R: Behavioral psychotherapy of anxiety disorders. *Psychiatr Ann* 21:358–367, 1991.

Ballenger JC (ed): *Clinical Aspects of Panic Disorder, Frontiers of Clinical Neuroscience,* vol. 9. Wiley-Liss, New York, 1990.

Bell CJ, Nutt DJ: Serotonin and panic. *Br J Psychiatry* 172:465–471, 1998.

Braestrup C, Nielsen M: Neurotransmitters and CNS disease: Anxiety. *Lancet* 2:1030–1034, 1982.

Bridges PK, Bartlett JR, Hale AS, Poynton AM, Malizia AL, Hodgkiss AD: Psychosurgery: Stereotactic subcaudate tractotomy, an indispensable treatment. *Br J Psychiatry* 165:599–611, 1994.

Cassano GB, Rotondo A, Maser JD, Shear MK, Frank E, Mauri M, Dell'Osso L: The panic-agoraphobic spectrum: Rationale, assessment, and clinical usefulness. *CNS Spectrums* 3:35–48, 1998.

Crits-Christoph P: The factor structure of the cognitive-somatic anxiety questionnaire. *J Psychosom Res* 30:685–690, 1986.

den Boer JA, Ad Sitsen JM (eds): *Handbook of Depression and Anxiety, A Biological Approach.* Marcel Dekker, New York, 1994.

Eaton WW, Keyl PM: Risk factors for the onset of diagnostic interview schedule/DSM-III agoraphobia in a prospective population-based study. *Arch Gen Psychiatry* 47:819–824, 1990.

Eison MS: Serotonin: A common neurobiological substrate in anxiety and depression. *J Clin Psychopharmacol* 10 *(suppl* 3):26S–30S, 1990.

Frank E, Cassano GB, Shear MK, Rotondo A, Dell'Osso L, Mauri M, Maser J, Grochocinski V: The spectrum model: A more coherent approach to the complexity of psychiatric symptomatology. *CNS Spectrums* 3:23–34, 1998.

Gelder MG: Psychological treatment of agoraphobia. *Psychiatr Ann* 21:354–358, 1991.

Goisnan RM, Goldenberg I, Vasile RG, Keller MB: Comorbidity of anxiety disorders in a multicenter anxiety study. *Compr Psychiatry* 36:303–311, 1995.

Gray JA: *The Neuropsychology of Anxiety: An Enquiry into the Functions of the Septo-Hippocampal System.* Oxford University Press, Oxford, 1982.

Helzer JE, Robins LE, McEvoy L: Post-traumatic stress disorder in the general population: Findings of the epidemiologic catchment area survey. *N Engl J Med* 317:1630–1634, 1987.

Hoehn-Saric R, McLeod DR (eds): *Biology of Anxiety Disorders.* American Psychiatric Press, Washington, DC, 1993.

Jacob RG, Furman JM, Durrant JD, Turner SM: Panic, agoraphobia, and vestibular dysfunction. *Am J Psychiatry* 153:503–512, 1996.

Katon W: *Panic Disorder in the Medical Setting.* National Institute of Mental Health DHHS Pub No. (ADM) 89-1629. U.S. Government Printing Office, Washington, DC, 1989.

Keck PE Jr, McElroy SL, Friedman LM: Valproate and carbamazepine in the treatment of panic and post-traumatic stress disorders, withdrawal states, and behavioral dyscontrol syndromes. *J Clin Psychopharm 12 (Suppl 1)*:365S–415S, 1992.

Kendler KS, Neale ML, Kessler RC, Heath AC, Eaves LJ: Major depression and generalized anxiety disorder. Same genes (partly) different environments? *Arch Gen Psychiatry 49*:716–722, 1993.

Klass ET, Di Nardo PA, Barlow DH: DSM-III-R personality diagnoses in anxiety disorder patients. *Compr Psychiatr 30*:251–258, 1989.

Lepola U, Nousiainen U, Puranen M, Riekkinen P, Rimon R: EEG and CT findings in patients with panic disorder. *Biol Psychiatry 28*:721–727, 1990.

Londborg PD, Wolkow R, Smith WT, DuBoff E, England D, Ferguson J, Rosenthal M, Weise C: Sertraline in the treatment of panic disorder: A multi-site, double-blind, placebo-controlled, fixed-dose investigation. *Br J Psychiatry 173*:54–60, 1998.

Nivista C, Petracca A, Akiskal HS, Galli A, Gepponi I, Lassano GB: Delimitation of generalized anxiety disorder: Clinical comparisons with panic and major depression. *Compr Psychiatry 31*:409–415, 1990.

Noyes R Jr, Reich JH, Suelzer M, Christiansen J: Personality traits associated with panic disorder: Change associated with treatment. *Compr Psychiatry 32*:283–294, 1991.

O'Sullivan G, Marks I: Follow-up studies of behavioral treatment of phobic and obsessive compulsive neuroses. *Psychiatr Ann 21*:368–373, 1991.

Pitts FN Jr, McClure JN Jr: Lactate metabolism in anxiety neurosis. *N Engl J Med 277*:1329–1336, 1967.

Pollack MH, Otto MW, Rosenbaum JF, Sachs GS: Personality disorders in patients with panic disorder: Association with childhood anxiety disorders, early trauma, comorbidity, and chronicity. *Compr Psychiatry 33*:78–83, 1992.

Rainey JM Jr, Pohl RB, Williams M, Knitter E, Freedman RR, Ettedgui E: A comparison of lactate and isoproterenol anxiety states. *Psychopathology 17(suppl)*:74–82, 1994.

Skre I, Onstad S, Torgersen S, Lygren S, Kringlen E: A twin study of DSM-III-R anxiety disorders. *Acta Psychiatr Scand 88*:85–92, 1993.

Torgersen S: Genetic factors in anxiety disorders. *Arch Gen Psychiatry 40*:1085–1089, 1983.

Uhde TW, Kellner CH: Cerebral ventricular size in panic disorder. *J Affect Disord 12*:175–178, 1987.

Weilburg JB, Schachter S, Worth J, Pollack MH, Sachs GS, Ives JR, Schomer DL: EEG abnormalities in patients with atypical panic attacks. *J Clin Psychiatry 56*:358–362, 1995.

Welkowitz LA, Popp LA, Cloitre M, Liebowitz MR, Martin MS, Gorman JM: Cognitive-behavior therapy for panic disorder delivered by psychopharmacologically oriented clinicians. *J Nerv Ment Dis 179*:473–477, 1991.

Wright JH, Borden J: Cognitive therapy of depression and anxiety. *Psychiatr Ann 21*:424–428, 1991.

Wu JC, Buchsbaum MS, Hershey TG, Hazlett E, Sicotte N, Johnson JC: PET in generalized anxiety disorder. *Biol Psychiatry 29*:1181–1199, 1991.

16

Aches and Pains, Sex and Sleep, and Violence

Patients with behavioral disorders often complain of sleep problems, headache, and other aches and pains. Sexual dysfunction is a side effect of many psychotropic drugs, and sexual dysfunction is both a sign of disease (e.g., some frontal lobe and epileptic conditions) and a DSM category (e.g., paraphilia). Violence is also a feature of several behavioral syndromes, but may also be a primary behavioral pattern. Each of these topics could fill books, but are covered together here for brevity and because of their common diagnostic challenge: Do they represent a primary condition, or are they features of another disorder? Successful management hinges on knowing the answer to this question. Persistent complaints of headache, other aches and pains, and sleep problems also lead to suffers being labeled "cranks" or "hypochondriacs." Occasionally, however, these isolated complaints are caused by a debilitating condition. Table 16.1 provides an overview of this chapter, displaying some of the common associations between these complaints and diseases.

HEADACHES

Close to 70% of patients seeing primary care physicians cite headache as a major complaint, but only 1% of headaches relate to serious brain disease or dysfunction. Headaches you have to worry about are typically associated with (1) a patient under age 5 or over 50; (2) recent onset is nocturnal or during situations associated with increased intracranial pressure or increased blood pressure (coitus, sneezing, exercise, straining, coughing); (3) pain that is crescendo or thunderclap in nature (aneurysms); (4) pain that is localized (e.g., retro-orbital as with aneurysm), behind right ear (e.g., lung cancer), facial (e.g., posterior fossa tumors), unilateral (e.g., migraines); (5) features of an endocrinopathy (e.g., pituitary tumor); and (6) neurologic signs (e.g., unilateral weakness).

Among the elderly, common causes of headache are (1) cerebrovascular dis-

TABLE 16.1. Examples of Pain, Sex and Sleep Problems, and Violence, Representing Primary Conditions and Signs of Other Behavioral Disorders

Example	Primary Condition	Sign of Another Syndrome
Headache	Neurovascular (e.g., migraine), traction and inflammatory (e.g., tumor), and neuralgic (e.g., sinusitis) headache disorders	Anxiety disorders, depressions, somatization disorder, Cluster B and C personality disorder, side effect of many psychotropic and other prescription drugs
Pain	Primary pain disorder	Depression, stroke, somatization disorder, Cluster B and C personality disorder, multiple sclerosis
Sexual dysfunction*	Paraphilias, gender identity disorders, stress-related disorders of arousal	Depression, bipolar mood disorder, anxiety disorder, alcohol and substance abuse, side effects of many psychotropic and other prescription drugs, OCD, many general medical conditions, Cluster A, B, and C personality disorders, dementia, stroke, traumatic brain injury, epilepsy, venereal disease, white matter degenerative disease
Sleep problem	Sleep apnea, somnambulism, pavor nocturnus, narcolepsy, restless leg syndrome	All axis I conditions, many general medical conditions, side effect of many psychotropic and other prescription drugs, dementia, delirium, stroke
Violence	Predatory, intermale, sex related, territorial	Antisocial personality disorder, bipolar mood disorder, alcohol and substance abuse, traumatic brain disorder, psychotic disorders, epilepsy, depression

*Sexual arousal and aversion disorders are almost always secondary to another behavioral condition, a general medical problem, or a drug.

ease; (2) diseases of the head, neck, eyes, ears, and nose; (3) medication related; (4) general medical disease producing headache with malaise; (5) intracranial mass lesions; (6) temporal arteritis; and (7) trigeminal neuralgia.

Headaches can be classified as (1) neurovascular (migraine, tension, and cluster); (2) traction and inflammatory (due to infection, trauma, stroke, tumors); and (3) neuralgic, involving structures outside the cranial cavity such as joint, dental, sinus, and eye disorders.

Most headaches are benign. Those that are dull, described as "a pressure feeling," generalized, and constant for several consecutive days are rarely associated with brain disease. Those that begin suddenly, awaken the patient, or are unilateral are often associated with pathology.

CLINICAL PRESENTATION:
NEUROVASCULAR HEADACHES—MIGRAINE/TENSION HEADACHES

Seventeen percent of women and 6% of men in the United States have migraine. More than 11 million experience substantial disability, costing 10 billion dollars annually. Most sufferers, however, are neither diagnosed nor treated with prescription drugs. Onset is typically before puberty. Prevalence peaks between 35 and 40 years for women and somewhat earlier for men.

Tension headaches are more common in women, usually starting between ages 20 and 40. Tension headaches are characterized by a steady ache (not pulsating); bilateral pain; moderate intensity; no nausea, vomiting, and photo- or phonophobia; and are often associated with localized muscle tenderness. Nevertheless, about one third of patients also experience migraine-like features, and the pathophysiology of tension headache appears similar to that of migraine. Think of tension headache as a migraine variant and treat for migraine.

Migraine is a neurovascular reaction to internal (e.g., hormonal) and external (e.g. stress) stimuli that begins with an unstable trigeminovascular reflex affecting pain control pathways, resulting in excessive discharge in the spinal nucleus of the trigeminal nerve and its thalamic connections. This leads to midbrain and pontine failure to inhibit subthreshold afferent stimuli from cervical blood vessels that then results in cranial blood vessel changes causing migraine symptoms. Serotonin (5-HT) plays a role in migraine by its action on blood vessels (vasoconstriction) and on central pain pathways. Migraine's triad is episodic headaches with neurologic, gastrointestinal, and autonomic signs. Migraine has four phases.

The *prodrome*, occurring in 60% of migraineurs, may last for hours or days. Features include nonmelancholic depression with dysphoria, irritability, restlessness and hypoactivity, fatigue, drowsiness, photophobia, phonophobia, hyperosmia, stiff neck, feeling cold, sluggishness, increased thirst, urinary or fluid retention, anorexia or food craving, and diarrhea or constipation. Cortical (mostly one-sided) depression of neuronal firing rates spreading from a specific, initially excitatory focus is an explanation for the initiating prodrome.

The *aura*, occurring in 20% of sufferers, develops over 5–20 minutes and may last an hour. Symptoms reflect widespread intracranial vasoconstriction. Migraine auras are characterized by positive (scintillations, fortification spectra, photopsia) and negative (scotoma) visual phenomena. Fortification spectra (teichopsia) are common, consisting of arcs of scintillating light that form a herringbone pattern or geometric shape in one visual field. Numbness or tingling of one side of the face and upper extremity, hemiparesis, dysphagia, or aphasia also can occur. The aura can be associated with mood changes, depersonalization, and derealization and can mimic psychosensory seizures and transient ischemic attacks (TIAs). The aura of migraine is longer than that of epilepsy, and the post-aura EEG is nonepileptic. Patients with TIAs develop more prolonged disorientation. Intracranial vasoconstriction is followed by extracranial vasodilation and headache.

The *headache* is throbbing and unilateral, although it can begin bilaterally. It is aggravated by physical activity. Although it can occur any time, it most commonly occurs upon awakening in the morning. Headache onset is gradual, peaks, and then subsides, and it lasts from several hours to 2–3 days. Associated with the headache phase are anorexia, nausea and vomiting, and sensory hyperexcitability (photophobia, phonophobia, osmophobia). Sufferers seek a dark quiet room. Other features include blurred vision, nasal stuffiness, abdominal cramps and diarrhea, polyuria, facial pallor, hot or cold sensations, sweating, localized scalp, face, or periorbital edema, scalp tenderness, temple vein and artery prominence, and neck stiffness. Impaired concentration is common and is associated with non-melancholic, atypical, or brief depressions, fatigue, anxiety and irritability, light-headedness, and feeling faint.

The *postdrome* occurs gradually, with fatigue, irritability, apathy, impaired concentration, scalp tenderness, and mood changes. It may last for hours or days.

Diagnosis of the classic form requires at least five attacks without an aura or two attacks with an aura that last several hours to several days. Attacks longer than 3 days are termed *status migrainous*. The modal migraineur has one to three headaches monthly.

There are several migraine variants: ophthalmoplegic (or retinal), hemiplegic, basilar artery, and "confusional." Ophthalmoplegic migraine headache lasts for days or weeks, and there are eye signs that include extraocular paresis, ptosis, and oculomotor nerve pupillary changes and transient loss of visual acuity. Hemiplegic migraine is associated with transient (<1 hour) aphasia, inability to think clearly, and sudden hemiparesis. Basilar artery migraine is associated with vertigo, tinnitus, dysarthria, ataxia, unsteadiness, syncope, bilateral visual blurring, and parasthesias, all of which can last several hours. Confusional migraine, or "epileptic migraine," is associated with loss of consciousness or disorientation and sensorimotor abnormalities.

Migraine can be triggered by lack of sleep; alcohol; high tyramine foods; sudden weather changes; glare or prolonged exposure to flickering of computer screens, televisions, or fluorescent lights; premenstrual hormonal changes; pungent odors; and high altitude. Migraine is influenced by sex hormones, particularly estrogen. Migraine often (1) begins at menarche (33% of women patients), (2) exacerbates during phases of the menstrual cycle (14% have headaches exclusively during menses, and 60% have headaches at, just before, after, or during menses or at ovulation), (3) gets worse during the first trimester of pregnancy (75%) and remits during the last trimester, (4) changes in frequency and character during menstrual cycles or with oral contraceptives, and (5) exacerbates during postmenopausal estrogen replacement therapy. Migraine is associated with dysmenorrhea and fluctuations in estrogen levels. Estrogen modulates 5-HT, and progesterone is vasoactive (works on the hypothalamus by arterial spasm), and these relationships may explain estrogen's effect on migraine.

In addition to its association with epilepsy, migraine is also associated with mood disorder. Migraineurs are two to three times as likely as controls to suffer from nonmelancholic depression and bipolar spectrum disorders. Commonly, however, the anorexia, sleep disturbance, and demoralization of migraine are misdiagnosed as depression, and antidepressants are given rather than more specific migraine treatments. Atypical depressive features (e.g., fluctuating mood, episodes of days rather than weeks), no melancholic features, and complaints of "tension headaches" or frank migraine symptoms indicate that the mood disorder is secondary and migraine the most likely cause.

There is also an association between migraine and anxiety disorder, particularly panic disorder. Exaggerated fears associated with migraine triggers (e.g., situations in which alcohol is typically consumed) can be mistaken for a phobic disorder. If a patient with suspected anxiety disorder also complains of headache, first rule out migraine. Migraineurs are also at greater risk for stroke (migrainous infarction), and about 10% of strokes in people under age 50 are associated with migraine. Platelet hyperaggregation, common in migraine, may play a role, and prophylactic aspirin (one baby aspirin daily) may reduce the migraineur's risk for stroke. Pharmacotherapy focuses on acute headache relief and prophylaxis. Table 16.2 displays these treatments. Triggers of episodes should also be identified and avoided.

Acute migraine relief usually requires more than aspirin or acetaminophen, which have most likely already been tried with minimal success by these patients. Combining these analgesics and adding caffeine and a low dose (5–10 mg) of diazepam works for many patients. If these fail, sumatriptan (although expensive) subcutaneously or orally can bring relief in 70%–80% of patients within 1–2 hours, respectively. About 40% of patients need a second dose within 24 hours. Dizziness and drowsiness are the most common side effects. Ergot preparations are less effective, but are still used if sumatriptan's high cost per dose is a problem. Breathing pure oxygen (over 15–20 minutes) at the start of an aura (only helpful if aura is typically long) may abort some attacks.

For patients with menstrual migraine, treatments include nonsteroidal anti-inflammatories or ergotamine (both reduce neurogenic inflammation), perimenstrual use of standard migraine prophylactic drugs (see Table 16.2), and short courses of corticosteroids or dopamine agonists (e.g., bromocriptine). For migraine exacerbated by postmenopausal estrogen replacement, treatment includes reducing the dose, changing from the conjugated estrogen to pure estradiol or synthetic estrone, converting from interrupted to continuous dosing, converting from oral to parental dosing, or adding androgens.

Consider prophylaxis if (1) two or more attacks occur per month, with disability lasting three or more days per attack; (2) when symptomatic medications are contraindicated or ineffective; (3) when acute treatment is required twice weekly; or (4) if infrequent attacks are nevertheless intense and disabling. Preventative medication is based on side effect profile and co-occurring conditions, with the drug begun at a low dose and increased slowly. A full therapeutic trial takes 2–6 months.

Other antimigraine agents are dihydroergotamine (alpha-adrenergic blocker that vasoconstricts and helps about 70% of patients), metoclopramide (a nonphenothiazine central dopamine antagonist, antiemetic with analgesic properties used with nonsteroidal anti-inflammatories), ketorolac (a parenteral nonsteroidal and analgesic inhibitor of prostaglandin synthesis), and butorphanol tartrate (an opioid with mixed agonist and antagonist properties with lower abuse potential).

Co-morbid neuropsychiatric conditions must also be resolved to achieve successful migraine prophylaxis. Twenty to 30% of migraineurs develop major depression (mostly nonmelancholic). Nortriptyline is a safe antidepressant for migraine. Patients with anxious-fearful personality disorders may be helped by the addition of a specific serotonin reuptake inhibitor (SSRI). In addition to medication, biofeedback, and relaxation training, patients should avoid well-documented triggers: poor sleep habits, alcohol, high caffeine intake and caffeine withdrawal, bright flashing lights, foods high in monosodium glutamate, nitrites, and perhaps tyramine, and very cold food and drink, such as ice cream. Drugs that can trigger migraine include oral contraceptives, indomethacin, cimetidine, thyroid, and nitroglycerine.

CLINICAL PRESENTATION: CLUSTER HEADACHE

Symptoms

Cluster headaches take two forms, episodic and chronic. Episodic cluster affects 80% of sufferers. It is characterized by periods of 1–3 months of headaches followed by attack-free periods of 6 months to several years. In chronic cluster, remissions are always shorter than 1 year. Cluster headache is unilateral (typically retro-orbital), severe, and, in 85% of patients, always on the same side. About 85% of patients are men, and among men with cluster headache many are smokers and heavy drinkers. Head pain, ipsilateral autonomic features, and behavioral changes typify the attack.

Typical onset age is in the late 20s to early 30s. About 1% of the population is affected. Diagnosis requires at least five attacks of severe unilateral orbital, supra-orbital, or temporal pain lasting—if untreated—15 minutes to 3 hours (average 45 minutes) *and* with at least one of the following: conjunctival injection, lacrimation, nasal congestion, rhinorrhea, forehead and facial sweating, meiosis, ptosis, or eyelid edema. Often, there is a prodrome of fullness in the ears, dull discomfort at the base of the skull, moodiness, and irritability. This is followed by sudden incapacitating, stabbing, burning, throbbing, or boring pain and autonomic and neurologic signs. A typical attack peaks in about 30 minutes, during which the patient cannot sit still. As the attack wanes, dull pain replaces stabbing pain. Neck stiffness can occur, the scalp over the pain area feels sensitive, and the patient feels washed out and may sleep.

Attacks occur about twice daily, but can occur up to 10 or more times daily. Most often they occur during sleep (50%–75% of patients), usually at the first REM period about 90 minutes after sleep onset. Attacks can be provoked by even small amounts of alcohol, drugs with vasodilating properties, allergic reactions that release histamine, or high altitude. The cluster period lasts 2–4 months, is often cyclic (associated with diminishing or lengthening hours of daylight), and peaks during the 2 weeks after the longest and shortest days of the year. During remissions, there are no spontaneous attacks, and attacks cannot be provoked. In addition to sharing a similar pathophysiology with migraine, cluster headache is also believed to involve hypothalamic dysfunction that impairs circadian and autoregulatory functions such as chemoreceptor oxygen concentration.

TABLE 16.2. Migraine Treatments

Drug	Indications/Contraindications	Mechanism of Action/Comments
<div align="center">ACUTE MIGRAINE RELIEF</div>		
Aspirin	Effective for many patients combined with caffeine more than 60 mg per dose (as high as 200 mg)	1. Analgesia, mild anti-inflammatory effect 2. Blocks prostaglandin E synthesis, which increases norepinephrine release 3. Also reduces neurogenic inflammation
Nonsteroidal anti-inflammatory agents (e.g., acetaminophen, naproxen)	Effective in high doses (1,200 mg ibuprofen stat, naproxen sodium 550–775 mg stat)	Must be taken with food, as it can cause gastric distress
Caffeine adjuvant	Avoid if cluster headache suspected	
Combined acetaminophen or aspirin, metoclopramide, or diazepam		1. Analgesic, antiemetic, and anxiolytic effects 2. Frequent use (once or more weekly) or use for several days can cause rebound headaches and resistance to prophylactic treatment
Codeine	If milder analgesics fail, can add in limited supply (not recommended)	Analgesia
Ergotamine, dihydroergotamine, or isometheptene	1. Contraindicated with pregnancy, hypertension, renal or hepatic disease, cerebral and peripheral vascular disease 2. Used less than in the past; 3. Combination of 1 mg ergotamine and 100 mg caffeine (1–2 tablets) every 30 minutes; up to six doses can work	1. Vasoconstriction 2. Blocks transmission in unmyelinated C fibers and reduces neurogenic inflammation
Domperidone	1 mg TID daily for several days can block symptoms if taken during the earliest prodrome signs, but only for prodrome that lasts several days	A peripheral dopamine antagonist
Sumatriptan	Substantial relief within 10 minutes of headache	1. Serotonin agonist ($5HT_{1D}$) prevents vasodilation of

TABLE 16.2. (*continued*)

Drug	Indications/Contraindications	Mechanism of Action/Comments
	ACUTE MIGRAINE RELIEF (*continued*)	
	and other features (6 mg SC [rapidly absorbed, <20% protein bound, liver metabolized 2-hour half-life]); oral dose (100 mg) relief in 30–60 minutes	cranial blood vessels and thus release of inflammatory mediators; costs $75 per dose 2. Contraindicated in patients with ischemic heart disease, angina pectoris, angina variant, previous myocardial infarction, and uncontrolled hypertension or who took ergotamines in past 24 hours 3. Benefits 70%–80% of patients within 4 hours
Oxygen	100% at >7 L/min by mask, usually works in 15 minutes	Patient keeps a tank at home and in car or at work
	PROPHYLACTIC MIGRAINE RELIEF	
Propranolol, nadolol, timolol	1. Most commonly used migraine prophylaxis 2. Useful in patients with hypertension or angina, more risky in patients with asthma, depression, congestive heart failure, Raynaud's disease, or diabetes (propanolol 60–360 mg, timolol 20–30 mg, atenolol 25–100 mg)	1. Beta-adrenergic blockers may alter vasular reactivity 2. Side effects at high doses include fatigue, bradyphrenia, hypotension, dizziness (do not use in older patients), weight gain, nightmares
Nonspecific and partially specific antidepressants	1. Useful when depression, chronic pain syndrome, or panic disorder co-morbid 2. Doses (given at night time) are usually less than those for depression	Nortriptyline has fewest side effects for most patients; amitriptyline has best evidence supporting efficacy
Methysergide	1. Useful if aura present 2. More risky if patient has angina or peripheral vascular disease 3. Never a first-line treatment because of risks (rare) of pleural, retroperitoneal, and endocardial fibrosis 4. More common side effects are epigastric discomfort	Serotonin antagonist; over 60% of patients benefit

TABLE 16.2. Migraine Treatments (*continued*)

Drug	Indications/Contraindications	Mechanism of Action/Comments
	PROPHYLACTIC MIGRAINE RELIEF (*continued*)	
	and muscle cramps; started low (0.5 mg) and slowly increased to 1–2 mg TID for 4 months, followed by at lease a 1-month period before restarting to avoid severe risks above	
Verapamil	1. Useful if aura present or if patient has angina, hypertension, or asthma 2. 40 mg TID up to 480 mg daily 3. Benefits 70% of patients	1. Calcium channel blocker; not as effective as above treatments 2 Can prevent vasoconstriction 3. Diltiazem (30–120 mg TID) may also work 4. Constipation and fluid retention most common side effects 5. Do not use if patient has heart disease
Valproate	1. Particularly useful if migraine co-occurs with epilepsy, panic disorder, or bipolar spectrum, but can be used for pure migraine 2. 500–1,000 mg daily	50%–65% of patients respond with 50% reduction at daily doses of 1,000–1,500 mg and blood levels between 70 and 120 mg/l

Differential Diagnosis

Cluster headache differs from migraine in that cluster attacks are (1) shorter, (2) always unilateral, (3) occur daily or several times daily, and (4) are not usually accompanied by nausea or vomiting. In contrast, the headache of *temporal arteritis* is persistent, and usually unilateral, burning, and throbbing. It is intensified by chewing, and may show point tenderness over a tortuous temporal artery. Patients with cluster and migraine headaches typically have had headaches for years. Patients with temporal arteritis more commonly develop their headaches later in life (after age 50), and the headache is perceived as different from past headaches.

Paroxysmal hemicrania resembles cluster headache in intensity, location, quality of pain, and autonomic symptomatology. Paroxysmal hemicrania differs from cluster headache by a 2–10-fold increased frequency of attacks, shorter duration of pain (several minutes), and complete dramatic response to indomethacin 200 mg daily for the acute attack and 25–100 mg daily for prophylaxis.

The episodic nature of cluster headache and the moodiness and irritability associated with the cluster prodrome can lead to misdiagnosis as primary depression or soft bipolar disorder, and mood stabilizers can help these patients (see below). Mood episodes, however, are almost always atypical, signaling a likely secondary condition.

Treatment

Sumatriptan, a serotonin agonist used for migraine, also aborts acute cluster attacks with relief in about 10 minutes in 75% of patients receiving 6 mg subcutaneously. Oxygen inhalation with the patient seated upright or leaning forward also aborts an attack safely and rapidly in 75% of patients. Prophylactic treatments include ergotamine, verapamil, lithium, prednisone, and methysergide. Prednisone 40–80 mg daily tapered over 3–4 weeks benefits 80% of patients and is often recommended as the first choice drug for patients whose clusters last less than 3–4 weeks. Verapamil 360–480 mg/day gives substantial relief to 70% of patients with both chronic and episodic forms. Lithium, in the same doses and with the same precautions as for mood disorders, is a good choice for the chronic form. Methysergide is rarely used because of its side effect of pleuropulmonary fibrosis. For older patients, verapamil 80 mg QID and ergotamine 2 mg 1 hour before bedtime is often used. Response rates are between 60% and 85%. Incomplete response to the verapamil–ergotamine combination can be enhanced with lithium 300 mg BID.

CLINICAL PRESENTATIONS: TRACTION AND INFLAMMATORY HEADACHE

Traction and inflammatory headaches result from distention, displacement, or inflammation of pain-sensitive structures (blood vessels and meninges) of the head. Brain masses (e.g., hematomas, abscesses, tumors), edema, and inflammations (e.g., meningitis, encephalitis, and intra- or extracranial arteritis or phlebitis) produce these headaches. Table 16.3 lists some common causes and characteristics of traction and inflammatory headaches.

Because the incidence of *brain tumor* is on the rise (peak age 40–60 years) and now annually effects 18,000 persons in the United States (almost as many as ovarian cancer), more than ever before you need to consider this as a cause of headache and neuropsychiatric disorder. In adults, 70% of brain tumors are supratentorial. In children (15%–20% of tumor patients), 70% of brain tumors are infratentorial. Table 16.4 lists some types of brain tumor. Common symptoms include headache (65% of patients, often retro-orbital, and due to increased intracranial pressure), visual signs (30%, visual blurring, diplopia, visual field defects), cranial nerve signs (IIIrd, IVth, and VIth nerves), seizures (30%), cognitive deficits and personality change (15%), and nausea and vomiting (10%). In children and young teens progressive headache associated with vomiting is a common presentation; in adults personality change is a common presentation. Ominous signs are impaired neurologic function with increased intracranial pressure signs in a person over age 40. Tumors involving ventral frontal cortex or temporoparietal cortex are more likely associated with abnormal mood states (anxiety, depression, irritability). Right-sided tumors may be slightly more likely to be involved. Mag-

TABLE 16.3. Common Causes of Traction and Inflammatory Headaches

Cause	Characteristics
Hypertension	1. Usually occipital, nagging, or throbbing, starting in the morning, diminishing when the patient is fully awake and standing
	2. Drowsiness and transient episodes of blurred vision can occur.
Transient ischemic attacks (TIAs)	1. Headaches during or immediately after an attack occur in 40% of TIAs, particularly vertebrobasilar (occipital)
	2. Carotid TIAs cause unilateral frontal headaches and transient neurologic signs (e.g., aphasia, paresis)
Aneurysm	1. Before rupture, headache or extraocular paresis due to oculomotor nerve compression, whereas rupture headache is felt in the eye or frontal area and may be associated with meiosis, ptosis, decreased vision, and neck bruit
	2. Subarachnoid hemorrhage, mostly due to a ruptured aneurysm in the posterior communicating artery, can produce thunderclap headache, orbital pain different from previous headaches within 1 week of rupture, meningismus, cranial nerve signs (IIIrd, IVth, Vth), nausea, vomiting
	3. Associated with heavy drinking
	4. 30%–45% mortality, 30% recover
Mass lesion (e.g., hemorrhage; brain tumor)	1. Headache due to increased intracranial pressure, and ipsilateral unilateral headache can occur with large lesions
	2. Headache due to brain tumor in onset and anatomic distribution typically similar to tension headaches, but so severe that the patient seeks medical care within 1–2 weeks
	3. Arteriovenous malformations mimic migraine and cluster
	4. Spontaneous cranial artery dissection (usually external or internal carotid) causes unilateral, focal nonthrobbing headache with meningismus, transient neurologic signs, bruits, and visual scintillations
Inflammation (cranial arteritis, infection, lupus erythematosis)	1. Severe and throbbing, lying flat may worsen pain, and meningeal signs may occur
	2. Polyarteritis nodosa involves multiple organ systems, so look for pathology outside central nervous system

TABLE 16.4. Common Brain Tumors

Type	Characteristics
Glioma (40%–60%)*	1. Astrocytomas and glioblastoma multiform most common
	2. Medulloblastoma tumor of childhood in the cerebellum
	3. Slow-growing forms in adults (e.g., benign astrocytoma) can cause psychoses (e.g., delusional disorder) or personality change
Meningioma (15%)	1. Slow-growing and encapsulated
	2. When near frontal lobe poles can cause manic depressive-like psychosis, which after many episodes (as tumor grows) results in frontal lobe dementia
Pituitary adenoma (5%–10%)	1. Endocrine active type (most common) produces typical endocrinopathy features
	2. Endocrine inactive type can produce intracranial mass effects and atypical mood disorders
Schwannoma (5%)	1. Often located at cerebellopontine angle
	2. No clear behavioral effects
Metastatic (30%)	1. Often multiple sites, and often in cerebral hemispheres
	2. Common sources are lung (50%), breast (15%), gastrointestinal tract (8%), genitourinary tract (6%), melanoma (6%)
	3. The brain receives 20% of blood flow from the heart and has an end-artery vascular pattern that traps cancer cells, leading to metastic deposit

*Percentages of total documented brain tumor patients combined from various surveys, so figures add up to over 100.

netic resonance imaging (MRI), computed tomography (CT) scan, and angiography are the best laboratory aids for identifying brain tumors.

CLINICAL PRESENTATIONS: CRANIAL NEURALGIAS

Cranial neuralgias include trigeminal and glossopharyngeal neuralgias, temporomandibular joint syndrome (TMJ), postherpetic neuralgia, and atypical neuralgias. Other headache causes include cervical osteoarthritis, eye pathology or visual acuity problems, dental pathology, and sinusitis.

Trigeminal neuralgia usually starts after age 50 and is twice as common in women. Onset before age 50, particularly in the 20s, suggests multiple sclerosis. Pain affects the face above the upper lip, is sharp and severe, and occurs in 20–30 second bursts. *Glossopharyngeal neuralgia* produces pain in the ear, tonsils, and pharynx and is triggered by swallowing, yawning, or eating. Carbamazepine is the treatment of choice for both, at doses below those for epilepsy.

TMJ is overdiagnosed. It is characterized by focal, usually unilateral facial pain in front of and behind the ear, muscle tenderness, TMJ crepitus, and limited jaw motion. Analgesics, muscle relaxants, and a bite plate usually relieve the pain.

Postherpetic neuralgia from herpes zoster infection may involve the gasserian ganglion of the ophthalmic division of the trigeminal nerve. Pain in the upper third of the face is unilateral, steady, burning, and aching and can interrupt sleep. Amantadine and analgesics are first-line treatments.

Atypical neuralgias are characterized by continuous steady aching with localized tenderness in various head locations. It may be associated with sweating, flushing, rhinitis, and pallor.

PAIN DISORDER

The DSM defines pain disorder as chronic pain in one or more sites that cannot be fully explained by a general medical or traditional neurologic condition. Pain syndromes are common, more so in women, peak in onset in the 30s and 40s, and are more frequent among blue-collar workers. Chronic pain disorders run in families. Nonmelancholic depressions, anxiety disorders, and substance abuse are also more common in the families of pain disorder patients.

The DSM pain disorder category represents a heterogeneous group of patients. Assessing the patient's prepain disorder personality helps discriminate subgroups tending to respond to certain treatments. The age of onset of the disorder may also help. Table 16.5 lists some patterns and their diagnostic and treatment implications. Analgesics, sedatives, and benzodiazepines usually do not help and may lead to dependence. Antidepressants are the most effective agents available.

TABLE 16.5. Pattern of Pain Disorder Patients

Characteristic	Diagnostic Implication	Treatment Implication(s)
Onset before puberty	Nonmelancholic depression	Antidepressant
Onset after age 60 years	Neurologic disease	Specific neurologic disease may respond to specific treatment
Anxious-fearful prepain personality disorder	Anxiety disorder, depression	Antidepressants, particularly SSRIs
Histrionic–high novelty seeking prepain personality disorder	Somatization disorder, substance abuse, antisocial behaviors	Comprehensive pain management program offers the best chance for improvement
Normal prepain personality	Idiopathic pain disorder	Antidepressants (nonspecific reuptake inhibitors may work the best if side effects can be tolerated)

Before attributing chronic pain to co-morbid behavioral syndromes, review the patient's medical records and do a detailed neurologic sensory system examination (pin prick and temperature perception are almost always impaired in neuropathic pain). Often, this modest reappraisal reveals the cause.

Neuropathic pain is likely with any of the following: (1) the pain has unusual referral patterns (e.g., unilateral to midline) and is associated with *allodynia* (pain from a non-noxious stimulus such as light stroking, a cold object) or *hyperalgesia* (exaggerated pain from a noxious stimulus such as a pick prick) and is exacerbated by emotion; (2) the pain is described as constant, burning, cramping, freezing, spasmodic, squeezing, electric, or jabbing; (3) the pain is exacerbated by activity, the wearing of certain clothing, and at certain times of the day (usually bedtime); (4) there is associated gait, coordination, or motor function problems suggestive of regional myofascial dysfunction from injury, disease, or a central lesion; (5) there are asymmetries in skin temperature, coloration, sweating patterns, hair and nail growth, edema or atrophy, weakness, or tremor; and (6) joint manipulation reproduces the patient's pain complaints (think of nerve entrapment).

Ninety percent of pain from central disease is due to stroke (8% of all stroke patients), and 78% of pain-producing strokes are supratentorial. Pain typically develops as motor and sensory losses improve. Although any stroke can cause a pain syndrome, strokes most likely to do so involve the lateral posterior thalamus or the parietal lobes. These strokes are often difficult to detect because mild hemiplegia (without spasticity) may be the only motor feature. Look for superficial hemianesthesia or hyperanesthesia, impaired deep sensation, mild hemiataxia (from proprioceptive problems), mild astereognosis, choreoathetosis, and sharp pain on the weak side. Among multiple sclerosis patients, 43% develop central pain syndromes due to spinal cord plaques. Other causes of central pain are spinal cord injury or disease, brain tumors, penetrating traumatic brain injury, epilepsy (parietal lobe focus), Parkinson's disease, and motor neuron disease.

Peripheral neuropathic pain may, after several years, lead to central nervous system cellular and gene expression changes. Receptive fields may be reorganized, changing the modulation of sensory perception, which in time enhances and maintains the perception of pain even after the peripheral pathology is corrected. Peripheral neuropathic pain can result from diabetes mellitus, alcohol abuse, HIV infection, hypothyroidism, vitamin deficiencies, anemia, trauma, vasculitis, and postherpetic neuralgia.

Patients with suspected neuropathic pain are best treated in pain programs where multiple treatment modalities are available. Nonspecific and partially specific monoamine reuptake-inhibiting antidepressants in doses typical for depression and carbamazepine can help even nondepressed patients.

SEXUAL DEVIATIONS

Sexually deviant behavior, recognized for centuries as characteristic of several medical conditions, remains stigmatized by legal codes of behavior and religious and social tradition. Some sexual behaviors considered medically normal (e.g., oral sex) remain criminal offenses in some parts of the United States. Homosexuality, traditionally viewed as a sexual deviation requiring treatment, was eventually dropped as a DSM diagnostic category. Homosexuality is likely a biologic variation with strong heritability that results in nonpathologic deviations in sexually dimorphic structures (e.g., the brains of male homosexuals are less masculinized).

The DSM has three categories of sexual deviation: (1) *sexual dysfunctions* (disturbances in arousal and performance), (2) *paraphilias* (inappropriate or dangerous sexual behaviors), and (3) *gender identity disorders* (classified among the childhood or adolescent onset conditions).

SEXUAL DYSFUNCTIONS

Sexual dysfunctions include disorders of *desire* (hypo or hyper, sexual aversion), arousal (female sexual arousal disorder, male erectile disorder), orgasm (inhibited female and male orgasm, premature ejaculation), and pain (dyspareunia, vaginismus, atypical [not otherwise specified]). This category is based on the idea that the sexual cycle can be divided into four phases: appetitive (fantasy and desire, libido), excitement (arousal), orgasm, and resolution.

Hyposexuality

Decreased sexual drive is common in neuropsychiatric disorders. It is typically observed in melancholia, schizophrenia with blunted affect, chronic psychosis, temporal lobe and other psychosensory epilepsies, hypothalamic and pituitary lesions,* alcohol and drug abuse, various endocrinopathies (particularly hypothyroidism, testosterone deficiency, diabetes), and many chronic general medical illnesses (e.g., heart, liver, kidneys).

Psychopharmacologic agents (commonly those with anticholinergic properties and SSRIs) also can impair sexual function. Table 16.6 lists some of the many drugs that cause sexual dysfunction. Hyposexuality is also fairly common in persons without psychiatric diagnosis, occurring in over 10% of adults of both genders. Some of this hyposexuality is related to stressful situations, while some may also result from personality trait patterns.

Hypersexuality

In neuropsychiatric clinical settings increased sexual arousal and activity is most commonly associated with mania. Frontal lobe lateral orbital lesions also cause inappropriate and increased sexual behavior. In primary mania and frontal lobe

---

* Most hypothalamic-pituitary disorders result in hyposexuality. Most common conditions are craniopharyngiomas, acromegaly, and pituitary adenoma (particularly when suprasellar), pituitary atrophy, or empty sella. Most become symptomatic between ages 16 and 35 years, and loss of libido may be the first sign. Look for visual disturbances (late), headache (late), features of acromegaly, and, in women, galactorrhea, menstrual irregularities and amenorrhea, and pain during coitus due to poor lubrication. Ten percent will have hyperprolactinemia.

TABLE 16.6. Some Drugs That Cause Sexual Dysfunction

ANTIHYPERTENSIVES* (MOST COMMON OFFENDERS)

Peripheral sympatholytics (quanadrel [Hydorel]): Impotence, ejaculatory failure

Centrally acting sympatholytics (clonidine [Catapres], methyldopa [Aldomet]): Loss of libido and impotence

Beta-blockers (propranolol [Inderal]): Loss of libido, impotence

PSYCHOTROPICS (NEXT MOST COMMON OFFENDERS)

Antidepressants: All types may cause loss of libido, impotence, delayed or difficult ejaculation, or anorgasmia, depending on the class of drug (see Chapter 7)

Antipsychotics: May cause loss of libido, impotence and ejaculatory problems; the more anticholinergic and D$_2$ tubulofundibular effects, the more likely are the sexual side effects (see Chapter 9); clozapine can cause priapism

Antianxiety agents: May cause delayed or no ejaculation or reduced libido, impotence (barbiturates, benzodiazepines); buspirone may cause priapism

Mood stabilizers: Can cause impotence and decreased libido (carbamazepine, lithium)

Stimulants and dopaminergic agents: May cause impotence (levodopa, methyldopa) or priapism (cocaine); bromocriptine may cause impotence and painful clitoral tumescence

OTHERS

Antacids may cause impotence and decreased libido (cimetidine [Tagamet], famotidine [Pepcid], ranitidine [Zantac])

Anti-inflammatories may cause impotence, ejaculatory failure (naproxen [Naprosyn])

---

*Angiotensin-converting enzyme and calcium channel blockers also can cause sexual dysfunction but are less likely.

dysinhibition syndromes, inappropriate verbal sexual behavior is most common (sexual jokes, solicitations of sexual activity), followed by attempts to fondle people or public masturbation. Actual copulation is uncommon, and planned sexual attacks are rare. Hypersexuality is also associated with seizure disorder, particularly post-ictally to a psychosensory fit from a temporal lobe focus. Other conditions associated with hypersexuality include the Kleine-Levin syndrome (hypothalamic dysfunction associated with periodic somnolence, hyperphagia, and hypersexuality) and the Kluver-Bucy syndrome.

Satyriasis (males) and *nymphomania* (females), not official diagnoses, most likely represent personality disorder or obsessive compulsive disorder (OCD) variants. However, when these behaviors begin abruptly in contrast to past behavior, or for the first time after age 35, look for neurologic disease.

Sexual aversion disorder is characterized by a persistent and recurrent aversion to sexual activity and avoidance of genital contact that is not due to other axis I conditions such as OCD, phobia, or depression. If you can eliminate these disorders as possibilities, and the sexual aversion is long standing, a personality disorder (Cluster B) is the most likely diagnosis.

Disorders of sexual arousal are fairly common, affecting 20% of all married men and 30% of married women during their life. Premature ejaculation is also common (30% of married men). Pain during sexual intercourse (*dyspareunia*) and painful vaginal contractions preventing or disrupting copulation (*vaginismus*) are less frequent. Once general medical and brain disease etiologies are eliminated (e.g., endocrinopathies, peripheral vascular disease, spinal cord disease, syphilis, multiple sclerosis, chronic renal or liver disease), most persons with these conditions will have a personality disorder or, anxiety disorder, or be under stress. *Impotence* also results from general medical disease (75% of cases most commonly resulting from diabetes), as well as anxiety disorder and substance abuse.

Paraphilias

Paraphilias include exhibitionism, fetishism, sadism, masochism, transvestism, voyeurism, pedophilia, and many others. These disorders are defined as recurrent, intense sexual urges or fantasies involving nonhumans, inanimate objects, children or other nonconsenting persons (rape is not included in DSM), or the suffering or humiliation of oneself or of others. The prevalence of paraphilias is unclear, but 3%–6% of the U.S. population may be affected. Most paraphilias develop during adolescence, and almost all occur in males. Most paraphiliacs are heterosexual.

When a paraphilia develops after age 35, suspect brain disease. Exhibitionism (particularly automatic disrobing), public or uncontrollable masturbation, and coital movements can occur during seizures. Temporal lobe epilepsy has been associated with ictal and interictal fetishism and transvestism and, in rarer instances, voyeurism, exhibitionism, sadism, masochism, pedophilia, frotteurism (rubbing against others), and genital self-mutilation. Postencephalic parkinsonism, frontal lobe lesions, and early Huntington's disease are also associated (though rarely) with paraphilia. Abnormal EEGs, cognitive dysfunction, abnormal cerebral blood flow and structure, and endocrine abnormalities have also been observed in individuals arrested for sexually related crimes. Gilles de la Tourette's syndrome and OCD are also, though rarely, associated with inappropriate sexual behavior, and some paraphilias may be variants of OCD.

Patients with borderline personality disorder also have an increased prevalence of paraphilias. Antisocial personality is more commonly associated with inappropriate, particularly aggressive and criminal, sexual behavior. Other persons with paraphilia have personality traits characterized by low cooperativeness, low reward dependence, and high harm avoidance. They are impulsive, hostile, have little warmth, and are prone to low grade nonmelancholic depression.

Gender Identity Disorders

DSM identifies four gender identity disorders: (1) gender identity disorder of childhood, (2) of adolescent or adult onset, (3) transsexualism, and (4) gender identity disorder not otherwise specified. Little is known about these conditions. Transsexualism has received the most media coverage because of the dramatic gender-change surgery associated with this condition, whereas transvestitism involves only cross-dressing.

Transsexualism entails a persistent discomfort and sense of inappropriateness about one's apparent gender (e.g., "I'm a woman in a man's body") and a persistent preoccupation with removing one's primary and secondary sex characteristics and acquiring the sex characteristics of the other gender. The DSM divides transsexualists into asexual, homosexual, and heterosexual subtypes. However, persons progressing from transvestitism to transsexualism are often bisexual and have gender dysphoria. They also have a history of childhood gender nonconformity behavior (e.g., a boy who ignores rough and tumble games, sports, and so forth, and prefers more traditional feminine role playing games). About 70% of transsexuals who undergo surgery are pleased with the outcome.

Transvestitism differs from transsexualism. The transvestite, almost always male, is typically heterosexual and initially cross-dresses to achieve sexual gratification (excitement and orgasm) but who in later life may cross-dress to relieve stress. Brain dysfunction has never been demonstrated in transvestites, and neurologic disease is usually not associated with it. Transvestites, however, typically have a low libido and a personality characterized by high novelty seeking and being less traditional and may meet criteria for a Cluster B personality disorder.

Differential Diagnosis

The basic steps in diagnosing sexual deviations are relatively straightforward. Usually the deviant behavior is clearly described, and so most often the issue is not the label, but the cause. In all cases, first make certain that the patient does not have a general medical or neurologic illness that explains the sexual deviation. If you find such a condition, it should be the focus of treatment. If no general medical or neurologic disorder is likely to explain the sexual deviation, then search for an axis I (particularly anxiety disorder and OCD) and an axis II (particularly antisocial personality) diagnosis. If you find an axis I diagnosis, it should be the focus of treatment. If you find a personality disorder as the only co-occurring condition, or no other DSM diagnosis is likely, focus treatment directly on the sexual deviation.

Treatment

One approach to the understanding of sexual deviation is that those that are compulsive in form are variants of OCD. A second view of sexual deviation applies an addiction model. Both of these views require significant scientific validation. Nevertheless, they are clinically helpful as they provide guidance for treatment.

Treatment Steps Based on Assumed Etiology

1. If you can identify a general medical or neurologic illness, treat the sexual dysfunction as if causally related to that condition. Thus, treating the general medical or neurologic disease should resolve the deviant sexual behavior.

2. If the sexual deviation remains despite successful treatment of the general medical or neurologic condition, or if there is no evidence of these, consider OCD or addiction as possible causes, and then treat for one or the other. In most cases this treatment will include pharmacotherapy and behavioral therapy.
3. If neither OCD nor an addiction seems the likely explanation for the sexual deviation, pharmacotherapy and behavioral therapy will still be the focus of management. These are best done, however, by specialists in sexual disorders. Behavioral approaches will involve the use of relaxation exercises and systematic desensitization. Additional techniques include vaginal dilators for vaginismus and local anesthetics for premature ejaculation. Treatments for hypo- or hypersexuality usually focus on couples. Seventy percent or more of patients completing a course of treatment significantly improve.

Paraphilias are more difficult to treat, but are also managed with behavioral and cognitive techniques, as well as social skills training. Aversive behavior therapy linking apomorphine-induced vomiting or a faradic shock to the paraphillic object or situation or to cross-dressing stimuli may reduce these behaviors, although results are mixed.

Triptorelin, a long-acting agonist analogue of gonadotropin-releasing hormone, given 3.75 mg IM monthly can substantially reduce paraphillic behaviors. Hot flashes, decreased facial and body hair, muscle tenderness, and injection site tenderness are common side effects. Because triptorelin may initially increase testosterone levels, increasing arousal, an antiandrogenic agent may be needed for the first month until testosterone levels drop. As osteoporosis may also occur, patients also receive supplementary calcium (carbonate is best absorbed, and citrate has less risk of renal stones) and vitamin D.

Antiandrogenic libido suppressants (synthetic progesterone) are also used to treat paraphiliacs. *Cyproterone acetate* (androcur) is a potent compound that blocks androgens at receptor sites, including those in the brain. Blocking reduces circulating testosterone and gonadotrophin. In the motivated patient, lower testosterone levels result in reduced sexual drive and reduced deviant sexual behavior. However, although testosterone blood levels need to be below 250 mg%, the correlation between blood level and therapeutic effect is only modest. Therapeutic doses are 100–500 mg orally/day or 100–500 mg depot/week. Side effects include reversible gynecomastia (20%) and infertility. Liver damage and thromboembolic disorders may also occur in an unknown but small percentage of patients.

Medroxyprogesterone acetate is another widely used agent for libido suppression that interferes with testosterone synthesis and target organ receptors. Depot doses are 400–600 mg/week. Side effects include hypertension, fatigue, edema, increased appetite and weight gain, and insomnia. Liver damage and thromboembolic disorders may also occur. Antiandrogenic agents may also decrease glucose tolerance, and treatment with either may result in depression. The nature of the depression is unclear. Reportedly, 40%–80% of patients have a significant benefit from treatment.

Surgery for sex offenders is the last resort. Castration has been done, but is not generally considered ethical. The effectiveness of stereotaxic hypothalamotomy is unproven. Other treatment strategies include (1) oral and implantable estrogens (side effects limit this approach) and (2) use of serotonergic-related agents, including SSRIs and buspirone (unclear if the paraphiliacs so treated had OCD or anxiety or mood disorder).

SLEEP DISORDERS

Sleep disorders include syndromes related to excessive daytime sleepiness (narcolepsy, sleep apnea), insomnias, and the parasomnias (somnambulism, night terrors).

CLINICAL PRESENTATION: EXCESSIVE DAYTIME SLEEPINESS

Excessive daytime sleepiness is common in the elderly. When onset occurs in younger people it may result from intense exertion at work or sports, environmental stress that causes poor or little nighttime sleep, the abuse of drugs or alcohol, or central nervous system or respiratory dysfunction.

Narcolepsy is characterized by unwanted sleep episodes, cataplexy, sleep paralysis, and hypnagogic hallucinations (vague, usually visual hallucinations experienced upon falling asleep). It affects 0.5% of the population, most often males, usually begins after puberty and before age 50, is probably heritable, and may be associated with histocompatibility complex antigen HLA-DR2, linking it in some cases to the short arm of chromosome 6. Because of their excessive and inopportune napping, narcoleptics may experience work, memory, and marital problems and accidents. Narcolepsy is a disorder of inopportune rapid eye movement (REM) sleep. Unwanted episodes of REM sleep (15–60 minutes) occur several times daily for 15–60 minutes; they are the only feature in about 25% of patients.

Associated *cataplexy* (sudden loss of muscle tone) can be mild or serious enough to cause falls and is often triggered by strong moods like laughter or crying. Cataplexy is the ambulatory equivalent of *sleep paralysis*, which is associated with a REM sleep episode partially intruding into wakefulness and lasting several minutes. Although frightening, sleep paralysis is benign. Hypnagogic (while falling asleep) and hypnopompic (while awakening) hallucinations and automatisms experienced by narcoleptics, although disturbing, should not be treated with neuroleptics. They resolve with the control of the narcolepsy with antidepressants and stimulants in doses used for anxiety disorders and dysthymias.

CLINICAL PRESENTATION: SLEEP APNEA

Obstructive sleep apnea affects 2%–4% of middle-aged men and 1%–2% of middle-aged women, causing excessive daytime sleepiness, fatigue, morning headaches, sexual dysfunction, impaired concentration and increased risks for traffic accidents, hypertension (60%), ischemic heart disease, and stroke. Interpersonal and job function can be affected because of cognitive problems and patients being misperceived as lazy or even demented. Obstructive sleep apnea may produce chronic hypoxia that results in personality changes, some patients becoming irritable and suspicious.

Obstructive sleep apnea is associated with some collapse of the pharyngeal airway leading to increased respiratory effort and snoring, some arousal and then sleep disturbance, hypertension, and the daytime problems listed above. Obesity, hypothyroidism, and alcohol or sedative use increase the risk for obstructive sleep apnea. The apnea need not be complete, however, and any substantial increase in upper airway resistance can cause the syndrome. During the full apnea, pulmonary and systemic arterial pressures rise, straining the heart, particularly its right side. The resulting bradycardia and hypoxemia (% saturation can range from the mid-80s to the high 60s) can lead to arrhythmias during sleep. The classic picture is of a thick-necked, large jowled man who dozes during the day and snores loudly at night. Confirming the diagnosis requires a one-night sleep laboratory study.

Treatments include weight loss; avoiding benzodiazepines, opiates, and alcohol; and, if the apnea is more severe, nasal continuous positive airway pressure. In severe cases, surgical correction of the airway (deviated nasal septum repair, removal of enlarged tonsils, tracheostomy) may be needed.

Central sleep apnea is more common in children. Caused by reduced medullary respiratory center responsivity to build up of carbon dioxide, it can result in sudden infant crib death. Most often, the child awakens in the morning with cyanosis that clears gradually by mid-day. Sleep laboratory testing documents the condition. In adults with central sleep apnea look for congestive heart failure, encephalitis, brain stem tumor or stroke, diabetes mellitus, or hypothyroidism. Patients complain of insomnia, frequent awakenings, morning headaches, and decreased libido. Snoring is less prominent than with obstructive sleep apnea, and atypical depression is a more likely co-morbidity. Treating the apnea usually resolves the depression. Treatment consists of theophylline, which increases respiratory center responsivity to carbon dioxide; or, if the patient is an infant, sleeping on the back and applying a chest-strap buzzer that rings if breathing stops, signaling the nurse or a parent to awaken the child immediately. Pediatric sleep specialists usually care for these patients.

Somnambulism (sleep walking) and *pavor nocturnus* (night terrors) occur in 15% and 6% of children, respectively. Each also occurs in about 1% of adults. Among persons with these conditions the risk is also higher for OCD and tic disorders. Somnambulism results from a disturbance in stage 4 sleep (deep sleep). The patient (amnestic for the event) rises from bed, walks, avoiding some obstacles, is unresponsive, and then returns to bed. Serious injury can occur. Treatment includes low doses of short- or intermediate-acting benzodiazepines for 6 months, protection from harmful objects, locking doors and windows, and patient and family education. Once the patient is asymptomatic, taper and then stop the benzodiazepine. Most children fully recover. Adult sleep walkers typically were childhood sleep walkers, and recurrence is usually associated with drug abuse.

Night terrors also results from a disturbance in stage 4 sleep. The patient (amnestic for the event) suddenly sits up, cries or screams, is inconsolable, and after several minutes returns to sleep. Treatment is the same as for sleep walking.

Clinical Presentation: Insomnia

Insomnia is a symptom. Most often, it results from environmental factors (stress, work shift changes, unfamiliar sleep setting), but it may also be due to depression, substance abuse and drug withdrawals, anxiety disorder, chronic pain syndromes, thyroid disease, and other sleep disorders. Treating the underlying condition resolves the insomnia, often an early sign of improvement.

When insomnia results from environmental or social stress rather than disease or is idiopathic (persistent sleep onset insomnia), behavioral management is preferable to sedative-hypnotics (including benzodiazepines), which may not be needed and if used may lead to dependence. Tell the patient:

1. Use your bedroom only for dressing, sex, and sleeping when drowsy. If you are not drowsy, do something else in another room. When you are drowsy, sleep in your bed. If you cannot fall asleep in 15 minutes, leave your bedroom.
2. Avoid stimulants (e.g., caffeine, nicotine) after the evening meal.
3. Keep the bedroom cool.
4. Establish, gradually if necessary, a routine bedtime and wake-up time that is followed on weekends.
5. Avoid falling sleep while reading or with the lights on.

If medication is needed, rapid onset, short-acting agents are best. Consider triazolam (Halcion), about 0.125–0.5 mg, or zolpidem (Ambien) 10 mg, and only use these for several weeks intermittently until the acute environmental problem is resolving.

Insomnia also can result from *restless leg syndrome* (nocturnal myoclonus), characterized by bilateral leg movements, occasionally violent, during lighter sleep stages. Patients with nocturnal myoclonus may benefit from bedtime administration of bromocriptine (2.5–5.0), clonazepam (0.5–1.5 mg) or levodopa with benserazide (50–100 mg).

Violence

Violence is ubiquitous in the animal kingdom. Patients with neuropsychiatric disorders are, as a group, more violence prone, and a substantial number of mental health workers are assaulted each year by a patient.

Although there is no fully satisfactory definition of violence, a reasonable one is behavior that results in injury to a person or object. *Self-injury* is included in the definition. Aggressive fantasies, dreams, and plans are not included in this definition, but persons with these subjective experiences are more likely to be violent. *Hostility* implies less specific behaviors such as temper tantrums, being irritable and verbally abusive, suspicious, or uncooperative. *Criminal violence* requires the violent act to violate criminal law and the perpetrator to have had intent and the "mental" capacity to understand the nature, wrongfulness, and consequences of the act. Violent crime includes murder, manslaughter, robbery, aggravated assault (the most frequent), forcible rape, and, sometimes, arson, extortion, kidnapping, hit and run auto accidents, and child abuse.

U.S. statistics about violent crime (arrest records and victimization reports) indicate that men are more likely than women to commit violent crimes (9:1 for murder, 8.5:1.5 for rape). Women murders typically kill a male who has victimized them. Violent crime peaks in persons aged 15–25 years. Arrest reports indicate that although the population ratio of European-Americans to African-Americans is almost 7 to 1, arrest rates for violent crime are about 1.2 : 1. African-Americans are arrested more often than European-Americans for violent crime. Victimization surveys, however, indicate that, based on their proportion of the U.S. population, European-Americans assault other European-Americans at about the predicted rate, European-Americans and African-Americans assault each other *below* the predicted rate, while African-Americans assault each other 800% *higher* than the predicted rate. Socioeconomic status accounts for most, but not all, of the reported racial differences in violent crime. What accounts for the remaining differences is unknown.

Alcohol and drug abuse plays a major role in violence. Fifty to 70% of murderers are intoxicated at the time of the murder, and 80%–90% of persons arrested after any major crime have substantial alcohol blood levels. Whether the alcohol led to the crime or ease of arrest is unclear. However, 50% of murder victims also had substantial alcohol blood levels at the time of their murder. Furthermore, 50% of men arrested for assaults and 65% arrested for robbery test positive for drugs (cocaine, marijuana). Phencyclidine is notorious for inducing a violent psychosis.

Among psychiatric patients, male outpatients are almost twice as likely to be violent than are women outpatients. However, women inpatients are more likely than men inpatients to be assaultive (20% of women and 10%–15% of men patients). The peak age for violence among psychiatric patients is a decade later than that of the general population. Psychiatric patients who are violent also tend to be under 40 or over 70, the former associated with drug abuse and psychosis, the latter with dementia. Among outpatients, increasing assaultiveness is correlated with decreasing education. African-American patients are more likely than European-American patients to be *readmitted* for violence. Among inpatients there are no racial differences in patients who have violent episodes. Figure 16.1 displays a rating scale widely used to assess violent or potentially violent patients and the monitoring of interventions to control and prevent violence. Among chronically hospitalized patients, 7% are assaultive. Among acutely hospitalized patients, assaults usually occur within the first 3 days of hospitalization.

Persons who recurrently injure themselves (7/1,000 in the general U.S. population) are more common among the institutionalized mentally retarded (10%–15% self-injure) and prisoners. Conditions associated with self-injury include de-

OVERT AGGRESSION SCALE (OAS)

Stuart Yudofsky, M.D., Jonathan Silver, M.D., Wynn Jackson, M.D., and Jean Endicott, Ph.D.

IDENTIFYING DATA

Name of patient	Name of rater
Sex of patient: 1 Male 2 Female	Date / / (mo/da/yr) Shift: 1 Night 2 Day 3 Evening

No aggressive incident(s) (verbal or physical against self, others, or objects) during the shift. (Check here) ☐

AGGRESSIVE BEHAVIOR (check all that apply)

VERBAL AGGRESSION	PHYSICAL AGGRESSION AGAINST SELF
☐ Makes loud noises, shouts angrily	☐ Picks or scratches skin, hits self, pulls hair (with no or minor injury only)
☐ Yells mild personal insults, e.g., "You're stupid!"	☐ Bangs head, hits fist into objects, throws self onto floor or into objects (hurts self without serious injury)
☐ Curses viciously, uses foul language in anger, makes moderate threats to others or self	☐ Small cuts or bruises, minor burns
☐ Makes clear threats of violence toward others or self (I'm going to kill you.), or requests to help to control self	☐ Mutilates self, makes deep cuts, bites that bleed, internal injury, fracture, loss of consciousness, loss of teeth

PHYSICAL AGGRESSION AGAINST OBJECTS	PHYSICAL AGGRESSION AGAINST OTHER PEOPLE
☐ Slams door, scatters clothing, makes a mess	☐ Makes threatening gesture, swings at people, grabs at clothes
☐ Throws objects down, kicks furniture without breaking it, marks the wall	☐ Strikes, kicks, pushes, pulls hair (without injury to them)
☐ Breaks objects, smashes windows	☐ Attacks others causing mild–moderate physical injury (bruises, sprains, welts)
☐ Sets fires, throws objects dangerously	☐ Attacks others causing severe physical injury (broken bones, deep lacerations, internal injury)
Time incident began: _____:_____ AM/PM	Duration of incident: _____:_____ (hours/minutes)

INTERVENTION (check all that apply)

☐ None ☐ Talking to patient ☐ Closer observation ☐ Holding patient	☐ Immediate medication given by mouth ☐ Immediate medication given by injection ☐ Isolation without seclusion (time out) ☐ Seclusion	☐ Use of restraints ☐ Injury requires immediate medical treatment for patient ☐ Injury requires immediate treatment for other person

COMMENTS

Figure 16.1. Overt Aggression Scale (OAS). (From Yudofsky SC, et al: The Overt Aggression Scale for the objective rating of verbal and physical aggression. *Am J Psychiatry* 143:35–39, 1986.)

pression, personality disorders (particularly Cluster B), developmental disorders, eating disorders, psychosis, post-traumatic stress disorder, OCD, epilepsy, and chronic drug abuse. Good ward management with a structured activity program, step system, and well-trained nursing staff can minimize violent and self-injurious incidents.

Predicting violence is the most important clinical issue, as it determines prevention. Table 16.7 lists behavioral disorders associated with increased violence risk. Although schizophrenia is also associated with an increased risk for violence, crime statistics are plagued by overdiagnosis of this condition. Among hospitalized schizophrenics who fit the behavioral pattern described in Chapter 9, violence is rarely planned and usually involves blindly striking out at another patient or staff member.

A general rule is that past violence and criminality predict future violence. For example, 90% of murdered children are previously abused or have a sibling who has been physically abused or neglected *before* the killings. Among Vietnam combat veterans receiving psychiatric evaluation, those most likely to act violently committed violent acts (e.g., tortured prisoners, attacked officers with grenades, mutilated the dead) in Vietnam. Among parolees, violence is three times more likely if the parolee has been previously arrested for a violent offense. Among a cohort of boys aged 10–18 years, most violent acts during the study period were committed by young male chronic offenders or by boys with a chronic history of arrests.

Table 16.8 lists behavioral examination features suggesting increased risk and imminent violence and the need for immediate intervention (see Chapters 5 and 8). Although studies of violence do not find consistent predictors, most clinicians take action when they observe a patient with "imminent risk" behavior. Table 16.9 lists clinical features associated with *low* risk.

The Neurobiology of Violence

The causes of violence are multiple. What makes some persons repeatedly violent appears to be an interaction among (1) genetic predisposition, (2) factors affecting neural development or function, and (3) experience that affects neural development or the learning of socialization behaviors.

Violence is familial. Monozygotic twin concordance rates for violence are greater than rates for dizygotic twins, and adoptees are more like their biologic than rearing parents in their tendency toward violence. The proportion of the heritability for violence due to antisocial personality is substantial. Some form of polygenic transmission seems likely. What is inherited is unclear, but may relate to some of the lower order personality traits associated with novelty seeking and harm avoidance, making repeatedly violent persons more impulsive, action prone, and inclined to perceive danger. Chromosomal anomalies (e.g., XYY, XXY), however, associated with low IQ, increased height, and acne, are *not* associated with increased violence.

Violence among nonhumans has relevance in understanding violence in humans. Table 16.10 lists types of nonhuman violence and their possible human counterparts. In addition, human violence is related to brain disease and to learned violence (e.g., assaults by one hockey player upon another, prize fighting, some gang-related violence, duels over "honor" in past eras). Most studies of nonhumans associate parts of the flight/fight system with aggression. Table 16.11 lists brain structures believed involved in violence. The neural systems for violence include structures responsible for flight/fight, emotional tone and expression, temperament, and appetitive and homeostatic behaviors. Which system initiates the violence probably determines what type of violent behavior will occur (e.g., fear induced, intramale).

Because 5-HT has been implicated in the mediation of violence, the median raphe nucleus and its projections to the limbic system (paralleling norepinephrine projections) may also be involved, and reduced median raphe nuclei activity increases limbic activity.

5-HT systems have some inhibitory control over aggression, and manipulating this system can alter aggressive behavior. Several findings implicate 5-HT in violence:

1. Lowering 5-HT brain activity increases violent behavior. This is done in laboratory animals by giving them a low tryptophan diet (tryptophan is the precursor of 5-HT, and males are particularly prone) blocking tryptophan decarboxylase (enzyme that converts tryptophan to 5-HT), or ablating 5-HT neurons.
2. Stressors (e.g., isolation) that increase violent behavior lower brain tryptophan.
3. Adult offspring of mice given alcohol during gestation have low 5-HT brain levels, increased locomotion, increased prepubertal play fighting, and postpubertal aggression.
4. Murderers (particularly those cruel to the victim) have low cerebral spinal fluid 5-HT metabolites and increased impulsiveness.

The brain, however, obviously works more as an integrated whole, so other neurochemical systems also play a role in aggression. Some relationships are (1) increased norepinephrine activity increases anxiety and then aggressive behavior (flight/fight), which can be blocked by beta adrenergic blocking agents; (2) central dopamine agonists (levodopa, apomorphine) increase aggressive behavior; and (3) chronic stimulant use increases aggressive behavior.

Because males are more prone to violence than are females, testosterone has been thought to mediate violence, and testosterone levels are high in aggressive primates and violent rapists, sex offenders, and other repeatedly violent persons. Aggressive behavior in adults is also increased when nonhuman and human fetuses are exposed to high testosterone levels (e.g., female rats gestating between two males or experimentally exposed to androgens; female human fetuses exposed to diethylstilbestrol or with an adrenogenital syndrome). However, although testosterone is a brain-organizing substance during gestation and perhaps at puberty, it is an activating substance at other times (it can only trigger what is already in place) and very sensitive to environmental feedback cues. Thus, the

TABLE 16.7. Behavioral Disorders Associated With
Increased Risk for Violence

ATTENTION DEFICIT HYPERACTIVITY DISORDER

When associated with behavioral features of developmental disorder

CONDUCT DISORDER

When associated with the antisocial personality child hood triad of cruelty to animals, fire setting, and enuresis

Intermittent explosive disorder may be a variant

HEAD INJURY

Particularly to frontal regions and anterior temporal lobe (right more than left), and nondominant hemisphere

Many will have abnormal EEGs with slowing over affected areas

Look for abnormal neurologic signs as predictors of violence: Visual field defects, unilateral Babinski sign, mild hemiparesis, clonus, macrocephaly, multiple soft signs

DRUG ABUSE

With chronic use of stimulants and inhalants

Acute phencyclidine intoxication and chronic anabolic steroid use also can cause violent behavior

ALCOHOLISM

With acute intoxication in a person with the early onset, highly heritable father to son type associated with impulsivity and criminality

BIPOLAR I DISORDER

Arrest records for unipolar patients and bipolar II patients are only slightly elevated and are accounted for by alcohol use

In about 50% of manic episodes, the patient is assaultive or threatening

SCHIZOAFFECTIVE DISORDER

Bipolar type: the more excitement and the more delusional, the more likelihood of violence

SCHIZOPHRENIA

Most likely in schizophrenics with preserved emotional expression, who also are irritable and

TABLE 16.7. (continued)

have persecutory delusional ideas (particularly
of being poisoned)

OTHER PSYCHOTIC DISORDERS

Delusional disorder

Nonaffective positive symptom psychosis

Violence in psychiatric patients is associated with abnormal EEG: frontotemporal slowing left more
than right; 50% of violent offenders have abnormal
EEG

EPILEPSY

Amygdala seizures cause rage

Mesial frontotemporal focus associated with violence

EPILEPTIC SPECTRUM DISORDER

Violence is more organized than that seen in post-ictal
states

EPISODIC DYSCONTROL SYNDROME

This is not a disease; look for drug abuse, head injury,
epilepsy, antisocial personality

TUMOR

Frontal pole slow-growing meningiomas

Ventromedial hypothalamic tumors (associated with
poor coordination and hyperphagia)

Anterior mesial temporal lobe tumors (right more
than left)

STROKE

Particularly when basal ganglia, frontal circuits, or
nondominant frontotemporoparietal cortex is
involved

ENCEPHALITIS

When impulsivity is increased

DEMENTIA

With frontal lobe dementias, associated with a disinhibited syndrome

ANTISOCIAL PERSONALITY DISORDER

Whenever you do not do exactly what they want

TABLE 16.8. Behavioral Indicators of Inpatient Violence

INCREASED RISK*

Persecutory delusions of being poisoned or of jealously

Fantastic persecutory delusions (e.g., possession, alien missions)

Angry command hallucinations

Experiences of alienation or control

Involuntary patient, or patient stating wishes to sign-out of the hospital against medical advice, each with a history of violence

Recent assaultiveness

Recent cognitive testing indicting frontal lobe dysfunction or disinhibition

IMMINENT RISK†

Irritability in previously violent person

Pacing and shouting

Pacing and punching the air or palm of hand

Menacing gestures

Extreme psychotic excitement

Current violent thoughts or statements

*Consider rapid initiation of definitive treatment (e.g., lithium or valproate loading).

†Sedation, seclusion, and restraint is likely at this point; intramuscular neuroleptic may be needed; do not delay response to these behaviors.

TABLE 16.9. Clinical Features of Low Violence Risk

Avolitional syndrome

Severe emotional blunting

Depression with psychomotor retardation

None of the following: psychosis, antisocial or borderline personality disorder, bipolar I disorder, chronic drug abuse

High IQ or education

Middle or upper socioeconomic background

No history of violence

TABLE 16.10. Nonhuman and Human Violence

Type of Violence	Nonhuman	Human
Predatory	Typically interspecies (e.g., lion hunting a zebra); but occasional cannibalism observed in some primates	Typically interspecies (e.g., deer hunting), but occasionally intra-species (e.g., nonritual cannibalism, some serial killers)
Intermale	Competition for access to females, often ritualized and can occur with or without injury	Competition for access to females (e.g., bar fights, "eternal triangle" violence, raids for females by hunter-gatherers)
Maternal aggression	Against intruders approaching young, typically during the period of lactation	Similar response, but flight more likely than fight, unless stimulus is intense (e.g., older person attacks child)
Male aggression	Typically directed at offspring of newly acquired female and leading to the death of those offspring, bringing the female back into heat	Step-children are several times more likely to be abused (sexually and physically) and killed (by stepfather) than are children biologically related to the father
Irritable aggression	More common in males than in females; associated with pain, hunger, or frustration; laboratory rats, birds, and primates may attack another animal when denied reward within a well-learned operant conditioning paradigm; crowding of rats may lead to increased incidence of violent attacks	The psychoanalytic idea of displacement; increased frequency of violence in situations of overcrowding, famine, summer heat waves
Sex related	Aggressive courtship leading to injury; attacks during courtship and mating by some species (e.g., female spotted hyena), forcible coitus (rape?) by male ducks of female partner who is likely to have or has recently mated with another male	Rape, sadomasochism
Territorial	Typically ritualistic and without injury, but occasionally injurious violence if one group invades another's territory; some chimpanzee groups go on premeditated raids to injure and drive off nearby groups; issue is not territory but resources: food, water (intragroup violence over "kills" is an extension of this)	Saber rattling by nations; war (e.g., Gulf War); violent migrations and immigrations over the centuries (e.g., Gothic tribes invading the Roman empire)
Fear-induced (defensive)	Many species of prey animals will defend themselves when flight is impossible or has not been successful (e.g., a deer will run from wolves, but if cornered will vigorously and sometimes successfully defend itself)	When attacked, many persons will fight back, sometimes successfully

TABLE 16.11. The Neurology of Violence

HYPOTHALAMUS

Lateral: Stimulation leads to attack and killing (predatory violence)
Medial: Stimulation leads to defensive display
Ventromedial: Stimulation increases likelihood of irritable aggression

AMYGDALA

Bilateral ablation disrupts ability to conform aggressive/submissive behaviors to established norms; predatory and fear-induced violence decrease, irritable aggression may increase

SUBCORTICAL GRAY MATTER (CENTRAL GRAY, LATERAL PREOPTIC AREA, PONTINE TEGMENTUM)

Stimulation leads to predatory attack, killing, threats depending on situational cues (inter-male; maternal)

HIPPOCAMPUS

Modulates violence as part of flight/fight processes (see Chapter 15)

CINGULATE GYRUS (ANTERIOR)

Influences rest of frontal lobes with increased arousal and emotion from other limbic structures; stimulation increases likelihood of irritable aggression

PREFRONTAL CORTEX

Modulates many forms of violence

BASAL GANGLIA/THALAMUS/CEREBELLUM (FASTIGIAL NUCLEUS AND ANTERIOR CEREBELLAR NEOCORTEX)

Provide the motor sequencing and procedural actions for violent behaviors

high testosterone levels in violent adult nonhuman primates and humans are more likely the consequences of their successful violent behavior than the cause. For example, alpha male primates have high testosterone levels. However, if you put the alpha male in with a new band who gangs up on him, his testosterone precipitously drops.

Table 16.12 offers a model for the above. Gestational and early childhood experience also plays a substantial role in the development of aggressiveness. These experiences fall into two categories: interpersonal and brain-damaging experiences. Table 16.13 lists examples of these experiences.

Prenatal factors that result in direct neural developmental abnormalities (teratogenesis) seem less important in a person becoming prone to violence than are

TABLE 16.12. A Model for Violence

Genetic predisposition to low 5-HT activity and low DA activity leads to traits such as impulsiveness

Genetic predisposition to increased norepinephrine activity leads to an overactive flight/fight system and the tendency toward irritability, or defensive or attack behaviors to environmental stress

An impulsive, flight/fight prone person with normal or high levels of testosterone (i.e., an adult male) is prone to aggressive action

Gestational and early childhood experiences moderate the above (ameliorating or exacerbating)

factors that reduce fetal blood supply or oxygen. Maternal drug use may be the worst case situation, as chronic heavy use has direct effects on the fetus and is also associated with the increased likelihood of poor maternal nutrition and prenatal care. Intravenous drug use also exposes the fetus to many of the risks faced by the mother (e.g., AIDS, hepatitis, syphilis). Maternal cocaine use (6%–17% of pregnant women, most of whom will be poor, unemployed, single, and African-American) may be the most likely drug abuse to increase offspring violence because cocaine (1) decreases uterine blood flow, which can cause fetal hypoxia and acidosis; (2) disrupts placental transportation of essential amino acids needed for fetal development; (3) disrupts fetal brain protein and DNA synthesis, myelin formation, and serotonergic system development; and (4) alters early transcription

TABLE 16.13. Experiences That Increase Violence Risk

Interpersonal*	Brain Damaging
Child abuse	Fetal exposure to alcohol
Violent parent	Fetal exposure to stimulant drugs†
Parent with abrasive, coercive parenting style	Childhood lead exposure
	Labor and delivery problems
Alcoholic parent	Childhood neuromotor deficits
Child neglect (providing no inhibition of the child's aggressive behavior and no reinforcement of positive social behavior, e.g., learning law-abiding behavior)	Childhood head injury, encephalitis, or epilepsy
	Use of drugs during critical developmental phases (e.g., puberty)
Observing violence (initially by parents, and then peers)	
Learning extreme male stereotyped behaviors (as in some street gang cultures)	

*Many of these factors are familial, also have genetic component, and can directly affect brain development.

†Disrupts serotonergic system development.

TABLE 16.14. Sequence of Events Increasing Violence Proneness

Genetic Predispositions	Prenatal Factors	Parental Factors	Prepubertal Childhood Factors	Adolescent Adult Factors
1. Impulsivity	1. Maternal drug (cocaine) and alcohol use	1. Poor mothering skills	1. Drug use	1. Drug and alcohol use
2. Easy arousibility	2. Other drug use	2. Maternal aloofness	2. Head injury*	2. Head injury*
3. High novelty seeking	3. Poor nutrition	3. Parental violence	3. Early onset psychiatric disorder	3. Peer violence
4. Specific behavioral conditions listed in Table 16.7	4. Poor prenatal care	4. Poor or absent non-violent role models	4. Poor environmental controls of child's violent behavior	4. Poor or absent nonviolent role models
5. Low brain reserve (IQ and cognition)	5. Prenatal factors increasing risk for prematurity and neurologic disease (e.g., difficult labor and delivery)	5. Psychiatric illness	5. No positive role models for nonviolent behavioral responses	
		6. Antisocial personality disorder	6. Learning disabilities	
			7. Peer violence	
			8. Conduct disorder	
			9. ADHD	

*Particularly to frontotemporal regions.

TABLE 16.15. Pharmacotherapy of Violence

Drug	Clinical Considerations
Carbamazepine	Best with epileptic patients, epilepsy spectrum disorder, nonepileptic patients with abnormal EEGs, and head injury patients, all in typical anticonvulsant doses (blood levels 8–12 mg/L)
Benzodiazepines	Oxazepam may be the safest, as the paradoxical reaction* has not been reported with it
Buspirone	When patient has a traumatic brain injury, dementia, or a developmental disorder
Beta-adrenergic blockers[†]	Best at high doses with head injury patients (e.g., propanolol above 320–520 mg daily)
Lithium	Best with mood disorder patients, persons with mental retardation and other developmental disorders, head injury patients, persons with conduct disorder, persons with blood levels in mid to low therapeutic mood disorder range
SSRI antidepressants	Best when violence associated with anxiety or depression, schizotypal and borderline personality disorders, obsessive features, self-injury or suicide
Bupropion	Best with patients who are impulsive or who have high novelty seeking behaviors
Nonspecific and partially specific monoamine-reuptake inhibitors	Useful for patients with emotional incontinence. Because anticholinergic side effects may increase irritability, before prescribing high doses, see if low doses of the nonspecific or modest doses of the partially specific agents work
Antiandrogens	Best with violent sex offenders
Antipsychotics	Only if the patient is psychotic and all other choices have not worked; for some patients ECT works better
Stimulants	Methylphenidate (20–60 mg daily) and to a lesser extent L-amphetamine can work for mild to moderate, but not severe aggressiveness; works best when ADHD co-morbid condition

*Excitement, hyperactivity, and agitation rather than sedation or tranquilization.

[†]*Propranolol* (Inderal) and *pindolol* (Visken), lipid-soluble nonselective B_1 and B_2 antagonists with 3–5-hour half-lives, and nadolol (Corgard) a water-soluble antagonist (14–18-hour half-life) have been used with modest success. If used, begin slowly and monitor pulse rate and blood pressure. Stop if severe dizziness, ataxia, or wheezing occurs. Treat for at least 8 weeks before declaring treatment resistance, and do not discontinue suddenly to avoid dramatic blood pressure changes.

factors and fos and jun genes, which may result in abnormal protein and enzyme production.

Women who use cocaine when pregnant are also more likely to use other illicit drugs, alcohol, and cigarettes and are less likely to get good prenatal care. Children whose mothers use cocaine (particularly crack) while pregnant are more likely to (1) be premature and to have low birth weight; (2) have a small head

TABLE 16.16. Behavioral Strategies To Control or Reduce Violence Risk

GOOD CARE AND COMMON SENSE

Provide good respectful care; have well structured inpatient and outpatient programs with low expressed emotion and friendly yet firm staff. Do not see alone those patients with violence indicators (see previous tables)

USE SECURITY

Have uniformed security in emergency room and an examining room with a panic button and easy access to the door

BE PREPARED

Do not confront patients who have violence indicators; that is what security personnel are for. If you must hospitalize or discharge from the emergency room against the patient's requests, do not tell the patient this until security personnel are present (5–6 persons) and ready to restrain, and the nurses and you are ready to sedate the patient who is to be involuntarily hospitalized

Keep the patient at a distance (10–15 feet)

Keep the patient talking

Get the patient to sit

Get the patient to eat or drink

LOOK FOR WEAPONS

All newly hospitalized patients with any of the conditions or behaviors associated with increased risk of violence should be in pajamas at least during the first 24 hours of hospitalization; street clothes should be removed in the admitting area, where security personnel are available and the clothes can be easily felt for weapons

---

circumference, a low Apgar score, congenital malformations (genitourinary, cardiac, cranial), and neuromotor and visual motor deficits; and (3) be colicky, inconsolable, and behaviorally less interactive. Mothers who continue to abuse drugs after delivery are less likely to provide adequate child care and maternal child contact and are more likely to be child abusers. Table 16.14 displays a sequence of events increasing violence proneness.

Management and Treatment of Violence

Tables 16.13 and 16.14 suggest that prevention may be the best treatment for violence. Programs that can *effectively* improve parenting skills and prenatal care and reduce drug and alcohol use should substantially help. Once identified as a child at risk, the earlier the interventions, the better the chances for reducing aggressive traits.

The treatment of adults who are repeatedly violent is based on the likely cause. The differential diagnosis of violence includes all conditions listed in Table 16.7. If you can identify a specific condition, treat for that.

Chapter 8 reviews the use of *antipsychotics* for manic excitement and psychosis. If a violent person has a condition that will respond to antipsychotics, then their use is reasonable. However, violence without psychosis does not respond to antipsychotics except as sedating agents. Use a sedative to sedate, not an antipsychotic. Benzodiazepines, however, may cause a paradoxic reaction with agitation and assaultiveness. Diazepam may be least likely to do this. Atypical antipsychotics (particularly clozapine) with their serotonergic effects may be particularly good choices for violent patients. Olanzapine, however, tends to be activating and may increase hyperactivity and aggression in psychotics with a history of these behaviors. Risperidone does not yet come in an intramuscular form, and above 8 mg daily (likely for violent patients) it may produce extrapyramidal side effects. Clozapine also has several limitations (e.g., agranulocytosis, sudden hypotensive collapse, salorrhea). Table 16.15 summarizes drug choices for violent patients. Table 16.16 lists some behavioral strategies to control or reduce the risk for imminent violence.

For self-injurious patients, if you can identify a specific condition (e.g., seizure disorder, OCD) treat for that. If you cannot identify a specific disorder, the following drugs work in some patients: carbamazepine, clonidine, lithium, opiate antagonists (e.g., naltrexone [Revia]), and antidepressants. Failure to respond to one drug does not mean the patient will not respond to another choice. Pharmacotherapy works best when combined with behavior therapy and counseling.

ADDITIONAL READINGS

Akbari HM, Kramer HK, Whitaker-Azmitia PM, Spear LP, Azmitia EC: Prenatal cocaine exposure disrupts the development of the serotonergic system. *Brain Res 572*:57-63, 1992.

Bailey J, Bell A: Familiality of female and male homosexuality. *Behav Genet 23*:313–322, 1993.

Berlin FS, Coyle GS: Sexual deviation syndromes. *Johns Hopkins Med J 149*:119–125, 1981.

Berlin FS, Meinecke CF: Treatment of sex offenders with antiandrogenic medication. *Am J Psychiatry 138*:601–607, 1981.

Birkett DP: Violence in geropsychiatry. *Psychiatr Ann 27*:752–756, 1997.

Blake PY, Pincus JH, Buckner C: Neurologic abnormalities in murderers. *Neurology 45*: 1641–1647, 1995.

Bodlund O, Kullgren G, Sundbom E, Hojerback T: Personality traits and disorders among transsexuals. *Acta Psychiatr Scand 88*:322–327, 1993.

Brennan PA, Mednick SA: Genetic perspectives on crime. *Acta Psychiatr Scand Suppl 370*: 19–26, 1993.

Brook JS, Whiteman MM, Finch S: Childhood aggression, adolescent delinquency, and drug use: A longitudinal study. *J Gen Psychol 153*:369–383, 1991.

Brown GR, Wise TN, Costa PT Jr, Herbst JH, Fagan PJ, Schmidt CW Jr: Personality characteristics and sexual functioning of 188 cross-dressing men. *J Nerv Ment Dis 184*:265–273, 1996.

Brunner HG, Nelen M, Breakefield XO, Ropers HH, van Oost BA: Abnormal behavior associated with a point mutation in the structural gene for monoamine oxidase A. *Sci 262*:578–580, 1993.

Buzan RD, Thomas M, Dubovsky SL, Treadway J: The use of opiate antagonists for recurrent self-injurious behavior. *J Neuropsychiatry 7*:437–444, 1995.

Byne W, Parsons B: Human sexual orientation: The biologic theories reappraised. *Arch Gen Psychiatry* 50:228–239, 1993.

Cadoret RJ, Yates WR, Troughton E, Woodworth G, Stewart MA: Genetic–environmental interaction in the genesis of aggressivity and conduct disorders. *Arch Gen Psychiatry* 52:916–924, 1995.

Campbell M, Gonzalez NM, Silva RR: The pharmacologic treatment of conduct disorders and rage outbursts. *Psychiatric Clin North Am Pediatr Psychopharmacol* 15:69–85, 1992.

Cases O, Seif I, Grimsby J, Gaspar P, Chen K, Pournin S, Muller U, Aguet M, Babinet C, Shih JC, DeMaeyer E: Aggressive behavior and altered amounts of brain serotonin and norepinephrine in mice lacking MAOA. *Science* 268:1763–1766, 1995.

Christiansen KO: A review of studies of criminality among twins. In Christiansen KO, Mednick S (eds): *Biosocial Bases of Criminal Behavior*, Gardner, New York, 1977.

Clark DJ: Psychopharmacology of severe self-injury associated with learning disabilities. *Brit J Psychiatry* 172:389–394, 1998.

Clark GT, Takeuchi H: Temporomandibular dysfunction, chronic orofacial pain and oral motor disorders in the 21st Century. *CDA J* 23:41–50, 1995.

Clarke DJ: Psychopharmacology of severe self-injury associated with learning disabilities. *Br J Psychiatry* 172:389–394, 1998.

Clauw DJ: The pathogenesis of chronic pain and fatigue syndromes, with special reference to fibromyalgia. *Med Hypoth* 44:369–378, 1995.

Coccaro EF: Impulsive aggression and central serotonergic system function in humans: An example of a dimensional brain–behavior relationship. *Int Clin Psychopharmacol* 7:3–12, 1992.

Coccaro EF, Bergeman CS, Kavoussi RJ, Seroczynski AD: Heritability of aggression and irritability: A twin study of the Buss-Durkee aggression scales in adult male subjects. *Biol Psychiatry* 41:273–284, 1997.

Coccaro EF, Bergeman CS, McClearn GE: Heritability of irritable impulsiveness: A study of twins reared together and apart. *Psychiatry Res* 48:229–242, 1993.

Coccaro EF, Kavoussi RJ: Fluoxetine and impulsive aggressive behavior in personality-disordered subjects. *Arch Gen Psychiatry* 54:1081–1088, 1997.

Coderre TJ, Katz J, Vaccarino AL, Melzack R: Contribution of central neuroplasticity to pathological pain: Review of clinical and experimental evidence. *Pain* 52:259–285, 1993.

Couch JR: Headache to worry about. *Med Clin North Am* 77:141–167, 1993.

Croop RS, Faulkner EB, Labriola DF, for the naltrexone usage study group: The safety profile of naltrexone in the treatment of alcoholism: Results from a multicenter usage study. *Arch Gen Psychiatry* 54:1130–1135, 1997.

Culebras A (ed): The neurology of sleep. *Neurology* 42(*suppl* 6):1–94, 1992.

DiLalla LF, Gottesman II: Biological and genetic contributors to violence—Widom's untold tale. *Psychol Bull* 109:125–129, 1991.

Elliott FA: Violence. The neurologic contribution: An overview. *Arch Neurol* 49:595–603, 1992.

Fagan PJ, Wise TN, Schmidt CW Jr, Ponticas Y, Marshall RD, Costa PTJ: A comparison of five-factor personality dimensions in males with sexual dysfunction and males with paraphilia. *J Pers Assess* 53:434–448, 1991.

Fava M, Rappe SM, West J, Herzog DG: Anger attacks in eating disorders. *Psychiatry Res* 56:205–212, 1995.

Gingras JL, Weese-Mayer DE, Hume RF Jr, O'Donnell KJ: Cocaine and development: Mechanisms of fetal toxicity and neonatal consequences of prenatal cocaine exposure. *Early Hum Dev* 31:1–24, 1992.

Green WH, Kowalik SC: Violence in child and adolescent psychiatry. *Psychiatr Ann* 27:745–751, 1997.

Harrison PJ, Everall IP, Catalan J: Homosexual behaviour hard-wired? Sexual orientation and brain structure [editorial]. *Psychol Med* 24:811–816, 1994.

Hodgins S: Mental disorder, intellectual deficiency, and crime: Evidence from a birth cohort. *Arch Gen Psychiatry 49*:476–483, 1992.

Hodgins S, Mednick SA, Brennen PA, Schulsinger F, Engberg M: Mental disorder and crime: Evidence from a Danish birth cohort. *Arch Gen Psychiatry 53*:489–496, 1996.

Hulter B, Lundberg PO: Sexual function in women with hypothalamo-pituitary disorders. *Arch Sex Behav 23*:171–182, 1994.

Kandel E: Biology, violence, and antisocial personality. *J Forensic Sci 37*:912–918, 1992.

Kavey NB, Whyte J, Resor SR Jr, Gidro-Frank S: Somnambulism in adults. *Neurology 40*:749–752, 1990.

Krakowski M, Czobor P, Carpenter MD, Libiger J, Kunz M, Papezova H, Parker BB, Schmader L, Abad T: Community violence and inpatient assaults: Neurobiological deficits. *J Neuropsychiatry Clin Neurosci 9*:549–555, 1997.

Kudrow L: Diagnosis and treatment of cluster headache. *Med Clin North Am 75*:579–594, 1991.

Kumar KL: Recent advances in acute management of migraine and cluster headaches. *J Gen Int Med 9*:339–348, 1994.

Levi R, Edman GV, Ekbom K, Waldenlind E: Episodic cluster headache I: Personality and some neuropsychological characteristics in male patients. *Headache 32*:119–125, 1992.

Levi R, Edman GV, Ekbom K, Waldenlind E: Episodic cluster headache II: High tobacco and alcohol consumption in males. *Headache 32*:184–187, 1992.

Lewis DO: From abuse to violence: Psychophysiological consequences of maltreatment. *J Am Acad Child Adolesc Psychiatry 31*:383–391, 1992.

Lipton RB, Pfeffer D, Newman LC, Solomon S: Headaches in the elderly. *J Pain Symptom Manage 8*:87–97, 1993.

Lyons MJ, True WR, Eisen SA, Goldberg J, Meyer JM, Faraone SV, Eaves LJ, Tsuang MT: Differential heritability of adult and juvenile antisocial traits. *Arch Gen Psychiatry 52*:906–915, 1995.

Madden DJ, Lion JR, Penna MW: Assaults on psychiatrists by patients. *Am J Psychiatry 133*:422–425, 1976.

Manzoni GC, Micieli G, Granella F, Tassorelli C, Zanferrari C, Cavallini A: Cluster headache—course over ten years in 189 patients. *Cephalalgia 11*:169–174, 1991.

Mattis JA, Fink M: A family study of patients with temper outbursts. *J Psychiatr Res 21*:249–255, 1987.

Mauskop A (ed): Neurobiology of migraine. *Clin Neurosci 5*:1–59, 1998.

Moller SE, Mortensen EL, Breum L, Alling C, Larsen OD, Boge-Rasmussen T, Jensen C, Bennicke K: Aggression and personality: Association with amino acids and monoamine metabolites. *Psychol Med 26*:323–331, 1996.

Nester PG: Neuropsychological and clinical correlates of murder and other forms of extreme violence in a forensic psychiatric population. *J Nerv Ment Dis 180*:418–423, 1992.

Odens ML, Fox CH: Adult sleep apnea syndromes. *Am Fam Phys 52*:859–866, 1995.

Overpeck MD, Brenner RA, Trumble AC, Trifiletti LB, Berendes HW: Risk factors for infant homicide in the United States. *N Engl J Med 339*:1211–1216, 1998.

Pihl RO, Hoaken PNS: Clinical correlates and predictors of violence in patients with substance use disorders. *Psychiatr Ann 27*:735–740, 1997.

Raine A, Brennan P, Mednick SA: Birth complications combined with early maternal rejection at age 1 year predispose to violent crime at age 18 years. *Arch Gen Psychiatry 51*:984–988, 1994.

Raine A, Brennan P, Mednick B, Mednick SA: High rates of violence, crime, academic problems, and behavioral problems in males with both early neuromotor deficits and unstable family environments. *Arch Gen Psychiatry 53*:544–549, 1996.

Reiss D, Hetherington EM, Plomin R, Howe GW, Simmens SJ, Henderson SH, O'Connor TJ, Bussell DA, Anderson ER, Law T: Genetic questions for environmental studies. Differential parenting and psychopathology in adolescence. *Arch Gen Psychiatry 52*:925–936, 1995.

Rosler A, Witztum E: Treatment of men with paraphilia with a long-acting analogue of gonadotropin-releasing hormone. *N Engl J Med 338*:416–422, 1998.

Rowbotham MC: Chronic pain: From theory to practical management. *Neurology 45(suppl 9)*:S5–S10, 1995.

Sastry BVR: Placental toxicology: Tobacco smoke, abuse drugs, multiple chemical interactions, and placental function. *Reprod Fertil Dev 3*:355–372, 1991.

Schievink WI: Intracranial aneurysms. *N Engl J Med 336*:28–39, 1997.

Schramm E, Hohagen F, Kappler C, Grasshoff U, Berger M: Mental comorbidity of chronic insomnia in general practice attenders using DSM-III-R. *Acta Psychiatr Scand 91*:10–17, 1995.

Simeon D, Stanley B, Frances A, Mann JJ, Winchel R, Stanley M: Self-mutilation in personality disorders: Psychological and biological correlates. *Am J Psychiatry 149*:221–226, 1992.

Singer L, Farkas K, Kliegman R: Childhood medical and behavioral consequences of maternal cocaine use. *J Pediatr Psychol 17*:389–406, 1992.

Stein DJ, Hollander E, Cohen L, Frenkel M, Saoud JB, DeCaria C, Aronowitz B, Levin A, Liebowitz MR, Cohen L: Neuropsychiatric impairment in impulsive personality disorders. *Psychiatry Res 48*:257–266, 1993.

Tiefer L: Critique of the DSM-III-R nosology of sexual dysfunctions. *Psychiatr Med 10*:227–245, 1992.

Tong S, McMichael AJ: Maternal smoking and neuropsychological development in childhood: A review of the evidence. *Dev Med Child Neurol 34*:191–197, 1992.

Tonkonogy JM: Violence and temporal lobe lesion: Head CT and MRI data. *J Neuropsychiatry 3*:189–196, 1991.

Treiman DM: Psychobiology of ictal aggression. In Smith D, Treiman D, Trimble M (eds): *Advances in Neurology: Neurobehavioral Problems in Epilepsy*, vol 55. Raven Press, New York, 1991 pp 341–356.

Trestman RL: Clinical correlates and predictors of violence in patients with personality disorders. *Psychiatr Ann 27*:741–744, 1997.

Van de Poll NE, Van Goozen SHM: Hypothalamic involvement in sexuality and hostility: Comparative psychological aspects. In Swab DF, Hofman MA, Mirmiran M, Ravid R, van Leeuwen FW (eds): *Progress in Brain Research*, vol 93. Elsevier Science, New York, 1992.

van Praag, HM, Plutchik R, Apter A: *Violence and Suicidality: Perspectives in Clinical and Psychobiological Research*. Brunner/Mazel, New York, 1990.

Virkkunen M, Eggert M, Rawlings R, Linnoila M: A prospective follow-up study of alcoholic violent offenders and fire setters. *Arch Gen Psychiatry 53*:523–529, 1996.

Volavka J: Aggression, electroencephalography and evoked potentials. A critical review. *Neuropsychiatry Neuropsychol Behav Neurol 3*:249–259, 1990.

Volavka J: *Neurobiology of Violence*. American Psychiatric Press, Washington, DC, 1995.

Volavka J, Martell D, Convit A: Psychobiology of the violent offender. *J Forensic Sci 37*:237–251, 1992.

Walling AD: Cluster headache. *Am Fam Phys 47*:1457–1463, 1993.

Wiggins RC: Pharmacokinetics of cocaine in pregnancy and effects on fetal maturation. *Clin Pharmacokinet 22*:85–93, 1992.

Wise TN: Transvestitic fetishism: Diagnosis and treatment. *Psychiatr Med 8*:75–84, 1990.

Index

Page references followed by the letter *f* are for figures.
Page references followed by the letter *n* are for notes.
Page references followed by the letter *t* are for tables.